A Practical Guide to Obstetrics

SECOND EDITION

A Practical Guide to Obstetrics

SECOND EDITION

Edited by

Gita Arjun, FACOG

Obstetrician and Gynecologist
Former Director, E V Kalyani Medical Centre
Chennai, India

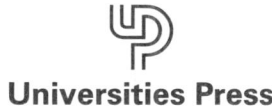

Universities Press

A PRACTICAL GUIDE TO OBSTETRICS, SECOND EDITION

UNIVERSITIES PRESS (INDIA) PRIVATE LIMITED

Registered Office
3-6-747/1/A & 3-6-754/1, Himayatnagar, Hyderabad 500 029, Telangana, India
info@universitiespress.com; www.universitiespress.com

Distributed by
Orient Blackswan Private Limited

Registered Office
3-6-752, Himayatnagar, Hyderabad 500 029, Telangana, India

Other Offices
Bengaluru, Chennai, Guwahati, Hyderabad, Kolkata
Mumbai, New Delhi, Noida, Patna, Visakhapatnam

© Universities Press (India) Private Limited 2013, 2022
First published 2013: Reprinted 2013, 2014
Second edition 2022

ISBN 978 93 93330 08 6

Cover and book design
© Universities Press (India) Private Limited 2022

501843

Typeset in Life BT 10.5/13.5 pt *by*
ELITE Graphics, Hyderabad 500 039

Printed in India at
Rasi Graphics Pvt Ltd., Chennai 600 014

Published by
Universities Press (India) Private Limited
3-6-747/1/A & 3-6-754/1, Himayatnagar, Hyderabad 500 029, Telangana, India

Contents

Foreword to the Second Edition

The second edition of *A Practical Guide to Obstetrics* is an encyclopedia of obstetrics and an excellent reference book for practising obstetricians and midwives in India. This book presents the most up-to-date information of practical relevance in a crisp and reader-friendly style. The book is well-illustrated with an ample number of photographs, figures and tables. Evidence-based facts are presented as bullet points. The use of lightbulb boxes for important pieces of information and thumbs up or down boxes to denote good and harmful practices makes it easy for the clinician to focus on the most crucial details.

The book opens with a preconception checklist for women planning pregnancy, which is followed by guidelines for early antenatal care and nutritional advice in the second and third trimesters. Common problems in the antenatal period and their management are described, followed by antepartum surveillance, prenatal screening, and diagnostic tests for genetic disorders. Ultrasound in the first trimester, the detection of abnormal pregnancies in the early first trimester, and ultrasound examination in the second and third trimesters are described with clear scan photographs. The chapter on respectful maternity care as a human right is a welcome feature of this book. A comprehensive description of normal labour and delivery is followed by an evidence-based approach to episiotomy and the prevention and repair of perineal trauma. Pain relief in labour, fetal surveillance, induction of labour, abnormal progress of labour, and operative vaginal delivery are described with no ambiguity. The chapters on breech and cesarean deliveries are followed by important topics such as reducing cesarean section rates and vaginal birth after cesarean delivery.

Maternal care in the puerperium and complications and issues related to lactation and breastfeeding are described well. Obstetric (antepartum hemorrhage, postpartum hemorrhage, preterm labour, Rh alloimmunisation, multiple pregnancy, intrauterine growth restriction, intrahepatic cholestasis, and stillbirths), medical (asthma, antiphospholipid syndrome, thyroid, hypertensive disorders, gestational and pregestational diabetes, high maternal BMI, pregnancy with PCO and after ART, and anemias) and infective (HIV, COVID-19) disorders and immunisation in pregnancy are covered in depth.

The amount of work that has surely gone into producing this book is certainly commendable; I congratulate the editor of this edition on preparing this unique evidence-based practical guide to obstetrics. A copy should be available in every medical library, ward and clinic. I would strongly recommend this book as an essential read for trainees, consultants, and midwives who provide maternity care.

Sir Sabaratnam Arulkumaran, PhD, DSc, FRCS, FRCOG
Professor Emeritus of Obstetrics and Gynaecology, St George's University of London
Past President of the British Medical Association, Royal College of Obstetricians and Gynaecologists and the International Federation of Obstetrics & Gynaecology

Preface to the Second Edition

The first edition of *A Practical Guide to Obstetrics* resonated with busy practitioners who struggle to keep up with the latest medical information essential for their practice. Postgraduate students of obstetrics found its systematic and evidence-based approach invaluable for applying theory to practice.

A major issue faced by obstetricians is adapting international guidelines to Indian circumstances, which is problematic in that these guidelines may not always be relevant because of differing healthcare delivery systems and limited resources. This may drive practitioners to adopt local practices that are not entirely evidence-based. The expectations of women may also vary based on cultural and social contexts.

The current edition of *A Practical Guide to Obstetrics* focuses on Indian data available for various clinical conditions. Since 2005, the Government of India, along with other agencies, has brought out guidelines for maternal healthcare. These are sound clinically and present the scope and purpose with clarity. However, a task force convened by the Ministry of Health and Family Welfare (MoHFW) found that Indian guidelines have weak documentation about their development process and are unclear on how they were adapted to local conditions. We have made recommendations in this book based on Indian conditions, resources and ease of applicability. This should help practitioners to relate these to various clinical situations and be able to practice with confidence.

The SARS-CoV-2 pandemic changed the world in many ways. Obstetricians had to rapidly learn about the disease and its impact on both the mother and her baby. Practices had to be adapted that would also ensure the safety of healthcare providers. To address these challenges, the second edition of *A Practical Guide to Obstetrics* includes a chapter on COVID-19 and the current recommendations for preventing and managing the disease in pregnant women.

Like the first edition, this book has a unique format which highlights clinical recommendations that are backed by strong evidence and practice points that should be adopted or avoided. We hope that these features, along with the clear and succinct style used, will make this book a handy reference tool for obstetricians.

Gita Arjun, FACOG
Obstetrician and Gynecologist
Former Director, E V Kalyani Medical College, Chennai, India

How to use this book

Important information is set apart from the text in three types of boxes:
- Light bulb (💡): This indicates an important piece of information based on strong evidence.
- Thumbs up (👍): This indicates a good practice point and is a recommendation for incorporation into practice.
- Thumbs down (👎): This indicates practices that should be avoided or may be harmful.

Preface to the First Edition

The practising clinician has limited time to spend on reading scientific literature, analysing the evidence and interpreting it correctly. The mantra for many years has been evidence-based medicine. However, randomised controlled trials and meta-analyses have their own problems: they require a clinician to have the capacity for rigorous scientific reasoning. Most of us do not have the time or the expertise to do that. Dr Richard Horton, Editor of *The Lancet*, called it learning 'the grammar of interpretive medicine'.

The obstetrician or gynecologist is no stranger to complications. In obstetrics, emergencies can arise with no warning. Complications in pregnancy can be a nightmare since obstetricians have to deal with the safety of two lives. Obstetrics is rife with situations where quick thinking and rapid intervention can prevent a catastrophe.

Faced with unexpected problems and complications, knowledge and experience come into play to ensure a favourable outcome.

The obstetric practitioner, therefore, needs to be armed with the current recommendations for a specific problem (knowledge). 'Evidence-based medicine (EBM)' could be a study that has examined that particular problem, or it could be a systematic review of all the studies done in that area. The practitioner then depends on the experience gained over years of focussed practice and applies this knowledge to the clinical situation. This is how theory is applied to practice or, in other words, evidence-based medicine is converted to evidence-based care (EBC) or management.

At the same time, evidence-based medicine has to be cost-effective and safe. *A Practical Guide to Obstetrics* has compiled cost-effective and safe EBM-based practices, truly converting theory to practice. This book incorporates the spirit behind the PROGRESS (Practical OG Congress) series of conferences. It is a practical handbook for students, postgraduates and practitioners.

The editors have published this book with the hope that it will become a well-thumbed reference book for any practitioner of obstetrics who wants to know the correct procedure to follow in a particular obstetric situation. To this end, we have used a unique format which makes for easy reading and have highlighted practice points.

Gita Arjun
Lakshmi Seshadri
Uma Ram

Chapter 1

Preconception Checklist for Women Planning Pregnancy

INTRODUCTION

- Preconception care has a positive impact on maternal and child health outcomes (WHO, 2013). Not only does preconception counselling and care reduce maternal morbidity and mortality, it also prevents poor pregnancy outcomes like low birth weight, premature birth, and infant mortality. Implementing preconception care whenever possible can be a major determinant in improving reproductive health outcomes, with the potential for reducing the economic burden on society.
- Optimising a woman's health and knowledge before she plans and conceives a pregnancy may eliminate or reduce the risk of poor outcomes in the mother, fetus, or neonate (ACOG, 2005).
- Nearly 50 per cent of pregnancies in India are unplanned or unintended (Singh et al., 2018). Consequently, it may be too late for appropriate health interventions in pregnancy by the time a couple seeks them. Therefore, every encounter with a woman who can potentially become pregnant must be used as an opportunity to initiate preconceptional care (Johnson et al., 2006).
- In India, the high prevalence of diabetes, hypertension, and dyslipidemias must be borne in mind when counselling a couple on preconception care.

The chief aims of preconception counselling and care include:
- Screening for risk factors
- Initiating preventive health measures
- Identifying and addressing individual health issues

DEFINITION OF PRECONCEPTION CARE

- The World Health Organization defines preconception care as the provision of biomedical, behavioural, and social health interventions to women and couples before conception occurs (WHO, 2013).
- By improving a woman's health status before she gets pregnant and by reducing risk factors that contribute to poor maternal and child health outcomes, the health of mothers and children can be impacted positively, in both the short and the long term.
- Preconception care comprises more than a single visit to a healthcare provider and includes preventive and primary care services for women before their first pregnancy or between pregnancies (also known as *interconception care*).

INITIATING PRECONCEPTION CARE

- Every woman of reproductive age should be asked at every healthcare encounter: 'Are you planning to get pregnant?' and 'Could you possibly become pregnant?' (Berghella et al., 2016). If the woman is not planning to get pregnant, giving her contraceptive advice can prevent an unintended pregnancy.
- Asking every woman about her intention to get pregnant promotes the idea that pregnancies should be intended and planned (Dunlop et al., 2007).
- It also promotes the initiation of preconception care strategies for women if and when they do desire to become pregnant.
- Women in the reproductive age group should also be made aware that health conditions and medications can affect pregnancy outcomes and conversely, that a pregnancy can affect a woman's health (Dunlop et al., 2008).

Opportunities to initiate preconception care

The opportunities available to initiate a conversation about preconceptional care include the following:

- Any visit to a doctor during the reproductive years
- nnual ob-gyn examination
- Postpartum checkup, which should include family planning, prescribing of contraception, and counselling
- A visit for a pregnancy test (especially if negative)
- Emergency visit
- Visit for infertility treatment
- Premarital counselling

 Most women do not consult the obstetrician for preconceptional advice prior to pregnancy. Therefore, all available opportunities should be utilised by the obstetrician/physician to initiate preconception counselling and care.

SPECIFIC GOALS OF PRECONCEPTION CARE

- **Screening for risk**
  - Personal and family history, physical examination, and laboratory screening
- **Preventive health**
  - Nutritional advice, supplements, weight management, exercise, and indicated vaccinations
- **Specific individual issues**
  - *Chronic diseases:* Aim to optimise control of disease and switch to safe medications
  - *Medications:* Discussion of current medications with the aim of changing or eliminating potential teratogens

INTERVENTIONS TO BE IMPLEMENTED IN THE PRECONCEPTION PERIOD

Evidence supports specific preconception interventions in all women in the reproductive age group (Table 1.1). These interventions improve the outcome of pregnancy.

Table 1.1 Recommended preconception interventions for all women

Intervention	Proven health benefit

• Folic acid supplementation (400 µg) initiated at least 1 month prior to conception
• A higher dose of 4 mg, may be considered for the following groups of women:
  – Those who are taking antiseizure medications and other drugs that might interfere with folic acid metabolism
  – Those who are obese
  – Those who have had a previous baby with NTD
	Reduces occurrence of neural tube defects by 70 per cent

Screening for anemia and instituting iron therapy for women who are anemic	Reduces risks of PPH, low birth weight, small-for-gestational age babies, maternal and perinatal death
HIV/AIDS screening and treatment	Allows for appropriate treatment and provides women (or couples) with additional information that can influence the timing of pregnancy and treatment
Hepatitis B vaccination for at-risk women	Prevents transmission of infection to the infant
STI screening and treatment	• Reduces the risk of ectopic pregnancy, infertility, and chronic pelvic pain associated with *Chlamydia trachomatis* and *Neisseria gonorrhoeae* • Reduces the possible risk to the fetus of death, and physical and developmental disabilities including intellectual disability and blindness
Indicated vaccination	• Rubella vaccination to protect against congenital rubella syndrome • Influenza vaccination to prevent serious complications in pregnancy • Tdap to prevent neonatal pertussis (if not immunised in the past two years) • Td booster
Optimising weight in underweight or overweight and obese women	Reaching a healthy weight before pregnancy reduces the following risks: • Low-birth-weight babies in underweight women • Neural tube defects, preterm delivery, diabetes, cesarean section, and hypertensive disease associated with obesity (See **Chapter 44**, *High BMI: Obstetric implications*)
Smoking cessation	Smoking cessation before pregnancy prevents smoking-associated preterm birth and low birth weight
Eliminating alcohol use	Controlling alcohol consumption before pregnancy prevents fetal alcohol syndrome and other alcohol-related birth defects

AIDS, acquired immunodeficiency syndrome; *BMI*, body mass index; *HIV*, human immunodeficiency virus; *NTD*, neural tube defect; *PPH*, postpartum hemorrhage; *STI*, sexually transmitted infections; *Td*, tetanus-diptheria vaccine; *Tdap*, tetanus, diphtheria, and pertussis vaccine

Several medical disorders may affect women before or during their pregnancy. These women need counselling regarding the effects of these disorders on pregnancy, complications they are prone to, and the special precautions to be initiated. Therefore, women with particular risk factors require individualised and specific recommendations (Table 1.2).

Table 1.2 Recommended preconception interventions for women with specific risk factors

Risk factor	Intervention	Proven health benefit
Antiepileptic drug use	Changing to a less teratogenic treatment regimen	Decreases risk of fetal malformations; NTD
Diabetes	Achieving and maintaining hemoglobin A1C <6.5 per cent (48 mmol/mol)	Decreases risk of miscarriages and preterm birth; congenital anomalies, length of NICU admission, perinatal mortality, and long-term health consequences in the infant
Hypertension	Discontinue angiotensin-converting enzyme inhibitors and angiotensin-receptor blockers; switch to methyldopa, labetalol or calcium channel blocker (nifedipine); if long-standing HTN, assess for renal disease, ventricular hypertrophy, and retinopathy	Decreases congenital anomalies, HTN complications, cesarean section, FGR, placental abruption, preterm birth, and perinatal death
Hypothyroidism	Thyroxine supplementation to maintain TSH level at <3.0 μIU/mL	Decreases infertility, preterm birth, low birth weight, fetal death, and possibly neurological problems in the infant
Hyperthyroidism	PTU to maintain FT4 in high normal range, and TSH in low normal range	Decreases spontaneous pregnancy loss, preterm birth, preeclampsia, fetal death, FGR, maternal congestive heart failure, thyroid storm, and neonatal Graves' disease
Asthma	Management with inhalation therapy (bronchodilators/glucocorticoids)	Decreases preterm birth, low birth weight, preeclampsia, and perinatal mortality
Systemic lupus erythematosus	≥6 months of quiescence on stable therapy	Decreases risk of HTN, preeclampsia, preterm birth, fetal death, FGR, neonatal lupus

FGR, fetal growth restriction; *FT4*, free thyroxin; *HTN*, hypertension; *NICU*, neonatal intensive care unit; *NTD*, neural tube defects; *PTU*, propylthiouracil; *TSH*, thyroid-stimulating hormone

All-or-none period of embryogenesis
The first two weeks after conception are a remarkable period for the embryo. At this stage, exposure to teratogens can result in one of the following consequences:
- **Complete loss of pregnancy** (spontaneous miscarriage) due to severe cellular insult or
- **No damage at all** because pleuripotent embryonic cells can replace the cells destroyed or damaged by the teratogen
  This is referred to as the 'all-or-none' period of embryogenesis.

MEDICATIONS THAT CAN BE TERATOGENIC IN PREGNANCY

- Any time a woman in the reproductive age group presents to a physician is an excellent opportunity to review whether she is on any potentially teratogenic medications.

- If the woman is on a teratogenic drug, it should be substituted with a safer one. For example, if a hypertensive woman in the reproductive age group is on an angiotensin-converting enzyme (ACE) inhibitor (e.g., enalapril or captopril), she must be advised to switch to a safer drug (e.g., methyldopa, labetalol, or nifedipine).

- It is unfortunate that many women (and occasionally their general physicians) feel compelled to stop effective and essential medications as soon as pregnancy is diagnosed. This jeopardises the health of both the woman and her baby.

- A few drugs are proven teratogens and must be avoided (see box below).

- In rare circumstances, a teratogenic drug may be continued, e.g., a woman with mechanical cardiac valves who accepts the risk of warfarin may be kept on the medication.

> **When prescribing drugs in pregnancy:**
> - Minimise the number of medications prescribed.
> - Choose a drug that has been available for a long time and has an established safety profile. Pregnancy is not the time to prescribe the newest drug available in the market.
> - Use the drug at the lowest dose and for the shortest duration that is effective.

Teratogenic prescription drugs contraindicated in pregnancy
- Androgens and testosterone derivatives (e.g., danazol)
- Angiotensin-converting enzyme (ACE) inhibitors (e.g., enalapril and captopril) and angiotensin II receptor blockers
- Coumadin derivatives (e.g., warfarin)
- Carbamazepine
- Diethylstilbestrol
- Folic acid antagonists (e.g., methotrexate and aminopterin)
- Statins
- Lithium
- Phenytoin
- Primidone
- Streptomycin and kanamycin
- Tetracycline
- Thalidomide and leflunomide
- Trimethadione and paramethadione
- Valproic acid
- Vitamin A above recommended daily allowance (RDA) and its derivatives (e.g., isotretinoin, etretinate, and retinoids)

(Modified from Berghella, 2016)

- The US Food and Drug Administration (FDA) safety rating system was a widely used tool for evaluating drug safety during pregnancy.

- This system rated medication risk using categories A, B, C, D, and X, based on the available data in human and animal studies.

- However, in 2015, the FDA replaced the former pregnancy risk letter categories with the **Pregnancy and Lactation Labelling Rule** (PLLR), with effect from June 2015.

- This has descriptive subsections for:
  - Pregnancy
  - Lactation
  - The effect of various drugs on females and males of reproductive potential

In cases where the woman conceived while on a teratogenic drug, termination of the pregnancy is usually not required, since most drugs only marginally increase the risk of congenital malformations.

EXPOSURE TO IONISING RADIATION

- In women who can potentially become pregnant, diagnostic X-rays must preferably be done in the first 14 days of the menstrual cycle to avoid inadvertent exposure to radiation.

Effect of radiation on the fetus

- The human embryo and fetus are particularly sensitive to ionising radiation. High radiation doses may lead to growth restriction, malformations, impaired brain function, and cancer. Fortunately, most common diagnostic radiological procedures do not expose the fetus to significant levels of radiation.
- The effect of radiation on the fetus depends on the gestational age and the dose of ionising radiation:
  - First 14 days after conception, >0.1 Gy (or 10 rad)
    - Death of embryo or no effect (**all-or-none** principle)
  - At all gestational ages, <0.05 Gy (or 5 rad)
    - No adverse effect
  - After 16 weeks, <0.50 Gy (or 50 rad)
    - No effect
- The following imaging studies performed on the mother have no effect on the fetus:
  - Diagnostic X-rays of the head, neck, chest, and limbs
  - Ultrasound and magnetic resonance imaging (MRI)
  - Dental X-rays
  - CT scans not involving the abdomen or pelvis

Safety precautions
A lead apron should be used over the abdomen of any pregnant woman undergoing non-abdominopelvic radiological imaging. This minimises fetal exposure.

References

1. American College of Obstetricians and Gynecologists. 2005 (reaffirmed 2017). ACOG Committee Opinion No. 313. The importance of preconception care in the continuum of women's health care. *Obstet Gynecol.* 106:665–6.
2. Berghella V (Ed). 2016. *Obstetric Evidence Based Guidelines,* Third Edition. CRC Press.

3. Dunlop AL, Gardiner PM, Shellhaas CS et al. 2008. The clinical content of preconception care: The use of medications and supplements among women of reproductive age. *Am J Obstet Gynecol.* 12:s367–s372.

4. Dunlop AL, Jack B, Frey K. 2007. National recommendations for preconception care: The essential role of the family physician.*J Am Board Fam Med.* 20(1):81-4.

5. Johnson K, Posner SF, Biermann J, Cordero JF, Atrash HK, Parker CS, Boulet S, Curtis MG. 2006. CDC/ATSDR Preconception Care Work Group, Select Panel on Preconception Care. Recommendations to improve preconception health and health care--United States. *MMWR Recomm Rep.* 55(RR-6):1.

6. Singh S, Shekhar C, Acharya R et al. 2018. The incidence of abortion and unintended pregnancy in India, 2015. *The Lancet Global Health.* 6 (1), pp. e111-e12C.

7. World Health Organization. 2013. Meeting to develop a global consensus on preconception care to reduce maternal and childhood mortality and morbidity, WHO, Geneva.

Chapter 2

Antenatal Care: Initial Assessment

INTRODUCTION

- Antenatal care (ANC) is the care provided by skilled healthcare professionals (nurses, midwives, general practitioners, or obstetricians) to pregnant women in order to safeguard the health of both mothers and babies during pregnancy. Antenatal care also aims to ensure an optimal outcome for both mother and baby.

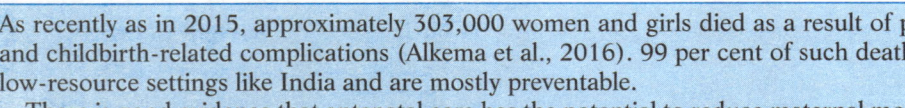

> As recently as in 2015, approximately 303,000 women and girls died as a result of pregnancy- and childbirth-related complications (Alkema et al., 2016). 99 per cent of such deaths occur in low-resource settings like India and are mostly preventable.
> There is good evidence that antenatal care has the potential to reduce maternal morbidity and mortality, as well as to improve newborn survival, especially in developing countries (Carroli et al., 2001; Bergsjo, 2001).

- ANC was originally instituted to reduce the incidence of low-birth-weight and preterm infants. Currently, its aims are broader and include the following:
  - To accurately estimate gestational age as early as possible
  - To identify pregnancies with maternal or fetal conditions associated with the potential for morbidity/mortality
  - To provide interventions to prevent or treat such complications
  - To provide education support and health promotion that can have lasting effects on the health of an entire family; this last component is a vital one and is essential in promoting and maintaining women's health (WHO, 2016)

> **How does ANC reduce maternal and perinatal morbidity and mortality?**
> - Directly
>   - Through the detection and treatment of pregnancy-related complications
> - Indirectly
>   - Through the identification and stratification of risk factors in pregnant women
>   - Through the implementation of preventive and therapeutic measures for complications during labour and delivery

- Global uptake of ANC varies widely and is influenced by the value women place on the service they receive.
- In the 1990s, the WHO introduced the **four-visit focused ANC** (FANC) model (WHO, 2002) for healthy women with no medical complications in low-resource areas. However, the reduced number of visits (typically fewer than five visits) was associated with 15 per cent more perinatal deaths for women with low-risk pregnancies in middle-

and lower-income countries when compared to women who had more visits (Doswell et al., 2015).

- Moreover, women prefer the standard number of visits, which usually varies from 8-12 visits during a pregnancy. The new WHO recommendations on antenatal care for a positive pregnancy experience recommend at least eight visits (WHO, 2016).

> The four-visit focused ANC model does not offer women adequate contact with healthcare practitioners and is no longer recommended. The new WHO guidelines recommend at least eight visits (WHO, 2016).

> **Number and timing of visits**
> ANC usually consists of 8–12 visits per pregnancy:
> - *Booking visit* at 10–14 weeks; aneuploidy screening can performed at this time (see **Chapter 7**, *Prenatal screening for genetic disorders*)
> - *Follow-up visits*
>   - About every four weeks at approximately 16, 20, 24, and 28 weeks
>   - About every two weeks from 32–36 weeks
>   - Then weekly until delivery

- In India, antenatal care is delivered partly by the public sector and partly by the private sector, and there is a large variation in the way women access antenatal care across socio-economic groups. The central and state governments have implemented extensive antenatal care packages across the country. Bookings can be made by the medical officers or by the village health nurse on the field. Women who have no risk factors are referred to the Primary Health Centre (PHC) for further antenatal care. Those who have one or more risk factors are referred to institutional care.
- It is imperative that ANC be protocol-driven and evidence-based, and that it involves the mother in decision-making by providing her with ample information.

THE FIRST OR BOOKING VISIT

> **What matters to women?**
> Downe et al. (2015) undertook a systematic review across 41 countries and found that women want and need a positive pregnancy experience from ANC staff and services. The theme that emerged globally, across all cultural and socio-demographic strata, is that women worldwide request the same four things:
> - Maintaining physical and socio-cultural normality
> - Maintaining a healthy pregnancy for mother and baby (including preventing and managing risks, illness, and death)
> - Transitioning effectively to positive labour and birth
> - Achieving positive motherhood
>
> It is essential for all providers of antenatal care to realise that it is the basic human right of a woman to be treated respectfully, to be involved in decision-making, and to be given empathetic and compassionate care.

- The first or booking antenatal visit is ideally initiated before 12 weeks of pregnancy. Less than 50 per cent of women in developing countries receive early antenatal care, whereas in developed countries, over 80 per cent of women receive such care (Moller et al., 2017).

- For antenatal care to be effective, women should be given information based on current available evidence in a manner that is easy to understand to enable them to make informed choices about their care (NICE, 2008). This includes information on the following:

> The first visit is an opportunity to earn the trust of the mother/couple and hence it should be a positive experience. The emphasis should be on courteous treatment and clear communication. There should be reinforcement of the fact that pregnancy is a normal, physiological event. The most important message to be conveyed to the mother is that the majority of pregnancies proceed without a complication. A confident mother will have a positive outlook and will participate in her pregnancy in an assured manner.

- Iron and folic acid supplementation with additional vitamin B12 and vitamin D supplementation when appropriate
- Lifestyle advice including exercise and activity
- Diet and nutrition advice with special emphasis on appropriate weight gain
- Antenatal screening tests for anemia, hemoglobinopathies, Down syndrome and fetal structural defects, diabetes, and hypertension
- The baby's growth and development
- Subsequent visits and place of delivery
- Antenatal classes focused on educating the couple about childbirth
- Discussion of mental health issues/safety in the domestic or workspace

The five components of the booking visit
1. Evaluation
   - History
   - Examination
2. Gestational age calculation and assessment
3. Risk stratification for subsequent management
4. Testing and screening
   - Blood investigations
   - Ultrasound
   - Aneuploidy screen
   - Gestational diabetes/gestational hypertension screen
5. General advice
   - Diet
   - Exercise
   - Travel
   - Work
   - Common symptoms and management

Evaluation

- The aim of prenatal care is the identification of women at increased risk of medical complications, pregnancy complications, or fetal abnormalities.

- A structured proforma such as that presented in Table 2.1 is useful as it minimises errors of omission.

Table 2.1   Structured proforma for the first booking visit

Parameters	Components
Demographics	• Name and age • Contact number • Address
Menstrual history	• Pattern of periods • Last menstrual period (LMP)

Obstetric history	• Prior pregnancy outcomes
	• Mode of conception
	• Antenatal problems
	  – Maternal
	  – Fetal
	• Intrapartum problems
	• Mode of delivery
	  – Spontaneous/instrumental
	  – Cesarean section
	• Indication
	• Birth weight and gender
	• Postnatal period
	• Lactation

Medical history	• Allergies to medications • Diabetes • PCOS • Chronic hypertension • Bronchial asthma • Tuberculosis • Recurrent urinary tract infection • Thyroid disorders • Gastrointestinal dysfunction • Neurological disorders • Pelvic infection/sexually transmitted infections • Risk for venous thromboembolism
Surgical history	• Cervical surgeries • Abdominal surgeries • Pelvic surgery for infertility
Family history	• Diabetes • Hypertension • Genetic disorders (pedigree chart if needed) • Psychiatric/mood disorders • Bleeding disorders • Babies with congenital abnormalities
Personal/drug history	• Diet • Current medications

(Continued)

(Continued)

Parameters	Components
	• Immunisation status for rubella
	• Smoking
	— Active/Passive
	• Alcohol
Psychosocial history	• Major depression
	• Domestic violence
	• Socio-economic status
	• Support systems

- The importance of a detailed history and examination cannot be overemphasised. It helps in the **stratification of risk** and in making a plan for pregnancy management, especially when high-risk factors are identified.
- An ANC record should be maintained for documenting care during the pregnancy. Structured records with reminder aids help ensure that ANC providers incorporate evidence-based protocols into their practice (Saccone and Sendek, 2016). This prevents errors arising from the overlooking of important patient data.

Initial examination

- Maternal height and weight should be documented at the booking visit, and body mass index (BMI) calculated. Calculating BMI helps to identify at-risk populations and enables counselling for appropriate weight gain in pregnancy. Both underweight and obese women should be counselled about their specific risks in pregnancy.

> **Calculating BMI**
> BMI = Weight (kg)/height squared (m²)
> BMI should be based on weight at the time of conception or the earliest known weight in pregnancy.

- The woman's weight should be recorded at every subsequent visit since optimal weight gain is associated with better outcomes (Saccone and Sendek, 2016). Both suboptimal weight gain and excessive weight gain are a cause for concern.
- Baseline blood pressure should be documented. Further evaluation is required if the baseline blood pressure is high (chronic hypertension).
- A complete physical examination should be performed.
- A pelvic examination should be performed to assess uterine size and shape. The adnexae should also be evaluated at this time (Lockwood and Magriples, 2018). When the uterine size on physical examination differs from that predicted by menstrual dating, an ultrasound evaluation of the uterus is indicated.
- Routine breast examination during antenatal care is not recommended solely for the prediction of successful breastfeeding (Lee and Thomas, 2008). In the past, it was thought that breast

> If a woman expresses concerns about flat or inverted nipples, she should be examined and her fears should be dispelled. She should be reassured that lactational assistance and education during breastfeeding initiation will help her effectively feed her infant.

examination at the initial antenatal appointment could help identify flat or inverted nipples, for which remedial nipple exercises could be prescribed. However, there is good evidence that neither flat nor inverted nipples prevent women from breastfeeding successfully.

Gestational age assessment

- Accurate assessment of gestational age is vital to the management of pregnancy.

> Though a routine ultrasound examination is not required at the initial visit, indications for accurate gestational age assessment include the following:
> - A history of irregular menses
> - Unknown or uncertain last menstrual period
> - Patients who conceived while taking oral contraceptive pills
> - Uterine size discordant with menstrual dates

- Assessing and assigning the correct estimated date of delivery (EDD) is useful for timing tests, monitoring fetal growth, and planning intervention and delivery in high-risk situations. It also significantly reduces the frequency of

> An ultrasound at $11–13^{+6}$ weeks helps in:
> - Confirming viability
> - Establishing gestational age accurately
> - Determining the number of viable fetuses
> - Evaluating fetal gross anatomy and risk of aneuploidy

labour induction for postterm pregnancy (Caughey et al., 2008) and the use of tocolysis for suspected preterm labour.

- In women with regular cycles (28–30 days), Naegele's rule is a simple method of pregnancy dating (EDD = LMP minus 3 months plus 7 days). This method assumes that the patient has a 28–30-day menstrual cycle with fertilisation occurring on day 14–16.

- Gestational age assignment using ultrasound is ideally done between $11–13^{+6}$ weeks, and the crown–rump length (CRL) is used for the purpose of dating (see **Chapter 9**, *Ultrasound in the first trimester*). At this time, aneuploidy screening can also be done in tandem. If the CRL is >84 mm, then the head

> **Assigning EDD in pregnancy resulting from assisted reproductive technology (ART)**
> If a pregnancy resulted from ART, the ART-derived gestational age should be used to assign the EDD. For example, the EDD for a pregnancy resulting from in vitro fertilisation should be established using the age of the embryo and the date of transfer.

circumference (HC) is used to determine the EDD (NICE, 2008; ISUOG, 2013).

- Gestational age assessment by ultrasound done before 20 weeks is more accurate than that estimated by menstrual history alone, especially in women with irregular cycles or those uncertain about the dates.

Stratification of risk

- **Pre-existing risk factors** that place the mother in a high-risk category may include the following:
    - Simple determinants (e.g., maternal age, height, or parity)
    - Medical conditions (e.g., asthma, diabetes, hypertension, or severe anemia)
    - Obstetric history of complications (e.g., previous stillbirth or cesarean section)

- **Risk factors that develop in the current pregnancy** may include the following:
  - Hypertension/diabetes
  - Multiple pregnancy
  - Antepartum hemorrhage
  - Abnormal lie
- A pregnant woman may be high-risk for a particular problem at booking (e.g., at risk for Down syndrome due to her age). If such a risk is ruled out by testing, the woman can subsequently revert to normal care.
- On the other hand, if a mother has a medical problem such as diabetes mellitus, chronic hypertension, or antiphospholipid syndrome (APS), she will remain high-risk not just through her pregnancy but also intra- and postpartum.
- Risk stratification helps in planning the appropriate level of care. Once a detailed history is taken, including that of family history of genetic disorders, all risk factors are documented and the pregnancy is assigned to one of four risk categories (Table 2.2).
- The difficulty with risk assessment lies in category II, in which the baby is unexpectedly compromised. The likelihood of predicting all adverse outcomes is limited; several scoring systems have been used for this purpose, but have failed to consistently identify this group.

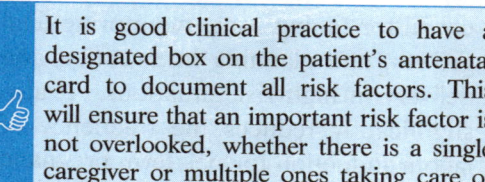

It is good clinical practice to have a designated box on the patient's antenatal card to document all risk factors. This will ensure that an important risk factor is not overlooked, whether there is a single caregiver or multiple ones taking care of the woman.

Table 2.2 Pregnancy risk categories

Category	Description
I	Low-risk mother with a low-risk fetus, i.e., normal pregnancy, mother and baby well
II	Low-risk mother with a high-risk fetus, e.g., normal pregnancy, mother well but baby unexpectedly compromised
III	High-risk mother with a low-risk fetus, e.g., maternal asthma
IV	High-risk mother with a high-risk infant, e.g., severe hypertension with fetal growth restriction

Testing and screening at the booking visit

Blood investigations

- ***Complete blood count (CBC; inclusive of hemoglobin, hematocrit, and other blood indices)*** is recommended for all pregnant women at their first antenatal visit. It helps in the early diagno-

Available evidence does not support routine screening of pregnant women for chlamydia, cytomegalovirus, toxoplasmosis and herpes simplex in pregnancy.

sis of anemia (hemoglobin <11 g/mL), the incidence of which has been reported to be as high as 85 per cent among pregnant women in India (Toteja et al., 2006).

A mean corpuscular volume (MCV) <80 fL is suggestive of iron deficiency anemia and an MCV >115 fL is suggestive of B_{12}-deficiency anemia. An MCV <80 fL in the absence of iron deficiency anemia is suggestive of hemoglobinopathy and should be investigated. If the hemoglobin is low and does not respond to adequate doses of hematinics, further testing using serum ferritin, total iron-binding capacity, and serum B12 level may be required.

 An MCV <80 fL in the absence of iron deficiency suggests thalassemia. In such cases, further testing with hemoglobin electrophoresis is indicated (see **Chapter 47**, *Anemia and hemoglobinopathies in pregnancy*).

- **Blood grouping and Rh typing** is recommended for all pregnant women at their first prenatal visit. If a woman is identified to be Rh (D)-negative, her husband/partner should be tested for Rh type because an Rh (D)-positive husband/partner places an Rh-negative woman at risk for Rh alloimmunisation.

  Antibody screening is recommended at the booking visit for all Rh (D)-negative women (Lockwood and Magriples, 2020). In the presence of antibodies, prevention of severe fetal anemia and fetal death is possible with specific interventions.

- **Screening for syphilis** should be offered to all pregnant women at an early stage in antenatal care because universal screening and treatment of syphilis prevent complications in the mother and her baby (Cheng et al., 2007).

- **Serological screening for hepatitis B surface antigen (HBsAg)** should be offered to all pregnant women so that effective postnatal interventions can be offered to infected women. Passive and active immunisation of the newborn within 12 hours of delivery can reduce the risk of HBV transmission by more than 95 per cent.

 Pregnant women need not be offered routine screening for hepatitis C virus unless they are at high risk for having the infection (NICE, 2008; Lockwood and Magriples, 2020). Hepatitis C status in pregnancy does not affect treatment, route of delivery, or breastfeeding.

- **Screening for HIV infection** should be offered early in antenatal care, and should be performed only after the woman's informed consent has been obtained.

  Advantages of universal screening for HIV
  - Informed decision to continue or terminate pregnancy
  - Initiation of early treatment for the mother
  - Prevention of transmission to partner or identification of infected partner
  - Prevention of vertical transmission to the newborn by appropriate antenatal interventions

- **Screening for gestational diabetes** is recommended at the booking visit for all Indian women since they are at intermediate/high risk of developing gestational diabetes. If the first-trimester screening test is negative, the test should be repeated at 24–28 weeks. Either fasting plasma glucose or plasma glucose two hours after the administration of 75 g glucose is acceptable as a screening test. Screening for diabetes in pregnancy is discussed in detail in **Chapter 40**, *Gestational and pre-gestational diabetes*.

- **Rubella susceptibility screening** should be offered early in antenatal care (if not done preconceptionally) to identify women at risk of contracting rubella infection and to enable vaccination in the **postnatal** period for the protection of future pregnancies (NICE, 2008; Lockwood and Magriples, 2020). It is safe for breastfeeding women to receive MMR vaccination.

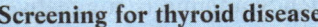

> **Screening for thyroid disease**
> Since there is insufficient evidence that the identification and treatment of subclinical hypothyroidism in pregnant women improves maternal or infant outcomes, universal screening for subclinical hypothyroidism by TSH or thyroid peroxidase (TPO) antibody is not currently recommended (Ross, 2018).

- *Screening for asymptomatic bacteriuria*, which is an established risk factor for preterm delivery, low birth weight, and acute pyelonephritis (Smaill and Vazquez, 2015), is recommended in high-resource countries. It occurs in approximately 9 per cent of pregnant women worldwide (WHO, 2016). Identification and treatment of asymptomatic bacteriuria reduces the risk of such complications. Ideally, screening for bacteriuria should be done with a culture of a clean-catch urine specimen. However, this test is not a part of routine antenatal care in India because of the cost involved and the requirement for laboratory facilities. In under-resourced areas, nitrite dipsticks may be used for screening (Jayalakshmi and Jayaram, 2008), and if positive, may be followed-up with a urine culture and sensitivity test to confirm significant bacteriuria. If the culture shows significant growth, appropriate antibiotics are prescribed.

- *Screening for aneuploidy (including Down syndrome)* should be offered to all women at booking wherever resources are available. After explaining the test, the decision to have the screening test should be left to the couple. The test that should ideally be offered is a combined first-trimester screening (done at $11-13^{+6}$ weeks); the second-trimester quadruple test (or triple test) should be reserved for women who book later in pregnancy (see **Chapter 7**, *Prenatal screening for genetic disorders*).

General advice and information to be given at the initial visit

Dietary advice and nutritional supplements

This is dealt with in detail in **Chapter 3,** *Dietary advice and nutritional supplements.*

Exercise in pregnancy

- In low-risk pregnancies, exercise is not only safe but also beneficial. Women should be encouraged to initiate or continue exercise to derive the health benefits associated with such activities.

> Structured physical exercise during pregnancy in low-risk pregnancies is associated with a significantly higher incidence of vaginal delivery and a significantly lower incidence of cesarean delivery (Domenjoz et al., 2014).

  At least 30 minutes of moderate exercise, 4–5 days a week, is recommended. Brisk walking is the best form of aerobic exercise that is accessible to all pregnant women.
- A recent review and meta-analysis (Di Mascio et al., 2016) found that aerobic exercise for 35–90 minutes, 3–4 times per week during pregnancy in normal-weight women with singleton, uncomplicated gestations lowers the incidence of gestational diabetes mellitus and hypertensive disorders, and therefore, should be encouraged.

- Exercise is not associated with an increased risk of preterm birth.
- Yoga in pregnancy is associated with decreased pain, discomfort, lowering of perceived stress, and improved quality of life (Babbar et al., 2012).
- Women with complicated pregnancies are discouraged from participating in intensive exercise activities. They can be educated about undertaking appropriate exercise.

Work

- Women with uncomplicated pregnancies may be allowed to carry on with their normal activities.
- Women can continue to go to work until they go into labour. The only planning required is to ensure that the mother can reach the healthcare facility from her place of employment in a reasonable amount of time.

 Working women and their caregivers should be aware of the rules regarding maternity leave at their workplace. As of March 2017, the Maternity Benefit (Amendment) Act increased maternity leave from 12 weeks to 26 weeks. Prenatal leave has also been extended from six weeks to eight weeks.

Travel

- Travel by two- and three-wheeler vehicles, cars and trains is safe in pregnancy.
- While most women are low-risk and can expect no problems with air travel during pregnancy, long-distance air travel is associated with an increased risk of venous thrombosis. This problem can be avoided by walking and exercising during the flight.

Sexual intercourse

- Pregnant women should be reassured that sexual intercourse in pregnancy is not known to be associated with any adverse outcomes.
- There is no evidence that sexual activity increases the risk of preterm birth between 29 and 36 weeks (Sayle et al., 2001).
- There is not enough evidence to suggest that sexual intercourse is effective for the induction of labour and should not be suggested as a form of induction (Saccone et al., 2016).

Smoking and alcohol intake

- Though smoking among Indian women is not common, enquiries about the habit should be made during history taking with respectful and sensitive questions.
- Smoking during pregnancy has been associated with numerous adverse pregnancy outcomes, including spontaneous pregnancy loss, placental abruption, preterm premature rupture of membranes, placenta previa, preterm labour and delivery, low birth weight, and ectopic pregnancy.
- Alcohol is a known teratogen at all stages of gestation. The most severe consequences of prenatal alcohol exposure are stillbirth (an 8-fold increase in the risk of stillbirth) and fetal alcohol spectrum disorder (FASD), which includes physical, mental, behavioural, and cognitive effects (Chang, 2018).

Though the effects vary with different factors, alcohol is best avoided throughout pregnancy.

Immunisation in pregnancy

The schedule for immunisation in pregnancy (including tetanus and influenza) is detailed in **Chapter 50**, *Immunisation in pregnancy*.

SCHEDULE FOR FURTHER VISITS

- Traditionally, the frequency of antenatal visits has been once a month until 28 weeks, once in two weeks until 36 weeks, and weekly thereafter. However, there have been no randomised trials to confirm the benefit of this schedule.
- The WHO antenatal care guidelines suggest a minimum of eight antenatal visits for all women, regardless of parity. The WHO advises at least one visit in the first trimester, two in the second trimester, and five in the third trimester.
- High-risk pregnancies are advised more frequent visits, depending on the risk factors.

References

1. Alkema L, Chou D, Hogan D, Zhang S, Moller A-B, Gemmill A et al. 2016. United Nations Maternal Mortality Estimation Inter-Agency Group – Collaborators and Technical Advisory Group. Global, regional, and national levels and trends in maternal mortality between 1990 and 2015, with scenario-based projections to 2030: A systematic analysis by the UN Maternal Mortality Estimation Inter-Agency Group. *Lancet.* 387(10017):462–74.

2. American College of Obstetricians and Gynecologists. 2018. ACOG Committee Opinion No. 732. Influenza vaccination during pregnancy. *Obstet Gynecol.* 131:e109–14.

3. Babbar S, Parks-Savage AC, Chauhan SP. 2012. Yoga during pregnancy: A review. *Am J Perinatol.* 29:459–464.

4. Bergsjo P. 2001. What is the evidence for the role of antenatal care strategies in the reduction of maternal mortality and morbidity? *Studies in HSO & P.* 17. 387–414

5. Blencowe H, Lawn J, Vandelaer J, Roper M, Cousens S. 2010. Tetanus toxoid immunization to reduce mortality from neonatal tetanus. *Int J Epidemiol.* 39 (Suppl. 1):i102–i109

6. Carroli G, Rooney C, Villar J. 2001. How effective is antenatal care in preventing maternal mortality and serious morbidity? An overview of the evidence. *Paediatr Perinatol Epidemiol.* 15 (Suppl. 1):1–42.

7. Caughey AB, Nicholson JM, Washington AE. 2008. First- vs second-trimester ultrasound: The effect on pregnancy dating and perinatal outcomes. *Am J Obstet Gynecol.* 198, 703.e1–703.e6.

8. Centers for Disease Control and Prevention. 2011. Updated recommendations for use of tetanus toxoid, reduced diphtheria toxoid and acellular pertussis vaccine (Tdap) in pregnant women and persons who have or anticipate having close contact with an infant aged <12 months—Advisory Committee on Immunization Practices (ACIP), 2012. 60:1424–6.

9. Chang G. 2018. Alcohol intake and pregnancy. Lockwood CJ (Ed). *UpToDate*: Waltham, MA.

10. Cheng JQ, Zhou H, Hong FC et al. 2007. Syphilis screening and intervention in 500,000 pregnant women in Shenzhen, the People's Republic of China. *Sex Transm Infect.* 83:347.

11. Di Mascio D, Magro-Malosso ER, Saccone G, Marhefka GD, Berghella V. 2016. Exercise during pregnancy in normal-weight women and risk of preterm birth: A systematic review and meta-analysis of randomized controlled trials. *Am J Obstet. Gynecol.*

12. Domenjoz I, Kayser B, Boulvain M. 2014. Effect of physical activity during pregnancy on mode of delivery. *Am J Obstet Gynecol.* 211(4): 401.e1–11.

13. Downe S, Finlayson K, Tuncalp Ö, Metin Gülmezoglu A. 2016. What matters to women: A systematic scoping review to identify the processes and outcomes of antenatal care provision that are important to healthy pregnant women. *BJOG.* 123:529–539.

14. Dowswell T, Carroli G, Duley L et al. 2015. Alternative versus standard packages of antenatal care for low-risk pregnancy. *Cochrane Database Sys Rev.* Issue 7. Art. no.: CD000934.

15. ISUOG. 2013. Practice Guidelines: Performance of first-trimester fetal ultrasound scan. *Ultrasound Obstet Gynecol.* 41:102–113.

16. Jayalakshmi J, Jayaram VS. 2008. Evaluation of various screening tests to detect asymptomatic bacteriuria in pregnant women. *Indian J Pathol Microbiol.* 51:379–81

17. Lee SJ, Thomas J. 2008. Antenatal breast examination for promoting breastfeeding. *Cochrane Database of Sys Rev.* Issue 3. Art. no.: CD006064.

18. Lockwood CJ, Magriples U. 2018. Prenatal care: Initial Assessment. Berghella V (Ed). *UpToDate.* Waltham, MA.

19. Moller AB, Petzold M, Chou D, Say L. 2017. Early antenatal care visit: A systematic analysis of regional and global levels and trends of coverage from 1990 to 2013. *Lancet Glob Health.* 5:e977.

20. NICE. 2008. Clinical Guideline no. 62. Routine care for the healthy pregnant woman.

21. Ross DS. 2018. Overview of thyroid disease in pregnancy. Cooper DS, Lockwood CJ (Eds). *UpToDate.* Waltham, MA.

22. Saccone G, Sendek K. 2016. *Prenatal* Care in Obstetric Evidence-Based Guidelines. Berghella V, Taylor and Francis (Eds). CRC Press.

23. Sayle AE, Savitz DA, Thorp JM Jr. et al. 2001. Sexual activity during late pregnancy and risk of preterm delivery. *Obstet & Gynecol.* 97:283.

24. Singh A, Pallikadavath S, Ogollah R, Stones W. 2012. Maternal tetanus toxoid vaccination and neonatal mortality in rural North India. PLoS ONE. 7(11):e48891.

25. Smaill FM, Vazquez JC. 2015. Antibiotics for asymptomatic bacteriuria in pregnancy. *Cochrane Database Sys Rev.* Issue 8. Art. no.: CD000490.

26. Toteja GS, Singh P, Dhillon BS, Saxena BN, Ahmed FU, Singh RP et al. 2006. Prevalence of anaemia among pregnant women and adolescent girls in 16 districts of India. *Food Nutr Bull.* 27:311–5.

27. World Health Organization. 2002. WHO antenatal care randomised trial. Manual for the implementation of the new Model. WHO, Geneva.

28. World Health Organization. 2016. WHO recommendation on the method for diagnosing asymptomatic bacteriuria in pregnancy (December 2016). The WHO Reproductive Health Library. WHO, Geneva.

29. World Health Organization. 2016. WHO recommendations on antenatal care for a positive pregnancy experience. WHO, Geneva.

Dietary Advice and Nutritional Supplements

INTRODUCTION

- Maternal physiological changes that occur during pregnancy require the right input of calories and a balanced diet. Macronutrients and micronutrients are also required to promote adequate fetal growth and development.
- Undernutrition and overnutrition are both associated with adverse pregnancy outcomes. Therefore, it is important to evaluate, monitor, and, when appropriate, make changes to improve maternal nutrition, both before and during pregnancy.

EFFECT OF MATERNAL WEIGHT ON PREGNANCY OUTCOMES

- Undernourished mothers (BMI <18 kg/m²), particularly low-income women, need special attention and focused dietary advice to meet their dietary needs. Unless they gain adequate weight during pregnancy, they are at risk of preterm labour and delivering low-birth-weight infants.
- For women whose BMI is >30 kg/m² at the initial visit, information should be provided on the impact of overweight and obesity on maternal and fetal well-being (see **Chapter 44**, *High maternal BMI: Obstetric implications*).
- Women who gain excessive weight in pregnancy are at an increased risk of preeclampsia, failed induction, cesarean delivery, and a macrosomic infant (DeVader et al., 2007).
- Olson and colleagues (2003) found that women who gained more weight than the recommended amount during pregnancy were three times more likely to retain 5 kg or more at one year postpartum (particularly low-income women).

DIETARY ADVICE

- Dietary advice is a very important part of the initial antenatal visit. The booking visit is an excellent opportunity to provide a dietary plan to the mother and to dispel cultural myths that interfere with proper nutrition.
- This is the best time to discuss and set weight gain goals that are appropriate for the individual. The mother must be given specific weight gain goals based on her weight and BMI at the initial visit (Table 3.1). This must be done with great sensitivity and without shaming the mother or sounding judgmental.

Avoiding excessive weight gain in pregnancy
There is good evidence to show that women who are given *dietary and/or exercise advice* to prevent excessive gestational weight gain as part of their antenatal care are less likely to gain excessive weight (WHO, 2016).

- Women should be educated about the ideal monthly weight gain. Women with a normal BMI should gain 1.0–1.5 kg per month after the initial three months. The maximum weight gain occurs after 20 weeks.

Table 3.1 Recommended weight gain based on pre-pregnancy BMI (Asian women)

Pre-pregnancy BMI (kg/m²)	Recommended weight gain (kg)
Normal (18.5–23)	11–15
Overweight (23–27.5)	10–12
Class I obese (27.5–31)	8–10
Class II obese (31–35)	5–7
Class III obese (≥35)	4

BMI, body mass index

Dietary advice for the first three months

- Most women struggle to maintain a balanced diet in the first three months of their pregnancy due to nausea and/or vomiting (see **Chapter 5**, *Common problems in the antenatal period and their management*).
- Pregnant women should be reassured that eating less, or suboptimally, will not affect the fetus.
- The mother must be advised to eat frequent, small, bland and low-fat snacks/meals. She must also be advised to avoid dehydration.

Healthy eating in pregnancy

- A healthy diet should provide adequate energy (from carbohydrates and fats) and a balanced combination of protein, vitamins, and minerals obtained through the consumption of a variety of foods including green and orange vegetables, meat, fish, beans, nuts, whole grains, and fruits.
- Though there is an increase in the daily caloric requirement during pregnancy, it can be met easily without excessive caloric load.
- In case the mother has difficulty in meeting, maintaining, or curtailing her caloric intake, she should be referred to a nutritionist who is specifically trained to advise pregnant women.

High-protein food supplements
High-protein food supplements are not recommended for pregnant women to improve perinatal and neonatal outcome. There is no evidence to support the prescribing of expensive protein powders (WHO, 2016).

Increased dietary requirements in pregnancy
- *Calories:* The recommended increase in daily caloric intake is 300 kcal/day in the second trimester and 400 kcal/day in the third trimester.
- *Carbohydrate:* The recommended daily allowance for carbohydrates is 175 g/day.
- *Protein:* Protein requirement in pregnancy is 1.1 g/kg/day.
- *Vitamins and minerals:* These are provided by the ingestion of fresh fruits and vegetables. However, supplements are essential.

Caffeine

- Moderate caffeine consumption (<200 mg/day) does not appear to be a major contributing factor in miscarriage, preterm birth, or low birth weight (Jahanfar and Jaafar, 2015).
- Two average cups of coffee or tea per day are safe in pregnancy.

ADVICE ON DIETARY SUPPLEMENTS

Iron

- Iron deficiency anemia may be related to puerperal sepsis, low birth weight, and preterm birth.
- Iron supplements (usually in combination with folic acid) are recommended for all pregnant women (WHO, 2018), especially in countries such as India where the prevalence of anemia (hemoglobin <11 g/mL) is as high as 85 per cent among pregnant women (Toteja et al., 2006).
- A systematic review of the Cochrane Database (Peña-Rosas, 2015), showed that routine iron and folic acid supplementation reduces the risk of maternal anemia and iron deficiency in pregnancy.

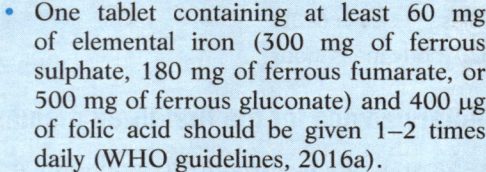

Recommended dosage of iron in pregnancy
- One tablet containing at least 60 mg of elemental iron (300 mg of ferrous sulphate, 180 mg of ferrous fumarate, or 500 mg of ferrous gluconate) and 400 µg of folic acid should be given 1–2 times daily (WHO guidelines, 2016a).
- Other iron salts are not more effective and are expensive.
- If the Hb is <7.0 g/dL, the dosage should be doubled.

Administering oral iron
- The dose should be taken on an empty stomach and with citrus juice for optimal absorption.
- The iron tablet should not be taken with calcium tablets, milk, tea, or coffee.

Folic acid

- Women should be informed that dietary supplementation with folic acid before conception and throughout the first 12 weeks of pregnancy reduces the risk of having a baby with a neural tube defect. The recommended dosage of folic acid is 400 µg per day.
- Mothers who are high-risk (previous baby with a neural tube defect, those on anti-convulsants, and those with pre-gestational diabetes) should be prescribed 4 mg daily.

Calcium

- Currently, there is no consensus on the role of routine calcium supplementation for pregnant women other than for preventing hypertension. In women with adequate dietary intake of calcium, a review of the Cochrane Database

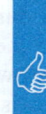

Women who do not take or do not tolerate dairy products should be prescribed calcium supplementation. Such women should be advised calcium supplementation with calcium carbonate or calcium citrate. The recommended dietary intake in pregnancy and lactation is 1000–1300 mg/day.

showed no additional benefits of calcium supplementation in the prevention of preterm birth or low infant birth weight (Buppasiri et al., 2015).

- Indian women with poor dietary calcium intake may be advised calcium supplementation with calcium carbonate or calcium citrate.
- In populations with low dietary calcium intake, daily calcium supplementation (1500–2000 mg oral elemental calcium) is recommended for pregnant women to reduce the risk of preeclampsia. When high dosage of calcium is not possible, even 500 mg daily seems to reduce the risk (Hofmeyr et al., 2018).
- Fetal skeletal development requires approximately 25–30 g of calcium during pregnancy, especially in the last trimester. Most of this calcium can be mobilised from the maternal stores.
- Calcium absorption increases during pregnancy and allows progressive retention throughout gestation.
- Dividing the dose of calcium may improve acceptability, with the total dosage divided into three doses, preferably taken at mealtimes. Calcium and iron should be taken at different times, several hours apart.

Vitamin D

- Routine vitamin D supplementation is **not routinely recommended** for pregnant women to improve maternal and perinatal outcomes (WHO guidelines, 2016). Instead, women should be advised that exposure to sunlight is the most important source of vitamin D. However, the amount of time of exposure required for it to be effective is not clear. It should be borne in mind that dark skin synthesises less vitamin D than light skin.

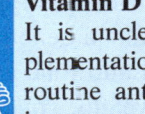

Vitamin D supplementation
It is unclear whether vitamin D supplementation should be given as part of routine antenatal care to all women to improve maternal and infant outcomes. Therefore, vitamin D need not be prescribed as a separate supplement (De-Regil et al., 2016, Cochrane Database).

- Vitamin D deficiency in pregnancy (<20 ng/mL or <50 nmol/L) may be associated with an increased risk of preeclampsia, gestational diabetes, preterm birth, and small-for-gestational-age infants (Wei et al., 2013).
- Vitamin D deficiency has a high prevalence among Indian pregnant women and coexists with other nutritional deficiencies, particularly calcium deficiency. However, there is insufficient evidence to support a recommendation for screening all pregnant women for vitamin D deficiency (ACOG Committee Opinion No. 495, 2011, reaffirmed 2017).
- For pregnant women thought to be at an increased risk of vitamin D deficiency (obesity, little or no exposure to sunlight), measuring maternal serum 25-hydroxyvitamin D levels can be considered. When vitamin D deficiency is identified during pregnancy, 1000–2000 IU of vitamin D per day is safe. Higher dose regimens used for the treatment of vitamin D deficiency have not been studied during pregnancy.

- There is limited data to assess any benefit of vitamin D supplements for total vegetarians, vegans, and women with extremely limited exposure to sunlight.

Other vitamins and micronutrients

- The following are not recommended routinely for a pregnant woman as they have not been shown to improve maternal and perinatal outcomes (WHO, 2016):
  - Vitamin A (unless in a geographic area with high prevalence of night blindness)
  - Vitamin B6 (pyridoxine)
  - Vitamins E and C

- A systematic review of the Cochrane Database on **zinc supplementation** (Ota et al., 2015) showed a small reduction in preterm births in women living in low-income areas who had taken such supplements. However, the authors felt that this reduction was a reflection of the overall poor nutrition and not specifically the deficiency of zinc.

Fish oil capsules or docosahexaenoic acid (DHA) supplements
There is no evidence to support the routine use of DHA supplementation during pregnancy. Supplementation has no impact on the child's cognitive development or other maternal and fetal outcomes (Saccone et al., 2015).

- The World Health Organization (WHO, 2016) does not recommend routinely prescribing **multiple micronutrient (MMN) supplementation**. However, a recent Cochrane review (Keats et al., 2019) suggests a benefit in the use of multiple micronutrient supplements (in combination with iron and folic acid) in low- and middle-income settings to reduce outcomes like low birth weight, small-for-gestational age babies, and possibly, preterm births. The optimal formulation for MMN supplements has not been determined.

References

1. American College of Obstetricians and Gynecologists. 2011 (reaffirmed 2017). ACOG Committee Opinion No. 495. Vitamin D: Screening and supplementation during pregnancy. *Obstet Gynecol.* 118:197–8.

2. Buppasiri P, Lumbiganon P, Thinkhamrop J, Ngamjarus C, Laopaiboon M, Medley N. 2015. Calcium supplementation (other than for preventing or treating hypertension) for improving pregnancy and infant outcomes. *Cochrane Database Syst Rev.* Issue 2. Art. no.: CD007079.

3. De-Regil LM, Palacios C, Lombardo LK, Peña-Rosas JP. 2016. Vitamin D supplementation for women during pregnancy. *Cochrane Database Syst Rev.* Issue 1. Art. no.: CD008873.

4. DeVader SR, Neeley H, Myles TD, Leet TL. 2007. Evaluation of gestational weight gain guidelines for women with normal pre-pregnancy body mass index. *Obstetrics & Gynecology.* 110, 745–751.

5. Hofmeyr G, Lawrie TA, Atallah ÁN, Torloni M. 2018. Calcium supplementation during pregnancy for preventing hypertensive disorders and related problems. *Cochrane Database Syst Rev.* Issue 10. Art. no.: CD001059.

6. Jahanfar S, Jaafar SH. 2015. Effects of restricted caffeine intake by mother on fetal, neonatal and pregnancy outcomes. *Cochrane Database Syst Rev.* Issue 6. Art. no.: CD006965.

7. Olson CM, Strawderman MS, Hinton PS, Pearson TA. 2003. Gestational weight gain and postpartum behaviors associated with weight change from early pregnancy to 1 y postpartum. *International Journal of Obesity*. Volume 27. 117–127.

8. Ota E, Mori R, Middleton P, Tobe-Gai R, Mahomed K, Miyazaki C et al. 2015. Zinc supplementation for improving pregnancy and infant outcome. *Cochrane Database Syst Rev*. Issue 2. Art. no.: CD000230.

9. Peña-Rosas J, De-Regil L, Garcia-Casal MN, Dowswell T. 2015. Daily oral iron supplementation during pregnancy. *Cochrane Database Syst Rev*. Issue 7. Art. no.: CD004736.

10. Saccone G, Saccone I, Berghella V. 2015. Omega-3 long chain polyunsaturated fatty acids and fish oil supplementation during pregnancy: Which evidence? *J Matern Fetal Neonatal Med*.

11. Toteja GS, Singh P, Dhillon BS, Saxena BN, Ahmed FU, S ngh RP et al. 2006. Prevalence of anaemia among pregnant women and adolescent girls in 16 distr cts of India. *Food Nutr Bull*. 27:311–5.

12. Wei SQ, Qi HP, Luo ZC et al. 2013. Maternal vitamin D status and adverse pregnancy outcomes: A systematic review and metaanalysis. *J Matern Fetal Neonatal Med*. 26:889–899.

13. World Health Organization. 2016. WHO recommendation on counselling on healthy eating and physical activity during pregnancy. The WHO Reproductive Health Library. WHO, Geneva.

14. World Health Organization. 2016. WHO recommendation regarding vitamin D supplementation during pregnancy for the prevention of pre-eclampsia. The WHO Reproductive Health Library. WHO, Geneva.

15. World Health Organization. 2018. WHO recommendation on daily oral iron and folic acid supplementation. The WHO Reproductive Health Library. WHO, Geneva.

Chapter 4

Antenatal Care: Second and Third Trimesters

INTRODUCTION

After the initial prenatal contact, the mother is given a schedule for follow-up visits. These subsequent visits monitor maternal and fetal health. Every visit is focused on the following:

- Identifying any problems that might arise
- Modifying risk stratification
- Implementing interventions that will help improve outcomes

All pregnant women want and deserve respectful and positive interactions with their healthcare provider.

At each visit, it is best to put the pregnant woman at ease by asking her general questions such as, "How are you feeling today?", "How is the baby?" and, in the third trimester, "Is the baby moving well?"

Further maternal and fetal investigations may also be required during specific trimesters of pregnancy. Follow-up visits most importantly provide ongoing opportunities for educating the mother and her family, answering her doubts, and allaying her fears. Communication is key to a successful and satisfying childbirth experience.

SCHEDULE OF VISITS

The typical schedule for prenatal visits for women with uncomplicated pregnancies as suggested by the American Academy of Pediatrics/American College of Obstetricians and Gynecologists (2017) is as follows:

- About every four weeks until 28 weeks of gestation
- About every two weeks from 28–36 weeks
- Then, weekly until delivery
  This is the schedule most commonly used and also the one followed by the author.
- If the first antenatal visit is around 12 weeks, it works out to approximately 12 visits for a term pregnancy. The number of visits will be more if the first visit is around six weeks of pregnancy.
- The World Health Organization's (WHO) antenatal care guidelines (2016) suggest a minimum of eight antenatal visits for all women, regardless of parity. The WHO advises at least one visit in the first trimester, two in the second trimester, and five in the third trimester. This was a revision of WHO's former recommendations called **Focused Antenatal Care (FANC),** which advocated four visits in a pregnancy. The changed recommendation was in response to a systematic review of the Cochrane Database (Doswell et al., 2015) that reported a 15 per cent increase in perinatal deaths in women with low-risk pregnancies in middle- and lower-income countries who had fewer antenatal visits (typically fewer than five visits) than those who had more visits.

- The Federation of Obstetric and Gynaecological Societies of India (Gole, 2015) suggests a similar schedule as the WHO, with the first visit preferably before 12 weeks.

Low-risk pregnancies

In women with low-risk pregnancies, no differences in neonatal intensive care unit admissions, five-minute Apgar score <7, neonatal demise, or small-for-gestational age infants were demonstrated between women who had more than 10 prenatal visits and those who had 10 or fewer prenatal visits (Carter et al., 2016).

High-risk pregnancies

High-risk pregnancies may require more visits depending on the specific problem and the need for frequent monitoring.

PHYSICAL EXAMINATION AT SUBSEQUENT VISITS

The focus of physical examination during each antenatal checkup has traditionally been on the following aspects:

- Maternal weight
- Blood pressure
- Fetal heart tones
- Uterine size and Leopold's manoeuvres
- Pelvic examination at term

Advantages of regular physical examinations

Apart from being simple, non-invasive, and inexpensive, the aforementioned tests have the following advantages:

- They detect up to 50 per cent of fetuses with growth restriction
- They prevent 70 per cent of cases of eclampsia by early detection of preeclampsia (Carolli et al., 2001)
- They reduce the requirement of cesarean section for breech by identifying 80 per cent of breech presentations prior to labour, when external cephalic version can still be performed
- They reduce the chance of postterm pregnancy since cervical assessment at term allows stripping (or sweeping) of membranes

Maternal weight

The maternal weight should be recorded at every antenatal visit since optimal weight gain is associated with better outcomes (Saccone and Sendek, 2016). Both suboptimal weight gain and excessive weight gain are a cause for concern (see **Chapter 3**, *Dietary advice and nutritional supplements*).

Blood pressure

- Though 120/80 mm of Hg is considered to be normal blood pressure, it is important to recognise that young Indian women may very well have lower blood pressure

In the absence of hemorrhage or shock leading to hemodynamic instability, there is no entity known as 'low blood pressure'.

readings, ranging from 90/60 to 110/70 mm of Hg, in the absence of any significant circulatory disturbances.

- Blood pressure decreases slightly in the second trimester and then rises at term in normal, uncomplicated pregnancies.
- The diagnosis of hypertension in pregnancy is made in a previously normotensive woman with new onset of hypertension—systolic blood pressure ≥140 mmHg or diastolic blood pressure ≥90 mmHg on two occasions at least four hours apart (see **Chapter 39**, *Hypertensive disorders in pregnancy*).

> **Accurate assessment of blood pressure**
> - Blood pressure is recorded after five minutes of rest.
> - Position: Any of the following positions are recommended since there is no substantial difference in the readings (August and Sibai, 2018):
>   – Seated with feet on the ground and legs uncrossed or
>   – In a semi-reclining position with back supported or
>   – Left lateral recumbency, with the cuff on the left arm
> - The arm should be supported and at the level of the heart.
> - An appropriately sized cuff should be used in obese women with large upper arm circumference.
> - Mercury manometers, though the most accurate, are not recommended anymore because of the restriction on mercury use. Aneroid devices can be used but should be calibrated regularly.
> - The first audible sound (Korotkoff I) is the systolic pressure, and the disappearance of sound (Korotkoff V) is the diastolic pressure. In pregnant women, sounds may still be audible with the cuff deflated, so Korotkoff IV (abrupt muffling) should be used (Pickering et al., 2005).

Fetal heart tones

- Fetal heart tones should be checked and recorded at every antenatal visit after the first trimester.

> In the early months of pregnancy, fetal heart tones are usually heard around the midline in the lower pole. As pregnancy progresses, they are heard better on the side of the abdomen where the fetal spine is palpable.

- Between 12 and 20 weeks, fetal heart tones are difficult to identify with anything other than a handheld Doppler device. After 20 weeks, fetal heart tones may also be picked up with a fetoscope or, with practice, with a regular stethoscope.

Uterine size and Leopold's manoeuvres

- **Uterine size** can be determined by abdominal palpation and comparing fundal height to anatomical landmarks such as the pubic symphysis, umbilicus, and xiphisternum. It may also be determined by measuring the *symphysio-fundal height (SFH)*. At present, there is no evidence to prove the superiority of one method over the other. Both are acceptable in clinical practice.
- A systematic review of the Cochrane Database (Robert et al., 2015) found insufficient evidence that measuring the SFH with a tape measure is effective in detecting fetal growth restriction. However, in low-resource areas where access to ultrasound (the most accurate

method of detecting fetal growth restriction) is limited, the WHO (2016) recommends SFH measurement as a low-cost method of detecting growth abnormalities.

> For fetuses growing normally, from 24 weeks of gestation, the SFH measurement in centimetres should correspond to the number of weeks of gestation. A difference of ±2 cm is considered normal. The measurement of SFH may raise a suspicion of fetal growth restriction (FGR) when the fundal height in centimetres is at least 3 cm below the gestational age in weeks.

- **Leopold's manoeuvres** performed in the third trimester help in determining the lie of the fetus, presentation, and engagement. When an abnormal presentation is suspected, for example, a breech, ultrasound can be used to confirm the findings. Offering an intervention like external cephalic version, in this case, can reduce the chance of a cesarean section (Hofmeyer and Kulier, 2012).

Pelvic examination at term

- A vaginal examination may be performed at or after 38 weeks of gestation. It provides information about the cervix, presenting part, engagement, membranes, and pelvis.
- A sterile glove should be used to avoid the risk of an ascending infection that may occur if the internal cervical os is open, or on occasion, if the membranes rupture during examination.

> Before performing a pelvic exam, the procedure should be briefly explained to the woman so that she is at ease. The examination should be done gently because, at term, the vagina is very hyperemic and tender. Adequate lubrication should be used. As always, the woman's modesty and privacy must be maintained.

- Cervical changes like effacement and dilatation do not help predict the exact date of delivery, but a ripe cervix (high Bishop score) indicates greater chances of vaginal birth. Similarly, a well-engaged head decreases the possibility of encountering cephalopelvic disproportion in labour.
- Though clinical pelvimetry is of limited value in predicting dystocia in labour, prominent ischial spines may alert the obstetrician to the possibility of mid-pelvic dystocia.

INVESTIGATIONS AT SUBSEQUENT VISITS

- **With every visit:** Urine dipstick for protein and sugar alerts the obstetrician to the presence of proteinuria or glucosuria.
- **11–13^{+6} weeks:** First-trimester bio-chemical screening for aneuploidy along with nuchal translucency screening by ultrasound should be offered to every pregnant woman, where facilities exist. Cell-free DNA aneuploidy testing

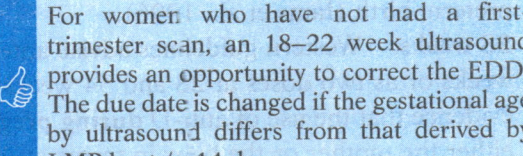

> For women who have not had a first-trimester scan, an 18–22 week ultrasound provides an opportunity to correct the EDD. The due date is changed if the gestational age by ultrasound differs from that derived by LMP by +/− 14 days.

(also called *non-invasive prenatal testing [NIPT]*) can be offered to high-risk women, though its cost may limit its usage (see **Chapter 7**, *Prenatal screening for genetic disorders*).

- **15–21 weeks:** If the mother has not had first-trimester aneuploidy screening, the quadruple test may be offered (see **Chapter 6**).

- **18–22 weeks:** A detailed ultrasound examination is offered between 18 and 22 weeks to rule out any fetal abnormalities (see **Chapter 11**, *Ultrasound in the second trimester*).

- **24–28 weeks:**
  - **Screening for gestational diabetes (GDM):** If the woman had screened negative for diabetes at her booking visit, screening is repeated at 24–28 weeks (see **Chapter 40**, *Gestational and pre-gestational diabetes*).
  - **Hemoglobin and hematocrit** are checked to assess anemia and modify iron supplementation if necessary.
  - **Antibody screening for Rh-negative women** is repeated at 28 weeks (in those who were antibody-negative at the booking visit).

Routine ultrasound in the third trimester
A systematic review of the Cochrane Database (Bricker et al., 2015) shows that routine late pregnancy ultrasound in low-risk or unselected populations does not confer any benefit on the mother or her baby. There was no difference in the primary outcomes of perinatal mortality, preterm birth at <37 weeks, cesarean section rates, and induction of labour rates among women who had ultrasound in their third trimester and those who had not.

Sovio et al. (2015), in the Pregnancy Outcome Prediction study, recommend universal third-trimester screening to improve the detection of small-for-gestational age (SGA) neonates and identify a subset at risk of morbidity. However, for every correct diagnosis of SGA, there were two false positives, i.e., neonates who were not SGA. Such screening, therefore, not only increases maternal anxiety but also leads to unnecessary interventions. Universal screening for SGA fetuses with ultrasound in the third trimester is still questionable (Romero and Deter, 2015).

INTERVENTIONS AT SUBSEQUENT VISITS

- **16–24 weeks:** Cervical length assessment by transvaginal ultrasound may be offered to women who have a **history of preterm birth**. A cervical length <25 mm at 22–24 weeks gestation is associated with a six-fold increase in the risk of preterm birth (Iams et al., 1996).

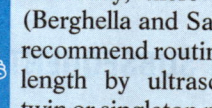

Currently, there is insufficient evidence (Berghella and Saccone, 2019) to recommend routine assessment of cervical length by ultrasound in asymptomatic twin or singleton pregnancies, or singleton pregnancies with preterm premature rupture of the membranes (PPROM).

- **28 weeks:** Western guidelines advise antenatal anti-D to be given as a single dose at 34 weeks or as two doses at 28 and 34 weeks. However, studies have shown no conclusive evidence that the use of anti-D **during pregnancy** (given at 28 and/or 34 weeks) benefits either the mother or the baby in terms of the incidence of RhD alloimmunisation during the pregnancy or postpartum, or the incidence of neonatal morbidity (see box).

> **Universal antenatal anti-D in India?**
> - Anti-D given postpartum effectively prevents 99 per cent of Rh alloimmunisation.
> - Antenatal anti-D given at 28 weeks shows a minor reduction in the rate of Rh alloimmunisation from 1 per cent to 0.2 per cent (Huchet, 1987).
> - Chilcott and colleagues (2002) calculated that 278 women would need to be treated antenatally with anti-D to avoid one case of sensitisation.
> - Crowther et al. (2013), in a systematic review of the Cochrane Database, expressed concerns that the cost and supply of anti-D would be a major consideration in some countries.
> Considering all these facts, universal anti-D may not be feasible or warranted in low-resource countries like India (WHO, 2016).

- **34–36 weeks**
  - **Maternal perception of fetal movement:** At every visit, the mother should be asked if she is feeling her baby move. Healthy pregnant women should be made aware of the importance of the following:
    - Fetal movements as an indicator of fetal health in the third trimester
    - Reporting reduced fetal movements

> In a low-resource country like India, daily fetal movement counting is a simple, effective, and low-cost antenatal intervention to assess fetal well-being (WHO, 2016). Feeling three movements within an hour is a reassuring sign.

  - The AFFIRM study (Norman et al., 2018) is a very large study that showed no decrease in stillbirth rate among women who were educated about fetal movements. However, the study included women who were at 24 weeks of gestation or more. Moreover, this study was done in the UK and Ireland, where the stillbirth rate is already very low.
  - All **healthy** pregnant women should be routinely educated about the importance of being aware of fetal movements, especially in the third trimester. This should be reinforced at each clinical visit (Gardener et al., 2017). Women should also be instructed on initiating a fetal movement count if they perceive decreased movements (Liston et al., 2018). See **Chapter 6,** *Antepartum fetal surveillance.*

> Teaching women how to count daily fetal movements has a positive effect on reducing their anxiety. Delaram and Shams (2016), found that women who performed fetal movement counting from 28 to 37 weeks' gestation reported less anxiety compared to those in the control group.

- **36 weeks:**
  - Fetal presentation is confirmed. If breech, external cephalic version is offered (NICE, 2008).
  - Antenatal classes should be offered to educate the woman/couple about the symptoms of labour and what to expect in labour. Pain relief options in labour can be discussed.
- **38 weeks: Sweeping (or stripping) of membranes** may be considered at or after 38 weeks if the cervix admits a finger.

- **39–40 weeks:**
  - Fetal surveillance can be started, if indicated.
  - Postterm pregnancy can be discussed.
- **41 weeks:** Induction of labour may be considered at 41 weeks for postterm pregnancy.

Compared with no sweeping, sweeping of membranes in low-risk pregnancies is associated with a lower number of postterm pregnancies (de Miranda et al., 2006). This is discussed in greater detail in **Chapter 19**, *Induction of labour*.

References

1. American Academy of Pediatrics Committee on Fetus and Newborn and American College of Obstetricians and Gynecologists Committee on Obstetric Practice. 2017. *Guidelines for Perinatal Care*, 8th Edition. Kilpatrick SJ, Papile L (Eds).

2. August P, Sibai BM. 2018. Preeclampsia: Clinical features and diagnosis. Lockwood CJ (Ed). *UpToDate*. Waltham, MA.

3. Berghella V, Saccone G. 2019. Cervical assessment by ultrasound for preventing preterm delivery. *Cochrane Database Syst Rev*. Issue 9. Art. no.: CD007235.

4. Bricker L, Neilson JP, Dowswell T. 2015. Routine ultrasound in late pregnancy (after 24 weeks gestation). *Cochrane Database Syst Rev*. Issue 6. Art. no: CD001451.

5. Carroli G, Rooney C, Villar J. 2001. How effective is antenatal care in preventing maternal mortality and serious morbidity? An overview of the evidence. *Paediatr Perinat Epidemiol*.15 Suppl 1:1.

6. Carter EB, Tuuli MG, Caughey AB et al. 2016. Number of prenatal visits and pregnancy outcomes in low-risk women. *J Perinatol*. 36:178.

7. Chilcott J, Lloyd Jones M, Wight J, Forman K, Wray J, Beverley C. 2002. A review of the clinical effectiveness and cost effectiveness of routine anti-D prophylaxis for pregnant women who are Rhesus (RhD)-negative. London: National Institute of Clinical Excellence.

8. Crowther CA, Middleton P, McBain RD. 2013. Anti-D administration in pregnancy for preventing Rhesus alloimmunisation. *Cochrane Database Syst Rev*. Issue 2. Art. no.: CD000020.

9. de Miranda E, van der Bom JG, Bonsel GJ et al. 2006. Membrane sweeping and prevention of post-term pregnancy in low-risk pregnancies: A randomised controlled trial. *BJOG*. 113:402–408.

10. Delaram M, Shams S. 2016. The effect of foetal movement counting on maternal anxiety: A randomised, controlled trial. *Journal of Obstet and Gynaecol*.

11. Dowswell T, Carroli G, Duley L et al. 2015. Alternative versus standard packages of antenatal care for low-risk pregnancy. *Cochrane Database Syst Rev*. Issue 10. Art. no.: CD000934.

12. Gardener G, Daly L, Bowring V et al. 2017. Clinical practice guideline for the care of women with decreased fetal movements. Centre of Research Excellence in Stillbirth. Brisbane, Australia.

13. Gole, S. 2015. Routine antenatal care for the healthy pregnant women. Good clinical practice recommendations. The Federation of Obstetric & Gynecological Societies of India.

14. Hofmeyr GJ, Kulier R. 2012. External cephalic version for breech presentation at term. *Cochrane Database Syst Rev*. Issue 10. Art. no.:CD000083.

15. Huchet J, Dallemagne S, Huchet C, Brossard Y, Larsen M, Parnet-Mathieu F. 1987. The antepartum use of anti-D immunoglobulin in rhesus negative women. Parallel evaluation of fetal blood cells

passing through the placenta. The results of a multi-centre study carried out in the region of Paris. *European Journal of Obstetrics, Gynecology, and Reproductive Biology.* 16:101–11.

16. Iams JD, Goldenberg RL, Meis PJ et al. 1996. The length of the cervix and the risk of spontaneous preterm delivery. *N Engl J Med.* 334:567–72.

17. Liston R, Sawchuck D, Young D. 2018. No. 197a. Fetal Health Surveillance: Antepartum Consensus Guideline. *J Obstet Gynaecol Can.*

18. NICE guideline 62. 2008. Routine care for the healthy pregnant woman.

19. Norman JE, Heazell AEP, Rodriguez A et al. 2018. Awareness of fetal movements and care package to reduce fetal mortality (AFFIRM): A stepped wedge, cluster-randomised trial. *Lancet.* Volume 392, Issue 10158.

20. Pickering TG, Hall JE, Appel LJ et al. 2005. Recommendations for blood pressure measurement in humans and experimental animals. Part 1: Blood pressure measurement in humans–a statement for professionals from the Subcommittee of Professional and Public Education of the American Heart Association Council on High Blood Pressure Research. Circulation. 111:697.

21. Robert PJ, Ho J, Valliappan RJ, Sivasankari. 2015. Symphysial fundal height (SFH) measurement in pregnancy for detecting abnormal fetal growth. *Cochrane Database Syst Rev.* Issue 9. Art. no.: CD008136.

22. Romero R, Deter R. 2015. Should serial fetal biometry be used in all pregnancies? *Lancet.* Nov 21. 86 (10008):2038–2040.

23. Saccone G, Sendek K. 2016. Prenatal Care in Obstetric Evidence-Based Guidelines. Vincenzo Berghella (Ed.). Taylor and Francis, CRC Press.

24. Sovio U, White IR, Dacey A et al. 2015. Screening for fetal growth restriction with universal third trimester ultrasonography in nulliparous women in the Pregnancy Outcome Prediction (POP) study: A prospective cohort study. *Lancet.*

25. World Health Organization. 2016. WHO recommendations on antenatal care for a positive pregnancy experience. WHO, Geneva.

Chapter 5

Common Problems in the Antenatal Period and their Management

INTRODUCTION

The physiological and mechanical changes that occur during pregnancy can result in minor or major problems for the mother. As pregnancy progresses, the body goes through a considerable number of changes; these changes may cause the woman significant discomfort, quite often requiring intervention. The same woman may have different symptoms and varying degrees of discomfort in different pregnancies. Women require an empathetic response to their problems. Their complaints should not be brushed off; rather, each woman should be reassured that these symptoms are experienced by most expectant mothers.

NAUSEA AND VOMITING OF PREGNANCY (NVP)

- This is perhaps the first and commonest symptom of pregnancy. Some degree of nausea, with or without vomiting, occurs in up to 80 per cent of women. This is a physiological response to the surge of β-hCG and possibly, estrogens, in the body.

 Although the term 'morning sickness' is commonly used, the symptoms may occur at any time of day; in 80 per cent of women, they persist throughout the day (Lacroix et al., 2000).

- The symptoms present usually at 5–6 weeks of gestation, and peak at about 8–9 weeks. Approximately one in five women reports symptoms even before she has positive pregnancy test results (Hinkle et al., 2016).

  Most women will experience abatement of symptoms by 16–20 weeks of gestation. Though the symptoms resolve by 20 weeks in 90 per cent of women, 15–20 per cent of women may have symptoms till the third trimester. A very small number (5 per cent) will have persistence of symptoms until delivery.
- The exact etiology of nausea and vomiting is poorly understood and is most probably multifactorial. The most likely etiology is the change in the hormonal milieu during pregnancy. Rising levels of β-hCG have been implicated, as has estradiol.
- Nausea and vomiting are more pronounced in pregnancies associated with the following:
  - Multiple gestation
  - Hydatidiform mole
  - Heartburn and acid reflux
- The general advice is to eat small, frequent meals with high protein, low fat and low carbohydrate content and to avoid iron supplements in the first trimester. The pregnant

woman should be advised to eat whatever foods appeal to her. Reassurance and explanation go a long way in ameliorating symptoms.

> **Are nausea and vomiting associated with a reduction in the risk of pregnancy loss?**
> Nausea with or without vomiting seems to be feto-protective. A recent study has shown that nausea alone or nausea with vomiting is associated with a 50–75 per cent reduction in the risk of pregnancy loss (Hinkle et al., 2016). Sapra et al. (2016), when studying the relationship between signs and symptoms of early pregnancy and pregnancy loss <20 weeks' gestation, found that nausea alone was not protective, but vomiting was.

Management of nausea and vomiting in pregnancy

Though nausea and vomiting are such common problems in pregnancy, not many management options are based on strong evidence. A systematic review of the Cochrane Database looked at many options and concluded that some interventions may be useful, though the evidence may not be consistent or of high quality (Matthews et al., 2015).

The Motherisk-Pregnancy Unique-Quantification of Emesis (**PUQE**) scoring index (Koren et al., 2002) is used for evaluating the severity of nausea and vomiting and may help in making clinical decisions for intervention. This scoring system is based on the mother's symptoms for the last 12 hours before the assessment (Table 5.1). The score assigns points for the following:
- The number of hours the woman feels nauseated
- The number of times she vomits
- The number of times she has dry heaves (retching) on a typical day

A high score of ≥13 indicates that the woman may need admission for intravenous fluids. She should also be evaluated for hypovolemia, and her serum electrolyte levels should be checked.

Table 5.1   The Pregnancy Unique-Quantification of Emesis (PUQE) scoring index

Symptom	1 point	2 points	3 points	4 points	5 points
Duration of nausea in the past 12 hours (in hours)	0	≤1	2–3	4–6	>6
Number of vomiting episodes in the past 12 hours	0	1–2	3–4	5–6	≥7
Number of episodes of dry heaves in the past 12 hours	0	1–2	3–4	5–6	≥7

Non-pharmacological measures

- **Dietary manipulation:**   Women should be advised to avoid the following:
  - An empty stomach: They can ensure this by consuming frequent, small snacks/meals
  - Food triggers: Spicy, oily, very sweet, acidic, strong-smelling food and coffee
  - Iron supplements (though folic acid may be continued)
- **Ginger:**   The consumption of ginger in any form (ginger tea, ginger added to food or ginger sweets) has been shown to reduce nausea and vomiting. However, a review of the Cochrane Database (Matthews et al., 2015) found that the evidence is limited and not very consistent.
- **Acupressure over the P6 point:**   The same review showed low-certainty evidence for the use of acupressure over the P6 point (located three-fingers' breadth proximal to the wrist,

on the inside of the wrist, in-between the two tendons, Figure 5.1), to relieve nausea and vomiting. It is not clear whether this is a placebo effect, but since the woman herself can apply the acupressure, it can be suggested as an option.

Pharmacological measures

When conservative measures fail, pharmacological intervention is the next acceptable step. The following are some such interventions (Table 5.2):

- **Vitamin B6 (pyridoxine)** is not recommended as a stand-alone drug for NVP (RCOG, 2016). A systematic review of the Cochrane Database (Matthews et al., 2015) concluded that there is a lack of consistent evidence to show that pyridoxine is an effective therapy for NVP. **It is useful in combination with doxylamine**.
- **Doxylamine succinate and pyridoxine (as a combination)** is the first-line treatment of choice for nausea and vomiting in pregnancy. It relieves symptoms in 70 per cent of women. 10 mg of doxylamine with 10 mg of pyridoxine can be given in a dosage of up to four tablets a day (i.e., two at bedtime, one in the morning, and one in the afternoon). The dosage and schedule are adjusted according to the severity of symptoms. The combination of doxylamine succinate (an antihistamine) and pyridoxine (a coenzyme involved in the metabolism of carbohydrates, proteins, and fats) is more effective than either drug

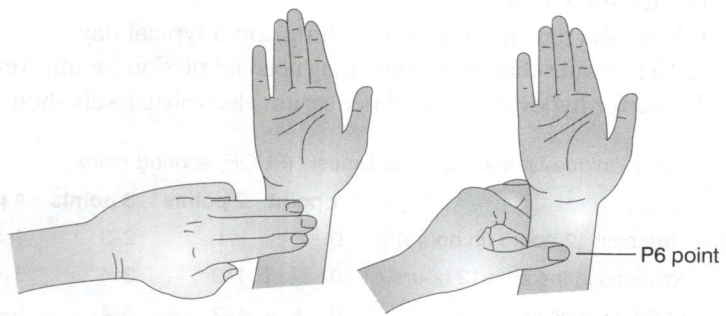

— P6 point

Figure 5.1   The P6 acupressure point is three fingers' breadth proximal to the wrist and on the inside of the wrist, in-between the two tendons. Pressure may be applied with the thumb for five minutes when nausea is present.

Table 5.2   Recommended dosages of drugs used in the treatment of nausea and vomiting in pregnancy

Drug	Dosage	Frequency
Doxylamine + pyridoxine	10 mg each	2 tablets at bedtime 1 tablet in the morning and 1 tablet in the afternoon can be given in addition (the number of doses can be modified depending on the severity of symptoms)
Meclizine	25 mg	1 tablet at bedtime 1 additional tablet in the afternoon, if required
Metoclopramide	5–10 mg	Every 8 hours IM or oral
Ondansetron	4–8 mg	Every 12 hours oral

alone and has a good safety record in pregnancy (Magee et al., 2002).

 It is a good idea to inform women that doxylamine, meclizine, and metoclopramide may cause drowsiness and dryness of the mouth.

- **Meclizine** has been shown to be effective in treating NVP. One dose of 25 mg is given at bedtime to prevent nausea in the morning and another dose can be given in the afternoon to prevent nausea in the evening. In case of severe vomiting, it can be given at intervals of 4–6 hours. Its safety record has been good, and the majority of studies have shown no association between prenatal antihistamine exposure and birth defects (Mitchell et al., 2011).

- **Metoclopramide** can be used as a second line of treatment if the above drugs are not effective (Matok et al., 2009). Drug-induced extrapyramidal symptoms and oculogyric crises can occur with the use of metoclopramide. These are treated by complete cessation of the drug.

 In women whose vomiting is worsened due to heartburn/acid reflux, antiemetic therapy in combination with antacids and H2 blockers results in significant improvement in symptoms and well-being 3–4 days after beginning therapy (Gill et al., 2009).

- **Ondansetron** is increasingly being used for the management of NVP though its safety has not been firmly established in pregnancy. It is recommended as a second line of therapy (ACOG, 2018).

HYPEREMESIS GRAVIDARUM (HG)

- Hyperemesis gravidarum is the severest manifestation of NVP, characterised by severe nausea and intractable vomiting sufficient to interfere with nutrition. It is characterised by dehydration, ketonuria, and weight loss. It affects about 0.3–3.6 per cent of pregnant women (RCOG, 2016).

 Evaluation for multiple pregnancy and hydatidiform mole is essential in the presence of intractable vomiting. An ultrasound will rule out or confirm these. Non-pregnancy-related causes of vomiting must also be excluded.

- Hyperemesis gravidarum may be defined as persistent and excessive vomiting starting before the end of the 22nd week of gestation and resulting in a weight loss of >5 per cent of body weight or >3 kg (Hod et al., 1994).

- Severe HG is associated with metabolic disturbances such as carbohydrate depletion, dehydration, and electrolyte imbalance. Hypokalemia can lead to continued vomiting, thus perpetuating the vicious cycle.

When is hospitalisation required?
- Persistent nausea and vomiting with inability to keep down oral antiemetics
- Continued nausea and vomiting associated with ketonuria and/or weight loss (>5 per cent of body weight or >3 kg) despite oral antiemetics
- Women showing signs of hypovolemia, which are:
  - Lethargy
  - Postural dizziness
  - Thirst
  - Tachycardia
  - Decreased urine volume and frequency

- Other unrelated causes of vomiting like appendicitis, gastroenteritis, acid peptic disease, torsion of an ovarian cyst, cerebral tumours, pyelonephritis, and uremia should be excluded.
- There is a 20 per cent *recurrence risk* of HG in women who had it in an earlier pregnancy (Dodds et al., 2006). One-third of women are reluctant to attempt another pregnancy because of the fear of recurrence.

Investigations

In women with persistent nausea and vomiting, laboratory evaluation helps to determine the severity of disease and exclude other diagnoses that could account for the symptoms. The following laboratory findings indicate or confirm the severity of the condition:

- **Urinalysis**
  - Oliguria
  - Dark colour
  - Increased specific gravity
  - Ketone bodies
  - Acidic pH
- **Hematological and biochemical findings**
  - Raised hematocrit
  - Raised blood urea
  - Hypokalemia and hypochloremic metabolic alkalosis from vomiting gastric secretions
  - Metabolic acidosis in severe cases
  - Liver function tests may be abnormal in 50 per cent of patients with HG (Abell and Riely, 1992). Alanine aminotransferase (ALT) and aspartate aminotransferase (AST) are only mildly elevated. Hyperbilirubinemia can occur, but rarely exceeds 4 mg/dL (Larrey et al., 1984).
  - Two-thirds of women with HG develop transient abnormal thyroid function tests with suppression of TSH (mild hyperthyroidism) that resolves completely when HG improves (Goodwin et al., 1992).

Possible complications of hyperemesis gravidarum
- Electrolyte imbalance
- Liver dysfunction and jaundice
- Acute renal failure
- Stress ulcers in the stomach
- Mallory-Weiss tears in the esophagus
- Esophageal rupture or Boerhaave syndrome
- Pneumothorax and pneumomediastinum
- Complications due to vitamin deficiency
  - Wernicke encephalopathy due to thiamine deficiency
  - Korsakoff psychosis
  - Peripheral neuritis
  - Vitamin K deficiency and bleeding disorders
- Depression

Management of hyperemesis gravidarum

Management depends on the severity of symptoms and consists of supportive and pharmacological measures, and counselling.

Women with hyperemesis who present with moderate-to-severe dehydration, ketosis, and electrolyte disturbances require prompt attention.

Supportive measures

- Prompt hospitalisation is mandatory to prevent complications.
- Replacement fluids (dextrose saline with added potassium) are given intravenously (IV) to correct dehydration, ketosis, electrolyte deficit, and acid–base imbalance.

 Thiamine replacement is indicated in hyperemesis gravidarum to prevent the development of Wernicke encephalopathy. Vitamin B1 (100 mg) should be added to the IV fluids for 3 days (Chiossi et al., 2006).

- Oral feeding is stopped to provide rest to the gastrointestinal tract.
- Enteral (tube feeding) or parenteral nutrition may be indicated in cases with significant weight loss.
- Most patients respond to therapy. An oral diet can be reintroduced gradually, beginning with fluids and then low-fat solids.

> **Nausea, vomiting, and hyperemesis in diabetic pregnant women**
> Women with pre-existing diabetes who develop nausea and vomiting of pregnancy must be advised on how to adjust their medications (especially insulin) to avoid a *hypoglycemic crisis*. If they take their usual dose but are unable to retain food, they may face repeated hypoglycemia. They should be educated on adjusting medication as necessary, and have biscuits, juice, or other snacks to help alleviate sudden hypoglycemia.

Pharmacological measures

- Oral medications are stopped if they are not tolerated, and parenteral drug therapy is started.
- Antiemetics like **promethazine** (12.5–25 mg 4 hourly rectal/intramuscular) or **metoclopramide** (10 mg 8 hourly intravenously) may be administered.

 A recent systematic review of the Cochrane Database compared promethazine, metoclopramide, and ondansetron and showed no clear superiority of one over the other in providing symptomatic relief (Boelig et al., 2016).

- **Ondansetron** (4–8 mg 8 hourly intravenously) is being used more often now but needs to be further evaluated (ACOG, 2018). It is more expensive than metoclopramide; this may influence use (Abas et al., 2014).
- **Methylprednisolone** (16 mg 8 hourly oral/IV for 3 days and tapered over the next two weeks) has been used in severe, intractable cases but data on its effectiveness is weak (Smith et al., 2018). There is a marginal increase in congenital malformations with

first-trimester use of steroids in experimental animals. For this reason, steroids should be avoided for this indication before 10 weeks.

Counselling

Counselling and behavioral therapy have been found to be effective in the early stages of HG as this condition is associated with some amount of psychological overlay.

ACID REFLUX DISEASE (HEARTBURN)

- Pregnancy is associated with decreased lower esophageal sphincter pressure, caused by both estrogen and progesterone. This results in acid reflux.
- Acid reflux (heartburn) occurs in 40–85 per cent of women during pregnancy (Ali and Egan, 2007). Rey and colleagues (2007) found that the incidence increases from the first to the third trimester with relief in the postpartum period. They also found that excess weight gain during pregnancy is associated with a higher risk of acid reflux in the third trimester.

Management of acid reflux in pregnancy

- **Lifestyle and dietary modification**
  - Elevation of the head of the bed
  - Avoiding lying down immediately after meals
  - Eating meals at least two to three hours before bedtime
  - Avoiding dietary triggers (oily and spicy foods, caffeine, chocolate, aerated beverages, and peppermint)
- **Medications**
  - If heartburn persists, *antacids* (magnesium carbonate, aluminium hydroxide, or calcium carbonate) are considered the first-line medical therapy (WHO, 2016). The effect is

 Antacids can interfere with the absorption of iron and, therefore, should not be taken within two hours of taking iron and folic acid supplements.

almost immediate because antacids neutralise gastric acid. However, relief is short-lived and the dosage needs to be repeated.
  - *Sucralfate* is safe and effective in pregnancy and can be given in a dose of 1 g three times daily.
  - *H₂ receptor antagonists* start working in 2.5 hours and their effect persists for 4–10 hours. Ranitidine has documented efficacy and safety profile in pregnancy, even in the first trimester (Larson et al., 1997). It can be taken in a dose of 150 mg at bedtime or twice a day.
  - *Proton-pump inhibitors (PPIs)* are the next line of management. Pasternak and Hviid (2010) found that the use of PPIs was not associated with an increased risk of major birth defects. Omeprazole, lansoprazole, and pantoprazole have been used in pregnancy and have a good safety record.

CONSTIPATION

- Circulating progesterone in pregnancy may be the cause of decreased small bowel and colonic motility in mid- and late pregnancy, which leads to constipation. After nausea, it is the second most common gastrointestinal complaint in pregnancy.
- Bloating and constipation are experienced by up to 24 per cent of pregnant women (Bradley et al., 2007). These symptoms may persist for 6–12 weeks postpartum. Often, constipation is complicated by hemorrhoids.
- Constipation may present as infrequent bowel movements or difficult evacuation or both.

Management of constipation in pregnancy

- **Lifestyle and dietary modification (WHO, 2016)**
  - Increasing the consumption of fibre (raw vegetables and green, leafy vegetables)
  - Consciously increasing the intake of water and other fluids
  - Moderate exercise, e.g., brisk walking
  - Avoiding iron preparations for a short while until constipation is relieved
- **Medications**
  - *Bulk-forming agents*: Fibre supplements (bran, psyllium husk) increase bulk and lead to softer stools and frequency of defecation. These may not always be effective.
  - *Stool softeners:* Docusate sodium is safe and effective in pregnancy.
  - *Lubricant laxatives:* Liquid paraffin is not absorbed and helps relieve constipation.
  - *Osmotic laxatives:* Lactulose may be used safely in pregnancy.
  - *Stimulant laxatives:* Bisacodyl suppository may be used in severe constipation. The oral form is better avoided because it may cause bloating and cramping.

- Laxatives should preferably be used only for short periods and only for symptomatic relief.
- Castor oil should **not** be used for constipation as it can result in severe diarrhea.

HEMORRHOIDS

- Hemorrhoids are varicosities in the anal canal caused by the increasing pelvic pressure from the growing uterus.
- Approximately 30–40 per cent of pregnant women have symptoms of pruritus, pain/discomfort, and/or bleeding due to hemorrhoids. The symptoms are exacerbated by constipation (Bianco, 2017).
- Hemorrhoids are usually more symptomatic in the last trimester of pregnancy, and immediately postpartum.
- Symptoms resolve spontaneously soon after birth. Surgical treatment is rarely required during pregnancy.

Management of hemorrhoids in pregnancy

- **Lifestyle and dietary modification**
  - Since constipation aggravates the discomfort of hemorrhoids, women should be advised to have a fibre-rich diet and increase the consumption of fluids.
  - Sitz baths can be advised for symptomatic relief.

- **Medications**
  - Local application of anti-inflammatory, antipruritic, and local anesthetic preparations are effective.

   Lidocaine 5% ointment should be prescribed for symptomatic relief. 2% gel is not as effective.

  - Stool softeners should be given concurrently to relieve or prevent constipation.

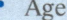

Anal fissure vs. hemorrhoids

Women may present with painful defecation in pregnancy. It is important to differentiate painful hemorrhoids from an anal fissure. Hemorrhoids may bleed but are usually not painful unless they are thrombosed.

- An anal fissure is usually a consequence of passing hard stools that cause a cut in the anoderm.
- The pain is exacerbated by passing motion and persists for several hours. It can interfere with daily work.
- An anal fissure can be identified by gently spreading the anal opening. A cut in the anoderm is usually seen at the 12 or 6 o'clock position. **A digital rectal exam should never be performed** because it will result in extreme pain.
- A stool softener or laxative may be prescribed to ease the pain by preventing constipation.
- Sitz baths help relieve pain.
- Nifedipine 0.3% ointment is effective as a local application 3–4 times daily. Often, the ointment is available in combination with lidocaine.
- Prompt treatment of an acute anal fissure will prevent it from progressing to a chronic anal fissure that requires surgical management.

LOW BACK PAIN (LBP)

- Low back pain is very common in pregnancy, and more than 60 per cent of pregnant women complain of it (Kovacs et al., 2012). The pain is usually localised to the lumbar region, above the sacrum.

Predictors for the occurrence of low back pain in pregnancy include the following (Wang et al., 2004):

- Age
- Low back pain during menstruation
- Previous history of back pain when not pregnant
- Low back pain during a previous pregnancy

- The physiological musculoskeletal changes that contribute to back pain include the following:
  - Weight gain
  - A shift in the centre of gravity
  - Exaggeration of lumbar lordosis
  - Widening and increased mobility of the sacroiliac joints and pubic symphysis in preparation for the passage of the fetus through the birth canal; increased laxity of the pelvic joints is caused by the hormone relaxin
- Low back pain can start at any point during pregnancy but is predominant in the second half of pregnancy when the lordosis gets more pronounced.

- Up to two-thirds of pregnant women find that low back pain interferes with their daily activities and affects their sleep patterns. Up to 10 per cent of women have to take time off from work because of low back pain.

Management of low back pain in pregnancy

- **Lifestyle changes**
  - Maintaining a good posture
  - Wearing comfortable, soft footwear with low-heels (completely flat slippers will aggravate the pain)
  - Sleeping on a firm mattress
  - Avoiding lifting heavy objects; it is better to squat to lift things from the floor
  - Lying in the lateral recumbent position, with the knees and hips bent and a pillow placed under the abdomen to support the weight of the uterus, or placed between the knees to reduce the mechanical burden on the back (Figure 5.2)
  - Applying hot or cold compress, along with massage
  - Regular exercise is thought to relieve back pain to some degree—a systematic review of the Cochrane Database (Liddle and Pennick, 2015) found that exercise may reduce the number of days of sick leave due to pregnancy-related low back pain
- **Medications**
  - Mild analgesics like paracetamol can be prescribed for relief of pain; if non-steroidal anti-inflammatory agents are used, e.g., ibuprofen, they are better restricted to between 12 and 30 weeks of gestation

LEG CRAMPS

Leg cramps commonly occur in the second half of pregnancy. These painful cramps usually occur over the calf muscles. Though they can occur at any time, they seem to be more common at night. The exact etiology of leg cramps is not known.

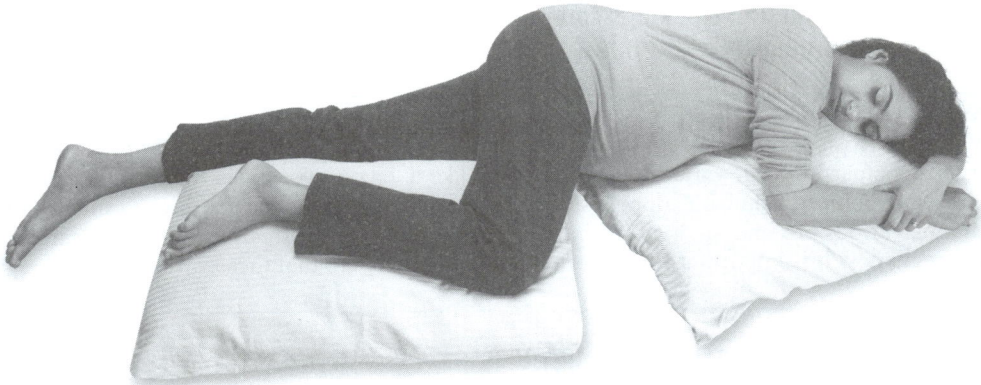

Figure 5.2 Recommended sleeping posture to avoid or relieve low back pain. Sleeping on the side with support for the abdomen and knees reduces the mechanical burden on the back.

Management of leg cramps in pregnancy

- **Exercise and stretches**
  - Stretches and stretching exercises not only relieve leg cramps, but they also reduce the frequency of occurrence.
  - Dorsiflexing the foot stretches the calf muscles and relieves cramping. This can be done by the pregnant woman herself or by her partner (Figure 5.3).
- **Medications**
  - A meta-analysis of the Cochrane Database (Young and Jewell, 2002) found no evidence to support the prescribing of calcium for the prevention of leg cramps.

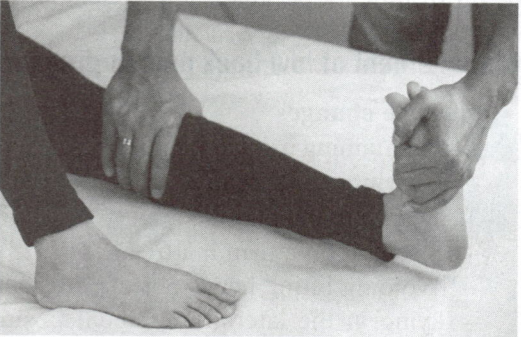

Figure 5.3 Cramping of the calf muscles can be relieved by dorsiflexing the foot.

  - In a very small trial (Dahle et al., 1995), magnesium was found to have some effect on the prevention of leg cramps, but it is difficult to make a recommendation based on this study.

VARICOSE VEINS

- Varicose veins are common in pregnancy and are a result of the pressure of the gravid uterus on the pelvic veins. Pregnancy is one of the reasons for the increased incidence of varicose veins in women.
- Varicose veins and edema in pregnancy may result in the following:
  - Leg pain
  - Night cramps
  - Feeling of heaviness
- Varicose veins need no treatment; simple rest with elevation of the legs usually resolves the issue. Compression stockings can improve the symptoms but do not prevent varicose veins from emerging (NICE, 2008).

> **Vulvar varicosities**
> Vulvar varicosities usually occur during pregnancy and typically regress spontaneously within six weeks postpartum. The varicosities may appear like a 'bag of worms' in the enlarged labia. Leg elevation, compression with support stockings, sleeping on the left side, exercise, and avoidance of long periods of standing or sitting have been suggested for the treatment of vulvar varicosities in pregnancy. It is important to reassure the pregnant woman that these varicosities will regress after delivery.

VAGINAL DISCHARGE AND VAGINITIS

- In pregnancy, there is a physiological increase in mucoid or watery vaginal discharge. This is not associated with itching and may become more pronounced closer to term.

- If vaginal discharge is associated with itching, soreness, offensive smell or dysuria, there may be an infective cause. In such cases, investigation should be considered for vaginitis.
- The commonest causes of vaginitis in pregnancy are vulvovaginal candidiasis, trichomoniasis, and bacterial vaginosis. These three infections account for over 90 per cent of vaginitis in pregnancy.

> Many pregnant women are distressed by the increased vaginal discharge in pregnancy. They must be reassured that this is a common physiological change due to the significantly increased volume of cervical secretions within the vagina. Vaginal discharge may present as a clear, watery discharge or a thick, mucoid discharge.

Vulvovaginal candidiasis

- Vulvovaginal candidiasis occurs more often in pregnancy because of the increased levels of circulating estrogens.

> The clinical diagnosis of candidiasis should be confirmed by the microscopic identification of the organism on a wet mount.

- Vulvar pruritus is the major feature of vulvovaginal candidiasis.
- The complaint of a thick, white, curdy discharge accompanied by pruritus is almost pathognomonic of candidiasis.
- Women may also complain of 'splash dysuria' (typically over the vulva after passing urine), soreness, irritation, and dyspareunia.

Management of vulvovaginal candidiasis in pregnancy

- **Lifestyle changes**
  - Avoidance of tight clothes
  - Avoidance of underwear made of synthetic material
  - Good control of diabetes (if present)
- **Medications for symptomatic relief**
  - Application of a topical imidazole (clotrimazole or miconazole) vaginally is the accepted mode of treatment for pregnant women with candidiasis.
  - Clotrimazole cream and vaginal suppositories are well tolerated by women in terms of local side effects like burning and irritation.
  - In addition, where vulvar candidiasis is more severe and associated with severe itching, a topical steroid (like beclomethasone) combined with an antifungal cream or ointment is useful for local application to the vulva. Intravaginal application of a steroid is not necessary.
  - Clotrimazole ointment or cream (with or without a topical steroid) can be applied for 3–6 days, depending on symptom relief.
  - Intravaginal clotrimazole suppositories (200 mg) can be used for 3–6 days, depending on the severity of the infection.

> **Intravaginal clotrimazole suppositories (200 mg)**
> The woman should be instructed on how to digitally insert the suppository as deep as possible into the vagina. The suppository is best inserted at bedtime.

- Oral azoles (fluconazole and ketoconazole) are not recommended in pregnancy because of the potential risks of birth defects.

 Administration of oral azoles during the first trimester has been associated with a set of birth defects (abnormalities of the cranium, face, bones, and heart) after first-trimester exposure to high-dose therapy (Lopez-Rangel and Van Allen, 2005).

Trichomonas vaginitis

- Trichomoniasis is caused by the protozoa *T. vaginalis*. Being the most common non-viral sexually transmitted infection worldwide, it is not surprising that it commonly presents in pregnancy.

- Trichomoniasis in pregnancy may present as a thin vaginal discharge (70 per cent of cases) associated with pruritus, or occasionally as a severe, acute, inflammatory disease.

T. vaginalis infection in pregnancy is associated with an increased risk of preterm birth, preterm, premature rupture of membranes and small-for-gestational age infants (Silver et al., 2014).

- There may be associated burning, dysuria, frequency, and dyspareunia.
- The diagnosis of *T. vaginalis* is made by taking a vaginal smear and identifying motile trichomonads on a wet mount.
- Since trichomoniasis is a sexually transmitted infection, it is mandatory to treat the woman's partner, even though most men are asymptomatic.

Management of trichomoniasis in pregnancy

Since trichomoniasis is associated with perinatal morbidity, it is important to treat it in pregnancy.

- **Lifestyle changes**
  - The woman should be instructed to avoid intercourse until she and her partner have completed treatment and are asymptomatic. This usually takes about a week.
- **Medication**
  - Metronidazole is the drug of choice for the treatment of symptomatic trichomoniasis in pregnancy. It is given in a dose of 400 mg twice daily for 5–7 days. It may be given as a single dose of 2 g but this is not well tolerated by women in the first trimester due to the nausea it may induce.

 Metronidazole therapy during the first or later trimesters of pregnancy has not been associated with preterm birth, low birth weight, or congenital anomalies (Koss et al., 2012).

- The woman's partner is treated with an oral single-dose regimen of 2 g of either tinidazole or metronidazole to maximise compliance. This treatment should be done simultaneously with the treatment of the pregnant woman.

 The woman's partner should be advised not to consume alcohol for 24 hours after metronidazole therapy and for 72 hours after tinidazole therapy as severe nausea and vomiting may occur as a reaction to the combination of metronidazole or tinidazole with alcohol.

- If a woman is unable to tolerate oral metronidazole, an alternative treatment is clotrimazole 1 per cent cream inserted vaginally at bedtime for seven consecutive days. This leads to symptomatic relief, but not the eradication of the organisms.
- In breastfeeding women, a 2 g single dose of metronidazole may be used, but the mother must be asked to express and discard milk for the next 12–24 hours. Women using tinidazole should be advised to avoid breastfeeding until three days after the last dose.

Bacterial vaginosis

- Bacterial vaginosis represents a change in the complex vaginal flora, leading away from lactobacilli towards an increase in concentration of other organisms, especially anaerobic gram-negative rods.

 Since there is no associated inflammation, this condition is called vaginosis, rather than vaginitis.

- It is characterised by the presence of a greyish, thin vaginal discharge with a 'fishy' odour.
- The diagnosis is based on the characteristic vaginal discharge with a fishy odour, elevated pH of >4.5, and the presence of *clue cells* on microscopy.

Management of bacterial vaginosis in pregnancy

Bacterial vaginosis in pregnancy is treated only when symptomatic. There is no evidence that screening and treatment of asymptomatic infection reduce the risk of preterm birth.

 Pregnant women do not commonly develop bacterial vaginosis after 16 weeks' gestation. Bacterial vaginosis also resolves spontaneously in up to 50 per cent of pregnant women (Hay et al., 1994).

- **Medication**
  Either one of the following regimens is effective:
  - Metronidazole 400 mg orally twice daily for seven days or
  - Clindamycin 300 mg orally twice daily for seven days
- There is no indication for treating the woman's partner.

POLYMORPHIC ERUPTION OF PREGNANCY (PEP)

- Polymorphic eruption of pregnancy (also known as pruritic urticarial plaques and papules of pregnancy [**PUPPP**]) is a dermatosis specific to pregnancy with no proven etiology.
- The incidence is 1/160 to 1/300 pregnancies (Vaughan Jones and Black, 1999).
- It is a benign, self-limiting skin disorder whose characteristic features are as follows:
  - An increased prevalence in primigravidas
  - Onset in the third trimester
  - Remission near the time of delivery
  - Distribution more prominently over the extremities and the abdomen, particularly over the striae, with no involvement of the face, palms, or soles

- There is an 8- to 12-fold increased association with multiple gestation.
- The skin lesions are extremely pruritic, erythematous papules that coalesce to form urticarial plaques, and progress to erythematous patches and vesicles.
- PEP generally lasts four to six weeks and resolves within two weeks postpartum.

 There are no associated maternal or fetal risks with PEP, and treatment is aimed at relieving the intense itching (Taylor et al., 2016).

Management of PEP

The main aim of treatment for PEP is relief from the intense pruritus. Early delivery for relief of symptoms is not required.

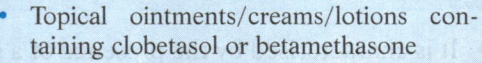 Both topical and systemic steroids have proven safety for use in pregnancy.

- **Topical steroid ointments or creams**
  - Betamethasone dipropionate or clobetasol propionate are the first line of treatment. They may be applied topically 1–2 times daily.
- **Oral medications**
  - Antihistamines like chlorpheniramine maleate (4 mg twice daily) or cetirizine (10 mg at bedtime) provide good symptom relief.
  - Systemic steroids, e.g., prednisone (0.5 mg/kg body weight per day) may be required if the pruritus is intense. It is usually given in a dose of 5–10 mg three times daily for 5–7 days and then tapered off over 7–10 days.

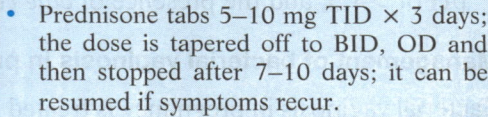

Treatment of PEP
- Topical ointments/creams/lotions containing clobetasol or betamethasone
- Chlorpheniramine maleate 4 mg BID or cetirizine 10 mg at bedtime
- Prednisone tabs 5–10 mg TID × 3 days; the dose is tapered off to BID, OD and then stopped after 7–10 days; it can be resumed if symptoms recur.

PIGMENTATION

- Most pregnant women develop some degree of skin pigmentation.
- Though the etiology is not clearly understood, one possibility is that estrogens and progesterone cause melanocytic stimulation (Geraghty and Pomeranz, 2011).
- Pigmentation is typically pronounced over the nipples, umbilicus, axillae, perineum, and linea alba, which darkens enough to be considered a *linea nigra*. Other pigmentation changes, such as palmar erythema, pseudoacanthosis nigricans, vulvar or dermal melanocytosis, or post-inflammatory hyperpigmentation secondary to specific dermatologic conditions of pregnancy are fairly common as well.
- Facial darkening, called *melasma*, is a diffuse macular facial hyperpigmentation. When melasma occurs as a result of pregnancy, it is known as *chloasma*. Because it is related to the hormones of pregnancy, it lessens after delivery.
- Melasma will usually disappear within a year after delivery, but for women in whom the chloasma persists after pregnancy, topical bleaching agents are the first line of therapy. A chemical peel may be considered if this approach fails.

As far as women are concerned, chloasma is the most disturbing of all skin pigmentations occurring in pregnancy. It affects up to 75 per cent of pregnant women. The distribution is usually malar but can be central or mandibular.

STRIAE GRAVIDARUM (STRETCH MARKS)

- Striae gravidarum or stretch marks are of great distress to pregnant women.
- Both hormonal and physical factors (distension of the abdomen and stretching of the skin) result in the attenuation of elastin fibres and fibrillin

 A systematic review of the Cochrane Database failed to show any evidence that commercially available topical creams have a role in the prevention or treatment of stretch marks (Brennan et al., 2012).

microfibrils in the dermis, leading to the appearance of stretch marks (Wong and Ellis, 1984).
- Usually occurring after the 24th week, stretch marks begin as dark red lines and progress into linear depressions. The skin over these depressions becomes soft and thinned out. The lines then become hypopigmented.
- They are most prominent on the abdomen, breasts, thighs, and buttocks, but in more severe cases, may also occur on the lower back, hips, upper arms and calves.
- Unfortunately, striae (stretch marks) cannot be prevented. The degree to which a woman experiences stretch marks is determined genetically since there appears to be a strong familial tendency. Excess weight gain during pregnancy also contributes to their severity.
- Fortunately, striae fade with time and the marks become silvery-white. However, the skin in those areas does not get back to its former condition.

INCONTINENCE

- A large number of women encounter their first episode of stress urinary incontinence (involuntary leakage of urine with a physical activity such as coughing or sneezing) during pregnancy (Handa, 2018).
- More than one-third of women experience stress incontinence in the second and third trimesters of pregnancy. Wesnes et al. (2007) reported that the prevalence of incontinence increased from 26 per cent before pregnancy to 58 per cent in week 30.
- Approximately one-third of pregnant women continue to have stress incontinence in the first three months postpartum (Woodley et al., 2017).

Pelvic floor muscle exercises (PFME)
Kegel's is a specific type of pelvic floor muscle exercises for the muscles that support the rectum, vagina, and the urethra.
 To teach a woman how to contract the right muscles, she is asked to try to stop the flow of urine when she is urinating. Once she knows how to squeeze the muscles to stop the flow of urine, she knows how to contract the right muscles. She should be instructed not to regularly stop the flow of urine midstream after she has learnt the exercise.

She can then start doing these exercises, anytime, anywhere, while she is sitting down. She is asked to squeeze the pelvic muscles at least 20–30 times at each attempt, at least three times a day. She should empty her bladder before doing the exercises. She should be instructed not to hold her breath or tighten her stomach, buttock, or thigh muscles at the same time.

- About 25 per cent of women have some anal incontinence (involuntary loss of flatus or feces) in late pregnancy.
- Both urinary and fecal incontinence are more common during pregnancy than before pregnancy.
- The majority of women with incontinence during pregnancy find complete resolution of symptoms after delivery. Even in those who have persistent symptoms postpartum, the severity and frequency reduces within a year (Hansen et al., 2012).
- There is some evidence that pelvic floor muscle exercises (PFME) in women having their first baby can prevent urinary incontinence in late pregnancy and postpartum. A systematic review of the Cochrane Database (Woodley et al., 2017) found that training continent women early in pregnancy with a structured PFME programme may prevent the onset of urinary incontinence in late pregnancy and postpartum.

References

1. Abas MN, Tan PC, Azmi N, Omar SZ. 2014. Ondansetron compared with metoclopramide for hyperemesis gravidarum: A randomized controlled trial. *Obstet Gynecol*.123:1272–9

2. Abell T, Riely C. 1992. Hyperemesis gravidarum. *Gastroenerol Clin North Am*. 21:835.

3. American College of Obstetricians and Gynecologists. 2018. ACOG Practice Bulletin 189. Nausea and vomiting of pregnancy. *Obstet Gynecol*. Vol. 131, No. 1.

4. Ali RA, Egan LJ. 2007. Gastroesophageal reflux disease in pregnancy. *Best Pract Res Clin Gastroenterol*. 21:793.

5. Bianco A. 2017. Maternal adaptations to pregnancy: Gastrointestinal tract. Lockwood CJ (Ed). *UpToDate*. Waltham, MA.

6. Boelig RC, Barton SJ, Saccone G, Kelly AJ, Edwards SJ, Berghella V. 2016. Interventions for treating hyperemesis gravidarum. *Cochrane Database Syst Rev*. Issue 5. Art. no.: CD010607

7. Bradley CS, Kennedy CM, Turcea AM, Rao SS, Nygaard IE. 2007. Constipation in pregnancy: Prevalence, symptoms, and risk factors. *Obstet Gynecol*. 110(6):1351–7.

8. Brennan M, Young G, Devane D. Topical preparations for preventing stretch marks in pregnancy. 2012. *Cochrane Database Syst Rev*. Issue 11. Art. no.: CD000066.

9. Chiossi G, Neri I, Cavazzuti M et al. 2006. Hyperemesis gravidarum complicated by Wernicke encephalopathy: Background, case report, and review of the literature. *Obstet Gynecol Surv*. 61:255.

10. Dahle LO, Berg G, Hammar M et al. 1995. The effect of oral magnesium substitution on pregnancy-induced leg cramps. *Am J Obstet Gynecol*. 173:175.

11. Dodds L, Fell DB, Joseph KS et al. 2006. Outcomes of pregnancies complicated by hyperemesis gravidarum. *Obstet Gynecol*. 107:285.

12. Geraghty LN, Pomeranz MK. 2011. Physiologic changes and dermatoses of pregnancy. *Int J Dermatol*. 50:771.

13. Gill SK, Maltepe C, Mastali K, Koren G. 2009. The effect of acid-reducing pharmacotherapy on the severity of nausea and vomiting of pregnancy. *Obstet Gynecol*. 2009:585269.

14. Goodwin TM, Montoro M, Mestman JH. 1992. Transient hyperthyroidism and hyperemesis gravidarum: Clinical aspects. *Am J Obstet Gynecol*. 2; 167:648–52.

15. Handa VL. 2018. Effect of pregnancy and childbirth on urinary incontinence and pelvic organ prolapse. Brubaker L (Ed). *UpToDate*, Waltham, MA.

16. Hansen BB, Svare J, Viktrup L et al. 2012. Urinary incontinence during pregnancy and 1 year after delivery in primiparous women compared with a control group of nulliparous women. *Neurourol Urodyn*. 31:475.

17. Hay PE, Morgan DJ, Ison CA et al. 1994. A longitudinal study of bacterial vaginosis during pregnancy. *Br J Obstet Gynaecol*. 101:1048.

18. Hinkle SN, Mumford SL, Grantz KL et al. 2016. Association of nausea and vomiting during pregnancy with pregnancy loss: A secondary analysis of a randomized clinical trial. *JAMA Intern Med*. 176:1621.

19. Hod M, Orvieto R, Kaplan B, Friedman S, Ovadia J. 1994. Hyperemesis gravidarum: A review. *J Reprod Med*. 39(8):605–12.

20. Koren G, Boskovic R, Hard M et al. 2002. Motherisk-PUQE (pregnancy-unique quantification of emesis and nausea) scoring system for nausea and vomiting of pregnancy. *Am J Obstet Gynecol*. 186:S228.

21. Koss CA, Baras DC, Lane SD et al. 2012. Investigation of metronidazole use during pregnancy and adverse birth outcomes. *Antimicrob Agents Chemother*. 56:4800.

22. Kovacs FM, Garcia E, Royuela A et al. 2012. Prevalence and factors associated with low back pain and pelvic girdle pain during pregnancy: A multicenter study conducted in the Spanish National Health Service. Spine (Phila Pa 1976). 37:1516.

23. Kuru O, Sen S, Akbayır O, Goksedef BP, Ozsürmeli M, Attar E, Saygılı H. 2012. Outcomes of pregnancies complicated by hyperemesis gravidarum. *Arch Gynecol Obstet*. 285(6):1517-21.

24. Lacroix R, Eason E, Melzack R. 2000. Nausea and vomiting during pregnancy: A prospective study of its frequency, intensity, and patterns of change. *Am J Obstet Gynecol*. 182:931.

25. Larrey D, Rueff B, Feldmann G et al. 1984. Recurrent jaundice caused by recurrent hyperemesis gravidarum. *Gut*. 25:1414.

26. Larson JD, Patatanian E, Miner PB Jr et al. 1997. Double-blind, placebo-controlled study of ranitidine for gastroesophageal reflux symptoms during pregnancy. *Obstet Gynecol*. 90:83.

27. Liddle SD, Pennick V. 2015. Interventions for preventing and treating low-back and pelvic pain during pregnancy. *Cochrane Database Syst Rev*. Issue 9. Art. no.:CD001139.

28. Lopez-Rangel E, Van Allen MI. 2005. Prenatal exposure to fluconazole: An identifiable dysmorphic phenotype. *Birth Defects Res A Clin Mol Teratol*. 73:919.

29. Magee LA, Mazzotta P, Koren G. 2002. Evidence-based view of safety and effectiveness of pharmacologic therapy for nausea and vomiting of pregnancy (NVP). *Am J Obstet Gynecol*. 186:S256–61

30. Matok I, Gorodischer R, Koren G, Sheiner E, Wiznitzer A, Levy A. 2009. The safety of metoclopramide use in the first trimester of pregnancy. *N Engl J Med*. 360:2528–35.

31. Matthews A, Haas DM, O'Mathúna DP, Dowswell T. 2015. Interventions for nausea and vomiting in early pregnancy. *Cochrane Database Syst Rev*. Issue 9. Art. no.: CD007575.

32. Mitchell AA, Gilboa SM, Werler MM, Kelley KE, Louik C, Hernandez-Diaz S. 2011. Medication use during pregnancy, with particular focus on prescription drugs: 1976–2008. National Birth Defects Prevention Study. *Am J Obstet Gynecol*. 205:51. e1–e8

33. National Institute for Health and Clinical Excellence (2008). Last updated January 2017. Antenatal care for uncomplicated pregnancies. NICE guideline (CG62).

34. Pasternak B, Hviid A. 2010. Use of proton-pump inhibitors in early pregnancy and the risk of birth defects. *N Engl J Med*. 363:2114.

35. RCOG Green-top Guideline No. 69. June 2016.

36. Rey E, Rodriguez-Artalejo F, Herraiz MA et al. 2007. Gastroesophageal reflux symptoms during and after pregnancy: A longitudinal study. *Am J Gastroenterol.* 102:2395.

37. Rhodes VA, McDaniel RW. 1999. the index of nausea, vomiting, and retching: A new format of the index of nausea and vomiting. *Oncol Nurs Forum.* 26:889.

38. Sapra KJ, Buck Louis GM, Sundaram R et al. 2016. Signs and symptoms associated with early pregnancy loss: Findings from a population-based preconception cohort. *Hum Reprod.* 31(4):887–896.

39. Silver BJ, Guy RJ, Kaldor JM et al. 2014. *Trichomonas vaginalis* as a cause of perinatal morbidity: A systematic review and meta-analysis. *Sex Transm Dis.* 41:369.

40. Smith JA, Fox KA, Clark S. 2018. Treatment and outcome of nausea and vomiting of pregnancy. Lockwood CJ (Ed). *UpToDate.* Waltham, MA.

41. Taylor D, Pappo E, Aronson IK. 2016. Polymorphic eruption of pregnancy. *Clin Dermatol.* 34:383.

42. Vaughan Jones SA, Black MMS. 1999. Pregnancy dermatoses. *J Am Acad Dermatol.* 40:233.

43. Veenendaal MV, van Abeelen AF, Painter RC, van der Post JA, Roseboom TJ. 2011. Consequences of hyperemesis gravidarum for offspring: A systematic review and meta-analysis. *BJOG.* 118(11):1302–13.

44. Wang SM, Dezinno P, Maranets I et al. 2004. Low back pain during pregnancy: Prevalence, risk factors, and outcomes. *Obstet Gynecol.* 104:65.

45. Wesnes SL, Rortveit G, Bø K, Hunskaar S. 2007. Urinary incontinence during pregnancy. *Obstet Gynecol.* 109:922.

46. Wong RC, Ellis CN. 1984. Physiologic skin changes in pregnancy. *J Am Acad Dermatol.* 10:929.

47. Woodley SJ, Boyle R, Cody JD, Mørkved S, Hay-Smith EC. 2017. Pelvic floor muscle training for prevention and treatment of urinary and faecal incontinence in antenatal and postnatal women. *Cochrane Database Syst Rev.* Issue 12. Art. No.: CD007471.

48. World Health Organization. 2016. WHO recommendation on interventions for the relief of heartburn during pregnancy. The WHO Reproductive Health Library. WHO, Geneva.

49. Young GL, Jewell D. 2002. Interventions for leg cramps in pregnancy. *Cochrane Database Syst Rev.* Issue 1. Art. no.: CD000121.

Chapter 6

Antepartum Fetal Surveillance

INTRODUCTION

- The primary aim of antepartum fetal surveillance is to prevent unexpected fetal demise (ACOG, 2014).
- In the presence of risk factors that may affect fetal well-being, antepartum fetal surveillance provides information about the intrauterine status of the fetus.
- Antepartum fetal surveillance may include inexpensive tests such as fetal kick counts or tests that require more resources such as non-stress tests, amniotic fluid evaluation, fetal biophysical profile, and Doppler assessments.
- The accuracy of a test depends on the underlying pathophysiologic condition that has prompted the surveillance. To make appropriate decisions, condition-specific fetal testing must be used (Kontopoulos and Vintzileos, 2004).
- A conscious effort must be made to match the test to the underlying pathological condition so that fewer tests are performed but at the same time, safety is not compromised.

Antepartum fetal surveillance techniques are useful in assessing the risk of fetal death in pregnancies complicated by the following:
- Pre-existing maternal conditions (e.g., hypertension)
- Newly developed complications (e.g., intrauterine growth restriction)

TESTS OF FETAL WELL-BEING

- The fetus responds to chronic hypoxemia with a sequence of biophysical changes that begin with physiological adaptation and may end with signs of physiological decompensation (Martin, 2008). Antepartum testing attempts to identify the changes that occur due to hypoxemia, thus allowing interventions before permanent damage has occurred.
- Biophysical tests that are used to assess fetal well-being in utero include the following:
  - Fetal movement count
  - Cardiotocography (CTG)/electronic fetal monitoring (EFM)
    - Non-stress test (NST)
    - Vibroacoustic stimulation
    - Contraction stress test (CST)
  - Ultrasonography
    - Amniotic fluid assessment
  - Biophysical profile (BPP), which combines ultrasonography and CTG
    - Fetal breathing
    - Fetal movement
    - Fetal tone

- Amniotic fluid index
- Non-stress test
- Doppler studies
  - Fetal umbilical artery
  - Fetal middle cerebral artery
  - Fetal ductus venosus

Indications for antenatal fetal surveillance
Previous obstetric history
Maternal
- Hypertensive disorders of pregnancy
- Placental abruption

Fetal
- Fetal growth restriction
- Stillbirth

Current pregnancy
Maternal
- Postterm pregnancy
- Hypertensive disorders of pregnancy
- Diabetes
  - Pre-gestational diabetes
  - Gestational diabetes requiring insulin
- Antiphospholipid antibody syndrome
- Advanced maternal age (elderly primigravida)
- Twin pregnancy
- Vaginal bleeding
- Preterm premature rupture of membranes
- Pregnancy after assisted reproductive technique

Fetal
- Decreased fetal movement
- Fetal growth restriction
- Oligohydramnios/polyhydramnios
- Multiple pregnancy (with significant growth discrepancy)
- Preterm labour

WHEN TO INITIATE ANTENATAL TESTING

- The initiation of antepartum fetal surveillance is individualised and depends on the severity of the risk factor or factors associated with the pregnancy. There is no gestational age cut-off at which it should be initiated. Initiating testing at 32–34 weeks of gestation is appropriate for most high-risk patients (Rouse et al., 1995).

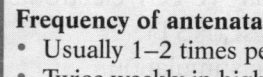

Frequency of antenatal testing
- Usually 1–2 times per week
- Twice weekly in high-risk pregnancies
- Every 24–48 hours in preterm cases where every day gained increases the chance of neonatal survival

- In pregnancies with multiple high-risk factors, testing might be initiated earlier (ACOG, 2014).

A general guideline for the timing of initiation of antenatal testing for common indications is presented in Table 6.1.

Table 6.1   Timing of initiation of antenatal fetal health surveillance

Indication	When to initiate fetal surveillance
Decreased or absent fetal movement in the 3rd trimester	Immediately
Adverse event in the previous pregnancy (e.g., stillbirth)	Two weeks before the gestational age at which the adverse event occurred in the previous pregnancy
Postterm pregnancy	40 weeks
Insulin-dependent or insulin-requiring pregnancies that are well-controlled and otherwise uncomplicated	34 weeks
Insulin-dependent or insulin-requiring pregnancies that are uncontrolled/associated with complications	32 weeks or earlier
Hypertensive disorders	32 weeks or earlier
Fetal growth restriction	At diagnosis and for follow-up

TESTS OF ANTENATAL FETAL SURVEILLANCE

I. FETAL MOVEMENT AWARENESS AND COUNTING

Rationale

- In the presence of fetal hypoxia and placental dysfunction, the fetus decreases gross body movements to conserve oxygen.
- A meta-analysis (Froen, 2004) demonstrated that women who report decreased fetal movement

 Maternal perception of *decreased* fetal movements is an indicator of pregnancies at increased risk of adverse outcomes (Fretts, 2018).

(DFM) are at an increased risk of adverse perinatal outcomes. In a case-control study of maternally perceived fetal movements in relation to late stillbirth, Heazell et al. (2018) found that DFM was associated with stillbirth.
- Early recognition of decreased fetal movement makes it possible to initiate interventions at a stage when the fetus is still compensated, thus preventing progression to fetal death.
- Up to 40 per cent of women experience DFM during their pregnancy, though most episodes are transient. Approximately 4–15 per cent of pregnant women seek medical attention because of persistent DFM in the third trimester.
- Though a review of the Cochrane Database (Mangesi et al., 2015) was unable to find enough evidence to recommend routine fetal movement counting, Delaram and Shams (2016) found that women who performed fetal movement counting from 28–37 weeks' gestation reported less anxiety than those in the control group.

Recommendations

- Daily monitoring of fetal movements starting at 26–32 weeks should be done in all pregnancies **with risk factors** for adverse perinatal outcome (Liston et al., 2018).

- All **healthy** pregnant women should be routinely educated about the importance of being aware of fetal movements, especially in the third trimester. This should be reinforced at each clinical visit

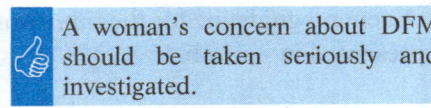
A woman's concern about DFM should be taken seriously and investigated.

(Gardener et al. 2017). They should also be instructed on initiating a fetal movement count if they perceive decreased movements (Liston et al., 2018).
- Women should be instructed to seek medical attention for persistent DFM. This should be done within two hours, especially if there are **<6 movements in two hours** or **absent fetal movements**.
- Women may be given any of the following guidelines (Fretts, 2018) to maintain a fetal movement count:
  - Perception of at least 10 fetal movements (FMs) over two hours when the mother is at rest and focused on counting ('count to 10' method)
  - Perception of at least 10 FMs during 12 hours of normal maternal activity
  - Perception of at least 4 FMs in one hour when the mother is at rest and focused on counting

Evaluation of decreased fetal movements

- Cardiotocography is done to record the fetal heart rate and to perform a non-stress test (NST). The presence of accelerations is reassuring (see section on *Non-stress test*).
- Ultrasound evaluation helps in:
  - Demonstrating fetal movements to the mother
  - Assessing amniotic fluid volume
  - Performing a biophysical profile, if needed (see section on *Biophysical profile*)
  The evaluation of DFM is summarised in Figure 6.1.

II. CARDIOTOCOGRAPHY (CTG) OR ELECTRONIC FETAL MONITORING (EFM)

The following tests may be done using a cardiotocograph (also known as electronic fetal monitor), though the non-stress test is the most commonly used test in routine obstetric practice.
- Non-stress test (NST)
- Vibroacoustic stimulation test (VAST)
- Contraction stress test (CST)

Non-stress test (NST)

The non-stress test is performed using a cardiotocograph (external CTG). The fetal heart rate is recorded in the absence of contractions. Accelerations of the fetal rate are looked for.

Rationale

- The heart rate of the healthy fetus will transiently accelerate with fetal movement.
- When there are accelerations associated with fetal movements, it is called a **reactive NST**. Heart rate reactivity is considered a good indicator of normal fetal autonomic function.

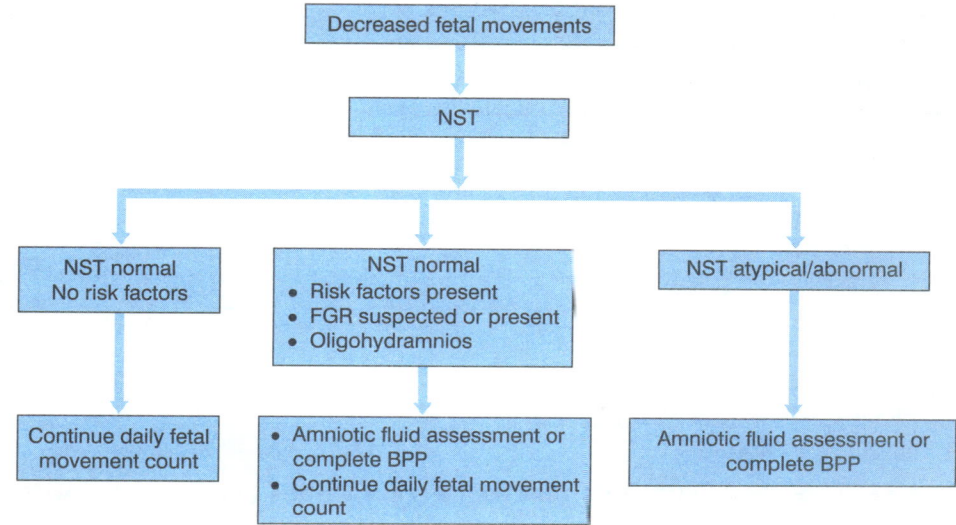

Figure 6.1 Summary of evaluation of decreased fetal movements reported by the pregnant woman. *BPP*, biophysical profile; *NST*, non-stress test

- Loss of reactivity (absent accelerations) is known as a **non-reactive NST**. This is associated most commonly with a fetal sleep cycle but may result from prematurity, sepsis, or any cause of central nervous system depression, including fetal acidosis.
- **Decelerations** may occur due to cord compression or hypoxia. Decelerations during an NST that persist for a minute or longer are significant and are associated with an increased risk of both cesarean delivery and fetal demise.

Procedure

- The test should preferably be done after the mother has eaten.
- After the transabdominal Doppler ultrasonic transducer and tocodynamometer are attached to her abdomen, the woman should be placed in the lateral recumbent or reclining position.
- She should be instructed to press the marker whenever she perceives fetal movements.

Interpretation

Reactive NST (Figure 6.2)

- Recorded over 20 minutes (the test should be extended to 40 minutes if there are no accelerations)
- Two or more accelerations that peak at least 15 beats per minute (bpm) above baseline and last at least 15 seconds each

Non-reactive NST (Figure 6.3)

- No accelerations in 40 minutes
- May be repeated after the mother has been fed

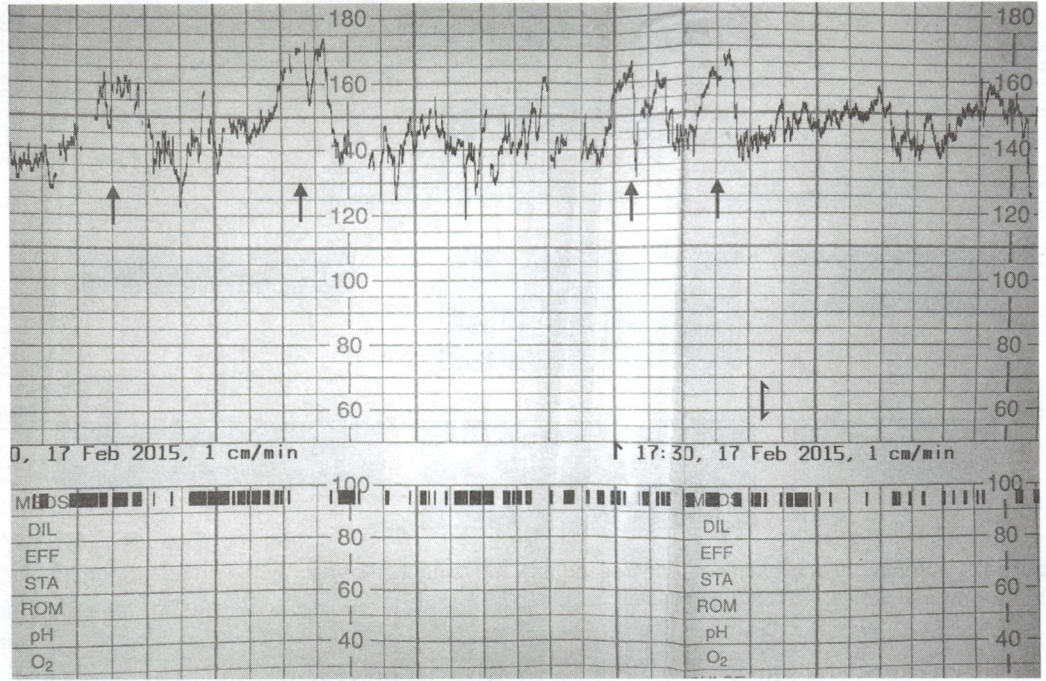

Figure 6.2   Reactive non-stress test showing accelerations (arrows). The waveform in the upper half of the graph represents the fetal heart rate.

- Vibroacoustic stimulation to elicit accelerations, or a complete biophysical profile (BPP) may be performed to confirm fetal status

Decelerations during an NST
- Significant if persisting for 1 minute or longer
- Associated with an increased risk of the following:
  - Cesarean delivery
  - Fetal demise

Other findings on NST
- *Bradycardia:*   Significant bradycardia is associated with increased perinatal mortality and morbidity and has a higher positive predictive value than a non-reactive NST. Further evaluation by biophysical profile is indicated.
- *Tachycardia:*   Preterm fetuses have a higher baseline FHR. In a term fetus, tachycardia may be due to maternal fever, fetal hypoxemia, or acidosis.
- *Loss of variability:*   This usually occurs along with baseline tachycardia. Loss of variability indicates fetal acidosis and requires further evaluation.

Recommendations

- Non-stress testing may be considered when risk factors for adverse perinatal outcomes are present.

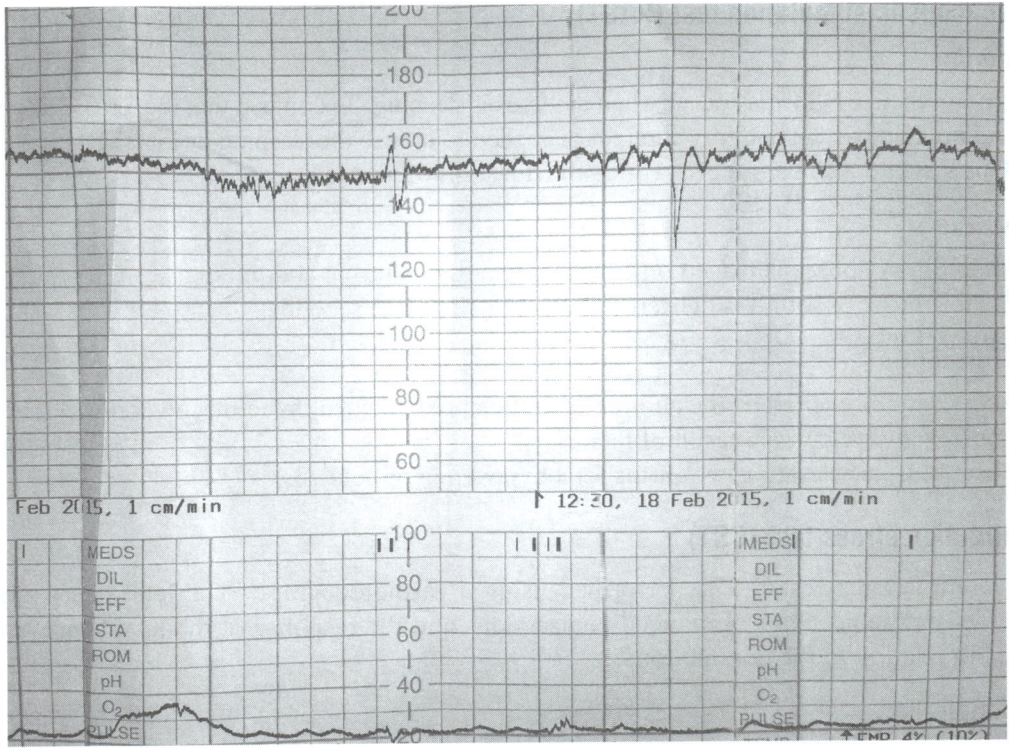

Figure 6.3 Non-reactive non-stress test showing absent accelerations. The waveform in the upper half of the graph represents the fetal heart rate.

- In the presence of a reactive non-stress test, usual fetal movement patterns, and absence of oligohydramnios, it is not necessary to proceed with further testing (Liston et al., 2018).
- A non-reactive NST requires further testing to confirm fetal compromise.

Predictive value of NST

- NST predicts the fetal status for the next 72 hours; therefore, in high-risk pregnancies like postterm pregnancy, insulin-dependent diabetes mellitus, or early-onset hypertension, the test should be performed twice a week.
- A reactive NST has a more accurate predictive value.
- A non-reactive NST has a false positive rate of 50 per cent. This means that half the fetuses

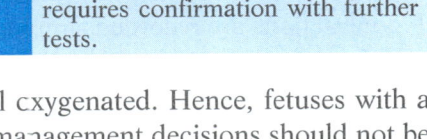

A reactive NST is 99.5 per cent accurate in predicting a healthy baby.

A non-reactive NST is only 50 per cent accurate in predicting a compromised fetus and therefore requires confirmation with further tests.

showing a non-reactive pattern may actually be well oxygenated. Hence, fetuses with a non-reactive NST should be evaluated further, and management decisions should not be based on the NST alone.

- NST cannot predict sudden events like placental abruption or cord accidents.

Vibroacoustic stimulation test (VAST)

Rationale

- A non-reactive NST may occur when the fetus is sleeping. To confirm that the fetus is sleeping and not hypoxic, an auditory stimulus is applied to arouse the sleeping or inactive fetus.
- This test can also be used to reduce the duration of an NST.

Procedure

- An auditory source is placed on or just above the maternal abdomen.
- A short burst of sound is delivered to the fetus for 1–2 seconds.

Interpretation

- Accelerations elicited by the auditory stimulus predict a healthy fetus and confirm that the non-reactive test was a result of fetal sleep.
- Absence of accelerations confirms fetal hypoxemia or acidosis.

Contraction stress test (CST)

The contraction stress test is performed using a cardiotocograph. The fetal heart rate is recorded in the presence of induced contractions and the response of the fetal heart rate is noted in relation to the contractions.

Rationale

- During a uterine contraction, there is a transient decrease in fetal oxygenation. If a fetus is already hypoxemic, the intermittent worsening of oxygenation during a uterine contraction will result in *late decelerations* (see **Chapter 18**, *Fetal health surveillance in labour*).
- Uterine contractions may also cause fetal umbilical cord compression in the case of decreased amniotic fluid (oligohydramnios) in a high-risk pregnancy. This can result in *variable decelerations* (see **Chapter 18**, *Fetal health surveillance in labour*).

Procedure

- The CST is recorded on a cardiotocograph after the transabdominal Doppler ultrasonic transducer and tocodynamometer are attached to the abdomen.
- The mother lies in the lateral recumbent position, and the fetal heart rate and uterine contractions are recorded simultaneously.

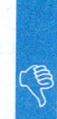 CST-induced contractions can lead to complications like the stimulation of regular uterine contractions and rupture of membranes. Hence it is not commonly performed in current obstetric practice.

- Contractions are induced with nipple stimulation or intravenous oxytocin until the mother has at least three contractions, each of 40 seconds' duration, within 10 minutes.

Interpretation

- *Positive (non-reassuring):* Late decelerations following 50 per cent or more of the contractions

- *Negative (reassuring):* No late or significant variable decelerations
- *Equivocal–suspicious:* Intermittent late decelerations or significant variable decelerations
- *Equivocal–hyperstimulatory:* Fetal heart rate decelerations that occur in the presence of contractions more frequent than every two minutes or lasting longer than 90 seconds
- *Unsatisfactory:* Tracing is uninterpretable or contractions are fewer than three in 10 minutes

III. BIOPHYSICAL PROFILE (BPP)

- The BPP is a non-invasive, accurate means of predicting the presence of significant fetal hypoxemia/acidosis (Manning, 1980).
- The complete BPP combines an NST with four biophysical variables measured by ultrasonography: **fetal movements**, **breathing**, **tone**, and **amniotic fluid volume**. Each variable is given a score of 2 (normal) or 0 (abnormal, absent, or insufficient). This test may take up to 30–60 minutes to perform, which often makes it difficult to conduct in a busy clinical practice.
- **The modified BPP (mBPP)** combines the NST with amniotic fluid volume assessment, the components of the BPP that are most predictive of fetal outcome. It is a faster method of assessing both acute and chronic fetal hypoxia.

 Modified BPP (NST with amniotic fluid assessment) appears to be as reliable a predictor of long-term fetal well-being as the complete BPP (Manning, 2018).

Rationale

- Fetal biophysical activities like body movements, breathing, and fetal heart rate and tone are regulated and controlled by discrete centres within the brain. The presence of these biophysical activities implies normal oxygenation of the fetal central nervous system.
- Fetal hypoxemia/acidosis causes loss of accelerations of the fetal heart rate (FHR), decreased breathing and body movements, and hypotonia. These four variables reflect *acute hypoxia*.

 The brain centres that develop earliest in gestation are the least sensitive to hypoxia. The fetal cardioregulatory centre develops last and is the most sensitive to hypoxia. The cascade of response to hypoxia follows a predictable course: loss of fetal heart rate accelerations, followed by fetal breathing, fetal movements, and lastly, fetal tone. This knowledge helps us understand the degree of hypoxia from the number of biophysical activities that have been affected.

- Decreased amniotic fluid volume reflects *chronic hypoxia* since it is a reflection of fetal renal function that decreases gradually with chronic hypoxia (Nicolaides, 1990).

Procedure

- An ultrasonographic examination is done, and gross body movements, fetal breathing movements, and fetal tone are noted. During this examination, the amniotic fluid volume is also measured. In mBPP, only the amniotic fluid volume is recorded with ultrasound.
- An NST is performed using a cardiotocograph.

Amniotic fluid index (AFI) vs. single deepest pocket (SDP) for fetal surveillance and preventing adverse pregnancy outcome

Amniotic fluid index (AFI) measurement: The uterus is divided into four quadrants using the linea nigra for the right and left divisions and the umbilicus for the upper and lower quadrants. Using ultrasound, the maximal vertical amniotic fluid pocket diameter in each quadrant (not containing cord or fetal extremities) is measured. The sum of the four measurements (in centimetres) is called AFI.

Single deepest pocket (SDP) measurement: Using ultrasound, the vertical dimension (in centimetres) of the largest pocket of amniotic fluid (not persistently containing umbilical cord or fetal extremities) is measured at a right angle to the uterine contour (Figure 6.4).

A systematic review of the Cochrane Database (Nabhan and Abdelmoula, 2008) concluded that the **SDP measurement in the assessment of amniotic fluid volume during fetal surveillance was a better choice.** The use of the amniotic fluid index leads to an overdiagnosis of oligohydramnios and an increase in the rate of induction of labour without improvement in perinatal outcomes. This recommendation was reinforced by the SAFE randomised controlled trial (Kehl et al., 2016).

Interpretation of the biophysical profile (BPP) score

In the case of a complete BPP, the score is assigned using the criteria presented in Table 6.2.

Management based on BPP scores

Based on BPP scores, clinical management is as presented in Table 6.3 (Manning, 2018).

Interpretation of the modified biophysical profile (mBPP)

Normal
- NST reactive
- Single deepest pocket ≥2 cm

Abnormal
- NST non-reactive
- Single deepest pocket <2 cm

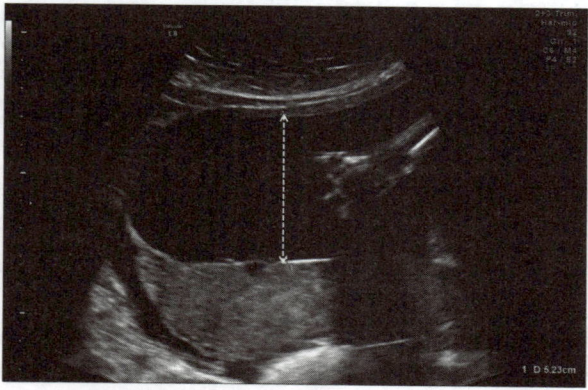

Figure 6.4   Measurement of single deepest vertical pocket (SDP) by ultrasound. The presence of an SDP ≥2 cm is reassuring.

Table 6.2   Scoring system for the complete biophysical profile

Criteria	Normal (score=2)	Abnormal (score=0)
Non-stress test	Reactive	Non-reactive
Fetal breathing movements	≥1 episodes, lasting at least 30 seconds within a 30-minute interval	No FBM in 30 minutes
Gross body movements	≥3 discrete body/limb movements in 30 minutes	Less than 3 in 30 min
Fetal tone	≥1 extensions of arm/leg or opening and closing of hand	No movements or slow movements or hand in constantly open position
Amniotic fluid volume using SDP	At least one pocket of amniotic fluid ≥2 cm	Largest SDP <2 cm

FBM, fetal breathing movements; *SDP*, single deepest vertical pocket

Table 6.3   Interpretation of BPP scores and recommended management

Score	Interpretation
10/10	Low risk of developing fetal asphyxia
8/10, normal AFV	Low risk of developing fetal asphyxia
8/10, low AFV	Consider chronic hypoxia—repeat test or deliver if at term
6/10	Significant possibility of developing fetal asphyxia
	– If AFV abnormal—deliver
	– If AFV normal, repeat test and consider delivery
4/10	High risk of fetal asphyxia within one week—delivery indicated
0–2/10	Certain fetal asphyxia—deliver

AFV, amniotic fluid volume

Recommendations

- BPP is not a first-line fetal surveillance test. It is considered the next step in the evaluation of women with an abnormal NST or CST.
- In pregnancies at increased risk of adverse perinatal outcome and where facilities and expertise exist, modified biophysical profile (mBPP) is recommended for the evaluation of fetal well-being.
- In situations where the mBPP is not conclusive, a complete BPP may be performed. However, a review of the Cochrane Database found that there was not enough evidence to support the routine use of BPP for the assessment of fetal well-being in high-risk pregnancies (Lalor et al., 2008).

> A review of the Cochrane Database found that there was not enough evidence to support the *routine* use of biophysical profile (BPP) for the assessment of fetal well-being in high-risk pregnancies (Lalor et al., 2008).

Predictive value of BPP

- A normal BPP is 99.9 per cent accurate in predicting a healthy baby and correlates well with good perinatal outcome.

- The earliest manifestations of acute hypoxia are an abnormal NST and the loss of breathing movements.
- A score of 6/10 without oligohydramnios is an equivocal test result and should be repeated within 24 hours if the mother is not delivered.
- A low BPP score has a high positive predictive value, and an abnormal BPP of <4 correlates with fetal asphyxia.

Predictive value of mBPP

- The predictive value of mBPP is as good as that of other biophysical tests.
- The mBPP has been found to be an excellent fetal surveillance tool.
- As an integral part of an mBPP, a reactive NST is 99 per cent accurate in predicting that the fetus is healthy.
- A non-reactive NST must be correlated with the amniotic fluid volume and may need to be followed-up with a complete BPP or delivery, depending on the gestational age and the maternal/fetal condition that prompted the fetal surveillance (ACOG, 2014).
- In the setting of otherwise uncomplicated, isolated, and persistent oligohydramnios, delivery at 36–37 weeks is recommended.
- Oligohydramnios in the presence of normal fetal growth may be less ominous than when it is associated with fetal growth restriction.

IV. DOPPLER VELOCIMETRY

- Doppler ultrasonography is a non-invasive technique used to measure blood flow in the placenta and fetal blood vessels.
- In high-risk pregnancies, abnormal blood flow patterns in fetal vessels detected by Doppler ultrasound may indicate poor fetal prognosis.

Umbilical artery Doppler velocimetry

- Abnormal placentation, such as in preeclampsia, results in vascular compromise. This leads to progressive hemodynamic changes in the fetoplacental circulation.

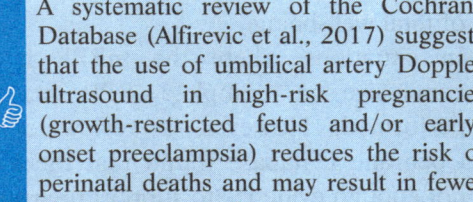

- In growth-restricted fetuses, umbilical artery Doppler velocimetry helps differentiate the compensated healthy fetus from the hypoxemic/acidotic fetus.
- When used in conjunction with standard fetal surveillance such as NST, mBPP, or complete BPP, it is associated with improved outcomes in growth-restricted fetuses.

A systematic review of the Cochrane Database (Alfirevic et al., 2017) suggests that the use of umbilical artery Doppler ultrasound in high-risk pregnancies (growth-restricted fetus and/or early-onset preeclampsia) reduces the risk of perinatal deaths and may result in fewer obstetric interventions.

Rationale

- Under normal conditions, the placenta offers little resistance to fetal and maternal blood flow, even during maternal diastole. A healthy, normally growing fetus will have a high-velocity diastolic flow in the umbilical artery.

- When 60–70 per cent of the placental vascular tree is compromised in the presence of fetal growth restriction and/or preeclampsia, umbilical artery Doppler indices increase (Thompson and Trudinger, 1990).
- In a growth-restricted fetus, as placental resistance increases, there is a decrease in the umbilical artery diastolic flow.
- With severe growth restriction, the diastolic flow may be absent or even reversed. This indicates severe hypoxia and acidosis.

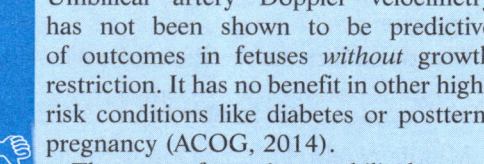

Umbilical artery Doppler velocimetry has not been shown to be predictive of outcomes in fetuses *without* growth restriction. It has no benefit in other high-risk conditions like diabetes or postterm pregnancy (ACOG, 2014).

 The use of routine umbilical artery Doppler ultrasound, or a combination of umbilical and uterine artery Doppler ultrasound in low-risk or unselected populations benefits neither mother nor baby (Alfirevic et al., 2015).

Umbilical artery flow indices

Systolic (S) and diastolic (D) peak blood flow in the fetal umbilical artery is measured, and various indices are calculated. As the diastolic flow decreases, the indices rise. Therefore, high indices indicate increased resistance to flow.

- Systolic to diastolic ratio (S/D)
- Resistance index or RI (S–D/S)
- Pulsatility index or PI (S–D/A)

A, mean peak frequency shift over the cardiac cycle; *D*, end-diastolic frequency shift; *S*, peak systolic frequency shift

Umbilical artery Doppler velocimetry in obstetric decision-making

- Umbilical artery Doppler velocimetry helps in deciding the time of delivery in the presence of fetal growth restriction, especially in preterm fetuses.
- The following are the recommendations regarding management:
  - *Normal indices:* Continue to observe with weekly Doppler studies, NST, and amniotic fluid volume assessment using single deepest vertical pocket (SDP).
  - *Absent end-diastolic flow:* This is an ominous finding with increased risk of perinatal mortality. Immediate delivery should be considered if beyond 34 weeks' gestation.
  - *Reversed end-diastolic flow:* This is a pre-terminal event associated with poor perinatal outcome. Immediate delivery is warranted.

Middle cerebral artery (MCA) Doppler

MCA Doppler velocimetry is an additional tool for the surveillance of pregnancies complicated by growth restriction.

Rationale

- When there is fetal hypoxia in the presence of growth restriction, there is preferential blood flow to preserve 'essential' organs such as the brain. Increased diastolic flow in the fetal middle cerebral artery indicates that the blood is being shunted to the brain. This is termed the 'brain-sparing effect' and is an early sign of fetal hypoxia.

- The pulsatility index (PI) of the MCA decreases in the presence of fetal hypoxia.

MCA Doppler velocimetry in obstetric decision-making

- Middle cerebral artery Doppler may be used as an adjunct to umbilical artery Doppler.
- An abnormal cerebroplacental (CP) ratio is an early predictor of adverse outcomes in growth-restricted fetuses.

> **The cerebroplacental ratio (CPR)**
> In the growth-restricted fetus, the CPR combines measurement of the placental resistance (UA Doppler) and the 'brain-sparing' effect (MCA Doppler).
>   The CPR is calculated by dividing the MCA PI by the umbilical artery PI. **It is considered abnormal if it is <1. An abnormal CPR is a good predictor of adverse outcome for the growth-restricted fetus.**
>   The CPR is also an earlier predictor of adverse outcome than the biophysical profile, umbilical artery, or middle cerebral artery (DeVore, 2015).

Ductus venosus Doppler

- **Ductus venosus (DV)** Doppler waveforms are biphasic in shape, with the first peak corresponding to ventricular systole, the second peak during passive filling in ventricular diastole, followed by a nadir in late diastole with atrial contraction.
- Continuous forward flow throughout the cardiac cycle is seen in the normal fetus.

Rationale

- DV waveforms reflect the physiologic status of the right ventricle.
- Decreased, absent, or reversed flow in the A wave (atrial contraction) may represent myocardial impairment and increased ventricular end-diastolic pressure resulting from an increase in right ventricular afterload.
- This abnormal waveform in the DV is linked to an increased neonatal mortality rate in growth-restricted fetuses (Baschat, 2004).
- Changes in the waveform pattern of the fetal ductus venosus occur late in hypoxia and indicate cardiac decompensation. It indicates a poor prognosis.

Predictive value of DV Doppler velocimetry

Ductus venosus Doppler is a good but late predictor of poor perinatal outcome. Its use is limited in the management of the growth-restricted fetus.

MANAGEMENT OF PREGNANCIES WITH NON-REASSURING ANTEPARTUM SURVEILLANCE TESTS

The management of abnormal results of antepartum surveillance tests depends both on the clinical condition and the clinical services available. The results must be correlated with certain fetal and maternal factors.

- **Gestational age** plays an important role in decision-making.
  - When the pregnancy is close to term, the decision to deliver is easier to make.
  - After 36–37 weeks gestational age, immediate delivery might be indicated to prevent further morbidity from worsening hypoxemia/acidosis.
  - When there is growth restriction with an abnormal test, the decision to deliver can be made if ≥34 weeks.
  - Management in the presence of prematurity has to be tailored to the individual pregnancy to optimise fetal outcome.
- **Severity of maternal disease**, especially worsening of the condition, tips the balance towards early delivery. Some clinical situations that may require early delivery in the face of abnormal tests are as follows:
  - Fetal growth restriction with oligohydramnios and abnormal umbilical artery Doppler flow
  - Diabetes with poor glycemic control
  - Worsening hypertensive disorder
- **The type of abnormality** found on the test may also guide management.
  - Repetitive late decelerations, prolonged deceleration, or severe variable decelerations on NST or CST generally mandate immediate delivery by cesarean section.
  - Absent or reversed end-diastolic flow in the umbilical artery is an indication of perinatal morbidity and mortality and requires intervention.

References

1. Alfirevic Z, Stampalija T, Dowswell T. 2017. Fetal and umbilical Doppler ultrasound in high-risk pregnancies. *Cochrane Database Syst Rev.* Issue 6. Art. no.: CD007529.
2. Alfirevic Z, Stampalija T, Medley N. 2015. Fetal and umbilical Doppler ultrasound in normal pregnancy. *Cochrane Database Syst Rev.* Issue 4. Art. no.: CD001450.
3. American College of Obstetricians and Gynecologists. 2014. ACOG Practice bulletin no. 145. Antepartum fetal surveillance. *Obstet Gynecol.* 124:182.
4. Baschat AA. 2004. Fetal responses to placental insufficiency: an update. *BJOG.* 111: 1031–1041.
5. Delaram M, Shams S. 2016. The effect of foetal movement counting on maternal anxiety: A randomised, controlled trial. *Journal of Obstet and Gynaecol.*
6. DeVore GR. 2015. The importance of the cerebroplacental ratio in the evaluation of fetal well-being in SGA and AGA fetuses. *Am J Obstet Gynecol.* 213:5.
7. Fretts RC. 2018. Decreased fetal movement: Diagnosis, evaluation, and management. Berghella, V (Ed). *UpToDate.* Waltham, MA.
8. Froen JF. 2004. A kick from within—fetal movement counting and the cancelled progress in antenatal care. *J Perinat Med.* 32:13–24. (Meta-analysis).
9. Gardener G, Daly L, Bowring V et al. 2017. Clinical practice guideline for the care of women with decreased fetal movements. Centre of Research Excellence in Stillbirth. Brisbane, Australia.
10. Heazell AEP, Budd J, Li M et al. 2018. Alterations in maternally perceived fetal movement and their association with late stillbirth: Findings from the Midland and North of England stillbirth case-control study. *BMJ Open.* 8(7):e020031.

11. Kehl S, Schelkle A, Thomas A et al. 2016. Single deepest vertical pocket or amniotic fluid index as evaluation test for predicting adverse pregnancy outcome (SAFE trial): A multicenter, open-label, randomized controlled trial. *Ultrasound Obstet Gynecol.* 47(6):674–9.

12. Kontopoulos EV, Vintzileos AM. 2004. Condition-specific antepartum fetal testing. *Am J Obstet Gynecol.* 191(5):1546–51.

13. Lalor JG, Fawole B, Alfirevic Z, Devane D. 2008. Biophysical profile for fetal assessment in high risk pregnancies. *Cochrane Database Syst Rev.* Issue 1. Art. no.: CD000038.

14. Liston R, Sawchuck D, Young D. 2018. Fetal health surveillance: Antepartum Consensus Guideline. *J Obstet Gynaecol Can.*

15. Mangesi L, Hofmeyr GJ, Smith V, Smyth RM. 2015. Fetal movement counting for assessment of fetal wellbeing. *Cochrane Database Syst Rev.* Issue 10. Art. no.: CD004909.

16. Manning FA, Platt LD, Sipos L. 1980. Antepartum fetal evaluation: Development of a fetal biophysical profile. *Am J Obstet Gynecol.* 136:787.

17. Manning FA. 2018. The fetal biophysical profile. Simpson LL, Levine D (Eds). *UpToDate.* Waltham, MA.

18. Martin CB Jr. 2008. Normal fetal physiology and behavior, and adaptive responses with hypoxemia. *Semin Perinatol.* 32:239.

19. Nabhan AF, Abdelmoula YA. 2008. Amniotic fluid index versus single deepest vertical pocket as a screening test for preventing adverse pregnancy outcome. *Cochrane Database Syst Rev.* Issue 3. Art. no.: CD006593.

20. Nicolaides KH, Peters MT, Vyas S et al. 1990. Relation of rate of urine production to oxygen tension in small-for-gestational-age fetuses. *Am J Obstet Gynecol.* 162:387.

21. Norman JE, Heazell AEP, Rodriguez A et al. 2018. Awareness of fetal movements and care package to reduce fetal mortality (AFFIRM): A stepped wedge, cluster-randomised trial. *Lancet.* Volume 392. Issue 10158.

22. Rouse DJ, Owen J, Goldenberg RL, Cliver SP. 1995. Determinants of the optimal time in gestation to initiate antenatal fetal testing: A decision-analytic approach. *Am J Obstet Gynecol.* 173:1357–63.

23. Thompson RS, Trudinger BJ. 1990. Doppler waveform pulsatility index and resistance, pressure and flow in the umbilical placental circulation: An investigation using a mathematical model. *Ultrasound Med Biol.* 16:449.

Chapter 7

Prenatal Screening for Genetic Disorders

INTRODUCTION

- Prenatal screening is aimed at assessing the risk of chromosomal abnormalities in individual pregnancies. Aneuploidy is the most common genetic abnormality detected by prenatal diagnosis. 90 per cent of aneuploidies involve chromosomes 21, 18, 13, X, or Y (Benacerraf, 2018).

> **Aneuploidy**
> Aneuploidy is the presence of an abnormal number of chromosomes in a cell. The number may be less (missing chromosome, e.g., XO or Turner syndrome) or more (extra chromosome, e.g., trisomies 21, 18, and 13) than the normal.
>
> Each chromosome contains a large number of genes and genetic material. When there is loss or gain of large chromosomal segments, the disruption of substantial amounts of genetic material often results in a non-viable pregnancy or early neonatal death because of birth defects incompatible with survival. A surviving newborn may present with congenital birth defects, failure to thrive, and functional abnormalities that include mild-to-severe intellectual disability, infertility, and shortened lifespan (ACOG, 2016).
>
> The incidence of aneuploidy increases with the following:
> - Increasing maternal age (though it may occur at any age)
> - History of a previous fetus with aneuploidy
> - Presence of fetal structural anomalies

- Since Down syndrome is the most common form of inherited intellectual disability, most prenatal screening focuses on identifying pregnancies at risk for this genetic disorder. The prevalence of Down syndrome is relatively high: approximately 1 in 800 live births (Nussbaum et al., 2016).
- It is important to understand that prenatal screening is limited to the identification of women with apparently healthy pregnancies who are at risk of an outcome that will warrant the next step: a prenatal diagnostic test (see **Chapter 8**, *Prenatal diagnostic testing for genetic disorders*).
- Thus, screening for Down syndrome does not aim to make a diagnosis of this condition, but rather helps to limit the use of invasive diagnostic procedures (chorionic villus sampling or amniocentesis), which would be too expensive and risky to offer without prior selection (Cuckle, 2014).
- Since its introduction in the 1990s, screening for Down syndrome has become more accurate and efficient. The combined first-trimester screen, which is currently more commonly used than second-trimester testing, has significantly decreased the number of invasive tests performed (Morgan et al., 2013).

- Serum screening is also extended to other aneuploidies, namely trisomy 18 (Edwards syndrome) and trisomy 13 (Patau syndrome) since the same biochemical markers are used to identify all three chromosomal abnormalities.
- Since prenatal screening utilises ultrasound, congenital anomalies such as cardiac defects and genetic syndromes can also be identified.

Who should be offered screening for aneuploidy?
Ideally, all pregnant women should be offered screening for aneuploidy. The burden of an affected child can be significant. Screening and diagnosis give the couple the opportunity to decide whether to continue with the pregnancy or to terminate it.

The availability of screening to a couple in India depends on a complex set of circumstances that involve the economics of screening as well as the availability of one or more of the screening modalities.

WHAT IS ANEUPLOIDY SCREENING?

- Aneuploidy screening is the process of surveying a pregnant population using specific anatomical and biochemical markers and defined screening cut-off levels to identify individuals in the population who are at high risk for having a fetus with aneuploidy.
- Aneuploidy screening tests help in stratifying the screened population into high- and low-risk groups for the condition in question, using a pre-defined cut-off. The high-risk group is then offered a diagnostic procedure.

Prenatal screening tests only provide a probability of the fetus being affected and cannot say whether the fetus is actually affected. Further diagnostic tests are required to confirm or rule out the probability.

COMMON SCREENING-RELATED TERMS

Screen-positive: A term that refers to the group which has been identified by the screening test as being at high risk for the condition. This does not necessarily mean that the fetus is affected (*false positive test*).

Screen-negative: A term that refers to the group which has been identified by the screening test as being at low risk for the condition. A small number of affected fetuses will be missed (*false negative test*).

Detection rate: The detection rate is the number of affected babies that the test will actually identify. The higher the detection rate, the better the test.

False positive rate (FPR): This is the number of women who have to undergo an unnecessary amniocentesis because the test was reported as screen-positive though the fetus was unaffected. The lower the FPR, the better the test.

Positive predictive value (PPV): This refers to the proportion of women with screen-positive results who have an affected fetus.

Odds of having an affected child given a positive result (OAPR): This is what the mother is actually interested in knowing. This is based on the PPV.

> The objective of **screening** for aneuploidy is to discover those among the apparently normal pregnancies who may in fact be carrying an affected fetus; screening is applied to the entire population. **Diagnostic tests** are applied at the individual level.

MATERNAL AGE AND THE RISK OF ANEUPLOIDY

- The risk of chromosomal problems such as trisomies increases with increasing maternal age. As the oocyte ages along with the woman, it is prone to non-disjunction errors in the meiotic division, which result in a fetus with aneuploidy.
- On the other hand, the risk of triploidy and Turner syndrome does not vary with maternal age.
- The risk of having a baby with Down syndrome at term in relation to increasing maternal age is presented in Table 7.1.
- Nearly 70 per cent of babies who have Down syndrome are born to mothers who are younger than 35 years. Hence maternal age in isolation is not recommended as a screening parameter (Nicolaides, 2003). However, it is a crucial component of screening strategies as it provides the pre-test risk for all screening tests.

> 95 per cent of cases of Down syndrome result from non-disjunction involving chromosome 21. Translocations or somatic mosaicism account for the remaining cases (Sherman et al., 2007).

Table 7.1   Risk of Down syndrome (DS) in the fetus in relation to maternal age (MA) at the estimated date of delivery (EDD) (adapted from Savva et al., 2010)

MA at EDD	Risk of DS	MA at EDD	Risk of DS	MA at EDD	Risk of DS
20	1:1475	30	1:935	40	1:85
21	1:1460	31	1:815	41	1:66
22	1:1440	32	1:695	42	1:54
23	1:1415	33	1:570	43	1:45
24	1:1380	34	1:455	44	1:39
25	1:1340	35	1:350	45	1:34
26	1:1285	36	1:265	46	1:31
27	1:1220	37	1:195	47	1:29
28	1:1140	38	1:145	48	1:27
29	1:1045	39	1:110	49	1:26

SCREENING TESTS FOR FETAL ANEUPLOIDY

The three screening modalities available are as follows:
- Maternal serum screening
  - First-trimester screening
  - Quadruple screen

- Triple screen
- Combined first- and second-trimester screening
- Ultrasonographic screening
- Cell-free DNA (cfDNA) screening

 Prenatal screening programmes based on maternal serum and ultrasound testing can detect up to 80–90 per cent of pregnancies affected by Down syndrome at a false positive rate of 5 per cent (ACOG, 2016).

MATERNAL SERUM SCREENING

- Since maternal age has an impact on the occurrence of trisomies, age is used to calculate the *pre-test risk,* and likelihood ratios are used to calculate the *final risk* from the screening.
- These likelihood ratios are derived from population-based statistics and, therefore, it is important to use local population-based statistics.
- The most widely used approach for screening measures maternal serum levels of specific **biochemical markers** associated with Down syndrome, trisomy 18, and trisomy 13. This is usually combined with the assessment of specific ultrasound markers, the most common being **nuchal translucency** (see the section on *Ultrasound screening for aneuploidy*).
- The following information is essential for all screening strategies for trisomies:
  - Maternal age
  - Maternal weight
  - Ethnicity

 In an IVF conception where a donor egg has been used, the donor's age has to be taken into account for risk estimation.

  - Maternal diabetic status (does not affect first trimester screening)
  - Type of conception (specifically, whether IVF)
  - Gestational age, which is calculated from CRL at 11–13^{+6} weeks or BPD/HC in second trimester fetuses
  - Whether the mother smokes
- The serum analytes that are measured show specific patterns with different trisomies. This helps in risk allocation (Table 7.2).

Table 7.2   Changes in levels of serum markers in the common trisomies

Serum markers	Trisomy 21	Trisomy 18	Trisomy 13
PAPP-A	Decreased	Decreased	Decreased
hCG	Increased	Decreased	Decreased
AFP	Decreased	Decreased	Decreased
uE3	Decreased	Decreased	Decreased
Inhibin A	Increased	Decreased	Increased

AFP, alpha-fetoprotein; *hCG*, human chorionic gonadotropin; *PAPP-A*, pregnancy-associated plasma protein A; *uE3*, unconjugated estriol

Dating scan for establishing accurate gestational age

All serum markers used for screening are gestational age-sensitive and vary with advancing gestation. It is therefore imperative that an accurate dating scan be carried out before any screening is offered to the woman. This is either established by an earlier scan or by obtaining an accurate CRL at the 11–13^{+6} weeks' scan. As the interpretation of nuchal translucency (NT) is based on CRL, it is important that the CRL be taken in the standard, neutral position and that the baby is not too flexed or extended when the measurement is taken.

First-trimester combined screening

- First-trimester screening (FTS) combines serum markers and ultrasound measurement of nuchal translucency (NT).
- The ideal time for screening is 11–13^{+6} weeks since the ultrasound and the blood tests can be done at the same sitting, increasing patient comfort and compliance (Nicolaides, 2011).
- First-trimester screening for Down syndrome has detection rates of 82–87 per cent at a 5 per cent false positive rate (FPR).
- The **advantages** of FTS are the following:
  - It enables early risk prediction for trisomy in pregnancy, so decisions can be made earlier.
  - Increased NT in the absence of chromosomal abnormality may be a marker for major cardiac defects, diaphragmatic hernia, renal anomalies, body stalk disruption, and abdominal wall defects, and requires follow-up.
  - Decreased PAPP-A or increased β-hCG may also be used to screen for preeclampsia.
  - Maternal diabetes does not affect the results.
- The disadvantages of FTS are the following:
  - It requires a specially trained ultrasonologist who can accurately measure nuchal translucency.
  - It cannot identify certain fetal anomalies and so a detailed second-trimester screening is required to screen for open neural tube defects and other fetal structural defects.

First-trimester combined screening

When:
- 11–13^{+6} weeks
- CRL should be between 45 and 84 mm

Serum analytes measured:
- Free β-hCG
- PAPP-A

Combined with:
- Nuchal translucency
- Other soft markers (depending on the expertise available at the centre performing the screening):
  - Absence or presence of nasal bone
  - Increased impedance to flow in the ductus venosus
  - Tricuspid regurgitation

Sensitivity:
- 82–87 per cent at a 5 per cent false positive rate

Second-trimester screening

Quadruple screen

- The quadruple screen is offered between 15 and 22^{+6} weeks of gestation and involves the analysis of four serum analytes.
- Accurate gestational dating by an early ultrasound is essential and improves risk accuracy determinations.
- It has almost the same detection rate as first-trimester screening: >80 per cent detection at a 5 per cent false positive rate for Down syndrome (ACOG, 2016).
- The levels of the analytes are interpreted as multiples of medians (MoMs) from the unaffected population, and a risk algorithm is created (Wald et al., 2003).
- The **advantage** of second-trimester screening is that it does not require specialised ultrasonographic measurements.
- The **disadvantage** of second-trimester screening is that the result may be available only after 20 weeks and may not leave the couple with the option to terminate the pregnancy since legal termination of pregnancy in India is not allowed beyond that gestational age.

> **Quadruple screen**
> **When:**
> - $15–22^{+6}$ weeks (accurate gestational dating is essential)
>
> **Serum analytes measured:**
> - Total hCG   • Alpha-fetoprotein (AFP)
> - Inhibin A   • Unconjugated estriol (uE3)
>
> **Sensitivity:**
> - 80 per cent at a 5 per cent false positive rate

Triple screen test

- The triple screen test is offered at $15–22^{+6}$ weeks of gestation and involves the analysis of three serum analytes: hCG, alpha-fetoprotein (AFP), and unconjugated estriol (uE3). **This test is now considered obsolete.**
- The triple screen is less sensitive for the detection of Down syndrome with a sensitivity of 69 per cent at a 5 per cent false positive rate (ACOG, 2016).
- The triple screen test may be offered when the laboratory facilities required for measuring inhibin A are not available.

> **Triple screen test**
> **When:**
> - $15–22^{+6}$ weeks (accurate gestational dating is essential)
>
> **Serum analytes measured:**
> - Total hCG
> - Alpha-fetoprotein (AFP)
> - Unconjugated estriol (uE3)
>
> **Sensitivity:**
> - 69 per cent at a 5 per cent false positive rate

Combined first- and second-trimester screening

- Combining first- and second-trimester screening provides a higher detection rate than a single-step test.
- The cost of two screening tests is prohibitive and hence this option is rarely offered in India.
- When offered, an integrated or sequential protocol can be used.
  - **Integrated protocol**
    - Both a first-trimester and second-trimester screening are done, but the report is only provided in the second trimester. The integrated test has detection rates of 85–95 per cent and the lowest false positive rate among Down syndrome screening tests.
  - **Sequential protocol**
    The sequential protocol may be stepwise or contingent.

    Stepwise sequential screening
    - First-trimester screening results are made known to the mother.
    - If the result is reported as low-risk, a quadruple screen is performed in the second trimester.
    - If the result is reported as high-risk, a diagnostic test or non-invasive prenatal testing (NIPT) using cell-free DNA is offered
    - The detection rate with this method is 92 per cent at a false positive rate of 5 per cent.

    Contingent protocol
    - The results are classified as low-risk (<1:1000), intermediate-risk (between 1:101 and 1:1000) or high-risk (e.g., ≥ 1:100).
    - The high-risk mothers are offered a diagnostic test or NIPT.
    - The low-risk mothers undergo no further tests.
    - Only those classified as intermediate-risk are offered a second-trimester screening test.

Screening for aneuploidy in multifetal pregnancy

- In twin pregnancies, a first-trimester combined screening test (FTS) is the best screening for Down syndrome and trisomy 18. However, no method of aneuploidy screening is as accurate as it is in singleton pregnancies (ACOG, 2016).
- In the presence of fetal demise or an anomaly in one fetus of a multiple gestation, serum-based aneuploidy screening should not be offered.
- The following are the choices available for aneuploidy screening in a multifetal pregnancy:
  - **Nuchal translucency** measurement allows independent screening of each fetus in a twin or high-order multifetal gestation. It has been recommended that greater reliance be placed on the nuchal translucency (NT) risk alone when counselling women about invasive testing (Spencer and Nicolaides, 2003).
  - **First-trimester combined screening** is the best option for twin pregnancies. It provides the risk for the entire pregnancy and not only for the individual fetus.

– **Second-trimester serum screening** of twin gestations can identify approximately 50 per cent of pregnancies affected with Down syndrome at a 5 per cent false positive rate.

– **NIPT** using cell-free DNA testing is **not recommended** for aneuploidy screening in women with twin or high-order multifetal gestations (ACOG, 2015).

Chorionicity in assessing risk for aneuploidy
- Establishing chorionicity is an important first step for offering screening in twin gestation.
- In monochorionic pregnancy, either both the fetuses will be affected or both the fetuses will be unaffected. In dichorionic pregnancy, each fetus will have its own risk for Down syndrome.

Interpretation of screening results

- The test results are reported in a specific format that takes into account the pre-test risk based on maternal age. Usually, both a numerical and a graphic representation are provided.
- The reporting of the screening test can be done in either of two ways: *conventional reporting* or *the reporting format introduced by the Fetal Medicine Foundation*.
  - **Conventional reporting** is followed by most reporting laboratories in India and uses a cut-off of **1:250**.
  - **The Fetal Medicine Foundation (FMF) reporting format** was introduced to reduce the number of invasive procedures that women undergo. This format classifies results as **high-risk** (>1:100), **intermediate-risk** (1:101 to 1:1000), or **low-risk** (<1:1000). Of the women undergoing screening for aneuploidy, 3–5 per cent will be classified as high-risk and 10–15 per cent will be classified as intermediate-risk.

Screen-negative test result

- About 80–85 per cent of women having the combined test are reported to be screen-negative. This is done using a specific cut-off. The commonly used cut-off is 1 in 250.
- A screen-negative test should be interpreted to mean that the fetus is at low risk of having Down syndrome, trisomy 18, or trisomy 13. In such a case, the mother is advised routine prenatal care and requires no further testing.
- In the example shown in Figure 7.1, the mother's risk of having a baby with Down syndrome is 1 in 1452 just based on her age. However, based on the NT and serum markers, her risk of having a baby with Down syndrome decreases to 1 in 80,992.
- The couple should be reassured that their risk for having a baby with Down syndrome is very low. The phrase, *"The baby is completely normal"*, should be avoided because a screen-negative test result does not rule out other chromosomal abnormalities and structural anomalies.
- With a screen-negative test result, no further tests are required for Down syndrome, trisomy 18, or trisomy 13.

 No further testing needs to be offered after a screen-negative result.

Screen-positive test result

- A screen-positive result (Figure 7.2) does not mean that the fetus is definitely affected. It should be interpreted to mean that the fetus is at high risk of having Down syndrome.

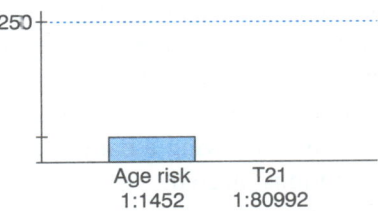

RISKS	
Disorder:	Down syndrome
Result:	Low
Final risk:	1:80992
Age risk:	1:1452
Cut-off:	1:250
Risk type:	Risk at term
Status:	Calculated

Figure 7.1 A screen-negative first trimester combined test for Down syndrome: the pre-test risk based on maternal age is 1:1452. The post-test risk has been reported as 1:80992. This is well below the cut-off risk of 1:250. Similar risks are estimated for Edwards syndrome and Patau syndrome. *T21*, trisomy 21

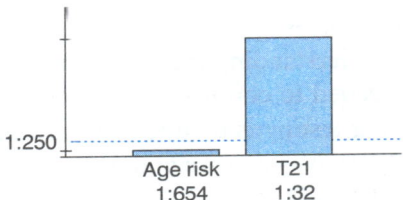

RISKS	
Disorder:	Down syndrome
Result:	Increased
Final risk:	1:32
Age risk:	1:654
Cut-off:	1:250
Risk type:	Risk at term
Status:	Calculated

Figure 7.2 A screen-positive first trimester combined test for Down syndrome: the pre-test risk based on maternal age is 1:654. The post-test risk is reported as 1:32. This is well above the cut-off of 1:250. Diagnostic testing should be offered for this pregnancy. *T21*, trisomy 21

Based on her age, this 33-year-old gravida has a 1:654 chance of having a baby with Down syndrome. After testing, she is reported to have a 1:32 risk of having a baby with Down syndrome. This means that if 32 women aged 33 had the same test results, 1 of them would have a baby with Down syndrome.

- With a screen-positive test result, a diagnostic test (chorionic villus sampling/amniocentesis) or secondary screening with cell-free DNA is offered (see section on *Counselling for screen-positive results*).

 There is no role for repeating a maternal serum screening in the presence of a screen-positive result.

Counselling for screen-positive results

- After a positive screening test, it is important to spend time with the couple to explain the results, offer further diagnostic testing, and answer their questions. A genetic counsellor, if available, is the ideal person to counsel the couple.
- **Conventional report (cut-off 1:250)**
  - If the risk is **more** than the cut-off (e.g., 1:50, 1:200), the couple is offered either of the following choices:
    - *Invasive testing:* CVS in the first trimester or amniocentesis in the second trimester can be offered.

- *Non-invasive prenatal testing (NIPT):* If a couple wants to avoid an invasive test, they can choose to undergo an NIPT with cell-free DNA (cfDNA). If the NIPT is positive, the couple can be advised to undergo an invasive test for definitive confirmation of aneuploidy.
  - If the risk is **less** than the cut-off (e.g., 1:400, 1:10000), the couple is informed that the risk of having a baby with Down syndrome is extremely low, and no further intervention is offered.
- **The FMF reporting convention:**
  - Women classified as **high-risk** (>1:100) are offered one of the following choices:
    - *Invasive testing* (chorionic villus sampling or amniocentesis): This will detect all chromosomal abnormalities, not just trisomies (see **Chapter 8**, *Prenatal diagnostic testing for genetic disorders*). This is the best option for follow-up.
    - *Secondary screening* with NIPT (see section on *Non-invasive prenatal testing*): If the couple is apprehensive about the risks of a diagnostic test, NIPT is offered, with the understanding that if that too comes back positive, a diagnostic test would still be needed to confirm or rule out a trisomy. If the NIPT is reported as negative, no further testing is required. It must be mentioned that:
      - NIPT is expensive and may not be affordable for most patients.
      - NIPT will miss 17 per cent of chromosomal abnormalities (Norton, 2014).
    - The couple may choose to continue the pregnancy with no further testing.
  - Women at **intermediate risk** (1:101 to 1:1000) are given the option of an NIPT with cfDNA, with invasive testing reserved for those whose results are positive.
  - Women classified as **low-risk** do not need any intervention and may return to routine antenatal care.

> The FMF method of classification and follow-up is more feasible in countries where the cost of NIPT is not a problem.

ULTRASOUND SCREENING FOR ANEUPLOIDY

- Some obstetric ultrasound findings that are considered normal variants are significant because they are associated with an increased risk of underlying fetal aneuploidy. These are known as **soft markers**. These should be considered distinct from major fetal anatomic malformations and/or growth restriction, which also indicate an increased risk of genetic disorders.
- A genetic sonogram (to look for soft markers) should ideally be incorporated into the mid-trimester anomaly scan.
- Isolated soft markers are present in 11–17 per cent of normal fetuses (Breathnach et al., 2007).
- Most fetuses with an isolated soft marker are chromosomally normal (Bethune, 2007). These markers are usually

Ultrasound contributes to aneuploidy screening in four important ways:
- Accurate gestational dating
- Detection of multiple gestation
- Identification of major structural abnormalities
- Identification of soft markers

transient, have no clinical consequences, and most often resolve with advancing gestation or after birth. However, since soft markers may be associated with fetal aneuploidy, further correlation with maternal serum screening is required.

- The **first-trimester soft markers** include:
  - Increased nuchal translucency (NT)
  - Absent nasal bone
  - Increased impedance to flow in the ductus venosus
  - Tricuspid regurgitation

The last three markers require higher expertise to image and so NT continues to be the most important ultrasound marker for Down syndrome. If serum screening is not available, NT alone may be used for screening for Down syndrome in a twin pregnancy.

- The **second-trimester soft markers** include (in descending order of likelihood ratio):
  - Absent or hypoplastic nasal bone
  - Aberrant right subclavian artery
  - Ventriculomegaly
  - Increased nuchal fold thickness
  - Hyperechoic bowel
  - Pyelectasis
  - Echogenic intracardiac focus
  - Short humerus
  - Short femur

Role of ultrasound in first-trimester screening for aneuploidy

- Anatomic markers used for aneuploidy screening in the first trimester include:
  - Increased nuchal translucency
  - Absent nasal bone
- Doppler markers used in the first trimester include:
  - Abnormal flow in the ductus venosus
  - Tricuspid regurgitation

Increased nuchal translucency (NT)

- Nuchal translucency is a small, thin, hypoechoic space present in the posterior fetal neck in normal first-trimester fetuses.

 Nuchal translucency need not be measured in the first trimester in women who have opted to undergo non-invasive prenatal testing and have screened negative.

- NT thickness increases with fetal crown–rump length (CRL). Normal NT ranges from 1.2 mm–2.1 mm at CRL of 45 mm to 1.9 mm–2.7 mm at CRL of 84 mm.
- Increased NT is a marker for aneuploidy as well as poor pregnancy outcomes.
- Increased NT in the first trimester is the most commonly used sonographic marker for Down syndrome. Measurement of NT is combined with maternal serum testing in first-trimester screening.

- The likelihood of aneuploidy increases with increasing nuchal translucency above the 95th centile (approximately 3 mm).
- Most fetuses with trisomy 21 have a nuchal thickness <4.5 mm, and most fetuses with trisomy 13, trisomy 18, or Turner syndrome have nuchal thickness ≥4.5 mm (Kagan et al., 2006).

Procedure for nuchal translucency (NT) measurement

There are specific criteria (as delineated by The Fetal Medicine Foundation) that should be satisfied to obtain an accurate NT. Certification for competency in measuring NT is available from The Fetal Medicine Foundation (https://fetalmedicine.org).

- The gestational period must be between 11–13 weeks[+6] days.
- The fetal crown–rump length should be between 45 and 84 mm.
- The magnification of the image should be such that the fetal head and thorax occupy the whole screen.
- A mid-sagittal view of the face should be obtained (Figure 7.3). This is defined by the presence of the echogenic tip of the nose and the rectangular shape of the palate anteriorly, the translucent diencephalon in the centre, and the nuchal membrane posteriorly. The zygoma should not be visualised.
- The fetus should be in a neutral position, with the head in line with the spine.
- The widest area of the nuchal fluid space is measured from its inner-to-inner borders in the midsagittal plane (Figure 7.3).
- Care must be taken to distinguish between fetal skin and the amnion (Figure 7.4).
- The umbilical cord may be around the fetal neck in about 5 per cent of cases, and this finding may produce a falsely increased NT. In such cases, the measurements of NT above and below the cord are different and, in the calculation of risk, it is more appropriate to use the average of the two measurements.
- Once an accurate NT is measured, the crown–rump length (CRL) and the NT measurement are entered in an online calculator that provides the NT percentile.

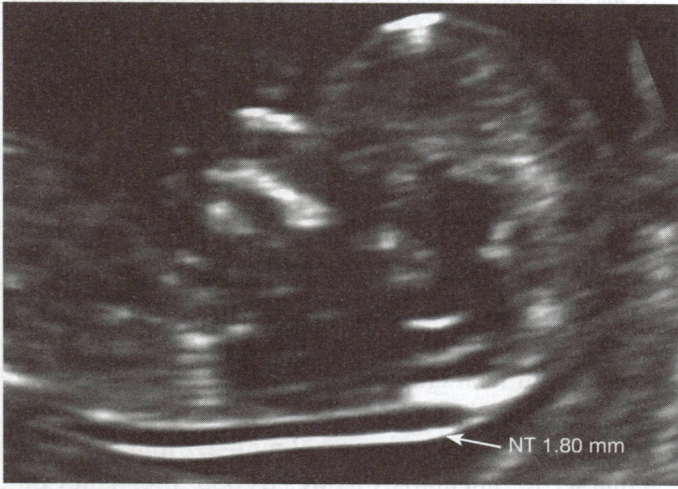

NT 1.80 mm

Figure 7.3   Measurements of the nuchal translucency should be taken with the inner border of the horizontal line of the callipers placed on the line that defines the nuchal translucency thickness; the crossbar of the calliper should be such that it merges with the white line of the border and not placed in the nuchal fluid (*Image courtesy:* Mediscan Systems, Chennai).

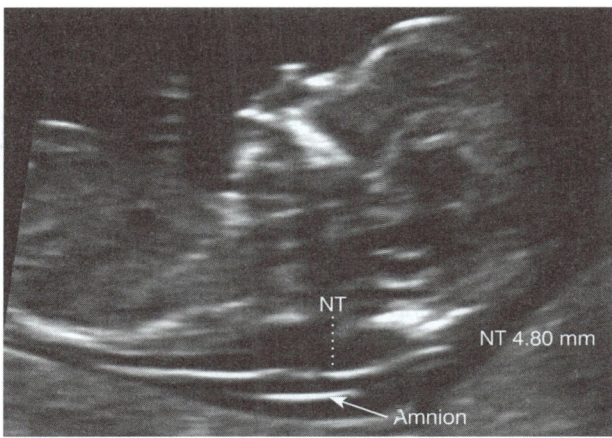

Figure 7.4 Increased nuchal translucency: care must be taken not to include the amnion (arrow) (*Image courtesy*: Mediscan Systems, Chennai).

Increased NT and risk of aneuploidy
Kagan et al. (2006), in a study of 11,315 pregnancies, found that the frequency of aneuploidy increased with increasing NT. The risk was as follows:
- 7 per cent   with NT of 3 mm–3.4 mm
- 50 per cent with NT of 5.5–6.4 mm
- 75 per cent with NT of ≥8.5 mm

Significance of increased NT in a chromosomally normal fetus

- Increased NT is an expression not only of chromosomal abnormalities, but also of fetal malformations and genetic syndromes. An NT >99th centile is significant in a chromosomally normal fetus.
- The initial NT thickness may indicate the prognosis of a poor pregnancy outcome—the greater the NT, the greater the chance of a poor outcome.

Increased NT and pregnancy outcome
In a review, De Domenico et al. (2011) stated that the chances of delivering a baby *with no major abnormalities* are as follows:
- 70 per cent for NT of 3.5–4.4 mm
- 50 per cent for NT of 4.5–5.4 mm
- 30 per cent for NT of 5.5–6.4 mm
- 15 per cent for NT of ≥ 6.5

- Several abnormalities have been reported in fetuses with enlarged NT, the most common being cardiac defects, diaphragmatic hernia, exomphalos, body stalk anomaly, skeletal defects, and certain genetic syndromes. Increased or dicordant NT measurements in monochorionic twins may be indicative of impending twin-to-twin-transfusion syndrome (TTTS).
- The risk of miscarriage and fetal death (especially before 20 weeks) is increased with an NT >99th centile.

- If the increased NT is also associated with a decreased PAPP-A value (<1st centile), the risk of fetal growth restriction increases.

Increased NT in monochorionic twins
Increased NT or >20 per cent discordance between NT measurements in monochorionic twins may predict twin-to-twin-transfusion syndrome (TTTS).

Management of pregnancy with increased NT

The management of a pregnancy with increased NT depends on the NT value. Figures 7.5 and 7.6 present algorithms of the approach to the management of NT.

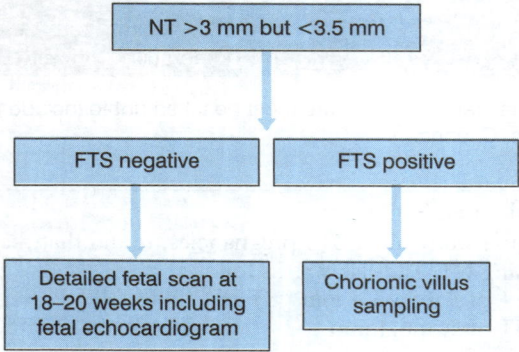

Figure 7.5   Nuchal translucency (NT) between 3 mm (90th centile) and 3.4 mm is assessed based on the result of first-trimester screening (FTS). If the FTS is negative (risk of aneuploidy is low), a detailed scan at 18–20 weeks along with a fetal echocardiogram should be performed to look for fetal structural abnormalities. If the FTS is positive (risk of aneuploidy is high), a chorionic villus sampling should be offered for definitive diagnosis.

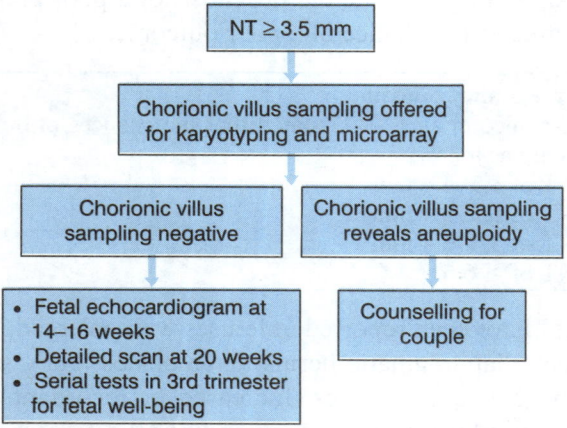

Figure 7.6   When the nuchal translucency (NT) is ≥3.5 mm (99th centile), diagnostic testing with chorionic villus sampling is offered (for karyotyping and microarray). If the fetus is euploid, careful monitoring for structural anomalies should be carried out. Serial tests for fetal well-being shoud be offered. If the fetus has aneuploidy, the couple should be counselled about further management.

> **Cystic hygroma**
> - The term cystic hygroma was previously used for significantly increased nuchal translucency, which also extended to the side of the neck or the entire length of the fetus.
> - However, following recent recommendations, this distinction is no longer made since a nuchal translucency >3.5 mm carries the same fetal implications and needs to be investigated and managed in the same way.
> - In the first trimester, NT >3.5 mm is associated with an increased risk for the following:
>   - Fetal aneuploidy (Down syndrome, trisomy 18, or trisomy 13)
>   - Structural malformations (especially cardiac defects)
>   - Miscarriage
>   - Hydrops
>   - Fetal demise and neonatal death

Absent nasal bone

- A small nose and mid-face hypoplasia are well-known components of the Down syndrome phenotype. This fact has made it feasible to use the absence of the nasal bone to screen for trisomy 21.

 Identifying an absent nasal bone increases the sensitivity of first-trimester screening for aneuploidy and should be included in FTS if possible.

- In pregnancies in which chorionic villus sampling was performed because of a positive first-trimester screen, Cicero et al. (2001) found that the nasal bone was absent in 73 per cent of fetuses with trisomy 21. Subsequently, over 12 studies have confirmed that the nasal bone is absent at 11–14 weeks in 70 per cent of fetuses with trisomy 21, and in only 1.5 per cent of unaffected fetuses.
- When added to FTS, it can increase the detection rate to about 95 per cent, decreasing the false positive rate to 2 per cent (Berghella, 2016).
- Nasal bone assessment requires advanced sonology skills but has the potential to decrease the false positive rates and improve the detection rate of Down syndrome (Rosen et al., 2007).

First-trimester Doppler markers for aneuploidy

Abnormal flow in the ductus venosus

- Increased impedance to flow in the fetal ductus venosus at $11-13^{+6}$ weeks' gestation is associated with:
  - Fetal aneuploidies
  - Cardiac defects
  - Adverse pregnancy outcomes
- When the a-wave is reversed, the risk of aneuploidy (trisomy 13, trisomy 18, or trisomy 21) increases significantly (Nicolaides, 2011).
- Inclusion of ductus venosus blood flow in first-trimester combined screening improves the detection rate of trisomy 21 to 95 per cent for a false positive rate of 3 per cent.

- Assessment of ductus venosus flow could be reserved for pregnancies with an intermediate risk after first-trimester combined screening.

Tricuspid regurgitation

- Tricuspid regurgitation at $11-13^{+6}$ weeks' gestation is a common finding in fetuses with trisomies 21, 18, and 13 and in those with major cardiac defects.
- Studies show that 55 per cent of fetuses with trisomy 21 have tricuspid regurgitation.
- Inclusion of tricuspid blood flow in first-trimester combined screening improves the detection rate of Down syndrome to 95 per cent at a false positive rate of 3 per cent.
- Like with ductus venosus flow, the assessment of tricuspid flow could be reserved for pregnancies with intermediate risk after first-trimester combined testing.

Role of ultrasound in second-trimester screening for aneuploidy

Second-trimester ultrasound markers for aneuploidy

- Second-trimester soft markers include (in descending order of likelihood ratio):
  - Absent or hypoplastic nasal bone
  - Aberrant right subclavian artery
  - Ventriculomegaly
  - Increased nuchal fold thickness
  - Hyperechoic bowel
  - Pyelectasis
  - Echogenic intracardiac focus
  - Short humerus
  - Short femur
- The sensitivity of individual soft markers is low unless associated with a fetal structural abnormality.
- The likelihood of aneuploidy is significantly increased when more than one marker is present. However, soft markers are ineffecient for screening or excluding fetal aneuploidy.
- Increased nuchal fold thickness is the most accurate marker and was associated with approximately a 17-fold increased risk of Down syndrome in a meta-analysis looking at second-trimester markers for trisomy 21 (Smith–Bindman, 2001). It is detected in 20–33 per cent of fetuses with Down syndrome and in only 0.5–2 per cent of euploid fetuses (Agathokleous et al., 2013). However, the overall sensitivity of this finding is too low for it to be a practical screening test for Down syndrome.
- Structural abnormalities such as omphalocele (not containing the liver), duodenal atresia, and atrioventricular septal defects carry a high risk of aneuploidy. In a clinical setting, the identification of any of these major markers should prompt a prenatal diagnostic test (see **Chapter 8**, *Prenatal diagnostic testing for genetic disorders*).

    The various likelihood ratios (LR) for individual soft markers are given in Table 7.3.

Table 7.3 Likelihood ratios for trisomy 21 based on second-trimester soft markers seen on ultrasound scan (Nicolaides, 2003)

Marker	Likelihood ratio (LR)
Increased nuchal fold thickness	9.8
Echogenic bowel	3
Short femur	1.6
Intracardiac echogenic foci	1.1
Pyelectasis	1.0

NON-INVASIVE PRENATAL DIAGNOSIS (NIPT) USING CELL-FREE DNA FOR FETAL ANEUPLOIDY

- Non-invasive prenatal testing (**NIPT**) for aneuploidy using cfDNA in the maternal blood has been available for clinical use since 2011.
- It is termed non-invasive because it uses a maternal blood sample and avoids fetal sampling.
- It is an expensive test and is not available freely in developing countries.
- The cell-free DNA (cfDNA) found in maternal circulation is derived from both the mother and the fetal–placental unit. The primary source of fetal cfDNA is thought to be apoptosis of placental cells (syncytiotrophoblast), while maternal hematopoietic cells are the source of most maternal cfDNA (Palomaki et al. 2018).
- Sequencing of cfDNA in the maternal circulation can be used for prenatal screening for trisomy 21, trisomy 18, and trisomy 13.
- NIPT can also be used for sex chromosome aneuploidies (monosomy X or Turner syndrome, Klinefelter syndrome, XXX, XYY).

 Clinical guidelines at present do not recommend routine NIPT for microdeletion or duplication syndromes since this has not been validated clinically.

- Though some laboratories offer NIPT for deletion/duplication syndromes (Cri-du-chat syndrome, Prader-Willi/ Angelman syndrome, Jacobsen syndrome, DiGeorge syndrome II, Van der Woude syndrome), currently there is no published clinical validation.

 Currently, NIPT with cell-free DNA screening is not recommended in multiple gestation. This recommendation may change with further validation studies.

- NIPT is not recommended as routine aneuploidy screening in the general obstetric population (ACOG, 2015). This is because of:
  - Increased false positive results in low-risk women
  - Decreased cost-effectiveness in comparison to conventional aneuploidy screening in the low-risk obstetric population
  - Concerns that a pregnancy with a positive screen may be terminated without prenatal diagnostic testing
- Though the detection rate of trisomy is 98–99 per cent, a positive NIPT must be followed-up with chorionic villus sampling or amniocentesis to confirm the diagnosis.

NIPT using cell-free DNA screening
When:
- After 10 weeks' gestation

For whom:
- Women 35 years or older at delivery
- Pregnancy with ultrasonographic findings indicative of an increased risk of aneuploidy
- Previous pregnancy with trisomy-affected baby
- Parent carrying a balanced Robertsonian translocation with an increased risk of trisomy 13 or trisomy 21
- Women with positive first-trimester or second-trimester screening test results

Not recommended for routine screening in general obstetric population
Sensitivity:
- Trisomy 21: 99 per cent at false positive rate of 0.05 per cent
- Trisomy 18: 97 per cent at false positive rate of 0.05 per cent
- Trisomy 21: 96 per cent at false positive rate of 0.05 per cent

Methodology

- 20 mL of blood is drawn from the maternal vein using a 21-gauge straight needle. Two collection tubes are filled with 8–10 mL of blood each.
- The tubes are left at room temperature and transported to the laboratory where the test is to be performed. Laboratories use several methods for cfDNA counting including massively parallel genomic sequencing, whole gene sequencing, and chromosome selective sequencing.
- The test results are usually available in 7–10 days.

Interpretation and follow-up of screening results

Screen-positive result (Table 7.4)

- Even though NIPT with cfDNA screening has high detection rates, invasive diagnostic testing must be offered to confirm screen-positive test results (Palomaki et al., 2018).
- Though chorionic villus sampling may be offered, an amniocentesis after 15 weeks' gestation may be appropriate as the analysis of amniocytes is more representative of the fetal genotype than the analysis of placental cells (Grati et al., 2015).

Table 7.4   A screen-positive result on non-invasive prenatal testing using cell-free DNA; the result shows a high risk (>1/20) of Down syndrome; diagnostic testing should be offered in this case

Conditions	Risk score	Risk assessment
Trisomy 21	>1/20	High risk
Trisomy 18	1/1179223486	Low risk
Trisomy 13	1/765978861	Low risk

Screen-negative result

- A screen-negative result places the fetus at low risk of the aneuploidy that has been targeted. It does not completely rule out the possibility of an affected fetus or the presence of a chromosomal abnormality not tested for.

- No further testing is offered for a screen-negative result.
- However, if a fetal structural abnormality is identified later in the pregnancy, a diagnostic test may be offered at that time. An isolated soft marker does not require a diagnostic test.

No call or no result

- 1–5 per cent of cfDNA tests do not yield a result. This is called an assay failure and may be due to a low fetal fraction in maternal blood. This can result from:
  - High maternal body mass index
  - Fetal aneuploidy (especially trisomy 18)
  - Sample collected at <10 weeks' gestation
  - Improper test tubes used for collection of sample
  - Maternal use of low-molecular-weight heparin before 20 weeks' gestation
- The options available after a *no call or no result* test are (Palomaki et al., 2018):
  - Repeat NIPT (if the lab offers a repeat test without charging for it)
  - Screening for aneuploidy using standard ultrasound and serum markers
  - Diagnostic testing (amniocentesis, CVS) and karyotyping using microarray

The last option may be especially appropriate if the mother is already at high risk for aneuploidy prior to cfDNA testing (e.g., advanced maternal age or abnormal ultrasound).

References

1. Agathokleous M, Chaveeva P, Poon LC et al. 2013. Meta-analysis of second-trimester markers for trisomy 21. *Ultrasound Obstet Gynecol.* 41:247.

2. American College of Obstetricians and Gynecologists. 2015 (reaffirmed 2017). ACOG. Committee Opinion No. 640. Cell-free DNA screening for fetal aneuploidy. *Obstet Gynecol.* 126: e31–7.

3. American College of Obstetricians and Gynecologists. 2016. ACOG Practice Bulletin 163. Screening for aneuploidy. *Obstet Gynecol.* 127(5): e123–37.

4. Benacerraf BR. 2018. Sonographic findings associated with fetal aneuploidy. Wilkins-Haug L, Levine D. (Eds). *UpToDate.* Waltham, MA.

5. Berghella V (Ed). 2016. *Obstetric Evidence Based Guidelines,* Third Edition. CRC Press.

6. Bethune M. 2007. Literature review and suggested protocol for managing ultrasound soft markers for Down syndrome: Thickened nuchal fold, echogenic bowel, shortened femur, shortened humerus, pyelectasis and absent or hypoplastic nasal bone. *Australas Radiol.* 51: 218.

7. Breathnach FM, Fleming A, Malone FD. 2007. The second trimester genetic sonogram. *Am J Med Genet C Semin Med Genet.* 145C: 62.

8. Cicero S, Curcio P, Papageorghiou A, Sonek J, Nicolaides K. 2001. Absence of nasal bone in fetuses with trisomy 21 at 11–14 weeks of gestation: An observational study. *Lancet.* 358: 1665–7.

9. Cuckle H. 2014. Prenatal Screening Using Maternal Markers. *J Clin Med.* 3(2): 504–20.

10. De Domenico R, Faraci M, Hyseni E, Di Prima FAF, Valenti O, Monte S, Giorgio E, Renda E. 2011. Increased nuchal translucency in normal karyotype foetuses. *J Prenat Med.* 5(2): 23–26.

11. Grati FR, Bajaj K, Malvestiti F et al. 2015. The type of feto-placental aneuploidy detected by cfDNA testing may influence the choice of confirmatory diagnostic procedure. *Prenat Diagn.* 35: 994.

12. Kagan KO, Avgidou K, Molina FS et al. 2006. Relation between increased fetal nuchal translucency thickness and chromosomal defects. *Obstet Gynecol*. 107: 6.

13. Morgan S, Delbarre A, Ward P. 2013. Impact of introducing a national policy for prenatal Down syndrome screening on the diagnostic invasive procedure rate in England. *Ultrasound Obstet Gynecol*. 41: 526–529.

14. Nicolaides KH. 2003. Screening for chromosomal defects. *Ultrasound Obstet Gynecol*. 21: 313–321

15. Nicolaides KH. 2011. Screening for fetal aneuploidies at 11 to 13 weeks. *Prenat Diagn*. 31: 7.

16. Norton ME, Jelliffe-Pawlowski LL, Currier RJ. 2014. Chromosome abnormalities detected by current prenatal screening and non-invasive prenatal testing. *Obstetrics & Gynecology*. 124(5):979–986.

17. Nussbaum RL, McInnes RR, Willard HF. 2016. Principles of clinical cytogenetics and genome analysis. *Thompson & Thompson Genetics in Medicine*. Elsevier, Philadelphia (PA). p. 57–74.

18. Palomaki GE, Messerlian GM, Halliday JV. 2018. Prenatal screening for common aneuploidies using cell-free DNA. Wilkins-Haug L. (Ed). *UpToDate*, Waltham, MA.

19. Rosen T, D'Alton ME, Platt LD et al. 2007. First-trimester ultrasound assessment of the nasal bone to screen for aneuploidy. *Obstet Gynecol*. 110: 399.

20. Savva GM, Walker K, Morris JK. 2010. The maternal age-specific live birth prevalence of trisomies 13 and 18 compared to trisomy 21 (Down syndrome). *Prenat Diagn*. 30:57.

21. Sherman SL, Allen EG, Bean LH, Freeman SB. 2007. Epidemiology of Down syndrome. *Ment Retard Dev Disabil Res Rev*. 13: 221–7.

22. Smith-Bindman R, Hosmer W, Feldstein VA, Deeks JJ, Goldberg JD. 2001. Second-trimester ultrasound to detect fetuses with Down syndrome: A meta-analysis. *JAMA*. 285: 1044–1055.

23. Spencer K, Nicolaides KH. 2003. Screening for trisomy 21 in twins using first trimester ultrasound and maternal serum biochemistry in a one-stop clinic: A review of three years' experience. *BJOG*. 110:276–80.

24. Wald NJ, Rodeck C, Hackshaw AK, Walters J, Chitty L, Mackinson AM. 2003. First and second trimester antenatal screening for Down's syndrome: The results of the Serum, Urine and Ultrasound Screening Study (SURUSS). *Health Technol Assess*. 7:i–iv,1–88.

Chapter 8

Prenatal Diagnostic Testing for Genetic Disorders

INTRODUCTION

- Once the screening for aneuploidy is reported as positive, an invasive diagnostic test is necessary to confirm or rule out the presence of an affected fetus.

 In the case of a screen-positive test for aneuploidy, the only way of confirming or ruling out fetal chromosomal abnormalities is by karyotyping fetal tissue obtained with an invasive test.

- The commonly used invasive tests for prenatal diagnosis are **chorionic villus sampling (CVS)** and **amniocentesis**.
- **Fetal blood sampling** (cordocentesis) may also be offered, but it carries a greater risk of pregnancy loss. For this reason, it is reserved for clinical situations in which amniocentesis, CVS, or maternal blood sampling do not provide adequate diagnostic information.
- **Percutaneous biopsy of organs** is another invasive diagnostic procedure.

INDICATIONS FOR INVASIVE TESTING

The common indications for invasive diagnostic testing include the following:
- Screen-positive test results in either the first- or second-trimester screening for aneuploidy (including non-invasive prenatal testing using cell-free DNA)
- Imaging of structural fetal abnormalities suggestive of an underlying genetic condition
- History of a previous child or fetus affected by chromosomal abnormality
- Either one or both parents carriers of any of the following:
    - A balanced translocation or other structural chromosome disorder
    - Single gene disorder
    - Autosomal recessive disease

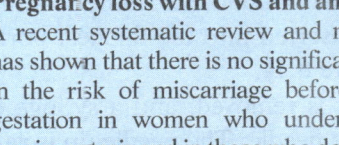 **Pregnancy loss with CVS and amniocentesis** A recent systematic review and meta-analysis has shown that there is no significant difference in the risk of miscarriage before 24 weeks' gestation in women who undergo CVS or amniocentesis and in those who do not undergo any invasive testing (Akolekar et al., 2015).

- Suspected or confirmed viral infections during pregnancy: Intrauterine infections with viruses such as parvovirus, rubella, cytomegalovirus, and herpes simplex virus or a parasite such as *Toxoplasma gondii* can give rise to congenital anomalies.

CHORIONIC VILLUS SAMPLING (CVS)

- Chorionic villus sampling is an invasive procedure done under continuous ultrasound guidance for the prenatal diagnosis of genetic disorders. Small samples of placental villi are obtained by the transabdominal or transcervical route.

- When aneuploidy is suspected, the tissue obtained is subjected to chromosomal analysis (see section below on *Processing of samples obtained by diagnostic testing*).
- Both amniocentesis and CVS, under continuous ultrasound guidance, have been available for more than two decades. They have a good safety record. Though pregnancy losses may result from these procedures, the timing of the procedure, technique, and operator experience can limit the loss rates.
- When there is reason to suspect that a fetus may be affected by a genetic disorder, DNA testing is carried out with a DNA probe specific for the mutation that causes the disease. Examples of single-gene disorders include sickle cell anemia, cystic fibrosis, and hemophilia.

Procedure

- The procedure is performed between 11–13 weeks. Early CVS before 10 weeks has been reported to be associated with oro-mandibular limb hypoplasia and isolated limb disruption defects and is therefore not recommended (Benn, 2016).
- CVS is performed as an out-patient procedure. Local anesthesia is used for transabdominal CVS.
- It can be performed either by a transabdominal or transcervical approach. The transabdominal route has come to be the preferred route in many centres for the following reasons:
  - The ease with which it can be performed as compared to the transcervical route
  - The greater sampling success at the first attempt (Smidt-Jensen et al., 1992)

 At least 5 mg of placental tissue should be obtained to consider it an adequate sample. The villi should be immediately separated from any blood clots clinging to them.

- A systematic review of the Cochrane Database showed that the risks are not significantly different with either approach (Alfirevic et al. 2017).
- For transabdominal CVS, under continuous ultrasound guidance, a 20-gauge needle with stylet is inserted into the thickest portion of the placenta, without entering the amniotic sac (Figure 8.1).
- The stylet is removed, and a syringe containing culture medium is then attached to the hub of the needle. The needle tip is rapidly moved with an up and down action inside the placenta until an adequate amount of the sample has been aspirated by the negative pressure created in the syringe. The negative pressure is maintained as the needle is withdrawn.

Post-procedure instructions

- Normal activity may be resumed after the procedure.
- Strenuous activity and sexual intercourse should be avoided for 48 hours after the procedure.
- A small amount of spotting is normal after the procedure but heavier bleeding, pain, and fever should be immediately reported.

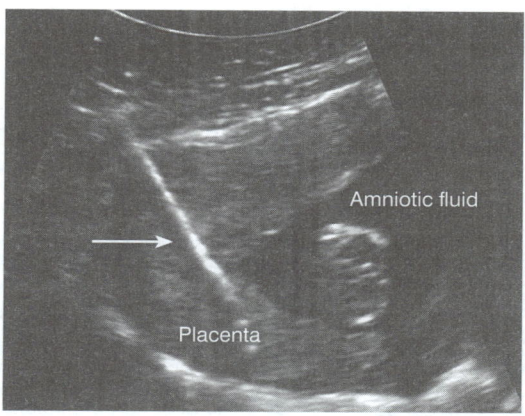

Figure 8.1 Chorionic villus sampling: Image of a needle inserted into the placenta transabdominally under ultrasound guidance. The arrow points to the needle in the substance of the placenta (*Image courtesy:* Mediscan Systems, Chennai).

Advantages of CVS

- Since CVS is done at 11–13 weeks, the results are available earlier in pregnancy. This reduces the period of anxiety that the at-risk couple faces while awaiting test results.
- In case of an abnormal result, termination of pregnancy is safer at this gestational age.
- The viable cells obtained by CVS for analysis allow for shorter specimen processing time (5–7 days vs. 7–14 days).
- The yield of fetal DNA from villi is higher than that from cells obtained at amniocentesis; hence CVS is the preferred procedure for DNA testing for genetic mutations.

Disadvantages of CVS

- It is sometimes more difficult to obtain adequate fetal tissue sample by CVS than it is by amniocentesis. Transcervical CVS has greater sampling failures as compared to transabdominal CVS (Alfirevic et al., 2017).
- Contamination with maternal cells is more frequent with CVS than it is with amniocentesis.
- Since placental tissue is analysed, there is a greater chance of *confined placental mosaicism*, a term that refers to a discrepancy between the genotype of the placenta and the genotype of the embryo/fetus. It is suspected when there is a structurally normal fetus with a CVS result showing an aneuploidy, often not compatible with life.

  When these differing results are obtained, amniocentesis is used to obtain the fetal karyotype to ensure that the fetus is chromosomally normal.

  CVS is compared with amniocentesis in Table 8.1.

AMNIOCENTESIS

- Amniocentesis is usually performed between 15 and 20 weeks of gestation, though it may be performed later.

- Several studies have confirmed the safety of the procedure as well as the accuracy of the cytogenetic diagnosis made from analysing the exfoliated fetal cells floating in the amniotic fluid (ACOG, 2016).
- Early amniocentesis (before 15 weeks) can lead to increased fetal loss, respiratory morbidity, and talipes deformity and is therefore not recommended (ACOG, 2016; RCOG, 2010).

Table 8.1   Chorionic villus sampling vs. amniocentesis

Features	Chorionic villus sampling	Amniocentesis
Timing	11–13 weeks	15–20 weeks
Route	Transabdominal or transvaginal	Transabdominal
Fetal loss rate	2/1000	1/1000
Diagnostic certainty	Lower (because of the possibility of confined placental mosaicism, see section on *Disadvantages of CVS*)	Higher

Procedure

- A 22- or 20-gauge needle with a stylet is passed transabdominally into the amniotic cavity (Figure 8.2) under continuous ultrasound guidance.
- Amniotic fluid is obtained from a pocket that is free of fetal parts and umbilical cord. Local anesthesia is not needed for the procedure.
- Though the placenta is generally avoided whilst inserting the needle, in some rare cases, a transplacental route may be the only window to access the amniotic cavity. Giarlandino and colleagues found no deleterious effects in cases where a transplacental route was the only option (1994).
- On removing the stylet, amniotic fluid will well up into the hub of the needle. The first 1 mL of fluid that is aspirated should be discarded since it may be contaminated with maternal cells.
- The next 20 mL of aspirated amniotic fluid is sent for testing.

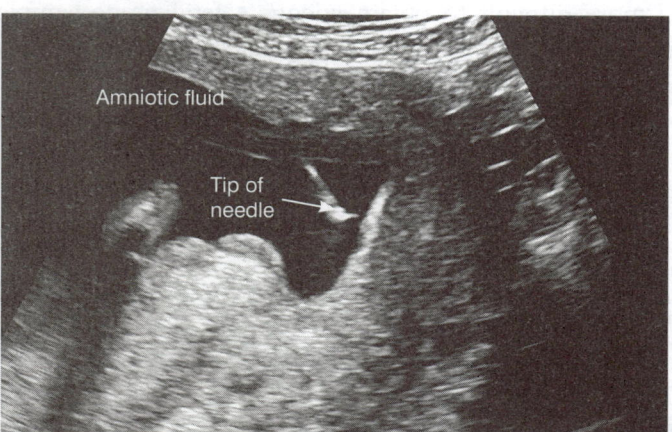

Figure 8.2   Amniocentesis: Image of a needle inserted into the amniotic cavity transabdominally under ultrasound guidance. The arrow points to the echogenic tip of the needle in the amniotic sac *(Image courtesy:* Cimar Hospital, Cochin).

> **CVS and amniocentesis in multiple gestation**
> - The procedure should be performed by a physician with a high level of expertise.
> - Only a single sample is required for monochorionic twins.
> - The placental positions should be mapped out clearly prior to CVS in a dichorionic pregnancy since a sample is required from each placenta.
> - Labelling of each fetus must be done meticulously so that chromosomal abnormality is not assigned to the wrong twin. The presence of a structural anomaly in one twin makes labelling easier.
> - Two separate punctures are used to access each individual placenta or amniotic sac. Two separate needles are also recommended to avoid cross-contamination.
> - The miscarriage rate is higher with these procedures than in singleton pregnancies (Yukobowich, 2001).

FETAL BLOOD SAMPLING

- Fetal blood sampling provides direct access to the fetal circulation. It is the procedure of choice when severe fetal anemia or thrombocytopenia is suspected.
- It is rarely performed for karyotyping and is done only if neither CVS nor amniocentesis is possible. The procedure-related pregnancy loss rate is <2 per cent.
- It is performed transabdominally after 18 weeks of gestation.

CONSIDERATIONS BEFORE PERFORMING AN INVASIVE TEST

- Informed consent should be obtained.
- The process should be explained with emphasis on the following:
  - The possibility of failure to obtain the sample
  - The possibility of failure to culture the cells
  - The risk of miscarriage
- Rhesus status needs to be documented and acted upon if the woman is Rh-negative.
- In cases where the mother is HIV or hepatitis B-positive, the risk of transmission of infection to the fetus during the procedure needs to be addressed.

> **CVS and amniocentesis in Rh-negative women**
> Maternal RhD status should be available or obtained in every case. Prophylaxis with anti-D immunoglobulin must be offered to an Rh-negative woman after each procedure.

- Heparin injections or aspirin or related anticoagulant medications should be stopped at least 24 hours prior to the procedure.

PROCESSING OF SAMPLES OBTAINED BY DIAGNOSTIC TESTING

- The laboratory techniques used to test fetal samples obtained through CVS or amniocentesis are as follows:
  - Conventional karyotype (KT) analysis
  - Rapid aneuploidy testing
    - Quantitative fluorescent polymerase chain reaction (QF-PCR)

- ♦ Fluorescence in situ hybridisation (FISH)
  - Chromosomal microarray analysis
  - Molecular DNA testing for genetic mutations
- The choice of laboratory testing performed to diagnose fetal genetic disorders depends upon the following:
  - The indication for the test
  - The gestational age at testing, especially if a decision has to be made about termination of pregnancy

Conventional KT

- Conventional KT involves the metaphase analysis of cultured cells. It takes 7–14 days to obtain a result. Conventional KT is only possible with viable cells.
- This method is adequate for the identification of all aneuploidies including the trisomies, 45, X (Turner syndrome), other sex chromosome aneuploidies such as 47, XXY (Klinefelter syndrome), and large rearrangements.
- The accuracy of KT in diagnosing aneuploidy and chromosomal abnormalities larger than 5–10 megabases is reported as being >99 per cent (Jackson, 1992).

Rapid aneuploidy testing

- **Quantitative fluorescent polymerase chain reaction (QF-PCR)** (or, more rarely, **fluorescence in situ hybridisation [FISH]**) may be carried out on chorionic villi or amniotic fluid to test for specific chromosomes (21, 13, 18, and sex chromosomes).
- These tests provide results in 24–48 hours.
- Abnormal results of rapid aneuploidy testing are always confirmed by conventional karyotyping. However, the decision to continue or terminate the pregnancy may be made on the basis of the results of rapid testing.

Chromosomal microarray analysis (CMA)

- Chromosomal microarray analysis may be performed on uncultured cells (turnaround time of 3–7 days) or cultured cells (turnaround time of 7–10 days).
- The major advantage is that it can be done on non-viable cells and is useful in cases of fetal death or stillbirth.
- It is more accurate in picking up submicroscopic changes that are too small to be detected by conventional karyotyping. 6–10 per cent of fetuses with a structural ultrasound anomaly and a normal karyotype will show a submicroscopic change on microarray analysis (Wapner, 2012; Hillman, 2013).
- CMA is recommended instead of karyotyping when the fetus has one or more major structural abnormalities identified on ultrasound (ACOG, 2016a).
- However, this technique cannot identify balanced translocations and triploidies.

Molecular DNA testing for genetic mutations

This is performed when a single-gene disorder is suspected based on familial history.

The indications, advantages, and disadvantages of the laboratory techniques used to test fetal samples obtained through CVS or amniocentesis are summarised in Table 8.2.

Table 8.2   Summary of prenatal genetic laboratory testing

Technique	Time to obtain result	Cells used	Conditions detected	Accuracy	Advantages	Disadvantages
Conventional KT	7–14 days	Cultured live cells in metaphase	All aneuploidies	>99 per cent for aneuploidy	• Very accurate for diagnosing common aneuploidies	• Long turnaround time for results • Culture failure in cases of fetal death or stillbirth
Chromosomal microarray analysis	3–5 days for uncultured tissue	Uncultured tissue/ cultured cells	Common chromosomal aneuploidy + submicroscopic changes too small to be detected by conventional KT	More accurate than KT in the presence of major structural fetal anomaly	• Shorter turnaround time with uncultured tissue • Non-viable cells can be tested; useful in cases of fetal death or stillbirth	• Cannot detect balanced rearrangements and some triploidies
Rapid aneuploidy tests (QF-PCR or FISH)	48 hours for uncultured tissue	Uncultured tissue/ cultured cells	Aneuploidy of chromosomes 13, 18, 21, X, and Y	Will miss other aneuploidies not covered by panel	• Shorter turnaround time with uncultured tissue • Useful for early decision making	• May require confirmation with conventional KT
Molecular DNA testing	3–14 days	Uncultured tissue/ cultured cells	Genetic mutations based on familial history or other findings in fetus	Accurate for the specific disorder	• Useful for single-gene disorders	• Expensive

DNA, deoxyribonucleic acid; FISH, fluorescent in situ hybridisation; KT, karyotyping; QF-PCR, quantitative fluorescent polymerase chain reaction

Breaking the news to the parents about an affected fetus
* Choose a time when you can speak one-on-one to the couple with minimal time constraints and interruptions.
* Initially, speak only to the couple. If they want you to speak to the rest of the family, have them come in after the couple has had time to process the news.
* Do not start the conversation with sentences like "I have bad news" or "I don't know how to tell you this".
* You may start by telling them that you have the results of the screening test and the baby has the condition that you were testing for.

(Continued)

(Continued)

- Give both verbal and written information about the condition and the challenges faced by the child and his parents.
- Allow them to ask questions and answer with empathy and sensitivity.
- Offer them the options available: continuing the pregnancy or terminating the pregnancy.
- Discuss possible pregnancy outcomes such as the increased risk of miscarriage and stillbirth.
- In the presence of a correctable structural anomaly, it is appropriate to provide referrals to other specialists (genetic counsellors, cardiologists, neonatologists, pediatric surgeons, etc.).
- If the parents want to continue the pregnancy after the fetus is diagnosed with Down syndrome, refer them to the Down Syndrome Foundation of India (www.downsyndrome.in).

References

1. Akolekar R, Beta J, Picciarelli G, Ogilvie C, D'Antonio F. 2015. Procedure-related risk of miscarriage following amniocentesis and chorionic villus sampling: A systematic review and meta-analysis. *Ultrasound Obstet Gynecol.* 45:16–26.

2. Alfirevic Z, Navaratnam K, Mujezinovic F. 2017. Amniocentesis and chorionic villus sampling for prenatal diagnosis. *Cochrane Database Syst Rev.* Issue 9. Art. no.: CD003252.

3. American College of Obstetrics and Gynecologists. 2016. ACOG Committee Opinion No. 682. Microarrays and next-generation sequencing technology: The use of advanced genetic diagnostic tools in obstetrics and gynecology. Committee on Genetics and the Society for Maternal-Fetal Medicine. *Obstet Gynecol.* 128(6):e262.

4. American College of Obstetrics and Gynecology. 2016. ACOG Practice Bulletin No. 162. Prenatal diagnostic testing for genetic disorders. *Obstet Gynecol.* 127: e108–22.

5. Benn PA. 2016. Prenatal diagnosis of chromosomal abnormalities through chorionic villus sampling and amniocentesis. Milunsky A, Milunsky JM (Eds). *Genetic disorders and the fetus: Diagnosis, prevention, and treatment.* 7th ed. Hoboken (NJ): Wiley Blackwell. 178–266.

6. Giorlandino C, Mobili L, Bilancioni E, D'Alessio P, Carcioppolo O, Gentili P et al. 1994. Transplacental amniocentesis: Is it really a higher-risk procedure? *Prenat Diagn.* 14:803–6.

7. Hillman SC, McMullan DJ, Hall G, Togneri FS, James N, Maher EJ, Meller CH, Williams D, Wapner RJ, Maher ER, Kilby MD. 2013. Use of prenatal chromosomal microarray: Prospective cohort study and systematic review and meta-analysis. *Ultrasound Obstet Gynecol.* 41: 610–620.

8. Jackson LG, Zachary JM, Fowler SE, Desnick RJ, Golbus MS, Ledbetter DH et al. 1992. A randomized comparison of transcervical and transabdominal chorionic-villus sampling. The U.S. National Institute of Child Health and Human Development Chorionic-Villus Sampling and Amniocentesis Study Group. *N Engl J Med.* 327:594–8.

9. Royal College of Obstetrics and Gynecology: 2010. Amniocentesis and chorionic villus sampling. Green-top guideline no. 8.

10. Smidt-Jensen S, Permin M, Philip J et al. 1992. Randomised comparison of amniocentesis and transabdominal and transcervical chorionic villus sampling. *Lancet.* 340:1237.

11. Wapner RJ, Martin CL, Levy B, Ballif BC, Eng CM, Zachary JM et al. 2012. Chromosomal microarray versus karyotyping for prenatal diagnosis. *N Engl J Med.* 367: 2175–84.

12. Yukobowich E, Anteby EY, Cohen SM, Lavy Y, Granat M, Yagel S. 2001. Risk of fetal loss in twin pregnancies undergoing second trimester amniocentesis. *Obstet Gynecol.* 98: 231–4.

Chapter 9

Ultrasound in the First Trimester

INTRODUCTION

- Advances in ultrasound technology, particularly high-frequency transvaginal scanning, have made imaging of the fetus in the first trimester a prerequisite to the delivery of good obstetric care in areas where resources are available and women can access these services.

- Ultrasound imaging in the first trimester has progressed rapidly to a level at which early fetal development can be assessed and monitored in detail (Salomon et al., 2013).

 Ultrasound at 11–13^{+6} weeks' gestation should be offered as a screening scan to all pregnant women, if resources allow it.

- The 11–13^{+6} weeks' scan has evolved over the past two decades from a scan done primarily to measure the crown–rump length (CRL) and fetal nuchal translucency (NT) to one that includes the examination of fetal anatomy for the diagnosis of major abnormalities. This allows parents the option of earlier and safer pregnancy termination if the fetus has lethal anomalies or anomalies that may lead to a major handicap (Syngelaki et al., 2011).

- Studies of the first-trimester anatomic survey have reported detection rates comparable with those achieved in the routine second- trimester anatomic survey (Timor-Tritsch et al., 2009).

- The 11–13^{+6} weeks' scan plays a role in assessing the following:
  - Fetal viability
  - Gestational age (dating)
  - Multiple gestation—viability, chorionicity, assignment of gestational age, screening for aneuploidy, structural abnormalities
  - Fetal anatomy
  - Screening for open neural tube defects
  - Screening for chromosomal abnormalities

 There is no indication for a 'routine' ultrasound just to confirm a pregnancy. Ultrasound is neither a clinically efficient nor cost-effective method to diagnose pregnancy in asymptomatic women (SOGC, 2003). A recent review of the Cochrane Database (Kaelin et al., 2021) concluded that early scans (before 11 weeks) may reduce short-term maternal anxiety. However, the evidence was unclear about its effect on reducing perinatal loss or induction of labour for postdated pregnancies.

FETAL VIABILITY

- Viability is the term used when cardiac activity is demonstrable in the embryo/fetus by transvaginal ultrasound examination (TVS).

- Embryonic cardiac activity has been documented in normal pregnancies at as early as 37 days of gestation, which is when the embryonic heart tube starts to beat.

- Cardiac activity is usually present when the embryo measures 2 mm or more (Levi et al., 1990), but may not be seen in around 5–10 per cent of viable embryos measuring between 2 and 4 mm (Goldstein, 1992; Brown et al., 1990). That is why non-viability is only confirmed with absent cardiac activity at a CRL length of 8 mm or more (see **Chapter 10**, *Ultrasound detection of abnormal pregnancy in early first trimester*).
- Around 2.8 per cent of pregnancies between 10 and 13 weeks are non-viable, representing early pregnancy failure. 45–70 per cent of such cases are chromosomally abnormal (Pandya et al., 1996).

ASSESSMENT OF GESTATIONAL AGE

- For women who have regular menstrual cycles and who have not used oral contraceptives just prior to pregnancy, dating of the pregnancy may be accurately done using Naegele's rule (see **Chapter 2**, *Antenatal care: initial assessment*). In these women, reconfirmation of gestational age by ultrasound may not be necessary (Olsen and Clausen, 1997).
- However, dating a pregnancy based on menstrual history may not be accurate in up to 40 per cent of women who are uncertain of their menstrual dates or in whom ovulation may not exactly correspond with the mid-menstrual cycle. In these women crown–rump length (CRL) at 8–12 weeks is the most accurate method to date pregnancy. This will predict the expected date of birth to within five days (2 standard deviations).
- Gestational age at the $11-13^{+6}$ weeks' scan is estimated from the fetal CRL. After the CRL is 84 mm or more, biparietal diameter (BPD) and head circumference are used.
- **Once assigned, the gestational age is not changed in subsequent scans.**

> When resources are available, it is recommended that all pregnancies be dated by ultrasound using CRL during the $11-13^{+6}$ weeks' scan. Accurate dating decreases the number of labour inductions for post-term pregnancy. It also provides a baseline in the event that fetal growth restriction occurs later. An accurate gestational age is also important in preventing iatrogenic prematurity in planned inductions or cesarean sections.

Crown–rump length

- The CRL is the longest straight-line measurement of the embryo, measured from the outer margin of the cephalic pole to the rump. CRL measurements can be carried out transabdominally or transvaginally.
- Crown–rump length has consistently been found to be the most accurate method of determining gestational age in the first trimester. CRL at $\leq 8-8^{+6}$ weeks of gestation is the most accurate biometric parameter for pregnancy dating (± 5 days). The accuracy of the CRL falls slightly with a margin of error of ± 7 days at 9^{+0} to 13^{+6} weeks' gestation.
- To obtain an accurate measurement, the following criteria should be met:
  - Adequate magnification to fill most of the width of the ultrasound screen, so that the measurement line between the crown and rump is at about 90° to the ultrasound beam (Salomon et al., 2009)
  - Midline sagittal section of the fetus (Figure 9.1) should be viewed, ideally with the embryo/fetus lying horizontally on the screen

- The fetus should be in resting or neutral position (i.e., neither flexed nor hyperextended)
- Clear visualisation of the endpoints of the crown and rump
- The distance between the farthest points on the crown and the rump (maximum straight-line length) is measured
- The extremities and the yolk sac are not included in the measurement

- Gestational age (GA) is directly calculated from the CRL using tables or the equipment software.
- When CRL is <25 mm, gestational age (in days) = CRL (mm) + 42 (Goldstein and Wolfson, 1994). The INTERGROWTH-21st Project has produced the first international standards for relating fetal crown–rump length to gestational age (Papageorghiou et al., 2014).
- If CRL is >84 mm (14^{+0} week of gestation), biparietal diameter (BPD) should be used for the assessment of gestational age.

> The expected date of delivery (EDD) derived from the earliest measurement of the CRL is assigned to the patient and is NOT changed in the subsequent scans. The CRL-assigned EDD forms the basis for:
> - Assessment of fetal growth
> - Timing of invasive procedures
> - Timing of planned induction or cesarean section

Biparietal diameter (BPD) and head circumference (HC)

- BPD and HC measurements are highly reproducible and are the most validated measurements for the assignment of gestational age (Figure 9.2).
- The biparietal diameter (BPD) and head circumference (HC) are measured on the largest true symmetrical axial view of the fetal head, on a plane that intersects both the third ventricle and the thalami.
- In cases where there are variations in the skull shape (e.g., dolichocephaly or brachycephaly), the HC is more dependable for assigning gestational age.

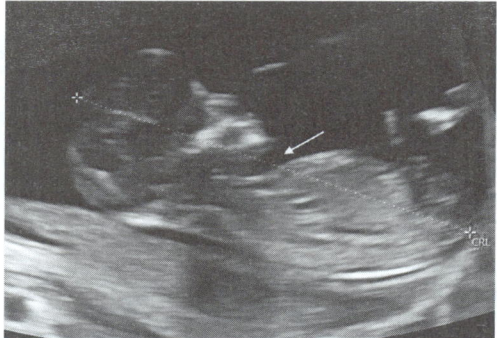

Figure 9.1 Midsagittal section and cursor placement for CRL measurement. After 10 weeks' gestation, in order to ensure that the fetus is not flexed, amniotic fluid should be visible between the fetal chin and chest (arrow) (*Image courtesy:* CIMAR, Cochin).

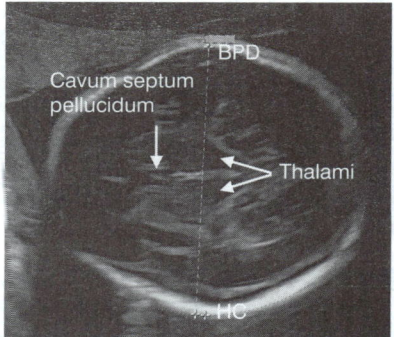

Figure 9.2 Measurement of biparietal diameter (BPD) and head circumference (HC) (*Image courtesy:* CIMAR, Cochin).

MULTIPLE GESTATION

Viability

First-trimester ultrasound is important for documenting the number of viable fetuses present in the uterus.

Chorionicity

- In the presence of multiple gestation, it is important to determine the chorionicity, which indicates the type of twinning that has occurred (see **Chapter 35**, *Multiple pregnancy*).
- Chorionicity is one of the chief predictors of higher perinatal mortality in twins. One-third of monochorionic (MC) twins are at a high risk of perinatal loss due to twin-to-twin transfusion syndrome (TTTS), selective fetal growth restriction, twin anemia–polycythemia sequence, congenital defects, or intrauterine demise (Lewi et al., 2010).
- Between 6 and 10 weeks' gestation, the presence of two gestational sacs indicates dichorionic (DC) twins. The dividing membrane is also thick in DC twins.
- A single sac with a single yolk sac but two fetuses indicates monoamniotic (MA) twins.
- Chorionicity determination is feasible and best seen at $11–13^{+6}$ weeks' gestation (Dias et al., 2011).
- The most accurate markers of chorionicity appear to be the combination of placental number with the use of the membrane *T sign* in monochorionic twins or *twin peak sign* in dichorionic twins (Figure 9.3a and b).
- Transvaginal scan also aids in the recognition of the thickness of the intertwin membrane.

Determination of chorionicity in the $11–13^{+6}$ weeks' scan
Accurate determination of chorionicity is mandatory in the routine care of twin pregnancies to distinguish which pregnancies are at high risk of perinatal complications. This is best done between 11 and 13^{+6} weeks' gestation.
- In monochorionic monoamniotic (MCDA) twins, there is no extension of tissue between the layers of the dividing membrane, and the membrane joins the placenta at right angles, giving rise to the *T sign* (Figure 9.3a).
- In dichorionic diamniotic (DCDA) twins, a triangular projection of placenta can be seen between the two layers of the dividing membrane, near the placental surface. This is called the *twin peak sign* or *lambda sign* (Figure 9.3b).
- In DCDA twins, the dividing membrane is ≥2 mm thick because it consists of the chorion and amnion of both twins (four layers). In MCDA twins, the membrane consists only of two amnions (two layers) and is <2 mm thick.
- Fetuses of different genders indicate dichorionicity.

It should be noted that the 'twin' in 'twin peak sign' refers not to the presence of two peaks, but to the twin fetuses.

CRL measurement and assignment of gestational age in multiple pregnancy

- CRL measurements in twin gestation are invariably not the same for both fetuses.
- The pregnancy is dated based on the larger CRL.

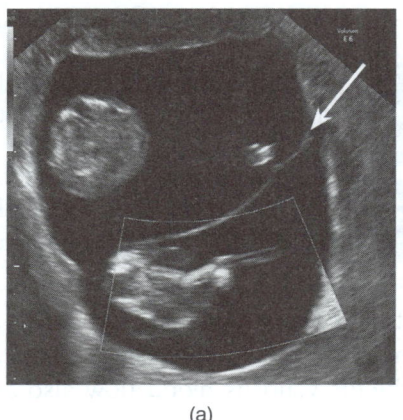
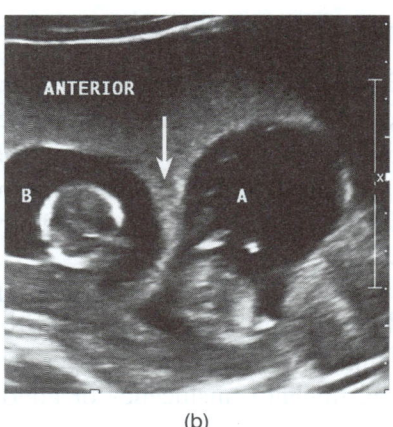

(a)   (b)

Figure 9.3   Ultrasound appearance of monochorionic and dichorionic twin pregnancies at 12 weeks of gestation. (a) T sign—there is no extension of placental tissue between the layers of the dividing membrane (arrow) in monochorionic diamniotic twins. (b) Twin peak sign or lambda sign—a triangular projection of the placenta (arrow) is seen between the layers of the membrane in dichorionic diamniotic twins (*Images courtesy:* Mediscan Systems, Chennai).

- CRL discordancy is said to be present if the difference between the two fetuses is more than 10 mm. The smaller fetus is considered abnormally small and is followed-up for interval growth, anomalies and if indicated, invasive testing.
- In monochorionic twinning, Lewi et al. (2010) demonstrated that a CRL difference of more than 12 mm is associated with a 50 per cent survival and an 80 per cent risk of adverse outcome.

Screening for aneuploidy in multiple pregnancy

See **Chapter 7**, *Prenatal screening for genetic disorders.*

Structural abnormalities in multiple pregnancy

- The incidence of congenital anomalies is three- to five-fold higher in monozygotic twins than it is in dizygotic twins or singletons, and higher in monozygotic monochorionic twins than it is in monozygotic dichorionic twins.
- In monochorionic twins, increased NT and abnormal ductus venosus Doppler are more predictive of twin-to-twin transfusion syndrome (TTTS) (10–15 per cent incidence) than chromosomal abnormalities (0.2 per cent incidence).
- Stagnati et al. (2017) reported that increased NT (>95th centile) in monochorionic twins is an important early predictor for the development of TTTS. Other predictors of TTTS in monochorionic twin pregnancies are as follows:
  - NT discrepancy > 20 per cent (the greater the NT discordance between monochorionic twins, the greater the risk of severe TTTS and early fetal death)
  - CRL discrepancy >10 per cent
  - Abnormal flow in the ductus venosus (DV) at the first-trimester scan

ASSESSMENT OF FETAL ANATOMY

- The 11–13^{+6} weeks' scan offers an early opportunity for the systematic study of fetal anatomy. Fetal anatomical assessment at a CRL of 42–84 mm yields the most structural information in the first trimester.

 50 per cent of major structural defects in low-risk pregnancies can be detected in the 11–13^{+6} weeks' scan. When in doubt regarding an anomaly in the first trimester, a repeat scan after 3–4 weeks should be recommended.

- While screening for major structural anomalies at the 11–13^{+6} weeks' scan, Souka et al. (2006) found that a structured approach to fetal anatomy could detect 50 per cent of major defects in low-risk pregnancies.
- Increased nuchal translucency or abnormal ductus venosus blood flow also appears to be associated with cardiac and skeletal defects. The presence of these markers should prompt a search for cardiac and skeletal anomalies (Grande et al., 2012).
- Syngelaki et al. (2011) divided anomalies at 11–13^{+6} weeks' gestation into detectable anomalies, potentially detectable anomalies, and undetectable anomalies (Table 9.1).

Requisites for a well-done anatomical survey

- **Equipment:** The equipment prerequisites for a first-trimester anomaly scan include the following:
  - Transabdominal curvilinear transducers with 3–7.5 MHz frequency
  - Transvaginal transducer with 3–9 MHz frequency
  - Supplementing transabdominal with transvaginal scan whenever needed
  - Liberal use of the zoom tool
  - Usage of 3D and colour Doppler whenever appropriate
- **Operator skills:** The operator should already be well-experienced in the mid-trimester detailed anatomical scan and well-informed regarding the embryologic aspects.
- **Checklist for a systematic approach:** Each organ system must be examined methodically, and a defined protocol must be adopted. Sagittal, axial, and coronal planes should be used to assess the intracranium, spine, orbits, premaxillary (retronasal) triangle, heart and thorax, kidneys, stomach, bladder, cord insertion, and limbs.

Table 9.1 Classification of structural anomalies in the 11–13^{+6} weeks' gestation ultrasound scan (Syngelaki et al., 2011)

Class	Anomalies
Detectable anomalies	Body stalk anomaly, anencephaly, alobar holoprosencephaly, exomphalos, gastroschisis, and megacystis
Potentially detectable anomalies	Absent hands or feet, polydactyly, posterior fossa defects, spina bifida, facial cleft, and cardiac and renal defects
Undetectable anomalies (Some defects are not detected because the fetus is small and the organs are not fully developed, and some defects develop later in pregnancy)	Microcephaly, agenesis of the corpus callosum, ventriculomegaly, sacrococcygeal teratomas, duodenal atresia and bowel obstruction, and severe hydronephrosis

Table 9.2 presents a sample checklist for a systematic approach to fetal anatomy in the 11–13^{+6} weeks' scan.

SCREENING FOR CHROMOSOMAL ABNORMALITIES

- The antenatal diagnosis of fetal aneuploidy is one of the major aims of prenatal screening programmes. The 11–13^{+6} weeks' scan is useful because fetuses with abnormal karyotypes often have anatomic changes or anomalies.
- In a given population, 70 per cent of trisomy 21 occur in mothers <35 years of age. 30 per cent of trisomy 21 occur in mothers >35 years of age. This fact underscores the importance of universal screening for Down syndrome, and not screening based on maternal age alone.
- First-trimester combined screening for aneuploidy is discussed in detail in **Chapter 7**, *Prenatal screening for genetic disorders*.

SCREENING FOR NEURAL TUBE DEFECTS

Anencephaly

- Anencephaly is the most common neural tube defect (NTD) and can be identified by 12 weeks' gestation by transvaginal ultrasonography (TVUS).

Table 9.2 Checklist for a systematic approach to fetal anatomy in the 11–13^{+6} week scan (adapted from the ISUOG Practice Guidelines: Performance of first-trimester fetal ultrasound scan, Salomon et al., 2013)

Organ/anatomical area	Present and/or normal	
Head	• Present • Midline falx	• Cranial bones • Choroid plexus-filled ventricles
Neck	• Normal appearance • Nuchal translucency measurement by a trained/certified operator	
Face	• Eyes with lens • Normal profile/mandible	• Nasal bone • Intact lips
Spine	• Vertebrae (longitudinal and axial) • Intact overlying skin	
Chest	• Symmetrical lung fields • No effusions or masses	
Heart	• Regular cardiac activity • Four symmetrical chambers	
Abdomen	• Stomach present in the left upper quadrant • Bladder • Kidneys	
Abdominal wall	• Normal cord insertion • No umbilical defects	
Extremities	• Four limbs, each with three segments • Hands and feet with normal orientation	
Placenta	• Size and texture	
Cord	• Three-vessel cord	

- The fetal face from the orbits to the chin is visualised in anencephaly, but the calvarium (skull) above the orbits anteriorly and above the cervical spine posteriorly is absent.

Spina bifida

- Closed spina bifida may be difficult to identify in the $11-13^{+6}$ weeks' scan.
- Open spina bifida can be detected by examining the posterior brain on the median plane of fetuses between 11 and 13^{+6} weeks. In a fetus without an open spina bifida, three anechoic spaces can be identified in the posterior brain: brainstem, intracranial translucency, and cisterna magna. The absence of one of the posterior brain spaces may be associated with a severe anomaly such as open spina bifida, cephalocele, Dandy–Walker sequence, and/or chromosomal aberrations (Volpe et al., 2015).

FIRST-TRIMESTER PREDICTION OF EARLY-ONSET PREECLAMPSIA AND FETAL GROWTH RESTRICTION

- A combination of maternal variables has been proposed to predict problems resulting from abnormal placentation, i.e., preeclampsia and fetal growth restriction (FGR).
- Markers in early pregnancy include the following:
  - Maternal history
  - Maternal mean arterial pressure
  - Increased pulsatility index in the uterine artery
  - Serum markers
    - Pregnancy-associated plasma protein-A (PAPP-A)
    - Placental growth factor (PLGF)
- Using these markers, Poon et al. (2009) developed an algorithm that they claim can predict 93.1 per cent of early-onset preeclampsia, 35.7 per cent of late-onset preeclampsia and 18.3 per cent of gestational hypertension.
- However, the American College of Obstetricians and Gynecologists does not recommend imaging and serum markers to predict preeclampsia. Their Committee Opinion Number 638 (2015, reaffirmed 2017) states that 'these tests require a large number of women to be identified as high-risk and to potentially undergo intensive surveillance in order to detect one case of early-onset preeclampsia'.
- ACOG continues to recommend using maternal history to categorise women as being high-risk or low-risk for early-onset preeclampsia.

References

1. American College of Obstetricians and Gynecologists. 2015. ACOG Committee Opinion No. 638. First-trimester risk assessment for early-onset preeclampsia. *Obstet Gynecol.* 126: e25–e27.
2. Brown DL, Emerson DS, Felker RE, Cartier MS, Smith WC. 1990. Diagnosis of early embryonic demise by endovaginal sonography. *J Ultrasound Med.* 9: 631–636.

3. Dias, T, Arcangeli T, Bhide A, Napolitano R et al. 2011. First-trimester ultrasound determination of chorionicity in twin pregnancy. *Ultrasound Obstet Gynecol.* 38: 530–532.

4. Goldstein SR, Wolfson R. 1994. Endovaginal ultrasonographic measurement of early embryonic size as a means of assessing gestational age. *J Ultrasound Med.* 13:27.

5. Goldstein SR. 1992. Significance of cardiac activity on endovaginal ultrasound in very early embryos. *Obstet Gynecol.* 80:670–672.

6. Grande M, Arigita M, Borobio V, Jimenez JM, Fernandez S, Borrell A. 2012. *Ultrasound Obstet Gynecol.* 39(2).

7. Kaelin Agten A, Xia J, Servante JA, Thornton JG, Jones NW. 2021. Routine ultrasound for fetal assessment before 24 weeks' gestation. *Cochrane Database Syst Rev.* Issue 8. Art. no.: CD014698.

8. Levi CS, Lyons EA, Zheng XH, Lindsay DJ, Holt SC. 1990. Endovaginal US: Demonstration of cardiac activity in embryos of less than 5.0 mm in crown–rump length. *Radiology.* 176: 71–74.

9. Lewi L, Gucciardo L, Mieghem TV, Philippe de Koninck, Beck V, Medek H, Van Schoubroeck D, Devlieger R, Luc De Catte, Jan Deprest. 2010. Monochorionic diamniotic twin pregnancies: Natural History and Risk Stratification. *Fetal Diagn Ther.* 27: 121–133.

10. Olsen O, Clausen JA. 1997. Routine ultrasound dating has not been shown to be more accurate than the calendar method. *Br J Obstet Gynaecol.* 104:1221–2.

11. Pandya PP, Snijders RJM, Psara N, Hilbert L, Nicolaides K. 1996. The prevalence of nonviable pregnancy at 10–13 weeks of gestation. *Ultrasound Obstet Gynecol.* 7: 170–173.

12. Papageorghiou AT, Kennedy SH, Salomon LJ et al. 2014. International standards for early fetal size and pregnancy dating based on ultrasound measurement of crown–rump length in the first trimester of pregnancy. *Ultrasound Obstet Gynecol.* 44:641.

13. Poon LC, Kametas NA, Maiz N, Akolekar R, Nicolaides KH. 2009. First-trimester prediction of hypertensive disorders in pregnancy. *Hypertension.* 53: 812–8.

14. Salomon LJ, Alfirevic Z, Bilardo CM, Chalouhi GE et al. 2013. ISUOG Practice Guidelines: Performance of first-trimester fetal ultrasound scan. *Ultrasound Obstet Gynecol.* 41: 102–113.

15. Salomon LJ, Bernard M, Amarsy R, Bernard JP, Ville Y. 2009. The impact of crown–rump length measurement error on combined Down syndrome screening: A simulation study. *Ultrasound Obstet Gynecol.* 33: 506–511.

16. SOGC Clinical Practice Guidelines No. 135. 2003. *J Obstet Gynaecol Can.* 25 (10):864–9.

17. Souka AP, Pilalis A, Kavalakis I, Antsaklis P, Papantoniou N, Mesogitis S, Antsaklis A. 2006. Screening for major structural abnormalities at the 11- to 14-week ultrasound scan. *Am J Obstet Gynecol.* 194:393–396.

18. Stagnati V, Zanardini C, Fichera A et al. 2017. Early prediction of twin-to-twin transfusion syndrome: Systematic review and meta-analysis. *Ultrasound Obstet Gynecol.* 49:573.

19. Syngelaki A, Chelemen T, Dagklis T et al. 2011. Challenges in the diagnosis of fetal non-chromosomal abnormalities at 11-13 weeks. *Prenat Diagn.* 31:90.

20. Syngelaki A, ChelemenT, Themistoklis D et al. 2011. Challenges in the diagnosis of fetal non-chromosomal abnormalities at 11–13 weeks. *Prenat Diagn.* 31: 90–102.

21. Timor-Tritsch IE, Fuchs KM, Monteagudo A, D'Alton ME. 2009. Performing a fetal anatomy scan at the time of first-trimester screening. *Obstet Gynecol.* 113: 402–407.

22. Volpe P, Muto B, Passamonti U et al. 2015. Abnormal sonographic appearance of posterior brain at 11–14 weeks and fetal outcome. *Prenat Diagn.* 35:717.

Chapter 10

Ultrasound Detection of Abnormal Pregnancy in the Early First Trimester

INTRODUCTION

- The use of transvaginal ultrasound (TVUS) has greatly facilitated the diagnosis and management of abnormal pregnancy in the early first trimester. This chapter deals with the use of ultrasound in the detection and follow-up of the following:
  - Early pregnancy failure
  - Ectopic pregnancy
  - Hydatidiform moles (molar pregnancy)

 Transvaginal ultrasound is the modality of choice for the diagnosis and follow-up of pathologic pregnancy in the early first trimester.

- Transvaginal ultrasound has enhanced the ability to detect and distinguish between the following possibilities in early pregnancy:
  - Viable versus non-viable intrauterine pregnancy (IUP)
  - IUP versus ectopic pregnancy
  - IUP of uncertain viability and pregnancy of unknown location
- In the era of highly sensitive urinary hCG assays, the easy availability of early ultrasound, and increased awareness among women and their doctors, there is a tendency to perform early scans even in the absence of abnormal symptoms.
- A scan done too early will result in an increased number of inconclusive scans that will only alarm the mother. Furthermore, repeat scans would be required to accurately determine both pregnancy location and viability.

> A scan done too early may result in the mistaken diagnosis of a non-viable pregnancy or a pregnancy in an unknown location. This may inadvertently result in interventions (e.g., methotrexate) that may disrupt an intrauterine pregnancy that might have had a normal outcome (Doubilet et al., 2013).

- It is recommended that the first ultrasound for a pregnant woman be performed at $11–13^{+6}$ weeks. Routine ultrasonogram (USG) is not recommended in the early first trimester.
- Symptoms that warrant a USG before the $11–13^{+6}$ weeks' scan are mainly the following:
  - Pain and bleeding
  - Previous history of early pregnancy loss, ectopic pregnancy, or molar pregnancy
  - Pregnancy following assisted reproductive techniques (ART)

EARLY PREGNANCY FAILURE

- Early pregnancy failure or loss is defined as a non-viable, intrauterine pregnancy within the first 12^{+6} weeks of gestation (NICE, 2012) diagnosed by the presence of the following:
  - An empty gestational sac or
  - A gestational sac containing an embryo or fetus without fetal heart activity.
- The terms miscarriage, spontaneous abortion, and early pregnancy loss are used interchangeably in the first trimester.
- Ultrasound diagnosis and the management of early pregnancy failure requires familiarity with the typical ultrasound appearances of normal early pregnancy development (Table 10.1) and the criteria for pregnancy failure.
- The use of obsolete terms such as *blighted ovum* and *anembryonic sac* should be abandoned. Such descriptions are of limited clinical usefulness and have therefore been largely replaced by ultrasound-based terminology (Table 10.2).

Table 10.1   Chronological landmarks in the development of the embryo (by transvaginal ultrasound examination)

Gestational age	Findings on ultrasound
5^{+0} weeks	Empty gestational sac (mean diameter 10 mm)
5^{+4} weeks	Gestational sac with yolk sac visible
6^{+0} weeks	Gestational sac (mean diameter 16 mm) and yolk sac with adjacent heartbeat but small embryo (3 mm)
8^{+0} weeks	Embryo with crown–rump length of 16 mm with separate amniotic sac and celomic cavity with yolk sac Fetal body movements visible, heart rate approximately 170 bpm

Table 10.2   Terminology for ultrasound description of early pregnancy (adapted from Doubilet et al., 2013)

Term	Description
Viable	A pregnancy that may potentially result in a live birth
Non-viable	A pregnancy that cannot result in a live birth
Intrauterine pregnancy of uncertain viability	TVUS shows an intrauterine gestational sac with no embryonic heartbeat but no findings of definite pregnancy failure
Pregnancy of unknown location	Positive urine or serum pregnancy test with no demonstrable IUP or ectopic pregnancy

IUP, intrauterine pregnancy; *TVUS*, transvaginal ultrasonography

Ultrasound diagnosis of early pregnancy failure

- Since the introduction of TVUS in the 1980s, the criteria for diagnosing pregnancy failure in an intrauterine pregnancy of uncertain viability have depended on the following indicators:
  - The absence of a visible embryo by the time the gestational sac has reached a certain mean sac diameter (MSD)
  - The absence of a visible embryo by a certain gestational age
  - The absence of cardiac activity by the time the embryo has reached a certain crown–rump length (CRL)

In this chapter, ultrasound refers to transvaginal US (TVUS) unless otherwise specified.

- The traditional discriminatory values that were earlier established to diagnose pregnancy failure have been revisited and modified to achieve as high a specificity and sensitivity as possible.
- To avoid mistakenly diagnosing pregnancy failure in an actually viable pregnancy, more stringent criteria were introduced in 2012 by the Society of Radiologists in Ultrasound Multispecialty Panel on Early First Trimester Diagnosis of Miscarriage and Exclusion of a Viable Intrauterine Pregnancy (Doubilet et al., 2013). These guidelines are based on studies that showed the limitations of the previous criteria using CRL and MSD (Abdallah et al., 2011; Abdallah et al., 2011a).
- For example, in the past, a CRL of 6 mm without cardiac activity fulfilled the criterion for pregnancy failure. However, it is well-known that interobserver variability exists in vaginal US measurements of CRL. Therefore, a 7 mm CRL is necessary to yield a specificity and positive predictive value of 100 per cent (Rodgers et al., 2015). The 6 mm CRL cut-off that was used previously has been abandoned.
- Similarly, the previously recommended MSD of 16 mm without an embryo as a criterion for pregnancy failure has been changed to an MSD cut-off of 25 mm. An MSD range of 16–24 mm without an embryo is considered suspicious of pregnancy failure.

 Embryos with a CRL of 6 mm and no cardiac activity have progressed to viable pregnancies (Hamilton, 2011). Similarly, gestational sacs with MSD between 17 and 21 mm and no visible embryo have continued as viable pregnancies (Abdallah et al., 2011).

 Fetal bradycardia and subchorionic hematoma
Other ultrasound findings that may be associated with pregnancy failure include:
- Slow fetal heart rate (<85 beats per minute at >7 weeks of gestation) may be associated with early pregnancy failure (Achiron et al., 1991). However, this requires evaluation after 7–10 days to conclusively diagnose pregnancy failure.
- Subchorionic hemorrhage also has been shown to be associated with early pregnancy loss but should not be used to make a definitive diagnosis; in such cases, a follow-up scan should be performed (Tuuli et al., 2011).

- The current criteria are divided into findings that are diagnostic of early pregnancy failure (see box on *Ultrasound findings diagnostic of early pregnancy failure*), and findings that are suggestive (but not diagnostic) of pregnancy failure (see box on *Ultrasound findings that are suggestive [but not diagnostic] of early pregnancy failure*).
- It must be kept in mind that the ultrasound criteria must be correlated with the mother's clinical symptoms and condition.

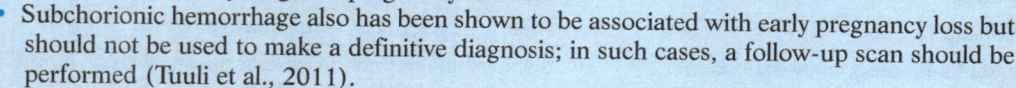

Ultrasound findings diagnostic of early pregnancy failure (adapted from Doubilet et al., 2013)
- Crown–rump length of ≥7 mm with no cardiac activity
- Mean sac diameter of ≥25 mm and no embryo
- Absence of embryo with heartbeat two weeks or more after a scan that showed a gestational sac without a yolk sac
- Absence of embryo with heartbeat 11 days or more after a scan that showed a gestational sac with a yolk sac

Ultrasound findings that are suggestive (but not diagnostic) of early pregnancy failure (adapted from Doubilet et al., 2013)
- Crown–rump length of <7 mm and no heartbeat
- Mean sac diameter of 16–24 mm and no embryo
- Absence of embryo with heartbeat 7–13 days after an ultrasound scan that showed a gestational sac without a yolk sac
- Absence of embryo with heartbeat 7–10 days after an ultrasound scan that showed a gestational sac with a yolk sac
- Absence of embryo for six weeks or longer after last menstrual period
- Empty amnion (amnion seen adjacent to yolk sac, with no visible embryo)
- Enlarged yolk sac (>7 mm)
- Small gestational sac in relation to the size of the embryo (<5 mm difference between mean sac diameter and crown–rump length)

Ectopic pregnancy

- Ectopic pregnancy is the implantation of the fertilised ovum outside the uterine cavity.

Locations of ectopic pregnancy in the first trimester
Though 96 per cent of ectopic pregnancies occur in the fallopian tube, they may occur in other locations (Bouyer et al., 2002). The distribution in different sites is as follows:
- Fallopian tube (96%)
  - Ampullary (70%)
  - Isthmic (15%)
  - Fimbrial (10%)
- Ovarian (3%)
- Cornual or interstitial (2.5%)
- Abdominal (1.5%)
- Hysterotomy/cesarean scar (0.5%)

- In the present era, the goal of good clinical practice should be to detect ectopic pregnancies at an early stage, when medical treatment is possible and surgical intervention may be avoided.
- Any woman with a possible pregnancy who has vaginal bleeding and/or abdominal pain in the first trimester should be evaluated for ectopic pregnancy.
- In a woman who is hemodynamically stable, the combination of TVUS and serum hCG level is the gold standard for the diagnosis of an ectopic pregnancy.
- The demonstration of an intrauterine pregnancy rules out an ectopic pregnancy since the incidence of heterotopic pregnancy is extremely low in spontaneously conceived pregnancies (SOGC Clinical Guidelines, 2016). However, care must be taken in an ART pregnancy to rule out a heterotopic pregnancy since its incidence is 1 in 100 (Dimitry et al., 1990).

 A negative serum hCG test rules out pregnancy, including ectopic pregnancy.

Ultrasound diagnosis of ectopic pregnancy

- Since 96 per cent of ectopic pregnancies are tubal, this chapter will focus on the ultrasound diagnosis of tubal ectopic pregnancy in the early first trimester.

- Once a pregnancy test (urine or serum) is reported as positive, TVUS helps in establishing whether it is an IUP or an ectopic pregnancy. Transabdominal ultrasound is only useful in a woman who has intra-abdominal bleeding due to a leaking or ruptured ectopic pregnancy.
- If the pregnancy test is positive but an IUP is not visualised and the adnexae are free, it may be labelled as *pregnancy of unknown location* (see box).

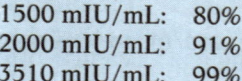

Pregnancy of unknown location
Pregnancy of unknown location is the term given to the transitory state of early pregnancy (with a positive pregnancy test) during which no definite IUP is visualised by TVUS and the adnexa are 'normal' (Mehta, 2018). The patient may have presented with bleeding and/or pain. In such a case, the three possible clinical conditions are the following:
- Early IUP
- Occult ectopic pregnancy
- Completed spontaneous abortion

A single hCG serum level does not allow reliable differentiation among these possibilities. In a hemodynamically stable patient, the strategies for follow-up include the following:
- Watchful expectancy
- Serial measurements of serum hCG
- Serial TVUS scans

- The **discriminatory zone** for hCG is the serum level above which a gestational sac should be visualised by TVUS if an IUP is present. Though a large majority of intrauterine pregnancies will be visualised with hCG levels of 1500–2000 mIU/mL, a level of 3500 mIU/mL is required to achieve a 99 per cent predictive probability of visualisation (Connolly, 2013).

Percentage of intrauterine pregnancies that will be visualised by TVUS at different hCG levels
1500 mIU/mL: 80%
2000 mIU/mL: 91%
3510 mIU/mL: 99%

- Therefore, in a stable patient with bleeding and/or pain in early pregnancy, serum hCG can be repeated every 48 hours to watch for a change in its levels. Seeber et al. (2006) found that 99.9 per cent of intrauterine pregnancies had an hCG rise of ≥35 per cent every two days. A serum hCG that does not rise appropriately is consistent with an abnormal pregnancy. The hCG concentration rises at a much slower rate in most, but not all, ectopic and non-viable IUPs (Silva et al., 2006).
- An ectopic pregnancy is suspected/diagnosed when an empty uterus is associated with the following:
  - Simple adnexal cyst
  - Complex adnexal mass
  - Solid adnexal mass

– Tubal ring
– Complex fluid in the pelvis

> **Cesarean scar ectopic pregnancy**
> With the indiscriminate rise in cesarean section rates, the incidence of ectopic pregnancies in the cesarean scar is increasing, currently being reported as 1 in 2000 pregnancies and accounting for 6 per cent of ectopic pregnancies among women with a prior cesarean delivery (Rotas et al., 2006). In women with a pregnancy of unknown location and a previous cesarean section, a high index of suspicion must be maintained to be able to make an accurate diagnosis. Almost all cesarean scar pregnancies are diagnosed and treated in the first trimester. The ultrasound image reveals an enlarged hysterotomy scar with an embedded mass that may bulge beyond the anterior contour of the uterus.

Figure 10.1 is a simple algorithm for the diagnosis of an unruptured ectopic pregnancy.

The role of colour Doppler in the diagnosis of ectopic pregnancy

- Colour Doppler may add useful information when the ultrasound findings are not definitive of an ectopic pregnancy. For example, with a complex adnexal mass, the finding of a low-impedance colour Doppler waveform or a ring of colour Doppler may strongly suggest an ectopic pregnancy (SOGC Clinical Practice Guidelines, 2016).
- Care must be taken not to mistake a corpus luteum for an ectopic pregnancy since both may have similar colour Doppler findings.
- The absence of a finding of colour flow using Doppler in a complex adnexal mass does not exclude an ectopic pregnancy (Kurjak et al., 1991).

> **Pregnancy of unknown location**
> Serum hCG >2000 mIU/mL
> Absent IUP on TVUS

> **High probability of ectopic pregnancy**
> Serum hCG >3500 mIU/mL
> Absent IUP on TVUS
> Adnexal mass or tubal ring on TVUS

> **Diagnostic of ectopic pregnancy**
> GS with live embryo seen
> inside fallopian tube on TVUS

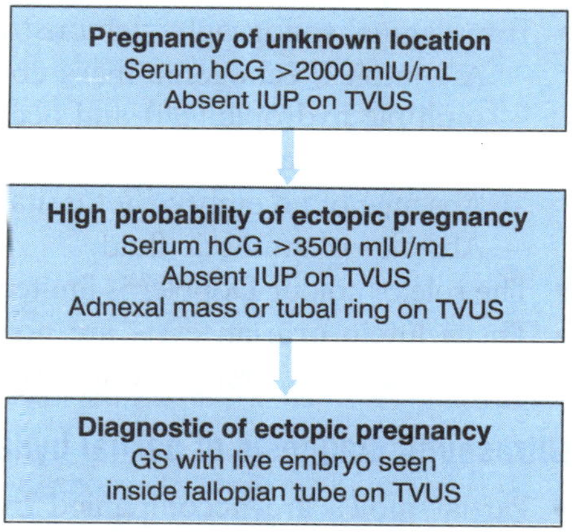

Figure 10.1 A simple algorithm for the diagnosis of an unruptured ectopic pregnancy in a hemodynamically stable woman. *GS* gestational sac; *IUP*, intrauterine pregnancy; *TVUS*, transvaginal ultrasonography

HYDATIDIFORM MOLE (MOLAR PREGNANCY)

- Ultrasonography is a sensitive and reliable method for diagnosing molar pregnancy (SOGC Clinical Practice Guidelines, 2003).
- Gestational trophoblastic disease presents most commonly as partial mole (incidence of 1 in 700) and complete mole (incidence of 1 in 1500–2000).
- Before the era of ultrasound, molar pregnancy was usually diagnosed in the second trimester with a presentation of vaginal bleeding, a uterus larger than gestational age and high levels of serum hCG. It could also be associated with preeclampsia, hyperemesis, hyperthyroidism, and respiratory distress.

- Though ultrasound has made the diagnosis of molar pregnancy easier, identification in the first trimester is difficult. A routine pre-evacuation ultrasound examination identifies less than 50 per cent of hydatiform moles, the majority presenting sonographically as missed or incomplete miscarriages (Fowler et al., 2006; Kirk et al., 2007).
- Partial moles are often diagnosed on histopathological examination after an evacuation.

Ultrasound diagnosis of complete hydatidiform mole

- The increasing use of ultrasound in early pregnancy allows for the detection of hydatidiform mole before the onset of systemic manifestations. Most cases are diagnosed in the first trimester, usually between 9 and 12 weeks.
- The diagnosis of molar pregnancy may be made in early first trimester even if the woman is asymptomatic. However, most often, it is made when a woman presents with vaginal bleeding.
- Transvaginal sonography demonstrates the following typical appearance:
  - A complex, echogenic mass containing many small cystic spaces (corresponding to multiple hydropic villi) and occasionally larger cystic spaces (Benson et al., 2000) in the uterine cavity
  - Absence of an embryo/fetus/its parts
  - Absence of amniotic fluid
- The role of colour Doppler is limited in the diagnosis of a complete mole (Jauniaux, 1998).
- Theca lutein ovarian cysts are not commonly seen when complete molar pregnancy is diagnosed in the first trimester (Benson et al., 2000; Kirk et al., 2007).

Ultrasound diagnosis of partial hydatiform mole

- Partial moles are accompanied by a fetus and amniotic fluid. Therefore, ultrasound examination usually leads to a partial mole being diagnosed as a missed or incomplete miscarriage in 15–60 per cent of cases (Berkowitz et al., 2018).
- Sonographic features suggestive of a partial molar pregnancy include the following:
  - A viable or non-viable fetus
  - Presence of amniotic fluid, though the volume may be reduced
  - Placenta with one or more of the following abnormal findings:
    - Enlarged, cystic spaces and/or
    - Increased echogenicity of chorionic villi
  - Ratio of transverse to anteroposterior dimension of the gestational sac >1.5 (Fine et al., 1989)
- Theca lutein cysts are usually absent.
- The detection rate of a partial mole by ultrasound is quite low (29 per cent) as compared to that of a complete mole (Kirk et al., 2007).

References

1. Abdallah Y, Daemen A, Guha S, Syed S, Naji O, Pexsters A et al. 2011. Gestational sac and embryonic growth are not useful as criteria to define miscarriage: A multi-center observational study. *Ultrasound Obstet Gynecol.* 38: 503–9.

2. Abdallah Y, Daemen A, Kirk E, Pexsters A, Naji O, Stalder C et al. 2011a. Limitations of current definitions of miscarriage using mean gestational sac diameter and crown–rump length measurements: A multicenter observational study. *Ultrasound Obstet Gynecol.* 38: 497–502.

3. Achiron R, Tadmor O, Mashiach S. 1991. Heart rate as a predictor of first trimester spontaneous abortion after ultrasound-proven viability. *Obstet Gynecol.* 78: 330–4.

4. Benson CB, Genest DR, Bernstein MR, Soto-Wright V et al. 2000. Sonographic appearance of first trimester complete hydatidiform moles. *Ultrasound Obstet Gynecol.* 16: 188–91.

5. Berkowitz RS, Goldstein DP, Horowitz NL. 2018. Hydatidiform mole: Epidemiology, clinical features, and diagnosis. Goff B (Ed). *UpToDate.* Waltham, MA.

6. Bouyer J, Coste J, Fernandez H et al. 2002. Sites of ectopic pregnancy: A 10 year population-based study of 1800 cases. *Hum Reprod.* 17: 3224.

7. Connolly A, Ryan DH, Stuebe AM, Wolfe HM. 2013. Re-evaluation of discriminatory and threshold levels for serum hCG in early pregnancy. *Obstet Gynecol.* 121(1): 65–70.

8. Dimitry ES, Subak-Sharpe R, Mills M, Maragara R, Winston R. 1990. Nine cases of heterotopic pregnancies in 4 years of in vitro fertilization. *Fertil Steril.* 53: 107–10.

9. Doubilet PM, Benson CB, Bourne T et al. 2013. Diagnostic criteria for nonviable pregnancy early in the first trimester. *N Engl J Med.* 369(15): 1443–1451.

10. Fine C, Bundy AL, Berkowitz RS et al. 1989. Sonographic diagnosis of partial hydatidiform mole. *Obstet Gynecol.* 73: 414.

11. Fowler DJ, Lindsay I, Seckl MJ et al. 2006. Routine pre-evacuation ultrasound diagnosis of hydatidiform mole: Experience of more than 1000 cases from a regional referral center. *Ultrasound Obstet Gynecol.* 27: 56–60.

12. Hamilton J. 2011. The 6 mm crown-rump length threshold for detecting fetal heart movements: What is the evidence? *Ultrasound Obstet Gynecol.* 38(suppl 1): 7.

13. Jauniaux E. 1998. Ultrasound diagnosis and follow up of gestational trophoblastic disease. *Ultrasound Obstet Gynecol.* 11(5): 367–77.

14. Kirk E, Papageorghiou AT, Condous G et al. 2007. The accuracy of first trimester ultrasound in the diagnosis of hydatidiform mole. *Ultrasound Obstet Gynecol.* 29: 70–75.

15. Kurjak A, Zalud I, Shulman H. 1991. Ectopic Pregnancy: Transvaginal color Doppler of trophoblastic flow in questionable adnexa. *J Ultrasound Med.* 10: 685–89.

16. Mehta TS. 2018. Ultrasonography of pregnancy of unknown location. Sharp HT, Levine D, Barbieri, RL (Eds). *UpToDate.* Waltham, MA.

17. National Institute for Health and Clinical Excellence. 2012. Ectopic pregnancy and miscarriage: Diagnosis and initial management in early pregnancy of ectopic pregnancy and miscarriage. NICE Clinical Guideline 154. Manchester (UK).

18. Rodgers SK, Chang C, DeBardeleben JT et al. 2015. Normal and abnormal US findings in early first-trimester pregnancy: Review of the Society of Radiologists in Ultrasound, 2012. Consensus Panel Recommendations. *Radiographics.* 35(7): 2135–48.

19. Rotas MA, Haberman S, Levgur M. 2006. Cesarean scar ectopic pregnancies: Etiology, diagnosis, and management. *Obstet Gynecol.* 107: 1373.

20. Seeber BE, Sammel MD, Guo W et al. 2006. Application of redefined human chorionic gonadotropin curves for the diagnosis of women at risk for ectopic pregnancy. *Fertil Steril.* 86: 454.

21. Silva C, Sammel MD, Zhou L et al. 2006. Human chorionic gonadotropin profile for women with ectopic pregnancy. *Obstet Gynecol.* 107: 605.

22. SOGC Clinical Practice Guidelines. No. 337, 2016. Ultrasound Evaluation of First Trimester Complications of Pregnancy. *J Obstet Gynaecol Can.* 38(10): 982–988.

23. SOGC Clinical Practice Guidelines No. 135, 2003. *J Obstet Gynaecol Can.* 25(10): 864–9.

24. Tuuli MG, Norman SM, Odibo AO, Macones GA, Cahill AG. 2011. Perinatal outcomes in women with subchorionic hematoma: A systematic review and meta-analysis. *Obstet Gynecol.* 117: 1205–12.

Chapter 11

Ultrasound in the Second Trimester

INTRODUCTION

- Ultrasound has become an integral and indispensable part of the prenatal evaluation and management of pregnancy.
- If only a single ultrasound examination is offered in pregnancy, it should be performed between 18 and 22 weeks of gestation. This gestational period allows a reasonably precise dating of pregnancy to within ±7–10 days (though an earlier dating is more accurate). It is also the ideal time to identify significant structural abnormalities and label a fetus as 'normal' with a good degree of accuracy.
- A properly performed second-trimester scan includes:
  - Confirmation of cardiac activity
  - Fetal number (and chorionicity in multiple pregnancy)
  - Fetal biometry to confirm gestational age (which is most accurate before 24 weeks)
  - Survey of fetal anatomy
  - Placental appearance and location
  - Maternal anatomy (cervix, uterus, and adnexa)

 **Timing of second-trimester scan in India**
The legal limit for the termination of pregnancy in India is 20 completed weeks of gestation. Based on this, the ideal time to perform a second-trimester target scan (in India) would be 18–20 weeks, which provides an opportunity to address any lethal anomaly requiring termination.

- Congenital malformations are abnormalities that have medical, surgical, or cosmetic significance. The majority of pregnancies result in the delivery of a structurally normal baby. However, approximately 2–4 per cent of live births have structural anomalies. In an Indian cohort, Bhide et al. (2016) found the prevalence of major congenital anomalies to be 2.3 per cent. Approximately 70 per cent of major anomalies and 45 per cent of minor anomalies can be identified by a good quality second-trimester ultrasound.

 In most countries, a routine scan between 18–22 completed weeks has been made a part of standard obstetric care (ACOG, 2016; SOGC, 2017). The National Health Mission, Government of India, has also made this recommendation (NHM, 2011). One ultrasound scan before 24 weeks of gestation is recommended by the World Health Organization (2018) to estimate gestational age, improve the detection of fetal anomalies and multiple pregnancies, reduce induction of labour for postterm pregnancy, and improve a woman's pregnancy experience.

IDEAL EQUIPMENT FOR THE SECOND-TRIMESTER SCAN

For routine screening, it is recommended (Salomon et al., ISUOG, 2011) that the equipment used should have at least the following:

- Real-time, greyscale ultrasound capabilities

- Transabdominal transducer (3–5 mHz range)
- Transvaginal transducer (5–10 mHz or higher) if the cervix needs to be evaluated
- Adjustable acoustic power output controls with output display standards
- Freeze-frame capabilities
- Electronic callipers
- Capacity to print/store images
- Regular maintenance and servicing, which are important for optimal equipment performance

- **Three dimensional (3D) ultrasonography** is an advancement in imaging technology. Though 3D capability is not mandatory, it can add value while evaluating malformations. In 3D ultrasonography, a volume of tissue is imaged and stored in multiple slices. The operator can look through, rotate, and process the volume of information in various ways to gain additional information about the anatomy of the fetus. 3D capability is an invaluable adjunct while evaluating malformations, e.g., cleft lip and palate, micrognathia, abnormal facial midline profile, agenesis of the corpus callosum and Dandy-Walker malformation, clubfeet, amputation defects, and skeletal dysplasia.
- **Four dimensional (4D) ultrasonography** is three dimensional ultrasound in real time (the fourth dimension). 4D ultrasonography has been evaluated for the diagnosis of anomalies but is not currently offered as a routine part of antenatal screening.

WHO SHOULD PERFORM THE SCAN?

- The second-trimester scan should be performed by an individual who has had adequate training in obstetric ultrasound and possesses a comprehensive knowledge of fetal growth and development. This could be a radiologist, an obstetrician, or a sonologist who has had structured, systematic training with certification.
- It is imperative to have adequate training in obstetric ultrasound, irrespective of the basic specialty. The diagnosis is not only dependent on the quality of imaging but also the knowledge of the operator—the more in-depth the medical knowledge (including pathophysiology and anatomy), the greater the chances of an accurate diagnosis. The images obtained during the real-time examination are critical since 'the one who holds the transducer makes the diagnosis' (Finberg, 2004).
- Periodic updating and implementation of evidence-based practice to keep abreast of advancements in the field ensure better diagnostic accuracy.

PERFORMING A TARGETED FETAL EXAMINATION (TAFE)

- The second-trimester scan should be performed in a systematic manner. To this end, several international societies like the AIUM, ISUOG, SOGC and others have issued guidelines for the examination of the fetus (AIUM, 2007; Salomon et al., ISUOG, 2011; SOGC, 2009).
- Several names have been given to the scan performed at 18–22 weeks:
  – Second-trimester anomaly scan
  – Targeted imaging for fetal anomalies (TIFFA)
  – Targeted scan

- Suresh and Suresh (2014) introduced the term 'TArgeted Fetal Examination' (TAFE) in the second trimester, as it is similar to clinically examining the developing fetus.

TAFE – The seven steps and the 'Rule of Three'

- TArgeted Fetal Examination is a simple method comprising seven steps to enhance the quality of examination and decrease the chances of missing a fetal problem.
- One of the steps is the 'Rule of Three' for the systematic, checklist-based evaluation of fetal anatomy. This ensures that all organs are examined for normalcy and increases the rate of identification of major anomalies.

THE SEVEN-STEP APPROACH TO TAFE

The following seven steps are performed in a sequential order to achieve maximum yield from the ultrasound examination in the least possible time.

1. History
2. Survey
3. Biometry
4. Targeted imaging
   using the 'Rule of Three'
5. Fetal environment
6. Fetal activity
7. Reporting

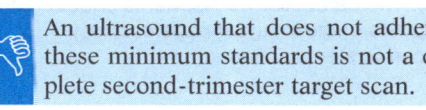 An ultrasound that does not adhere to these minimum standards is not a complete second-trimester target scan.

1. History

The primary objective of obtaining a relevant history is to determine whether the pregnancy is low-risk or to identify specific risk factors that will place the pregnancy in a high-risk category. In high-risk cases, the examination needs to be extended beyond the 'Rule of Three' approach (described below).

2. Survey

The survey scan is meant to provide a global picture of the gravid uterus. The information obtained during the survey is as follows:

- Number of fetuses
- Lie and position of the spine
- Viability of fetus(es)
- Location of the placenta
- Available space around the fetus and amniotic fluid

3. Biometry

Fetal biometry is done to assess the gestational age and determine whether the fetal size corresponds to gestational age by LMP. The minimum biometric parameters that should be measured are:

- Biparietal diameter (BPD) and head circumference (HC) (Figure 11.1)
- Abdominal circumference (AC) (Figure 11.2)
- Femur length (FL) (Figure 11.3)

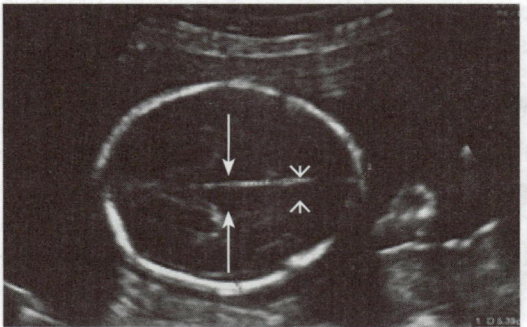

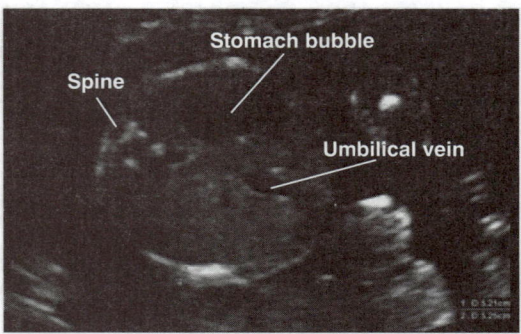

Figure 11.1 Biparietal diameter (BPD) and head circumference (HC)—the BPD should be measured on an axial plane that traverses the thalami (white arrows) and cavum septum pellucidum (arrowheads). The cerebellar hemispheres should not be in the plane of the image (*Image courtesy:* Mediscan Systems, Chennai).

Figure 11.2 Abdominal circumference is measured by a transverse section through the upper abdomen which should demonstrate the following fetal landmarks: fetal stomach, umbilical vein, and portal sinus. The kidneys and cord insertion should not be visible. The umbilical vein should not be seen extending to the skin line (*Image courtesy:* Mediscan Systems, Chennai).

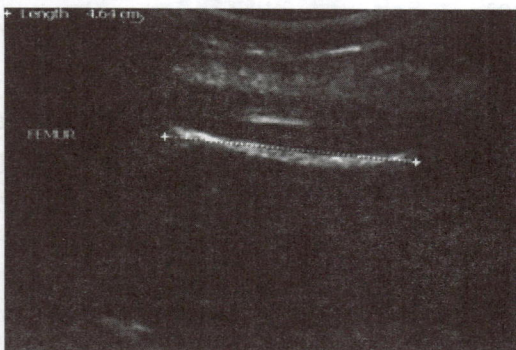

Figure 11.3 Femur length—the transducer should be aligned along the long axis of the bone so that the beam is perpendicular to the shaft. The measured ends should be blunt and not pointed (*Image courtesy:* Mediscan Systems, Chennai).

Assignment of gestational age in the 18–22 weeks' scan using biometry
- The gestational age (GA) and estimated date of delivery (EDD) are calculated based on the last menstrual period (LMP). This gives the presumptive menstrual age.
- If gestational age has been calculated using CRL in the first trimester and a due date has been assigned, the due date should not be changed in the second trimester.
- If an earlier ultrasound-based calculation of GA is not available, biometric parameters in the second trimester are used to confirm GA. In the second trimester, the best parameter for calculating gestational age is the *fetal head circumference*.
- The EDD should be corrected if there is a significant discrepancy between menstrual age and ultrasound GA.
- A discrepancy of >10 days between ultrasound dating and LMP dating supports reassignment of GA in the 18–22 weeks' scan.

4. Targeted imaging and the 'Rule of Three' approach

- This is the most crucial step, involving a detailed examination of the fetus in a systematic and reproducible manner.
- The 'Rule of Three' approach entails visualising three anatomical landmarks in each part of the fetus examined and in each plane through which the examination is performed. Similarly, the fetal environment also has three important structures to be evaluated. See the section on *Anatomical planes and structures to be examined using the 'Rule of Three'*.

5. Fetal environment

Examining the fetal environment is the 5th step in the seven-step process of TAFE. The placenta, the umbilical cord, and the amniotic fluid comprise the fetal environment. See section below on *Survey of fetal environment*.

6. Fetal activity

- There are no movement patterns specific to the second trimester. Normal fetuses typically have a relaxed position and show regular movements (Salomon et al., 2011).
- Temporary absence or reduction of fetal movements during the scan is not alarming at this stage of pregnancy.
- Abnormal fetal conditions such as arthrogryposis should be suspected in the presence of either of the following:
  – Abnormal positioning
  – Unusually restricted or persistently absent fetal movements
- The biophysical profile is not considered part of a routine mid-trimester scan.

The fetal examination is considered complete at the end of the above steps. If the examination is completed as per the protocol, reasonable reassurance can be given about the normalcy of the fetus.

7. Reporting

- This is the final step of TAFE.
- It is important to have a standardised and uniform reporting format that clearly presents all the findings.
- There must be constant communication between the obstetrician requesting the investigation and the person performing the ultrasound so that the mother gets the maximum benefit from the scan.

ANATOMICAL PLANES AND STRUCTURES TO BE EXAMINED USING THE RULE OF THREE

Head

The examination should be done in **three** planes with **three** structures identified in each plane:
1. *Transthalamic plane* (Figure 11.4)
   This plane is traditionally used to measure BPD and HC.
   i.   Midline falx, interrupted by the

   ii. Cavum septum pellucidum

   iii. Thalami, forming an arrow pointing to the occiput

2. *Ventricular plane* (Figure 11.5)

   i.   Lateral ventricles (LV)

   ii. Choroid plexus

   iii. Cavum septum pellucidum (CSP)

3. *Transcerebellar plane* (Figure 11.6)

   i.   Cerebellar hemispheres

   ii. Vermis

   iii. Cisterna magna

Spine

The spine is visualised in the sagittal and transverse axes (Figure 11.7). The coronal view of the spine is optional.

Sagittal axis

The **three** aspects of the spine that are looked for in the sagittal axis are as follows:

1. Cervical widening   2. Parallel thoracic and lumbar spine   3. Sacral tapering

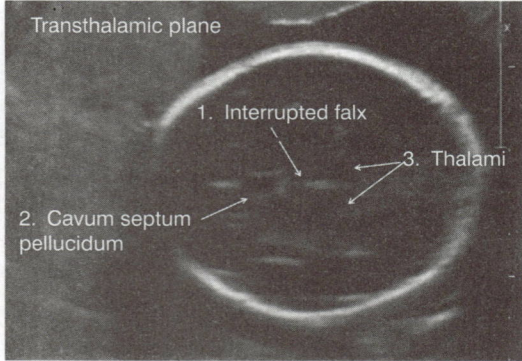

Figure 11.4 Transthalamic plane
(*Image courtesy:* Mediscan Systems, Chennai).

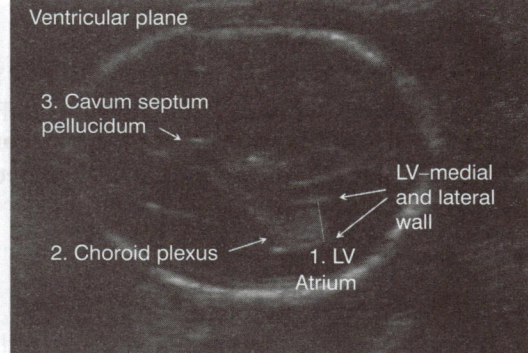

Figure 11.5 Ventricular plane
(*Image courtesy:* Mediscan Systems, Chennai).

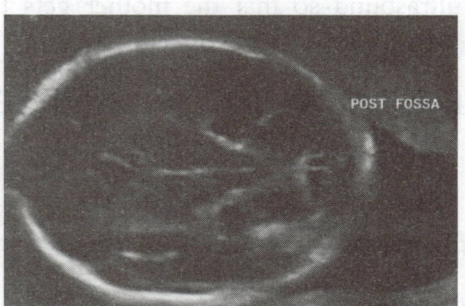

Figure 11.6 Transcerebellar plane.

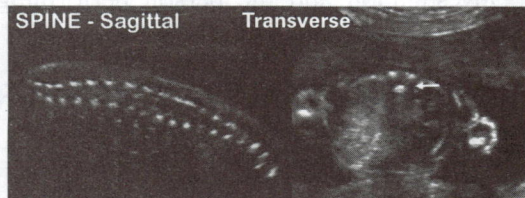

Figure 11.7 Spine in the sagittal and transverse axes. The arrow points to the three ossification centres.

Transverse axis

Three ossification centres forming a triangular shape are noted in the transverse axis of the spine.

Thorax

- The thorax comprises of three structures: the right lung, the left lung and the heart.
- Each structure occupies 1/3rd of the thorax.
- The heart is considered enlarged when it occupies more than 50 per cent of the thorax.

Heart

The three views of the heart that should be visualised are the four-chamber view, the outflow tracts and the three-vessel view.

1. *Four-chamber view* (Figure 11.8)

The following three need to be identified in this view:

i.   Crux of the heart formed by the interventricular septum (IVS), atrioventricular septum and the interatrial septum
ii. Chamber symmetry
iii. Movement of mitral and tricuspid valves in real time

2. *Outflow tracts* (Figures 11.9 and 11.10)

i)   At the origin, the outflow tracts are seen crossing each other with the pulmonary artery anteriorly and the aorta posteriorly.
ii) The anterior aortic root should be continuous with the interventricular septum and the posterior aortic root with the mitral valve.
iii) The crossing of the outflow tract can be appreciated in the transverse view ('circle sausage' view) which shows the cross section of the aorta and long section of the pulmonary artery with its bifurcation.

3. *Three-vessel view*

This is the most important view for identifying outflow tract anomalies (Figure 11.11).

i)   The three vessels seen from the left to right are the pulmonary artery, aorta, and superior vena cava.
ii) The three vessels are assessed in terms of number, alignment/arrangement, and size.

Abdomen

Three areas of the abdomen are examined: the upper abdomen, the mid-abdomen, and the lower abdomen.

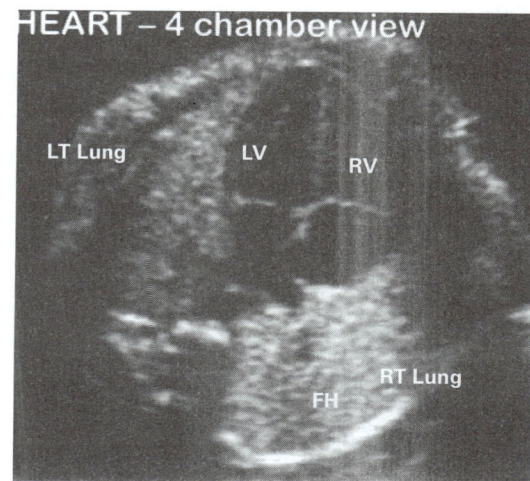

Figure 11.8   Four-chamber view of the heart.

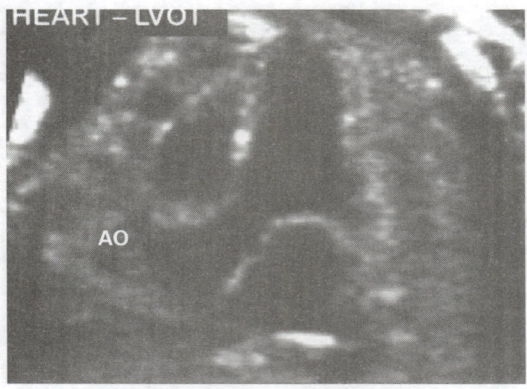

Figure 11.9   Left ventricular outflow.

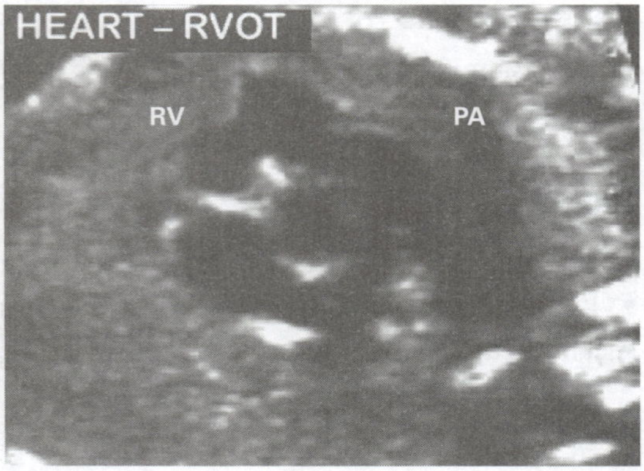

Figure 11.10   Right ventricular outflow.

1. *Upper abdomen* (Figure 11.12)

The **three** structures to be identified in the upper abdomen are as follows:

i) Stomach

ii) Portal vein

iii) Liver

    The gallbladder may be seen to the right of the abdomen within the liver echoes.

2. *Mid-abdomen* (Figure 11.13)

The **three** structures to be identified in the mid-abdomen are as follows:

i) Right kidney

ii) Left kidney

iii) Small bowel

    The AP diameter of the renal pelvis is measured in the transverse section of the kidneys. This can help identify hydronephrosis.

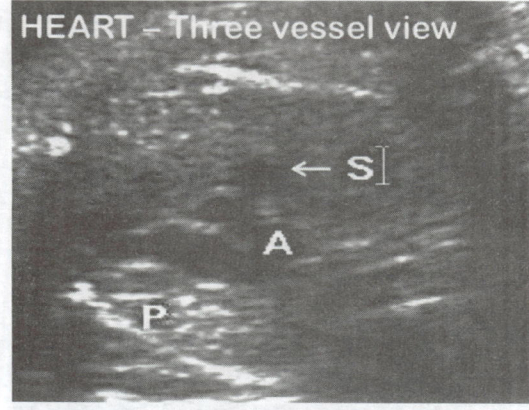

Figure 11.11   Three-vessel view—*P,* pulmonary artery; *A,* aorta; *S,* superior vena cava.

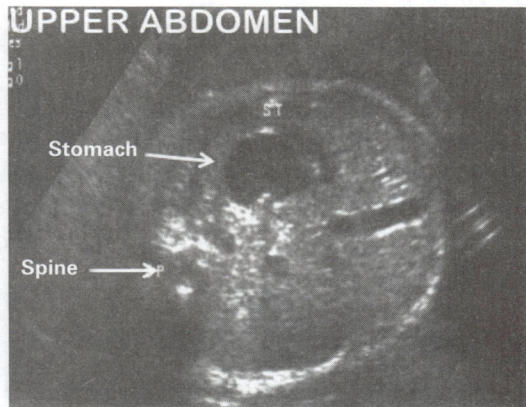

Figure 11.12   Upper abdomen.

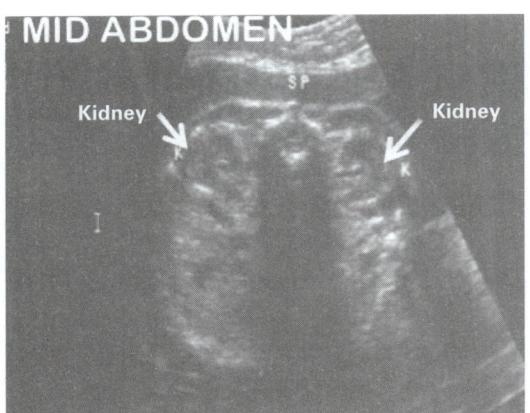

Figure 11.13   Mid-abdomen.

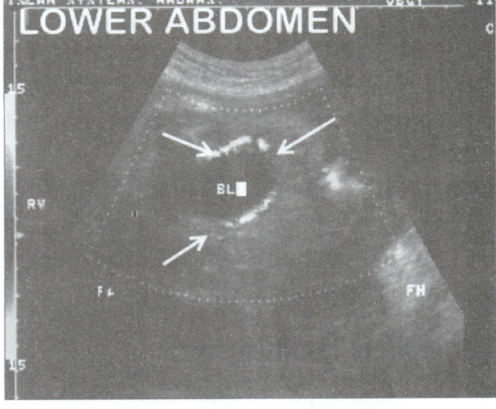

Figure 11.14   Lower abdomen.

3. *Lower abdomen* (Figure 11.14)

The **three** structures to be identified in the lower abdomen are as follows:

i)   Bladder

ii) Two umbilical arteries

iii) Genitalia

Colour Doppler is used to identify the two umbilical arteries, which are seen coursing along the sides of the bladder.

The extremities

All four limbs (Figures 11.15 and 11.16) should be visualised. In each limb, the following **three** are noted:

1. The **three** segments: proximal, mid, and distal

2. The **three** features: length, echogenicity, and shape

3. Subjective assessment of muscle mass

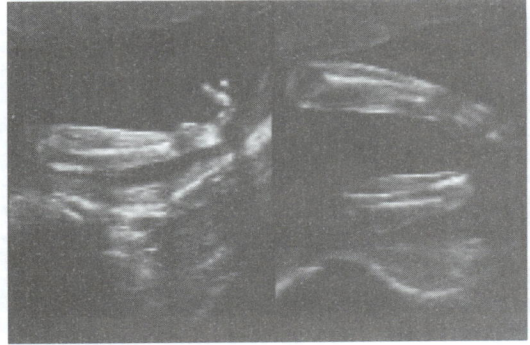

Figure 11.15   Upper limb.

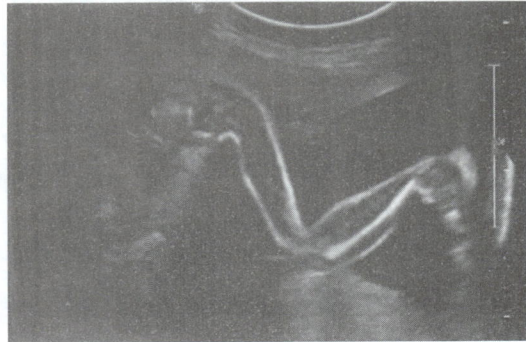

Figure 11.16   Lower limb.

Face

- The face is examined in **three** planes: axial, sagittal, and coronal.
- The **three** structures to be identified in the face are as follows:

> A normal premaxillary triangle assures the presence of intact lips and palate and helps rule out cleft lip and cleft palate.

  1. Orbits (in the axial view) (Figure 11.17)
  2. Nose and nasal bones (in the sagittal view)
  3. Mouth, including the lips and premaxillary triangle (in the coronal view) (Figures 11.18 and 11.19)

Soft markers for aneuploidy

An important step in the second-trimester scan is the identification of soft markers for aneuploidy (see **Chapter 7**, *Prenatal screening for genetic disorders*).

Second-trimester ultrasound markers for aneuploidy include (in descending order of likelihood ratio) the following:
- Absent or hypoplastic nasal bone
- Aberrant right subclavian artery
- Ventriculomegaly
- Increased nuchal fold thickness
- Hyperechoic bowel
- Pyelectasis
- Echogenic intracardiac focus
- Short humerus
- Short femur

SURVEY OF THE FETAL ENVIRONMENT

The placenta, the umbilical cord, and the amniotic fluid comprise the fetal environment. Their examination provides invaluable information regarding the fetal status.

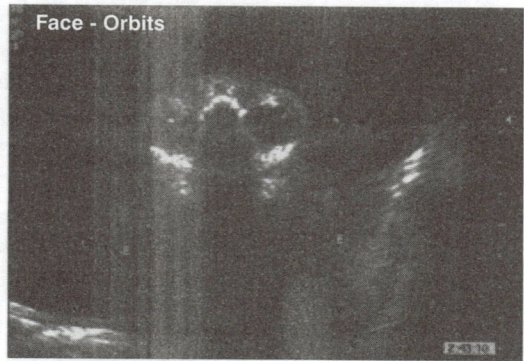

Figure 11.17   Face: axial view.

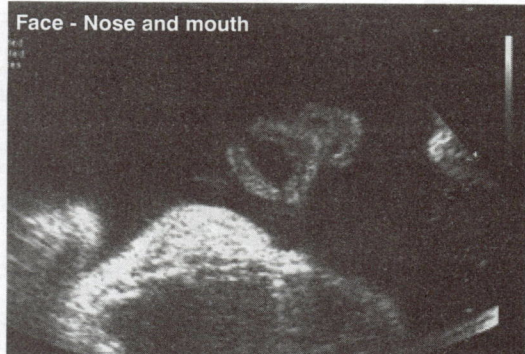

Figure 11.18   Face: coronal view showing lips and nostrils.

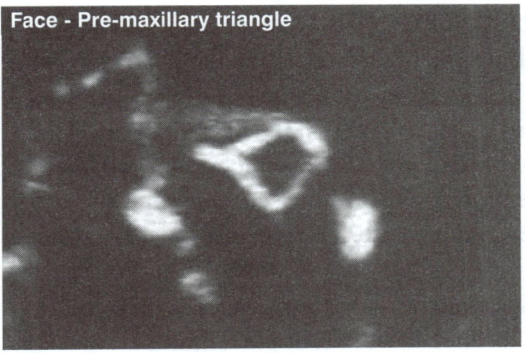

Face - Pre-maxillary triangle

Figure 11.19   Face: coronal view showing the pre-maxillary triangle.

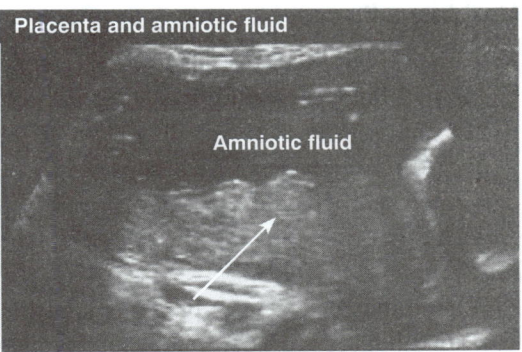

Placenta and amniotic fluid

Amniotic fluid

Figure 11.20   Posterior placenta (arrow).

Placenta

The placenta (Figure 11.20) is assessed in terms of the following:
- Location, with specific reference to its lower edge and its distance from the internal os
- The placental substance, for abnormal appearances or calcifications
- Identification of the subplacental complex of veins, visualised as a hypoechoic area behind the placenta

Placenta previa

- The most common presentation of placenta previa is as a finding on routine ultrasound examination at the second-trimester scan.
- Though 1–6 per cent of pregnant women are found to have evidence of placenta previa in the second trimester, the majority of these women are asymptomatic and 90 per cent of these early cases resolve (Oyelese et al., 2006).
- It is important to report the placental position with newer, accepted terms of classification:
  - *True placenta previa:* The internal cervical os is covered by the placenta completely or partially (this includes what was referred to as 'total' and 'partial' in the earlier classification).

 An over-distended bladder may stretch the placenta and lead to a misdiagnosis of previa. For this reason, the diagnosis of previa should be confirmed with an empty bladder.

  - *Low-lying placenta:* The placenta is in the lower segment, and the edge of the placenta is within 2 cm of the os but does not cover it.
- Placenta previa is best diagnosed with a transvaginal or translabial (perineal) ultrasound.

 Persistence until delivery
If the placenta extends ≥2.5 cm beyond the internal os at 20–24 weeks, vaginal delivery is almost certainly ruled out since there is a greater chance of persistence until delivery (Becker et al., 2001).

Morbidly adherent placenta (accreta, increta, percreta)

- With increasing rates of cesarean section, the risk of adherent placenta is increasing exponentially (Mazouni et al., 2007).
- Placenta accreta is present in almost 30 per cent of cases in which the placenta is implanted over the uterine scar as compared to 6.5 per cent of cases in which it is not. Among women with placenta previa, the risk of placenta accreta is almost 40 per cent in women with two or more previous cesarean deliveries and an anterior or central placenta previa (Miller et al., 1997).
- When anterior placenta previa is identified in a woman with a previous cesarean section, it is mandatory to document the presence or absence of adherent placenta.
- Ultrasound is associated with high sensitivity and specificity for the diagnosis of placenta accreta when specific defined criteria are used for the diagnosis.
- Greyscale ultrasound signs of adherent placenta are as follows (Pagani et al., 2018):
  - Loss of clear zone, defined as a loss or irregularity of the hypoechoic plane in the myometrium underneath the placental bed
  - Placental lacunae, often containing turbulent flow
  - Bladder wall interruption between the uterine serosa and bladder lumen
  - Myometrial thinning overlying placenta to <1 mm or undetectable
  - Focal exophytic mass of placental tissue breaking through the uterine serosa and extending beyond it; this is most often seen inside the filled urinary bladder
- Colour Doppler signs of adherent placenta include the following (Pagani et al., 2018):
  - Placental lacunar flow
  - Subplacental vascularity seen behind the placental bed
  - Uterovesical hypervascularity seen between the myometrium and posterior wall of the bladder

Amniotic fluid

- Subjective assessment of amniotic fluid is done in the mid-trimester stage and is not inferior to the quantitative measurement techniques. A quantitative assessment is performed in women if:
  - The qualitative assessment seems abnormal
  - If there is increased risk of pregnancy complications
- In the second trimester, if quantitative assessment is required, the single deepest pocket (SDP) measurement is preferred. The vertical dimension (in centimetres) of the largest pocket of amniotic fluid (not persistently containing umbilical cord or fetal extremities) is measured at a right angle to the uterine contour.

 A systematic review of the Cochrane Database showed that the single deepest vertical pocket measurement in the assessment of amniotic fluid volume during fetal surveillance seems a better choice (Nabhan et al., 2008).

- Women with deviations from the normal should undergo a more detailed examination of fetal structural anatomy and should be followed-up clinically.

Umbilical cord

- Examination of the umbilical cord should be an integral part of the second-trimester ultrasound scan.
- Some sonographic findings of the umbilical cord are associated with structural and chromosomal fetal anomalies, fetal growth restriction, and other pathological conditions that may lead to increased fetal morbidity and mortality. Identification of suspicious findings should prompt a thorough search for fetal structural and chromosomal anomalies (Weissman and Drugan, 2001).
- The umbilical cord is traced from the fetal insertion site to the placental insertion site. The following are noted:
  - Number of vessels—a single umbilical artery (SUA) should be documented
  - Presence of knots, cysts, and tumours
- **Nuchal cord:** An incidental finding of nuchal cord on ultrasound examination is very common. It does not warrant reporting, nor does it require a change in prenatal or intrapartum care. A nuchal cord appears to be a normal part of intrauterine life and is not associated with significant perinatal morbidity and mortality (Clapp et al., 2003).
- Doppler studies may be performed as indicated in a high-risk pregnancy.

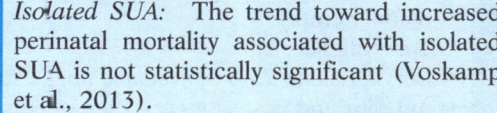

Single umbilical artery (SUA)
Isolated SUA: The trend toward increased perinatal mortality associated with isolated SUA is not statistically significant (Voskamp et al., 2013).
Non-isolated SUA: Perinatal morbidity and mortality are increased and depend on the underlying chromosomal and anatomic anomalies.

Routine Doppler during a second-trimester scan?
Current guidelines do not recommend Doppler studies as part of the routine second-trimester ultrasound examination. There is insufficient evidence to support the universal use of uterine or umbilical artery Doppler evaluation for the screening of low-risk pregnancies (Salomon et al., ISUOG, 2011).

After completion of the fetal examination, the fetus is classified under one of the following categories:
- Structurally normal for the period of gestation
- Soft marker detected
- Significant/lethal anomaly detected
- Suspicion of anomaly that warrants a consultation with a maternal–fetal or fetal medicine specialist

MATERNAL ANATOMY

Cervical length

- A short cervix has been associated with an increased risk of preterm birth.
- If cervical length is measured in all women undergoing a second-trimester scan,

A systematic review of the Cochrane Database (Berghella et al., 2019) found that currently, there is not enough high-quality research to show whether measuring cervical length in women with twin or singleton pregnancies has any effect on preventing preterm births.

the number of women who need to be screened to prevent one preterm birth has been estimated to be 913 (Miller et al., 2015).

- Therefore, a universal programme for the screening of cervical length is not recommended because it would require significant resources and also cause anxiety and unnecessary intervention (Salomon et al., 2011).
- However, the Society for Maternal–Fetal Medicine (2016) recommends routine cervical length screening during the second-trimester scan between 16 and 24 weeks of gestation for women with a singleton pregnancy and **history of spontaneous preterm birth**.

Criteria for measuring cervical length
- Bladder empty
- Transvaginal scan
- Cervix fills up 75% of available image space
- Anterior and posterior cervix are of equal thickness
- Internal and external cervical os are seen
- Endocervical canal is seen throughout
- Callipers placed at the internal and external os, where the anterior and posterior walls of the cervix meet
- If the endocervical canal curves, two or more linear measurements should be used and added to obtain the cervical length
- Shortest best measurement reported
- Dynamic cervical shortening examination time of 3–5 minutes and/or suprapubic/fundal pressure

Source: ACR–ACOG–AIUM–SMFM–SRU Practice Parameter for the Performance of Standard Diagnostic Obstetrical Ultrasound, American College of Radiology, 2018

Uterine fibroids and adnexal masses

- During the second trimester, ultrasound may identify uterine fibroids and adnexal masses. These should be documented.
- If the fibroids are likely to interfere with labour, a special note should be made as follow-up scans may be required.
- It is worth remembering that 70 per cent of women with fibroids 10 cm or larger achieve a vaginal delivery (Qidwai et al., 2006). This information is useful for preconception and prenatal counselling of women with fibroids (see **Chapter 38**, *Pregnancy in women with fibroids*).

LIMITATIONS OF A SECOND-TRIMESTER ULTRASOUND

- While most major malformations may be seen during the second trimester, some evolve with advancing gestational age.
- The overall detection rate of fetal anomalies in the second trimester is around 50 per cent, with approximately 35 per cent detection of cardiac defects and upto almost 90 per cent rate of detection of central nervous system and urogenital defects (Grandjean et al., Eurofetus Study, 1999). However, the detection rate for lethal abnormalities in the second trimester can be as high as 92 per cent (Hildebrand et al., 2010). In another study

(Rydberg and Tunón, 2017), the prenatal detection rate of chromosomal abnormalities by second trimester ultrasound screening in a non-selected population was found to be 60.7 per cent and, for structural malformations, 39.0 per cent.

- The accuracy of anomaly detection is limited by the following factors:
  - Gestational age at examination
  - High BMI of the mother, which makes visualisation difficult
  - Liquor volume and fetal position
  - Type of malformation
  - Operator experience and quality of equipment

 In low-risk pregnancies, the detection rate for fetal anomalies decreases from 66 per cent in women with normal weight to 25 per cent in overweight women (Dashe et al., 2009).

- Patients should be counselled adequately about these limitations. If specific parts of the fetal anatomy cannot be imaged, this should be mentioned in the report.

THE PRECONCEPTION AND PRENATAL DIAGNOSTIC TECHNIQUES (PCPNDT) ACT

- Female feticide rose alarmingly in India in the 1990s. Consequently, the child sex ratio (female: male) dropped. Though the adult sex ratio in the country has improved from 933 in 2001 to 940 in 2011, the child sex ratio dipped from 927 in 2001 to 918 in 2011. The disturbing decline in the child sex ratio is a matter of serious concern and prompted the Government of India to pass an Act of Parliament in 1994, which was amended in 2003 to the 'Preconception and Prenatal Diagnostic Techniques Act' (PCPNDT Act).

 Sex determination by ultrasound in any form is illegal and punishable by the PCPNDT Act. Divulging the sex of the baby in any form, written, oral, or by gesture is illegal in India.

- The Act has been primarily enacted to prevent sex determination by ultrasound as a means to combat sex-selective abortion.
- The main provisions in the Act are as follows:
  - Absolute prohibition of sex determination/selection
  - No communication can be made about the sex of the fetus in any manner
  - The prenatal screening and diagnostic techniques must be conducted by qualified persons only
  - Every centre/institute conducting these tests must be registered under the Act

Every centre/institute must prominently display a notice declaring that sex determination/selection is prohibited under the law and is not conducted at that centre.

  - Applications (form A) for permission to provide prenatal screening services should be sent for registration to the appropriate authority, the protocol being as follows:
    - Approved applicants receive form B as a certificate, which must be displayed in the centre; the certificate is valid for five years

♦ One month before the expiry of the certificate, a renewal request should be sent in form A to the appropriate authority

 All centres offering ultrasound examinations, all USG machines and all persons performing ultrasounds have to be registered with the appropriate authority in the respective state or district.

— Before conducting a test, the appropriate form must be filled, which in the case of sonography, is form F (patient details, indication of the test, patient's declaration that she does not want to know the sex of fetus, doctor's declaration that he/she has not determined/conveyed the sex of fetus, etc.)
   ♦ Form F specifies 23 indications under which sonography/sonographically-assisted invasive procedures can be performed
   ♦ A complete report of all such tests conducted in a month must be sent to the authorities by the 5th day of the subsequent month
— All the records (including referral slips) must be maintained
— Any change in equipment, employee or address must be informed to the appropriate authority
— Sale of equipment/machines is prohibited to anyone who is not registered under the Act
— Anyone not fulfilling the rules is punishable under the Act

Details of the Act are available at https://india.unfpa.org under Standard Operating Guidelines for District Appropriate Authorities on PCPNDT Act, 1994.

References

1. ACR–ACOG–AIUM–SMFM–SRU Practice Parameter for the Performance of Standard Diagnostic Obstetrical Ultrasound. American College of Radiology. 2018.

2. American College of Obstetricians and Gynecologists. 2016. ACOG Practice Bulletin No. 175. Ultrasound in pregnancy. *Obstet Gynecol.* 128: 241–56.

3. Becker RH, Vonk R, Mende BC et al. 2001. The relevance of placental location at 20–23 gestational weeks for prediction of placenta previa at delivery: Evaluation of 8650 cases. *Ultrasound Obstet Gyneco.* 17:496.

4. Berghella V, Saccone G. 2019. Cervical assessment by ultrasound for preventing preterm delivery. *Cochrane Database Syst Rev.* Issue 9. Art. no.: CD007235.

5. Bhide P, Gund P, Kar A. 2016. Prevalence of congenital anomalies in an Indian maternal cohort: healthcare, prevention, and surveillance implications. Eapen V (ed.). *PLoS ONE.*11(11): 0166408.

6. Clapp JF 3rd, Stepanchak W, Hashimoto K et al. 2003. The natural history of antenatal nuchal cords. *Am J Obstet Gynecol.* 189:488.

7. Dashe JS, McIntire DD, Twickler DM. 2009. Effect of maternal obesity on the ultrasound detection of anomalous fetuses. *Obstet Gynecol.* 113(5):1001–7.

8. Finberg HJ. 2004. Whither (Wither?) the ultrasound specialist? *Journal of Ultrasound in Medicine.* 23: 1543–1547.

9. Grandjean H, Larroque D, Levi S, and the Eurofetus team. 1999. The performance of routine ultrasonographic screening of pregnancies in the Eurofetus study. *Am J Obstet Gynecol.* 181: 446–454.

10. Hildebrand E, Selbing A, Blomberg M. 2010. Comparison of first and second trimester ultrasound screening for fetal anomalies in the southeast region of Sweden. *Acta Obstet Gynecol Scand.* 89(11):1412–9.

11. Mazouni C, Gorincour G, Juhan V, Bretelle F. 2007. Placenta accreta: A review of current advances in prenatal diagnosis. *Placenta.* 28: 599–603.

12. Miller DA, Chollet JA, Goodwin TM. 1997. Clinical risk factors for placenta previa–placenta accreta. *American Journal of Obstetrics & Gynecology.* Volume 177, Issue 1, 210–214.

13. Miller ES, Tita AT, Grobman WA. 2015. Second-trimester cervical length screening among asymptomatic women: An evaluation of risk-based strategies. *Obstet Gynecol.* 126:61.

14. Nabhan AF, Abdelmoula YA. 2008. Amniotic fluid index versus single deepest vertical pocket as a screening test for preventing adverse pregnancy outcome. *Cochrane Database Syst Rev.* Issue 3. Art. no.: CD006593.

15. National Health Mission (NHM), Ministry of Health and Family Welfare, Government of India. 2011. Standard guidelines on use of ultrasound during pregnancy.

16. Oyelese Y, Smulian JC. 2006. Placenta previa, placenta accreta, and vasa previa. *Obstet Gynecol.* 107:927.

17. Pagani G, Cali G, Acharya G et al. 2018. Diagnostic accuracy of ultrasound in detecting the severity of abnormally invasive placentation: A systematic review and meta-analysis. *Acta Obstet Gynecol Scand.* 97:25.

18. Qidwai GI, Caughey AB, Jacoby AF. 2006. Obstetric outcomes in women with sonographically identified uterine leiomyomata. *Obstet Gynecol.* 107: 376–382.

19. Rydberg C, Tunón K. 2017. Detection of fetal abnormalities by second-trimester ultrasound screening in a non-selected population. *Acta Obstet Gynecol Scand.* 96(2):176–182.

20. Salomon LJ, Alfirevic Z, Berghella V et al. 2011. Practice guidelines for performance of the routine mid-trimester fetal ultrasound scan. *Ultrasound Obstet Gynecol.* 37: 116–126.

21. Society for Maternal-Fetal Medicine (SMFM). McIntosh J, Feltovich H et al. 2016. The role of routine cervical length screening in selected high- and low-risk women for preterm birth prevention. *Am J Obstet Gynecol.* 215:B2.

22. SOGC Practice Guidelines No. 223. Cargill Y, Morin L et al. 2017. Content of a complete routine second trimester obstetrical ultrasound examination and report. *Journal of Obstetrics and Gynaecology Canada.* Vo. 39. Issue 8. e144–e149

23. Suresh S, Suresh I. 2014. The second trimester obstetric scan (7+3=10): A rational approach (including the 'rule of three'). *J Fetal Med.* 1:59–73.

24. Voskamp BJ, Fleurke-Rozema H, Oude-Rengerink K et al. 2013. Relationship of isolated single umbilical artery to fetal growth, aneuploidy and perinatal mortality: Systematic review and meta-analysis. *Ultrasound Obstet Gynecol.* 42:622.

25. World Health Organization. 2018. WHO Recommendations on antenatal care for a positive pregnancy experience: Ultrasound Examination. WHO. Geneva.

26. Weissman A, Drugan A. 2001. Sonographic findings of the umbilical cord: Implications for the risk of fetal chromosomal anomalies. *Ultrasound Obstet Gynecol.* 17: 536–541.

Chapter 12

Ultrasound in the Third Trimester

INTRODUCTION

- There is no doubt that ultrasound has contributed enormously to the management of both the low-risk and the high-risk pregnancy. It has also been established that if resources are available, every pregnant woman should have a scan at $11-13^{+6}$ weeks and at 18–22 weeks.
- However, the indication for a routine ultrasound in the third trimester for women with an uncomplicated pregnancy is still debated. Studies have not demonstrated any difference in the primary outcomes of perinatal mortality, preterm birth at less than 37 weeks, cesarean section rates, and induction of labour rates if ultrasound is introduced as a routine protocol in late pregnancy (Thornton, 2016).
- One of the reasons cited for a routine third-trimester ultrasound is the identification of fetal growth restriction (FGR). In a population-based study, Sylvan et al., (2005) found that routine third-trimester ultrasound screening in an unselected population does not reduce perinatal mortality or early neonatal morbidity for small-for-gestational age (SGA) neonates. Though the Pregnancy Outcome Prediction study (Sovio et al., 2015) advocated universal sonography in the third trimester because it triples the detection of small-for-gestational age (SGA) neonates, analysis of the study shows that universal ultrasound tends to overdiagnose SGA more often than clinically indicated ultrasound.
- In a resource-rich country, this examination may be offered routinely to all women (Ray and Grangé, 2016).
- In India, where resources are low and ultrasound is not available to all, third-trimester obstetric ultrasound may be confined to specific indications (Table 12.1).

 A systematic review of the Cochrane Database (Bricker et al., 2015) concluded that 'based on existing evidence, routine late-pregnancy ultrasound in low-risk or unselected populations does not confer a benefit on the mother or baby'.

INDICATIONS FOR ULTRASONOGRAPHY IN THE THIRD TRIMESTER

Certain maternal conditions may require monitoring of the fetus and its environment in the third trimester.

I. Evaluation of fetal growth disorders

Fetal growth restriction (FGR)

- Fetal growth restriction (also known as intrauterine growth restriction or IUGR) refers to a fetus that has failed to maintain the growth velocity predicted by earlier scans.

Table 12.1 Indications for ultrasound examination in the third trimester and the clinical reasons for performing it

Indication	Clinical reason
Evaluation of fetal growth disorders	Clinical suspicion of growth restriction/discrepancy between uterine size and clinical dates/suspected macrosomia
Evaluation of fetal well-being	Maternal or fetal complication/s requiring fetal surveillance (see **Chapter 6**, *Antepartum fetal surveillance*)
Follow-up evaluation of a fetal anomaly	Anomaly suspected or identified in the second-trimester scan
Screening for specific anomalies that can be identified only in the third trimester	Previous history of infant with microcephaly, achondroplasia, etc.
Amniotic fluid abnormalities	Oligohydramnios or polyhydramnios suspected/discrepancy between uterine size and clinical dates
Evaluation of premature rupture of membranes	Suspicion of leaking amniotic fluid
Evaluation/follow-up of placental location	Placenta previa or adherent placenta identified in the second-trimester scan
Evaluation of vaginal bleeding of placental etiology	To rule out placenta previa, or placental abruption
Determination of fetal presentation	Suspected breech presentation or transverse lie
Suspected fetal death	Absent fetal heart tones
Evaluation of multiple pregnancy	To rule out discordant growth; identify development of complications; decide on the best mode of delivery
Adjunct to external cephalic version	Helps with assessing amniotic fluid volume, fetal presentation and lie (see **Chapter 22**, *Breech delivery*)
Evaluation of abdominal or pelvic pain	Suspected uterine or extra-uterine pathology

The fetus does not achieve its growth potential due to factors that may be fetal, placental, maternal, or a combination of these factors (see **Chapter 36**, *Fetal growth disorders: growth restriction and macrosomia*).

 Currently, there is insufficient evidence to recommend universal screening for fetal growth restriction in the third trimester in low-risk women (Saccone et al., 2016).

- A clinical suspicion of growth restriction may be raised during an antenatal visit when the uterine size by palpation or tape measurement reveals a discrepancy with the gestational age. Alternatively, the mother may have a medical or obstetric condition that increases the risk of growth restriction. In either of these scenarios, ultrasonography in the third trimester is the modality of choice to identify FGR (see box).

- Though growth restriction is defined traditionally as weight below the 10th percentile for the gestational age, ultrasound diagnosis of FGR is significant when the growth and weight fall below the 5th percentile. The 5th percentile is a better cut-off than the 10th percentile in defining SGA because the risks of adverse outcomes increase substantially when the growth is <5th percentile (Zhang et al., 2011).

- Third-trimester screening for fetal growth restriction is principally for asymmetric growth restriction (see **Chapter 36**, *Fetal growth disorders: growth restriction and macrosomia*) and not for symmetric growth restriction, which manifests earlier in pregnancy. Since asymmetric growth restriction is primarily due to uteroplacental insufficiency caused by various factors, it presents itself in the third trimester.

Indications for screening women in the third trimester for fetal growth restriction
- Significant lag of the fundal height on physical examination
- Suboptimal growth on a prior ultrasound
- History of a prior birth of a small-for-gestational age infant
- Poor maternal weight gain
- Maternal conditions associated with fetal growth restriction
  – Hypertension/preeclampsia
  – Systemic lupus erythematosus
  – Antiphospholipid antibody syndrome

Ultrasound diagnosis of the fetus with growth restriction

Abdominal circumference (AC)
- Of the four biometric parameters (BPD, HC, AC, and FL), abdominal circumference is the single most sensitive parameter for the diagnosis of FGR.
- Since there is depletion of abdominal adipose tissue and decreased hepatic size caused by reduced glycogen storage in the liver in the growth-restricted fetus, the abdominal circumference will decrease in the third trimester.
- It has been well established that the sensitivity of AC in predicting growth restriction increases with increasing gestational age. It is most sensitive closer to term (Ferrazzi et al., 1986).
- AC is more sensitive when the interval between measurements is more than two weeks (Mongelli et al., 1998).

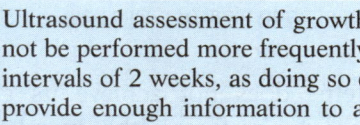
Ultrasound assessment of growth should not be performed more frequently than at intervals of 2 weeks, as doing so does not provide enough information to act upon (ACOG, 2016).

- Fetal growth is usually assessed with serial ultrasound examinations every 3–4 weeks. Interval growth assessment in the severely growth-restricted fetus may sometimes be indicated as frequently as every two weeks.

Estimated fetal weight (EFW)
- Fetal weight is estimated by using equations that incorporate two or more biometric parameters. Equations that incorporate AC, BPD, and FL seem to provide the most accurate estimates of fetal weight, especially in the growth-restricted fetus (Guidetti et al., 1990).
- Fetal weight estimation is one of the most common and reliable methods of identifying the growth-restricted fetus.

There are differences in birth weight among countries, e.g., India has significantly smaller neonates than other countries, even after adjusting for gestational age. It is therefore important to use country-specific charts (Kiserud et al., 2017).

- EFW varies with ethnicity and race. It is therefore important to calculate estimated fetal weight using charts specific to the racial background of the mother. The World Health Organization has published the World Health Organization's Fetal Growth Charts, which contain common ultrasound biometric measurements based on longitudinal data derived from 10 countries including India (Kiserud et al., 2017). The INTERGROWTH-21 growth chart is also becoming a global standard because it has incorporated the World Health Organization's recommendations (see box below). The standards and tools of the INTERGROWTH-21 project are available for clinicians at https://intergrowth21.tghn.org/standards-tools/.
- EFW is most sensitive for predicting FGR and adverse outcomes associated with FGR in infants with severe growth restriction, i.e., birth weight <3rd percentile. EFW <3rd percentile is consistently associated with adverse outcome (Divon, 2018).

> **Growth charts and growth velocity**
> *Growth charts:* To accurately diagnose fetal growth restriction, it is mandatory to place the biometric parameters (especially AC and EFW) on a standard growth curve. The INTERGROWTH-21 project produced the first comprehensive set of international standards for optimal fetal and newborn growth that perfectly match the existing World Health Organization's child growth standards (Papageorghiou et al., 2018). Using the growth chart for the fetus positions the growth parameters on the specific percentile and allows for the diagnosis of FGR.
>
> *Growth velocity:* The rate of interval growth is known as growth velocity. In FGR, the growth velocity of both the AC and EFW slows down (de Jong et al., 1999). This can be seen on the chart as plateauing or dropping (Figure 12.1).
>
> Growth charts help in differentiating a physiologically small fetus from a growth-restricted fetus. **The small but normal fetus will maintain its growth velocity** (Figure 12.2). In addition, there will be no changes in the amniotic fluid level and umbilical Doppler flow in these normal fetuses (see **Chapter 36**, *Fetal growth disorders: growth restriction and macrosomia*).

Macrosomia

- A macrosomic or large-for-gestational age (LGA) infant is one whose birth weight is equal to or greater than the 90th percentile for a given gestational age. This definition is based on the average birth weight at each gestational age, and is country-specific (see **Chapter 36**, *Fetal growth disorders: growth restriction and macrosomia*).
- An analysis of the World Health Organization's Global Survey on Maternal and Perinatal Health study data (Koyanagi et al., 2013), shows that even in developing countries, 4000 g is the threshold at or beyond which adverse maternal and neonatal outcomes occur.
- The common indications for ruling out macrosomia in the third trimester are as follows:
  - Uterine size larger than expected for gestational age
  - Gestational diabetes, especially if poorly controlled
  - Decision for trial of labour in a woman with a previous cesarean section
  - History of shoulder dystocia

Ultrasound prediction of macrosomia

- Although ultrasonography in the third trimester enables the direct measurement of various fetal body parts, its accuracy in predicting macrosomia is poor (Coomarasamy et al., 2005).

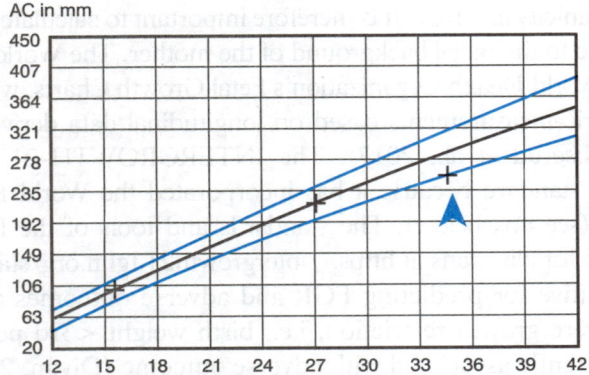

Figure 12.1 Fetal growth restriction: The three lines on the growth chart represent the 90th percentile (uppermost curve), the 50th percentile (middle curve), and the 5th percentile (lowermost line). In this chart, the abdominal circumference (AC) has not kept up the growth velocity and has fallen below the 5th percentile at 34–35 weeks (arrow).

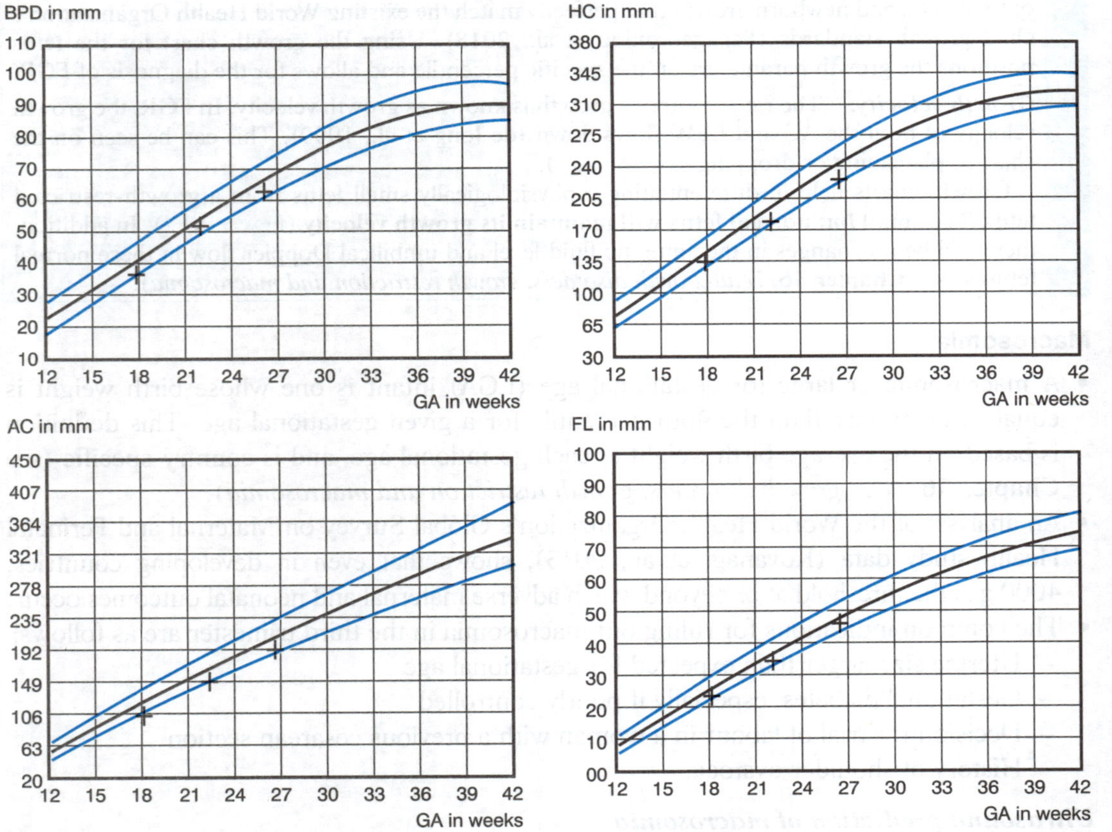

Figure 12.2 Low growth profile fetus: The fetal biometric parameters (BPD, HC, AC, and FL) are all at the low normal percentile but are maintaining growth velocity. This is the growth chart of a fetus that is constitutionally small but otherwise healthy.

- **Abdominal circumference** (AC) is the most common single parameter used to assess the risk of macrosomia.
- The formula for calculating estimated fetal weight (EFW) commonly includes a combination of biparietal diameter (BPD), head circumference (HC), AC, and femur length (FL). EFW is calculated using different formulas but almost all formulas have poor accuracy in predicting macrosomia of >4000 g (Hoopmann et al., 2010).
- The larger the fetus, the less accurate is the ultrasound estimation of fetal weight. Ultrasound is also a poor predictor of fetal weight in multiple gestation and diabetic pregnancies (Combs et al., 2000).
- Measurement of subcutaneous fat at the midhumerus, abdominal wall, thigh, and other areas has been evaluated but was found to be no more accurate than estimated fetal weight.

II. Evaluation of fetal well-being

- One of the commonest indications for ultrasound examination in the third trimester is to evaluate fetal well-being.
- Ultrasound is an important component of the biophysical profile (BPP), the modified biophysical profile (mBPP), and the evaluation of amniotic fluid as part of antepartum fetal surveillance.
- Doppler velocimetry of the fetal umbilical artery, the middle cerebral artery, and the ductus venosus also provides invaluable information about fetal well-being.
- All these tests are discussed in detail in **Chapter 6**, *Antepartum fetal health surveillance*.

III. Diagnosis and follow-up evaluation of fetal anomaly

- *Screening for anomalies that present in the third trimester:* Some anomalies, e.g., congenital heart defects, can be missed on ultrasound scanning at an earlier stage of pregnancy, while others such as duodenal atresia, microcephaly, or achondroplasia may not manifest before the third trimester (Dommergues et al., 1999).
- *Follow-up evaluation of a fetal anomaly:* In some fetal anomalies, although diagnosis is possible in the second trimester, third-trimester follow-up is required to establish the prognosis. For example, isolated dilatation of the cerebral ventricles in the second trimester may be a benign disorder, or it may be secondary to complex cerebral malformations that may not be diagnosed until the third trimester. Similarly, mild fetal hydronephrosis and congenital diaphragmatic hernia diagnosed in the second trimester may need a third-trimester ultrasound for follow-up and management decisions.

IV. Diagnosis and evaluation of suspected amniotic fluid abnormalities

- Ultrasound estimation of amniotic fluid volume is indicated in the third trimester to assess the effect of various physiological and pathological processes on the fetal environment. The common indications for evaluation are as follows:
    - Fetal congenital anomalies (both oligohydramnios and polyhydramnios)
    - Premature rupture of membranes (oligohydramnios)

- Pregnancy complications related to uteroplacental insufficiency (oligohydramnios)
- Diabetes in pregnancy (polyhydramnios)

- Amniotic fluid volume is also assessed along with other sonographic tests (BPP and mBPP) in the evaluation and management of complicated pregnancies.
- Amniotic fluid should be assessed subjectively during all ultrasound scans in the second trimester and followed with an objective measurement if the amniotic fluid volume seems abnormal. If a scan is done in the third trimester, it is best to document the amniotic fluid volume in all cases. The objective methods used to assess amniotic fluid volume are the single deepest pocket (SDP) technique and the amniotic fluid index (AFI).

Single deepest pocket (SDP) technique

- The single deepest pocket is the vertical dimension (in centimetres) of the largest pocket of amniotic fluid not persistently containing umbilical cord or fetal extremities. It is measured perpendicular to the uterine contour. 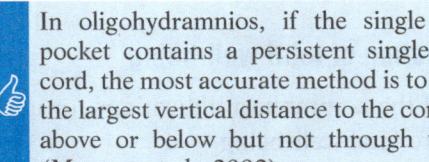 In oligohydramnios, if the single deepest pocket contains a persistent single loop of cord, the most accurate method is to measure the largest vertical distance to the cord, either above or below but not through the cord (Magann et al., 2002).

  The horizontal component of the vertical dimension must be at least 1 cm (See **Chapter 6**, *Antepartum fetal surveillance*).
- In multiple gestation, the SDP of each sac is measured to assess individual amniotic fluid volume.
- SDP is interpreted as follows (Reddy et al., 2014):
  - Oligohydramnios   ≤2 cm
  - Normal   ≥2 cm and <8 cm
  - Polyhydramnios   ≥8 cm

Amniotic fluid index (AFI) measurement

- The uterus is divided into four quadrants using the linea nigra for the right and left divisions and the umbilicus for the upper and lower quadrants.
- Using ultrasound, the maximal vertical amniotic fluid pocket diameter in each quadrant (not containing cord or fetal extremities) is measured. The sum of the four measurements (in centimetres) is called AFI.
- AFI is interpreted as follows:
  - Oligohydramnios ≤5 cm
  - Normal   >5 cm and <24 cm
  - Polyhydramnios   ≥24 cm

Single deepest pocket vs. amniotic fluid index: Which is the better technique?
A systematic review of the Cochrane Database (Nabhan AF and Abdelmoula YA, 2008) concluded that the **SDP measurement in the assessment of amniotic fluid volume during fetal surveillance was a better choice**. The use of the AFI leads to an overdiagnosis of oligohydramnios and an increase in the rate of induction of labour without improvement in perinatal outcomes. This recommendation was reinforced by the SAFE randomised controlled trial (Kehl et al., 2016).

Oligohydramnios

- Oligohydramnios refers to amniotic fluid volume that is less than expected for a particular gestational age. It is most often diagnosed in the third trimester and the majority of cases are due to an unknown etiology (Beloosesky, 2018).
- Oligohydamnios is defined as an SDP ≤2 cm or an AFI ≤5 cm.
- The common causes of oligohydramnios that require follow-up and management are as follows:
  - Growth restriction
  - Fetal congenital anomaly, especially of the urinary tract
  - Postdated pregnancy
  - Leaking membranes
- Abnormal umbilical and middle cerebral artery Doppler studies help corroborate the diagnosis of oligohydramnios resulting from poor placental function.
- Idiopathic oligohydramnios can be treated with oral or intravenous hydration with good results.

 Sildenafil should not be used in idiopathic oligohydramnios because of reports of higher than expected rates of lung disease and death of newborns in the intervention group (Hawkes, 2018).

Polyhydramnios

- Polyhydramnios is the excessive accumulation of amniotic fluid. It is associated with an increased risk of unfavourable pregnancy outcomes.
- An ultrasound is indicated in the third trimester to rule out polyhydramnios when the uterine size is significantly larger than the gestational age.
- Polyhydramnios is usually defined as an SDP ≥8 cm or an AFI ≥24 cm.

 Polyhydramnios is typically caused by conditions that lead to the following:
- Decreased fetal swallowing or
- Increased fetal urination

- Polyhydramnios is commonly caused by the following:
  - Fetal structural anomaly/anomalies that interfere with fetal swallowing
    - Anencephaly
    - Esophageal atresia
    - Congenital diaphragmatic hernia
    - Thoracic masses
  - Increased fetal urine production
    - Fetal anemia leading to cardiac failure
    - Fetal Bartter syndrome (associated with polyuria and sodium loss)
  - Fetal chromosomal abnormality (e.g., trisomy 18)
  - Twin–twin transfusion syndrome
  - Fetal neuromuscular disorders (e.g., arthrogryposis)
  - Fetal infection (e.g., parvovirus)

– Maternal diabetes mellitus—since fetal glycosuria is the underlying cause, polyhydramnios is more often associated with poor glycemic control

V. Evaluation/follow-up of placental location

Third-trimester follow-up of placenta previa

- Though 1–6 per cent of pregnant women are found to have evidence of placenta previa in the second trimester, the majority of these women are asymptomatic. 90 per cent of these early cases resolve spontaneously (Oyelese 2006).

> **Persistence till delivery**
> If the placenta extends ≥2.5 cm beyond the internal os at 20–24 weeks, vaginal delivery is almost certainly ruled out since there is a greater chance of persistence till delivery (Becker et al., 2001).

- It has been recommended that third-trimester scans to assess placenta previa be limited to cases where the placental edge either reaches or overlaps the internal cervical os at 20–24 weeks of pregnancy (Bhide and Thilaganathan, 2004).
- In a retrospective study, Dashe et al. (2002) concluded that the gestational age at which the previa was identified by ultrasound is a good indicator of persistence of placenta previa at term. The type of placentation (low-lying or complete) and prior cesarean delivery are important factors that modify the risk of previa complicating delivery (Table 12.2). Placenta previa identified in the third trimester tends to persist. The later the previa is identified, the greater the risk of persistence. After 28 weeks, the presence or absence of a prior cesarean scar does not seem to make a difference.
- At the 36 weeks' follow-up, if the placental edge is lying over the internal os, cesarean delivery is indicated. A trial of labour is a possibility if the placental edge is <2 cm but >1 cm from the internal os (low-lying), and but does not cover the internal os. The risk of bleeding increases as the distance between the placental edge and internal os decreases, and in the presence of vasa previa. When the distance between the placental edge and the internal os is ≤2 cm, the frequency of an emergency section for profuse bleeding is 45 per cent. The decision to attempt vaginal delivery in this situation should be taken after discussion with the couple and must be based on the availability of blood products and immediate access to a theatre with a surgical team, including an anesthetist (see **Chapter 31**, *Antepartum hemorrhage*).

Table 12.2   Risk of persistence of placenta previa at term in relation to identification in the third trimester (Dashe et al., 2002)

Placenta previa identified at	Risk of persistence at term with *no previous cesarean* (%)	Risk of persistence at term with *previous cesarean* (%)
24–27 weeks	56	84
28–31 weeks	88–89	88–89
32–35 weeks	89–90	89–90

In the presence of a persistent anterior placenta previa and a prior cesarean scar, it is mandatory to rule out morbidly adherent placenta (see **Chapter 11**, *Ultrasound in the second trimester*).

VI. Evaluation of vaginal bleeding of placental etiology

Placenta previa

- A high presenting part, an abnormal lie, and painless or provoked bleeding, irrespective of previous imaging results are suggestive of a low-lying placenta.
- While clinical acumen remains vitally important in suspecting and managing placenta previa, the definitive diagnosis of most low-lying placentas is now achieved with ultrasound imaging.
- *Transvaginal* scanning is superior to transabdominal ultrasound in providing a clearer image of the relationship between the edge of the placenta and the internal cervical os. *Translabial (perineal)* sonography is an excellent alternative in the presence of bleeding.

Placental abruption

- The diagnosis of placental abruption is primarily clinical, but ultrasonography can be used as a valuable adjunct in diagnosis and management of abruption.
- The appearance of abruption on ultrasonography varies depending on the size, location, and time elapsed since the onset of abruption.
- A retroplacental hematoma is the classic ultrasound finding and strongly supports the clinical diagnosis. However, this is absent in many patients with abruption.

Though the sensitivity of ultrasound for the detection of placental abruption is poor, it is highly specific. Identifying abruption on ultrasound invariably means that it is a significant bleed, and is associated with increased maternal morbidity, requires more aggressive obstetric management, and is associated with worse perinatal outcome, especially in preterm pregnancies (Shinde et al., 2016).

- An acute retroplacental hematoma may appear solid, complex, and hyper- or iso-echoic in comparison to the placenta. A hypoechoic appearance will result only after a few hours, when liquefaction of the hematoma has occurred.
- Location and extent of abruption correlate with fetal mortality. The volume of the hematoma (estimated by length × width × height/2) and the extent of placental detachment are the most accurate predictors of pregnancy outcome.
- A hematoma larger than 50 mL or a placental detachment greater than 50 per cent indicates a guarded neonatal prognosis.
- In the presence of placental abruption, ultrasound also helps in evaluating fetal lie and estimated fetal weight, which may play a role in management decisions.

VII. Determination of fetal presentation

- Fetal presentation should be assessed using clinical examination at each antenatal visit in the late second and third trimester. If a fetal malpresentation is suspected during clinical examination, it should be confirmed by ultrasound evaluation.

- In a breech presentation, ultrasonography can also establish the type of breech presentation by imaging the fetal femurs and their relationship to the distal bones.

 It has been shown that ultrasound in the third trimester is better than clinical evaluation in determining fetal presentation and should be used to confirm suspected malpresentation (Nassar et al., 2006).

- In case of malpresentations, it is important to exclude any causative factors (e.g., polyhydramnios, low-lying placenta, or fetal anomaly) that may influence management decisions and the mode of delivery.

VIII. Evaluation of suspected fetal death

- Auscultation of the fetal heart by a Pinard stethoscope or hand-held Doppler device is insufficiently accurate for the diagnosis of intrauterine fetal death (IUFD) because it can give false reassurance—

 Absent cardiac activity on direct visualisation of the fetal heart on ultrasound examination is the definitive test for confirming IUFD (Fretts, 2005).

maternal pelvic blood flow can result in an apparently normal fetal heart rate pattern.

- Imaging can be technically difficult, particularly in the presence of maternal obesity, abdominal scars, and oligohydramnios, but views can often be augmented with colour Doppler of the fetal heart and umbilical cord.

- In addition to the absence of fetal cardiac activity, other secondary features might be seen such as the collapse of the fetal skull with overlapping bones (Spalding sign), hydrops, or maceration resulting in an unrecognisable fetal mass.

- Intrafetal gas (within the heart, blood vessels, and joints) is a late feature when there is delay in recognising IUFD.

Previous history of stillbirth

- Third-trimester screening is recommended in otherwise healthy women with a history of a previous stillbirth.

- It is recommended that antepartum fetal surveillance be initiated two weeks before the gestational age at which the stillbirth occurred in the previous pregnancy (Spong, 2012).

IX. Evaluation of multiple pregnancies

- Serial ultrasound examination is recommended in multiple pregnancies.

- Third-trimester ultrasound examination helps to:
  - Assess growth (concordant or discordant)
  - Identify development of any complications
  - Decide on the best mode of delivery

See **Chapter 35**, *Multiple pregnancy* for further details.

X. Ultrasound as an adjunct to external cephalic version

- External cephalic version (ECV) is the manipulation of the breech fetus, through the maternal abdomen, to a cephalic presentation. It is best done at 37 weeks of gestation (RCOG, 2017; ACOG, 2016).
- This procedure decreases the number of breech presentations in labour and consequently decreases the frequency of cesarean delivery by approximately 40 per cent (Hofmeyr et al., 2015).
- Prior to the procedure, ultrasound examination is used to assess fetal position, amniotic fluid volume, placental location, and fetal weight to help determine if the procedure should be performed and the likelihood of success. After the procedure, ultrasound helps confirm the presentation and well-being of the fetus. The steps of ECV are described in greater detail in **Chapter 22**, *Breech delivery*.
- A meta-analysis (Grootscholten et al., 2008) showed that ECV is a safe procedure and successful in 58 per cent of cases.
- The procedure is well demonstrated on the World Health Organization's Reproductive Health Library website (*https://extranet.who.int/rhl/resources/videos/external-cephalic-version-why-and-how*).

References

1. American College of Obstetricians and Gynecologists. 2016 (reaffirmed 2018). ACOG Practice Bulletin No. 161. External cephalic version. *Obstet Gynecol.* 127:e54.

2. Becker RH, Vonk R, Mende BC et al. 2001. The relevance of placental location at 20–23 gestational weeks for prediction of placenta previa at delivery: Evaluation of 8650 cases. *Ultrasound Obstet Gynecol.* 17: 496–501.

3. Beloosesky R, Ross MG. 2018. Oligohydramnios. Simpson LL, Levine D (Eds). *UpToDate*. Waltham, MA.

4. Bhide A, Thilaganathan B. 2004. Recent advances in the management of placenta previa. *Curr Opin Obstet Gynecol.* 16:447–51.

5. Bricker L, Medley N, Pratt JJ. 2015. Routine ultrasound in late pregnancy (after 24 weeks' gestation). *Cochrane Database Syst Rev.* Issue 6. Art. no.: CD001451.

6. Combs CA, Rosenn B, Miodovnik M, Siddiqi TA. 2000. Sonographic EFW and macrosomia: Is there an optimum formula to predict diabetic fetal macrosomia? *J Matern Fetal Med.* 9:55.

7. Coomarasamy A, Connock M, Thornton J, Khan KS. 2005. Accuracy of ultrasound biometry in the prediction of macrosomia: A systematic quantitative review. *BJOG.* 112: 1461–1466.

8. Dashe JS, McIntire DD, Ramus RM, Santos-Ramos R, Twickle DM. 2002. Persistence of placenta previa according to gestational age at ultrasound detection. *Obstet Gynecol.* 99:692–7.

9. de Jong CL, Francis A, van Geijn HP, Gardosi J. 1999. Fetal growth rate and adverse perinatal events. *Ultrasound Obstet Gynecol.* 13:86.

10. Divon MY. 2018. Fetal growth restriction: Diagnosis. Levin D (Ed). *UpToDate*. Waltham, MA.

11. Dommergues M, Benachi A, Benifla JL, des Noettes R, Dumez Y. 1999. The reasons for termination of pregnancy in the third trimester. *Br J Obstet Gynaecol.* 106(4):297–303.

12. Ferrazzi E, Nicolini U, Kustermann A, Pardi G. 1986. Routine obstetric ultrasound: Effectiveness of cross-sectional screening for fetal growth retardation. *J Clin Ultrasound.* 14:17.

13. Fretts RC. 2005. Etiology and prevention of stillbirth. *Am J Obstet Gynecol.* 193:1923–35.

14. Grootscholten K, Kok M, Oei SG et al. 2008. External cephalic version-related risks: A meta-analysis. *Obstet Gynecol.* 112:1143.

15. Guidetti DA, Divon MY, Braverman JJ et al. 1990. Sonographic estimates of fetal weight in the intrauterine growth retardation population. *Am J Perinatol.* 7:5.

16. Hawkes N. 2018. Trial of Viagra for fetal growth restriction is halted after baby deaths. *BMJ.* 362:k3247.

17. Hofmeyr GJ, Kulier R, West HM. 2015. External cephalic version for breech presentation at term. *Cochrane Database Syst Rev.* Issue 4. Art. no.: CD000083.

18. Hoopmann M, Abele H, Wagner N et al. 2010. Performance of 36 different weight estimation formulae in fetuses with macrosomia. *Fetal Diagn Ther.* 27:204.

19. Kehl S, Schelkle A, Thomas A, Puhl A et al., 2016. Single deepest vertical pocket or amniotic fluid index as evaluation test for predicting adverse pregnancy outcome (SAFE trial): A multicenter, open label, randomized controlled trial. *Ultrasound Obstet Gynecol.* 47(6):674-9.

20. Kiserud T, Piaggio G, Carroli G et al. 2017. The World Health Organization fetal growth charts: A multinational longitudinal study of ultrasound biometric measurements and estimated fetal weight. *PLoS Med.* 14:e1002220.

21. Koyanagi A, Zhang J, Dagvadorj A, Hirayama F, Shibuya K, Souza JP et al. 2013. Macrosomia in 23 developing countries: An analysis of a multicountry, facility-based, cross-sectional survey. *Lancet.* 381(9865):476–483.

22. Magann EF, Chauhan SP, Washington W et al. 2002. Ultrasound estimation of amniotic fluid volume using the largest vertical pocket containing umbilical cord: Measure to or through the cord? *Ultrasound Obstet Gynecol.* 20:464.

23. Mongelli M, Ek S, Tambyraja R. 1998. Screening for fetal growth restriction: A mathematical model of the effect of time interval and ultrasound error. *Obstet Gynecol.* 92:908.

24. Nabhan AF, Abdelmoula YA. 2008. Amniotic fluid index versus single deepest vertical pocket as a screening test for preventing adverse pregnancy outcome. *Cochrane Database Syst Rev.* Issue 3. Art. no.: CD006593.

25. Nassar N, Roberts CL, Cameron CA, Olive EC. 2006. Diagnostic accuracy of clinical examination for detection of non-cephalic presentation in late pregnancy: Cross-sectional analytic study. *BMJ.* 333(7568):578–80.

26. Oyelese Y. 2009. Placenta previa: The evolving role of ultrasound. *Ultrasound Obstet Gynecol.* 34: 123-126.

27. Papageorghiou AT, Kennedy SH, Salomon LJ, Altman DG, Ohuma EO et al. 2018. The INTERGROWTH-21st fetal growth standards: Toward the global integration of pregnancy and pediatric care. *Am J of Obstet & Gynec.* Volume 218, Issue 2, S630–S640.

28. Ray C, Grangé G. 2016. Routine third trimester ultrasound in low-risk pregnancy confers no benefit: AGAINST: Arguments for a routine third trimester ultrasound: What the meta-analysis does not show! *BJOG: Int J Obstet Gy.* 123: 1122–1122.

29. RCOG Green-top Guideline No. 20a. 2017. External Cephalic Version and Reducing the Incidence of Term Breech Presentation.

30. Reddy UM, Abuhamad AZ, Levine D et al. 2014. Fetal imaging: Executive summary of a joint Eunice Kennedy Shriver National Institute of Child Health and Human Development, Society for Maternal-

Fetal Medicine, American Institute of Ultrasound in Medicine, American College of Obstetricians and Gynecologists, American College of Radiology, Society for Pediatric Radiology, and Society of Radiologists in Ultrasound Fetal Imaging workshop. *Obstet Gynecol.* 123:1070.

31. Saccone G, Sendek K. 2016. Prenatal care in obstetric evidence-based guidelines. Vincenzo Berghella (Ed.). Taylor and Francis, CRC Press.

32. Shinde GR, Vaswani BP, Patange RP et al. 2016. Diagnostic performance of ultrasonography for detection of abruption and its clinical correlation and maternal and foetal outcome. *J Clin Diagn Res.* 10:QC04.

33. Spong CY. 2012. Add stillbirth to the list of outcomes to worry about in a pregnant woman with a history of preterm birth or fetal growth restriction. *Obstet Gynecol.* 119:495.

34. Sylvan K, Ryding EL, Rydhstroem H. 2005. Routine ultrasound screening in the third trimester: A population-based study. *Acta Obstetricia et Gynecologica Scandinavica.* 84: 1154–1158.

35. Sovio U, White IR, Dacey A et al. 2015. Screening for fetal growth restriction with universal third trimester ultrasonography in nulliparous women in the pregnancy outcome prediction (POP) study: A prospective cohort study. *Lancet.* 386:2089.

36. Thornton J. 2016. Routine third trimester ultrasound in low-risk pregnancy confers no benefit. FOR: The benefits of routine third-trimester scanning are less clear cut. *BJOG.* 123: 1121–1121.

37. Zhang J, Mikolajczyk R, Grewal J et al. 2011. Prenatal application of the individualized fetal growth reference. *Am J Epidemiol.* 173:539.

Chapter 13

Respectful Maternity Care: A Human Right

INTRODUCTION

- For most couples, childbirth is a life-changing experience. Across all cultural, geographic, and economic strata, women who opt for motherhood want only one thing: a safe passage for themselves and their baby. They desire respectful and responsible care from their caregivers.

 It is a basic human right to receive a positive, evidence-based, equitable, compassionate, and respectful childbirth experience.

- In 2016, the World Health Organization released recommendations on antenatal care for a positive pregnancy experience (WHO, 2016). In 2018, it released similar guidelines on intrapartum care for a positive childbirth experience (WHO, 2018) to ensure that women not only survive childbirth but 'have a sense of control through involvement in decision-making, which leaves them with a sense of personal achievement'.

 It is well-established that substandard quality of care (including disrespectful and abusive behaviour) is a significant factor leading to maternal morbidity and mortality (Bowser and Hill, 2010).

- Disrespectful and abusive behaviour in labour rooms is a global problem (Bohren et al., 2015; Freedman and Kruk, 2014). It is the responsibility of the healthcare provider to ensure that she and her team consciously work towards showing compassion and respect to the birthing mother and allow her to go through the process with her dignity and modesty intact.
- The training for compassionate care should start in medical colleges and teaching institutions. The senior teachers should lead by example.

OVER-MEDICALISATION OF LABOUR AND CHILDBIRTH

- India is a country that suffers from enormous inequity in the delivery of healthcare to mothers and their babies.
- On one hand, we have areas (mostly rural and the urban poor) where the care offered is **too little, too late**. The lack of facilities (too little) leads to maternal as well as perinatal morbidity and mortality because of delay in appropriate interventions (too late).
- On the other hand, urban India has seen an explosion of interventions leading to the over-medicalisation of maternity care. This results in **too much, too soon**. The outcome of this

is the inappropriate use of unnecessary, non-evidence-based interventions (too much). Inductions, augmentation, and cesarean sections are carried out before allowing enough time for labour to progress (too soon).

- Since 2005, the Government of India, along with other agencies, has brought out guidelines for maternal healthcare. Though they are sound clinically and present the scope and purpose with clarity, Indian guidelines have weak documentation about their development process (Sonawane et al., 2015). They rely heavily on international recommendations and are unclear on how they were adapted to local conditions (Mehndiratta et al., 2017).
- Practitioners either choose international guidelines or develop local practices that are not evidence-based. Across most countries, there exists a large gap between the knowledge of appropriate care and the actual care delivered—the so-called 'know–do gap' (Miller et al., 2016).

DISRESPECTFUL AND ABUSIVE BEHAVIOUR IN LABOUR AND CHILDBIRTH

- Over recent years, one of the measures of good maternal healthcare is the evaluation of how many women in a state have institutional delivery. This rate has gone up in many states in India by demand generation, community mobilisation, education, financial incentives, and policy measures. Almost all state governments and the central government have created schemes to financially incentivise pregnant women to deliver in facilities.

- However, many women leave institutions (both public and private) where they have had their childbirth experience with bitter memories of disrespectful treatment that dehumanises them.

In India, most maternity care during labour is provided by women (obstetricians, midwives, nurses, and trained birth attendants). It is therefore doubly heartbreaking that it is women who abuse women in labour with such regularity, when in fact, they should be expected to have much more empathy and compassion for another woman undergoing so much pain and tribulation.

The reason for this norm is the insensitive treatment in the labour room that generations of nurses, medical students, and postgraduates are exposed to in teaching institutions. Unless the change comes from the top-down, women will continue to receive below par treatment.

- Disrespectful and abusive treatment during childbirth includes the following (WHO, 2014):
  - Outright physical abuse (slapping, pinching, manhandling)
  - Profound humiliation and verbal abuse
  - Gross violations of privacy
  - Lack of concern for a woman's modesty
  - Refusal to give pain medication
  - Refusal to allow a family member in the labour room for support
  - Lack of confidentiality
  - Coercive or unconsented medical procedures (including insertion of postpartum IUCDs and sterilisation)
  - Failure to get fully informed consent

- Refusal of admission to health facilities
- Neglecting women during childbirth, resulting in life-threatening but avoidable complications
- Refusal to discharge women and their newborns in facilities after childbirth due to an inability to pay
- Adolescent girls, unmarried women, women from low socio-economic groups, women from ethnic minorities, migrant women, and women living with HIV are particularly likely to experience disrespectful and abusive treatment (WHO, 2014).

MEASURES FOR RESPECTFUL AND HUMANE TREATMENT DURING LABOUR

Many of the measures discussed below have also been advocated in the LaQshya-Labour Room Quality Improvement Initiative by the National Health Mission, Ministry of Health and Family Welfare, Government of India (2018).

Preparing the couple for labour and childbirth

- It must be recognised that every woman approaches labour with fear and apprehension, and not just in her first pregnancy. Educating women about what to expect in labour goes a long way in making them less apprehensive.
- Some private hospitals offer classes/lectures/information for couples who will soon face labour. It is important for public facilities that cater to low-income communities to also provide information in the form of classes/graphic pamphlets to enable every woman and her husband/family to be prepared for labour.

Respectful care during labour

- All women want to be treated with kindness, empathy, and dignity during labour and childbirth.
- We talk about letting someone 'die with dignity' but unfortunately, the concept of letting a woman 'labour with dignity' is superseded by the caregiver's authority and decisions. The woman is often stripped of all autonomy when she enters the labour room.

Women will change their obstetrician/place of delivery and will also not recommend such healthcare providers to others if they have experienced degrading and unacceptable behaviour (D'Ambruoso et al., 2005).

- Humane and respectful procedures to follow while receiving the patient into the labour room include the following:
  - Greeting her with a smile
  - Introducing yourself, if the mother is seeing you for the first time
  - Being calm and polite
  - Using the respectful form of addressing (using formal pronouns typical of the vernaculam) even if she is younger than you
  - Explaining briefly what will happen next

- Explaining any procedure that will be carried out (e.g., amniotomy, local or regional analgesia, ventouse or forceps application) and gently warning her about the discomfort she will face during that procedure
- Being kind and gentle during pelvic examinations
- Listening to the woman as she expresses herself

> Women want to be treated with dignity. Several studies have shown that women across the globe believe that the nurse, midwife, or doctor should inform them and get their permission before performing a potentially embarrassing and painful procedure like a pelvic examination (Bhattacharyya et al., 2015; Ying Lai and Levy, 2002).

- Labouring women are at their most vulnerable. They are in pain and frightened beyond belief. They must be allowed to maintain their dignity in the face of the intense experience of labour.
- While attending to a woman in labour, do not:
  - Raise your voice or scold the mother
  - Use abusive language
  - Humiliate her verbally
  - Pinch or slap her
  - Threaten to walk out if she does not stop crying or screaming
  - Leave her half-naked/naked and exposed in the labour room

Communication with the mother and family

It is important for effective communication to be maintained between the maternity care providers and the woman in labour (WHO, 2018). There is no excuse for rudeness and meanness. The following are suggestions for ensuring clarity and promoting trust:

- Keep your explanations simple and use language that can be understood by the mother and her family.
- Avoid medical jargon and use pictorial and graphic materials when needed to communicate processes or procedures.
- Update the mother and her family about what is happening—this can be done as often as feasible, depending upon the work load.
- Do not be condescending; do not avoid explaining what is happening on the assumption that 'she/they won't understand anyway'.
- The language of kindness is universal; it is not what the patient understands that is always important, but the reassurance she feels. Women have repeatedly vocalised in several studies that they were reassured by the kindness and empathy shown even if they did not always understand the explanation offered by their caregiver.

> Nurses and doctors sometimes feel overwhelmed in overcrowded and busy labour facilities. Nevertheless, it is important that they spend time communicating with the patient. There is no excuse for rudeness and meanness. Reassurance with a few kind words goes a long way in alleviating the mother's discomfort.

Privacy in the labour room

- Privacy and the ability to maintain her modesty in the labour room is a basic human right that every mother should receive (Miltenburg et al., 2016).
- Even in the most low-resource areas, a curtain or screen should be provided to protect the woman's privacy.
- The woman should have the upper half of the body clothed and the lower half covered with a sheet. Even in the poorest setting, the woman can at least be covered with an old sari.
- Non-medical staff members (especially male) should not be allowed to wander in and out of the labour room.

Pain relief

- Women should be offered pain relief in labour (see **Chapter 17**, *Pain relief in labour*). They should not be made to feel ashamed for requesting pain relief.
- The type of analgesia offered depends on the resources available.
- If feasible, women should be offered early pain relief. Since opioids like pethidine may not be always available, intramuscular tramadol may be offered. Paracetamol 600 mg IM is proving to be useful in alleviating the pain of labour to a certain extent in low-resource areas where opioids are not available.
- Epidural analgesia is the best form of pain relief in labour but its availability is limited by the lack of the required facilities, trained personnel, and the expense. In hospitals with the available facilities, epidural analgesia has proven very successful in pain relief in labour.

Companionship and support during labour and childbirth

- Every woman deserves to have a person of her choosing by her side during labour and delivery.
- Though some private facilities in India have adopted the practice of allowing husbands/ family members in the labour room, most public facilities end up isolating the woman from her family.

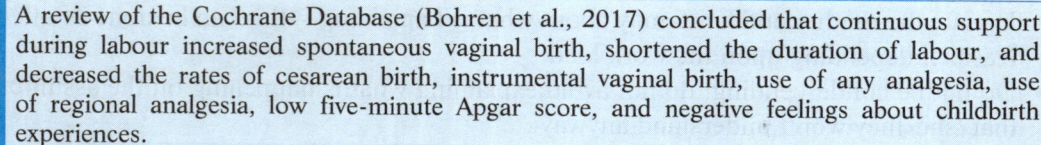

A review of the Cochrane Database (Bohren et al., 2017) concluded that continuous support during labour increased spontaneous vaginal birth, shortened the duration of labour, and decreased the rates of cesarean birth, instrumental vaginal birth, use of any analgesia, use of regional analgesia, low five-minute Apgar score, and negative feelings about childbirth experiences.

- The WHO recommends a companion who can be 'any person chosen by the woman to provide her with continuous support during labour and childbirth'. This may be someone from the woman's family or spouse/partner, a female friend or relative, or a community member.
- In low-resource areas, crowded facilities and the lack of space often limit the availability of a companion during labour. To protect the privacy of other mothers in the labour room, men are usually not allowed in as support companions in public hospitals in India.

In summary, training in medical colleges and postgraduate institutions should necessarily include sensitivity training to exhibit kindness, compassion, and respect for the labouring mother.

References

1. Bhattacharyya S, Issac A, Rajbangshi P, Srivastava A, Avan BI. 2015. Neither we are satisfied nor they–users and provider's perspective: A qualitative study of maternity care in secondary level public health facilities, Uttar Pradesh, India. *BMC Health Serv Res.* 15:421.

2. Bohren MA, Vogel JP, Hunter EC, Lutsiv O, Makh SK, Souza JP et al. 2015. The mistreatment of women during childbirth in health facilities globally: A mixed-methods systematic review. *PLoS Med.* 12:e1001847.

3. Bowser D, Hill K. 2010. Exploring evidence for disrespect and abuse in facility-based childbirth. Report of a landscape analysis. USAID-TRAction Project. Harvard School of Public Health: University Research Co., LLC.

4. D'Ambruoso L, Abbey M, Hussein J. 2005. Please understand when I cry out in pain: Women's accounts of maternity services during labour and delivery in Ghana. *BMC Public Health.* 5:140.

5. Freedman LP, Kruk ME. 2014. Disrespect and abuse of women in childbirth: Challenging the global quality and accountability agendas. *Lancet.* 384:e42–4.

6. LaQshya Guidelines. 2018. http://nhm.gov.in/New_Updates_2018/NHM_Components/RMNCH_MH_Guidelines/LaQshya-Guidelines.pdf

7. Mehndiratta A, Sharma S, Gupta NP et al. 2017. Adapting clinical guidelines in India: A pragmatic approach. BMJ (*Clinical research ed.*). 359, j5147.

8. Miller S, Abalos E, Chamillard M et al. 2016. Beyond too little, too late and too much, too soon: A pathway towards evidence-based, respectful maternity care worldwide. *Lancet.* 388(10056):2176-2192.

9. Miltenburg AS, Lambermon F, Hamelink C, Meguid T. 2016. Maternity care and human rights: What do women think? *BMC Int Health Hum Rights.* 16:17.

10. Sonawane DB, Karvande SS, Cluzeau FA et al. 2015. Appraisal of maternity management and family planning guidelines using the agree II instrument in India. *Indian J Public Health.* 59:264-71.

11. World Health Organization. 2014. The prevention and elimination of disrespect and abuse during facility-based childbirth. WHO, Geneva.

12. World Health Organization. 2016. WHO Recommendations on Antenatal Care for a Positive Pregnancy Experience. WHO, Geneva.

13. World Health Organization. 2018. WHO Recommendations: Intrapartum Care for a Positive Childbirth Experience. WHO, Geneva.

14. Ying Lai C, Levy V. 2002. Hong Kong Chinese women's experiences of vaginal examinations in labour. *Midwifery.* 18:296–303.

Chapter 14

Normal Labour and Delivery: Evidence-Based Management

INTRODUCTION

- Normal birth is defined as the spontaneous birth of an infant in the vertex position between 37 and 42 weeks of pregnancy after spontaneous onset of labour in a low-risk pregnancy that remains low-risk throughout labour and delivery. At the end of the process, the mother and baby are in good health. Giving birth to a healthy baby in a clinically and psychologically safe environment is an important part of a positive childbirth experience (WHO, 2018).
- This chapter deals with specific evidence-based recommendations for the management of normal labour and delivery.

ADMISSION TO HOSPITAL

- When a woman presents to the hospital in labour, an initial assessment should be performed to determine whether the mother is in labour or not.

 It is important that the labouring woman receives respectful, empathetic treatment and obstetric care right from her initial presentation to the facility (see **Chapter 13**, *Respectful maternity care: a human right*).

- If she is in labour (presence of regular, painful contractions, and cervical dilatation greater than 3 cm), the woman should be admitted to the hospital and supported appropriately, even in early labour. If the woman lives close to the hospital and wants to wait at home for active labour, the woman should be allowed to do so (WHO, 2018a).
- If it is not clear that the woman is in labour, she should be encouraged to walk around or relax, and the cervix should be reassessed after 2–4 hours, depending on how strong the uterine contractions are.

ADMISSION TO THE LABOUR ROOM/WARD

It is reasonable to delay admission to the labour room until the woman is in the **active stage of labour**. She can be observed in the room or ward until she is in active labour.

 The definitions of the latent and active phases of labour have undergone changes in the past decade. Data from the Consortium on Safe Labor (Zhang et al., 2010) and the WHO Recommendations for Intrapartum Care (WHO, 2018) provide the following definitions:

Latent phase: The latent phase is a period of time characterised by painful uterine contractions and variable changes of the cervix, including some degree of effacement and slow progression of dilatation up to 5 cm for the first and subsequent labours.

Active phase: The active phase of the first stage is a period of time characterised by regular and painful uterine contractions, a substantial degree of cervical effacement and more rapid cervical dilatation from 5 cm to full dilatation for first and subsequent labours.

The active phase is also the maximal slope in the rate of change of cervical dilatation over time and often does not start until at least 6 cm (ACOG, 2014).

The median duration of the active first stage is 4 hours in first labours and 3 hours in second and subsequent labours, when the reference starting point is 5 cm cervical dilatation.

INITIAL EXAMINATION ON ADMISSION

The aims of the initial examination are to determine:

- Maternal health (documentation of blood pressure, pulse rate, and temperature)
- Presence of fetal heartbeat and to assess fetal well-being
- Whether membranes are intact or ruptured
- Presence of normal or excessive vaginal bleeding
- Cervical dilatation and effacement
- Station of fetal presenting part
- Fetal lie, presentation, and position
- Fetal weight and clinical assessment of pelvic capacity (though clinical pelvimetry need not be done)

- The mother's antenatal records must be available in the labour room.
- Her blood group and Rh type must be clearly noted.
- Any medical/obstetric complications must be reviewed.

PREPARATION

- **Enema:** There is no evidence to support routinely administering an enema prior to delivery (Reveiz et al., 2013). However, if the mother is constipated and requests an enema, she may be given one for the sake of comfort during labour.

 If a mother complains of an urge to pass motion, a vaginal examination must be done to ensure that the urge is not due to the fetal head lying low in the vagina and causing rectal pressure.

- **Shaving of pubic hair and perineum:** There is no evidence to support the need to shave pubic hair or the perineum (Basevi and Lavender, 2014). The perineum alone may be shaved, in the area below the fourchette, if an episiotomy is being considered or deemed to be necessary, or if a tear is being sutured. This is only to make it easier to place sutures and prevent the discomfort caused by hair getting caught in sutures.
- **Bladder emptying:** The mother should be encouraged to empty her bladder as often as she wants during labour. Catheterisation is usually not indicated.

ORAL INTAKE

The Practice Guidelines for Obstetric Anesthesia (2016) and the ACOG (2019) recommend the following:

Liquids

- Women considered low-risk (no antenatal or intrapartum complications) may be allowed to have sips of water/non-particulate fruit juices during labour.
- If oral fluids are being restricted because of an increased risk of cesarean birth, then maintenance intravenous fluids with 5 per cent dextrose in 0.45 per cent saline, normal saline, or lactated Ringer's solution may be administered.
- The uncomplicated mother undergoing elective surgery (e.g., scheduled cesarean delivery or postpartum tubal ligation) may have moderate amounts of clear liquids up to two hours before induction of anesthesia.

 Earlier concerns about neonatal hypoglycemia and lower umbilical cord pH values with the use of 5 per cent dextrose-containing fluids have not been borne out by recent RCTs. 5 per cent dextrose in normal saline can be used safely in the labour room.

If a labouring woman requires an emergency cesarean section, she may be given H_2-receptor antagonists (e.g., ranitidine 50 mg IV) and/or metoclopramide to prevent complications of anesthetic aspiration.

Solids

- Solid foods should be avoided for women in labour (ACOG, 2019).
- The woman undergoing elective surgery (e.g., scheduled cesarean delivery or postpartum tubal ligation) should not have solids for 6–8 hours prior to surgery.

ANTIBIOTICS

Prophylactic antibiotics

- Vaginal delivery is not an indication for routine antibiotic prophylaxis (see **Chapter 26**, *Prophylactic antibiotics in obstetrics*).
- Endocarditis prophylaxis is not recommended in women with cardiac lesions since the rate of bacteremia is low with vaginal delivery.

Therapeutic antibiotics

- Antibiotics are indicated in the presence of suspected chorioamnionitis. The signs and symptoms may include the following:
  - Ruptured membranes >18 hrs
  - Maternal temperature of ≥38°C
  - Foul-smelling vaginal discharge
  - Maternal tachycardia >100/min
  - Fetal tachycardia >160/min
  - Uterine tenderness
- In the presence of these signs and symptoms, a high vaginal smear is recommended for culture and sensitivity. The mother should then started on any of the following (Tita, 2019):
  - Ampicillin 2 g IV every six hours PLUS gentamicin 5 mg/kg IV once daily OR
  - Cefuroxime 1.5 g IV every 8 hours OR

- Ampicillin-sulbactam 3 g IV every six hours OR
- Cefotetan 2 g IV every 12 hours

MATERNAL ACTIVITY

- The WHO recommendations for intrapartum care (2018) encourage mobility in women at low risk. They also discourage enforced confinement to the bed in these women. The mother should be allowed to walk, sit, or lie down according to her preference.
- Walking during the first stage neither improves nor worsens active labour but certainly is not harmful to the mother or the fetus (Bloom et al., 1998).

PAIN RELIEF

See **Chapter 17,** *Pain relief in labour.*

AMNIOTOMY

- Amniotomy (artificial rupture of membranes or AROM) by itself has not been shown to shorten the first or second stage of labour or reduce the rate of cesarean delivery in women who have spontaneous onset of labour (Smyth et al., 2013).
- In high-risk women, amniotomy allows the obstetrician to check for meconium which, when present, may warrant enhanced monitoring of fetal status.
- Women undergoing augmentation or induction of labour have been shown to benefit from the combination of oxytocin administration and amniotomy (see **Chapter 19,** *Induction of labour*).

Practical considerations for amniotomy
- Amniotomy should be performed under strict aseptic precautions.
- It is best done after 3–4 cm cervical dilatation and with an engaged presenting part.
- The author suggests using the left hand for the vaginal examination and the right hand to perform the amniotomy (for right-handed individuals) for better control over the instrument.
- An amniotomy hook may be used, but if it is not available, an Allis forceps may be used.
- **Controlled amniotomy:** When there is polyhydramnios or an unengaged presenting part, the examining fingers must be kept over the amniotomy site so that the fluid is released in a controlled manner. This minimises the risk of amniotic fluid gushing out rapidly and prevents umbilical cord prolapse. This also allows the operator to guide the unengaged head so that it drops gently into the pelvis as the fluid is released.
- The fetal heart must be monitored after the amniotomy. Prolonged bradycardia may indicate an occult umbilical cord prolapse.

MONITORING OF UTERINE CONTRACTIONS

- Monitoring of uterine contractions is a very important aspect of monitoring the progress of labour (see **Chapter 20,** *Abnormal progression of labour*).

- The easiest method of monitoring contractions is to place the palm of the hand flat on the uterine fundus and palpate the contraction. The contraction is timed from the onset of the hardening of the uterus to when the uterine muscle relaxes.
- The frequency of contractions is documented as the number of contractions over 10 minutes.
- In the late active phase, there are usually 3–4 contractions over 10 minutes, each lasting 45–60 seconds.
- If a CTG is available, uterine contractions are recorded with external tocodynamometry.

MONITORING OF CERVICAL CHANGES AND FETAL STATION

Gentle and respectful vaginal examination
- Vaginal examinations must be done under aseptic conditions.
- The mother should be informed about the procedure and her consent obtained.
- She should be prepared (with kind words) about the discomfort she will face during the procedure.
- The mother should be kept covered with a sheet during the examination and attention should be paid to maintaining her modesty.
- The vaginal examination should be done gently and with adequate lubrication (see **Chapter 13**, *Respectful maternity care: a human right*).

- Vaginal digital examination is done to assess the cervix (dilatation and effacement), fetal position, and fetal descent.
- The frequency and timing of intrapartum vaginal examination depends on how the labour is progressing. Commonly, vaginal examination is performed at the following stages:
  - On admission
  - At two- to four-hour intervals in the first stage (more frequently if labour seems to be progressing fast)
  - When the mother feels the urge to push (to determine whether the cervix is fully dilated)
  - At 15- to 30-minute intervals in the second stage
  - Prior to administering analgesia/anesthesia
  - If FHR abnormalities occur (to evaluate for complications such as cord prolapse or uterine rupture)

MONITORING OF FETAL RESPONSE TO LABOUR

See **Chapter 18**, *Fetal health surveillance in labour*.

PUSHING DURING SECOND STAGE OF LABOUR

- When the presenting part descends and presses against the rectum, the mother experiences an uncontrollable urge to bear down. Very often, the mother will say she 'wants to pass motion' because of the rectal pressure.

- If the vaginal examination reveals a fully dilated cervix, she may be allowed to begin pushing.
- If the cervix is not completely dilated, the mother may be asked to lie on her side and take deep breaths so that she does not push against the partially dilated cervix.

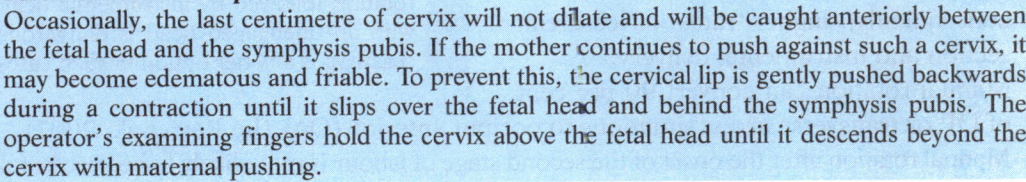

Persistent anterior lip of the cervix

Occasionally, the last centimetre of cervix will not dilate and will be caught anteriorly between the fetal head and the symphysis pubis. If the mother continues to push against such a cervix, it may become edematous and friable. To prevent this, the cervical lip is gently pushed backwards during a contraction until it slips over the fetal head and behind the symphysis pubis. The operator's examining fingers hold the cervix above the fetal head until it descends beyond the cervix with maternal pushing.

Position for pushing

- Two systematic reviews of the Cochrane Database compared the positions in which mothers pushed during the second stage of labour without epidural analgesia (Gupta et al., 2017) and with epidural analgesia (Walker et al., 2018). The reviews compared upright positions (sitting, squatting, kneeling) versus lying positions (lateral, semi-recumbent, lithotomy, Trendelenburg) and found that no single position was clearly superior.
- The lithotomy position is usually recommended when fetal manipulation is required or operative delivery is needed.

 Though upright positions may marginally decrease the duration of the second stage, they also increase the rate of second-degree tears and blood loss of >500 mL.

Technique for pushing

- Women are advised to pull back their knees, tuck in their chin, take a deep breath, bear down with a closed glottis at the start of a contraction (Valsalva pushing), and push for 10–15 seconds, with an average of 2–3 pushes per contraction.
- The duration of the second stage of labour is shorter with Valsalva pushing (Prins et al., 2011).

Perineal massage during pushing

- Perineal massage is performed with two fingers of the lubricated gloved hand moving from side to side over the fourchette with mild, downward pressure.
- This gentle stretching of the introitus during the second stage of labour reduces the incidence of third- and fourth-degree tears (see **Chapter 16**, *Prevention and repair of perineal trauma occurring in childbirth*).

MANUAL ROTATION OF FETAL HEAD IN THE SECOND STAGE OF LABOUR

- The frequency of fetuses in the occiput posterior (OP) position in labour is approximately 20 per cent and, of this, 5 per cent persistently remain posterior until the end of labour.

- Persistent occiput posterior (POP) is associated with increased rates of maternal and newborn morbidity.
- Persistent posterior positions and persistent transverse positions are associated with arrest of labour, and consequently, higher rates of cesarean section and instrumental delivery.

> Persistent occipitoposterior position may often be associated with significant moulding and caput formation. The vertex may appear to be low in the pelvis even though the biparietal diameter is still above the spine (unengaged). Manual/ digital rotation followed by instrumental delivery with an unengaged head is dangerous; a cesarean is a better option in such cases.

- Manual rotation can convert 90 per cent of OP or transverse arrest situations to occiput anterior (OA) (Le Ray et al., 2007).
- Manual rotation after the onset of the second stage of labour is more likely to be successful if it is performed before arrest occurs. Manual rotation is more successful in multiparous women.
- After manual rotation, delivery can occur spontaneously or with the use of forceps or ventouse (see **Chapter 21**, *Operative vaginal delivery*).

Technique for digital or manual rotation

- The bladder should be emptied before proceeding with manual rotation.
- It is best to drop the lower end of the labour bed and place the woman at the edge of the bed in a dorsal lithotomy position with her hips flexed and legs supported in stirrups. This allows the obstetrician to have better access to the fetal head (Barth, 2015).

Digital rotation

- The author prefers digital rotation as it is easy to perform and is less uncomfortable for the mother.
- The vertex must be carefully palpated to identify the posterior fontanelle and the parietal bones. This makes it easier to identify the exact position of the occiput.
- The index and middle fingers are used to locate and apply counterclockwise pressure to the posterior edge of the upper parietal bone at the lambdoid suture, and the fetal head is gently rotated till the occiput reaches the anterior position (Figure 14.1). The rotation is done during a contraction and with the mother pushing down so that the digital rotation assists the physiological rotation of the head.
- Quite often, as soon as the rotation is achieved, the vertex will descend rapidly and delivery will occur.
- The rotation may also be done to achieve an occiput anterior position for forceps or ventouse application.

Manual rotation

- For manual rotation from the left OP position, the operator's right hand is placed in the vagina, with the palm facing upwards. Four fingers are placed against the left side of the fetal head. The thumb is then placed on the right side of the opposite parietal bone (Figure 14.2). The fetal head is slightly pushed up, flexed, and rotated counterclockwise to left OA or OA by pronation of the right hand (Barth, 2015).

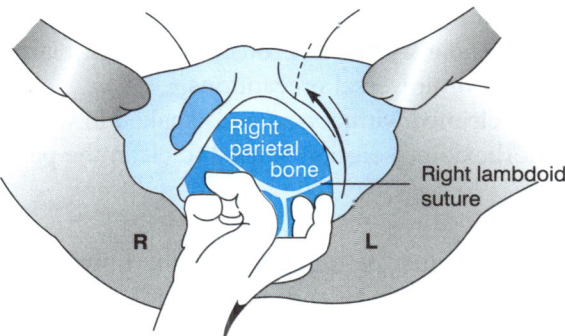

Figure 14.1   Digital rotation from the left occiput posterior to the left occiput anterior position. The index and middle fingers are used to locate and apply counterclockwise pressure on the posterior margin of the right parietal bone at the right lambdoid suture.

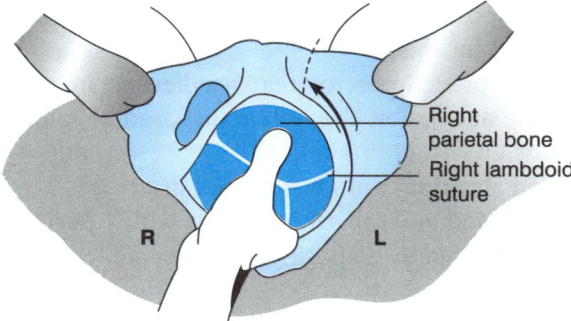

Figure 14.2   Manual rotation from left occiput posterior to left occiput anterior. With the palm of the right hand facing upwards, four fingers are placed along the left side of the fetal head with the thumb on the right parietal bone. While gently disengaging the fetal head, the operator rotates the occiput counterclockwise into the anterior segment of the pelvis.

- The operator's left hand is used if the fetal head is in the right OP position and the direction of rotation is exactly reversed.

EPISIOTOMY

Routine use of episiotomy is not recommended (see **Chapter 15**, *Evidence-based approach to episiotomy*).

SPONTANEOUS VAGINAL DELIVERY

Aseptic precautions

- The obstetrician should wear a waterproof apron underneath a sterile cloth gown or use a disposable waterproof gown.

- Sterile gloves are mandatory.
- A cap and mask are not mandatory but do protect the obstetrician from being splashed by bodily fluids and are a part of universal precautions.
- The perineum should be cleaned with cotton pads soaked in water. Following this, either povidone-iodine or chlorhexidine solution is used to clean the perineal area.

Universal precautions

- All staff in the labour room must be taught about the universal precautions to prevent infection or spread of HIV, hepatitis B, and other bloodborne infections.
- Universal precautions include:
  - Hand hygiene before and after contact with every patient, regardless of whether gloves are also used
  - Using protective barriers such as gloves, gowns/aprons, masks for direct contact with blood and other body fluids
  - Safe collection and disposal of needles and sharps (impervious containers that cannot be pierced are required for this)
  - Following the correct procedures to treat needlestick injuries (the area should be washed out with soap and water, the needle disposed of safely, and immediate post-exposure prophylaxis given)
  - Covering all cuts and abrasions with waterproof dressings
  - Cleaning up spills of blood and other body fluids with 1 part bleach in 10 parts water
  - Segregating waste and properly disposing contaminated waste

Precautions for SARS-CoV-2 (COVID-19)

- The following precautions have been recommended by the Ministry of Health and Family Welfare, Directorate General of Health Services, India (2020), and the US Centers for Disease Control and Prevention (2020):
  - Women should be screened for clinical manifestations of COVID-19 (e.g., cough, headache, sore throat, body pain, fever, shortness of breath, loss of taste/smell). A history should be elicited for close contact with a confirmed case prior to and upon entry into the labour room.
  - It should be ensured that all women admitted to the labour room are masked.
  - Healthcare workers should protect themselves by taking contact and droplet precautions (i.e., gown, gloves, N95 mask, face shield or goggles).
  - Special care should be taken (N95 mask for healthcare providers) during episodes of deep respiratory efforts made by the woman, and during the second stage of labour.

Maternal position for delivery

- If the mother is on a labour table, dropping the end flap will provide access to the perineum and fetus, especially if fetal manipulation is required.
- If the fetal heart rate has stayed normal and no fetal manipulation is required, the mother may deliver in the lateral or partial sitting position.

- Stirrups may or may not be used, according to the facilities available. Corton et al. (2012) found that the use of stirrups did not increase the severity of lacerations or obstetric outcomes

 The use of stirrups has not been shown to have any disadvantages as compared to delivering in bed without stirrups (Corton et al., 2012).

such as prolonged second stage of labour, forceps delivery, or cesarean birth. The study also found that infant outcomes were unaffected by the use of stirrups.

Delivery of fetus

The important techniques involved in spontaneous vaginal delivery are described below. Refer to **Chapter 21,** *Operative vaginal delivery* and **Chapter 23,** *Cesarean section: procedure and technique,* for further information on those techniques of delivery.

- Perineal support and the use of the modified Ritgen manoeuvre have been traditionally used to reduce the occurrence of significant perineal trauma during childbirth. Perineal support has been particularly found to be protective against obstetric anal sphincter injuries (Hals et al., 2010; Laine et al., 2012).
- When the head is crowning, the mother should be asked to take shallow and short breaths and to stop pushing. This prevents the uncontrolled expulsion of the fetal head. One hand is used to maintain the head in a flexed position and control the speed of crowning, and the other hand is used to gently ease the perineum away from the fetal face. Some obstetricians support the perineum with a surgical pad (Figure 14.3). Once the fetal head is delivered, external rotation (restitution) occurs spontaneously.

Delivery of shoulders

- Once the head is delivered, a hand is placed on either side of the head and gentle downward traction is applied toward the mother's sacrum as she pushes. The anterior shoulder will slip under the symphysis pubis and will be delivered.

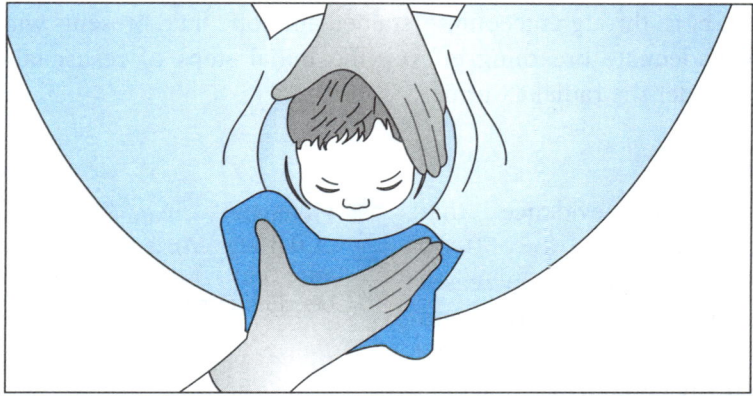

Figure 14.3 As the head is delivered, one hand controls the head and gently flexes it to avoid sudden expulsion. The other hand supports the perineum and gently slips the perineum away from the fetal face.

- The posterior shoulder is then delivered by upward traction. Care should be taken to perform these manoeuvres without undue stretching of the fetal neck to avoid perineal injury and/or traction injuries to the fetal brachial plexus.
- With uterine contractions, the delivery of the shoulders is followed by delivery of the rest of the fetus.

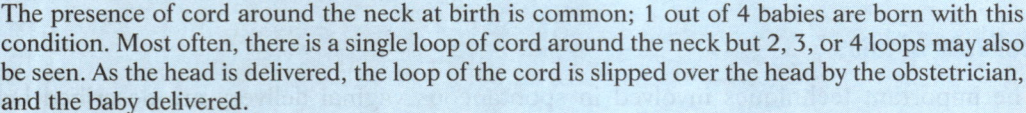

Nuchal cord (cord around the neck)
The presence of cord around the neck at birth is common; 1 out of 4 babies are born with this condition. Most often, there is a single loop of cord around the neck but 2, 3, or 4 loops may also be seen. As the head is delivered, the loop of the cord is slipped over the head by the obstetrician, and the baby delivered.

Occasionally, the cord may be tightly wrapped around the neck. In such a situation, two pairs of Allis clamps are used on the cord, and the cord is cut between the clamps. This allows the delivery of the fetal head.

IMMEDIATE CARE OF THE NEWBORN

Oropharyngeal suctioning

- For a baby born after 35 weeks, a towel may be used to wipe the nose and mouth at birth (Kelleher et al., 2013). This is an alternative (and equally effective method) to oronasopharyngeal suction, which is required only if the baby has excessive secretions.
- Traditionally, for a baby born through meconium-stained fluid, it was recommended that the mouth and nose be suctioned as soon as the head was delivered and before the shoulders are delivered. However, recent guidelines (ACOG, 2017) recommend the following:
  - An infant born through meconium-stained amniotic fluid can be delivered before proceeding to clear meconium from its nose and mouth with a bulb syringe.
  - If the infant is vigorous with good respiratory effort and muscle tone, the infant may stay with the mother while it receives the initial steps of newborn care.
  - If the infant born through meconium-stained amniotic fluid presents with poor muscle tone and inadequate breathing efforts, the initial steps of resuscitation should be completed under the radiant warmer.

Cord clamping

- There is growing evidence that delaying cord clamping for 30–60 seconds following delivery increases early hemoglobin concentrations and iron stores in infants and is therefore recommended (ACOG, 2017a; WHO, 2018a).

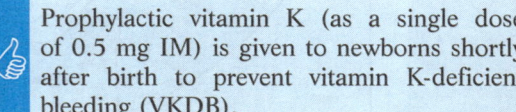

Prophylactic vitamin K (as a single dose of 0.5 mg IM) is given to newborns shortly after birth to prevent vitamin K-deficient bleeding (VKDB).

- However, delayed cord clamping causes a 40 per cent increase in neonatal jaundice, requiring phototherapy. Therefore, delayed cord clamping should be considered only as long as access to phototherapy is available (McDonald et al., 2013). Phototherapy increases the cost of hospitalisation, which is a consideration in low-resource countries.

Cleaning and bathing

- The baby should be dried with a towel and laid on the mother's chest.
- A bath can be given after six hours and can be delayed up to 24 hours.

MANAGEMENT OF THE THIRD STAGE OF LABOUR

- The placenta is delivered by *active management of the third stage of labour*.
- Active management consists of:
  - Prophylactic administration of an uterotonic agent before the delivery of the placenta
  - Controlled traction of the umbilical cord after cord clamping and transection
  - Uterine massage

Uterotonic agents (to be given after the delivery of the anterior shoulder or the placenta)
- Oxytocin 10 units IM or in an IV infusion
- Methylergometrine (Methergine) 0.2 mg IV or IM

References

1. American College of Obstetricians and Gynecologists (ACOG). 2014 (reaffirmed 2017). Safe prevention of the primary cesarean delivery. Obstetric Care Consensus No. 1. *Obstet Gynecol.* 123:693–711.
2. American College of Obstetricians and Gynecologists. 2019. ACOG Committee Opinion No. 766. Approaches to limit intervention during labor and birth. *Obstet Gynecol.*
3. American College of Obstetricians and Gynecologists. 2017. ACOG Committee Opinion No 689. Delivery of a newborn with meconium-stained amniotic fluid. *Obstet Gynecol.* 129:e33.
4. American College of Obstetricians and Gynecologists. 2017a. ACOG Committee Opinion No. 684. 2017a. Delayed umbilical cord clamping after birth. *Obstet Gynecol.* 129:e5.
5. Barth WH Jr. 2015. Clinical Expert Series. Persistent Occiput Posterior. *Obstet Gynecol.* 125:695–709.
6. Basevi V, Lavender T. 2014. Routine perineal shaving on admission in labour. *Cochrane Database Syst Rev.* Issue 11. Art. no. CD001236.
7. Bloom SL, McIntire DD, Kelly MA et al. 1998. Lack of effect of walking on labor and delivery. *N Engl J Med.* 339:76.
8. Corton MM, Lankford JC, Ames R, McIntire DD, Alexander JM, Leveno KJ. 2012. A randomized trial of birthing with and without stirrups. *Am J Obstet Gynecol.* 207(2):133.e1–133.e1335.
9. Gupta JK, Sood A, Hofmeyr GJ, Vogel JP. 2017. Position in the second stage of labour for women without epidural anaesthesia. *Cochrane Database Syst Rev.* Issue 5. Art. no.: CD002006.
10. Hals E, Øian P, Pirhonen T, Gissler M et al. 2010. A multicenter interventional program to reduce the incidence of anal sphincter tears. *Obstet Gynecol.* 116:901–908.
11. Kelleher J, Bhat R, Salas AA et al. 2013. Oronasopharyngeal suction versus wiping of the mouth and nose at birth: A randomised equivalency trial. *Lancet.* 382:326.

12. Laine K, Skjeldestad FE, Sandvik L et al. 2012. Incidence of obstetric anal sphincter injuries after training to protect the perineum: Cohort study. *BMJ Open*. 2(5). e001649.

13. Le Ray C, Serres P, Schmitz T et al. 2007. Manual rotation in occiput posterior or transverse positions: risk factors and consequences on the cesarean delivery rate. *Obstet Gynecol*. 110:873.

14. McDonald SJ, Middleton P, Dowswell T, Morris PS. 2013. Effect of timing of umbilical cord clamping of term infants on maternal and neonatal outcomes. *Cochrane Database Syst Rev*. Issue 7. Art. no.: CD004074.

15. Novel Coronavirus Disease 2019 (COVID-19): Additional guidelines on rational use of personal protective equipment (setting approach for health functionaries working in non-COVID areas). Available at https://www.mohfw.gov.in/pdf/ Additional guidelines on rational use of Personal Protective Equipment setting approach for Health functionaries working in non COVID areas.pdf.

16. Practice Guidelines for Obstetric Anesthesia: An Updated Report by the American Society of Anesthesiologists Task Force on Obstetric Anesthesia and the Society for Obstetric Anesthesia and Perinatology. 2016. *Anesthesiology*. 124(2): 270-300.

17. Prins M, Boxem J, Lucas C, Hutton E. 2011. Effect of spontaneous pushing versus Valsalva pushing in the second stage of labour on mother and fetus: A systematic review of randomised trials. *BJOG*. 118:662.

18. Reveiz L, Gaitán HG, Cuervo LG. 2013. Enemas during labour. *Cochrane Database Syst Rev*. Issue 7. Art. no.: CD000330.

19. Smyth RM, Markham C, Dowswell T. 2013. Amniotomy for shortening spontaneous labour. *Cochrane Database Syst Rev*. Issue 6. Art. no.: CD006167.

20. Tita ATN. 2020. Prenatal care: Intra-amniotic infection (clinical chorioamnionitis or triple I). Berghella V (Ed). *UpToDate*. Waltham, MA.

21. US Centers for Disease Control and Prevention. Coronavirus Disease 2019. Considerations for Inpatient Obstetric Healthcare Settings. Available at https://www.cdc.gov/coronavirus/2019-ncov/hcp/inpatient-obstetric-healthcare-guidance.html.

22. Walker KF, Kibuka M, Thornton JG, Jones NW. 2018. Maternal position in the second stage of labour for women with epidural anaesthesia. *Cochrane Database Syst Rev*. Issue 11. Art. no.: CD008070.

23. World Health Organization. 2018a. WHO recommendations: Intrapartum care for a positive childbirth experience. WHO, Geneva.

24. World Health Organization. WHO recommendation on labour ward admission policy. 2018a. WHO Press.

25. Zhang J, Landy HJ, Branch DW, Burkman R, Haberman S, Gregory KD et al. 2010. Contemporary patterns of spontaneous labor with normal neonatal outcomes. Consortium on Safe Labor. *Obstet Gynecol*. 116:1281-7.

Chapter 15

Evidence-Based Approach to Episiotomy

INTRODUCTION

- Episiotomy is a surgical incision on the perineum, made to enlarge the posterior aspect of the vagina. The incision is usually made during the second stage of labour, as the fetal head is crowning.
- It is still the most common surgical procedure performed by obstetricians though growing evidence has shown that episiotomy should be selective and restricted.
- Episiotomy was popularised in the 20th century and was performed almost universally for vaginal deliveries.
- Episiotomy was advocated because it was thought to:
  - Facilitate the second stage of labour
  - Reduce perineal trauma
  - Reduce pelvic floor dysfunction and prolapse, urinary and fecal incontinence, and sexual dysfunction
- It was also thought to benefit the fetus by:
  - Shortening the second stage
  - Reducing potential trauma to the fetal head
- In 1996, the World Health Organization (WHO) called for a reduction in the episiotomy rate to 10 per cent (WHO, 1996). Since then, there has been a global decline in the episiotomy rate.

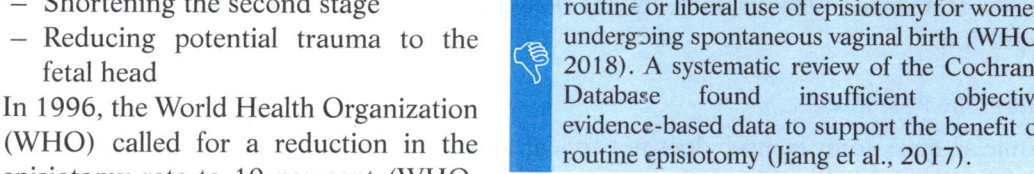

Currently, the WHO does not recommend routine or liberal use of episiotomy for women undergoing spontaneous vaginal birth (WHO, 2018). A systematic review of the Cochrane Database found insufficient objective evidence-based data to support the benefit of routine episiotomy (Jiang et al., 2017).

- Though the goal of 10 per cent may not be attainable, especially in nulliparas, the acceptable rate of episiotomy should not be more than 30 per cent. However, population-based studies in India continue to show high episiotomy rates (Singh et al., 2016; Sathiyasekaran et al., 2007).

The place of delivery and the person conducting the delivery have a significant impact on the rate of episiotomy. Private hospitals have much higher rates of episiotomy as compared to public hospitals. Trained birth attendants perform the least number of episiotomies, followed by nurses. Doctors perform the highest number of episiotomies (Sathiyasekaran et al., 2007).

SELECTIVE VERSUS ROUTINE USE OF EPISIOTOMY FOR VAGINAL BIRTH

- During spontaneous vaginal delivery, vaginal and perineal tears/lacerations may occur, which require suturing. Occasionally, these tears may extend to the rectum and increase the risk of anal sphincter injury.

- To avoid these severe tears, obstetricians traditionally resorted to an episiotomy to prevent severe tearing and to facilitate the birth.
- However, believing that routine episiotomy reduces perineal/vaginal trauma is not justified by current evidence. An episiotomy can actually increase severe perineal trauma.
- A systematic review of the Cochrane Database (Jiang et al., 2017) showed that avoiding routine episiotomy actually reduced severe perineal trauma by 30 per cent.

In women for whom no instrumental delivery is intended, routine episiotomy results in a higher number of severe perineal/vaginal trauma.

On the other hand, there is no clear evidence that selective episiotomy policies result in harm to the mother or baby (Rodis, 2018).

INDICATIONS FOR EPISIOTOMY

- An episiotomy is indicated when the obstetrician believes that enlarging the birth outlet will facilitate the delivery of the fetus and benefit the mother or baby.
- The clinical decision should also take into consideration the potential adverse outcomes associated with the procedure.
- Though there is not enough evidence to justify routine episiotomy, clinical judgement may dictate the need for an episiotomy in the situations listed below (ACOG, 2018).

Non-reassuring fetal heart rate

In the presence of a non-reassuring fetal heart rate (FHR) tracing, episiotomy helps shorten the second stage of labour and expedite delivery if perineal tissue is thought to be blocking expulsion.

Shoulder dystocia

While an episiotomy by itself does not appear to prevent shoulder dystocia or help release the impacted anterior shoulder, it may be used to make space for the operator's fingers and thus facilitate the delivery of the posterior shoulder and other internal procedures. A systematic review (Sagi-Dain and Sagi, 2015) had conflicting reports on the use of episiotomy in the presence of shoulder dystocia. However, performing an episiotomy immediately after failed downward traction (with and without McRoberts) and before attempting any of the vaginal manoeuvres seems to be a practical approach (Rodis, 2018).

Operative vaginal delivery

There is no consensus on whether episiotomy is indicated with operative vaginal delivery. Episiotomy may facilitate placement of the forceps or vacuum extractor in women with a narrow vaginal outlet. It may also prevent anal sphincter

A systematic review (Lund et al., 2016) showed that mediolateral or lateral episiotomy significantly reduced the risk of obstetric anal sphincter injury (OASIS) in vacuum-assisted deliveries in primiparous women.

damage in women with a short perineum who require operative vaginal delivery.

PROCEDURE OF EPISIOTOMY

- A mediolateral episiotomy is the commonest episiotomy performed. It should be performed under aseptic conditions.
- Though the episiotomy can be on either the left or right side, the repair of an incision on the woman's left side is mechanically easier for a right-handed obstetrician.
- The optimal time for an episiotomy is during the crowning of the head. An episiotomy done too early will increase blood loss.
- The fingers are inserted into the vagina between the head and the perineum. During a contraction, an incision is made at approximately a 45° angle from the midline to the perineal body.
- The apex of the incision should start in the exact midline of the perineum, not lateral to the midline.
- A Mayo's scissor or a straight scissor is used to make the incision in a single cut.
- The incision should extend approximately 4 cm into the perineum and may reach the ischiorectal fossa.

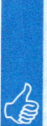 If the mother has not received epidural analgesia, a local anesthetic (5–10 mL of 1 per cent lidocaine) is injected into the planned episiotomy site. It should preferably be given during a contraction so that the mother does not perceive the pain of the injection.

REPAIR OF EPISIOTOMY

- The episiotomy is repaired after the placenta is delivered.
- Adequate pain relief should be provided before suturing. The level of analgesia should be tested and if required, the lidocaine given prior to making the incision can be topped up.

 When the mother is extremely uncomfortable and is crying with pain, ignoring her, taunting her or telling her to just put up with the pain is tantamount to abuse. This is one of the areas where respectful and compassionate care is mandatory in the delivery room.

- Good quality, focused lighting is essential for the repair of an episiotomy or vaginal/perineal lacerations.
- A quick survey must be done to look for periurethral, labial, and fourchette tears and also for the extension of the episiotomy into a third- or fourth-degree tear.
- Repair of an episiotomy is undertaken in three stages: *repair of the vaginal mucosa, repair of the muscle layer,* and *repair of the skin layer*.
- A rapidly absorbable synthetic suture material (2–0 polyglactin 910) is recommended to suture the perineum (Kettle et al., 2012). If cost is a constraint, 2–0 chromic catgut may be used.
- In a systematic review of the Cochrane Database, Kettle et al. (2012) recommended continuous suturing technique to appose the vaginal wall and muscle layers, and a continuous subcuticular technique for the skin layer. This results in less short-term pain, and reduces the need for analgesia and suture removal.

 Currently, there is no evidence to support the use of prophylactic antibiotics for episiotomy (Bonet et al., 2017). The WHO (2015) strongly recommends against routine antibiotic prophylaxis with episiotomy.

- It is good clinical practice to perform a rectal examination on completion of the repair to ensure that no suture material has been inserted through the rectal mucosa. This is particularly important after repairing third- and fourth-degree tears.

Procedure of episiotomy repair

- The vaginal epithelium is reapproximated first, with a continuous locked suture that provides hemostasis and approximation. The apex must be identified carefully and *the first suture should be placed 1 cm above the apex*.

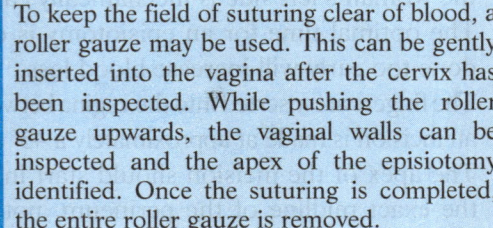

To keep the field of suturing clear of blood, a roller gauze may be used. This can be gently inserted into the vagina after the cervix has been inspected. While pushing the roller gauze upwards, the vaginal walls can be inspected and the apex of the episiotomy identified. Once the suturing is completed, the entire roller gauze is removed.

- The anatomical landmarks, such as the hymenal ring and the vermilion border (where the vaginal mucosa and the skin meet), should be identified and reapproximated accurately.

Individual cotton balls and tampons should not be used to keep the field clear since doing so may result in the inadvertent retention of one and consequently, foul-smelling discharge a few days later.

- Following the closure of the vaginal portion of the laceration down to the level of the hymenal ring, the same suture is passed through the vaginal layer and brought out in the middle, just below the hymen.
- The perineal body and bulbocavernosus muscle are then reapproximated with a continuous running suture. The suture is then placed through the superficial bulbocavernosus muscle on each side in a 'V' configuration, commonly referred to as the 'crown stitch'.
- The suture is then passed through the deep perineal tissue from side to side in a vertical direction until the lower end of the perineal tear is reached.
- The skin is approximated using a subcuticular suture and tied at, or just inside, the introitus. Interrupted mattress sutures should be avoided since they are more uncomfortable and painful than subcuticular sutures.

POSTPARTUM CARE OF THE PERINEUM

- All women who have had a vaginal delivery, with or without an episiotomy, should be given instructions on perineal care and hygiene.
- Emphasis must be laid on educating them on:
  - Perineal care and hygiene
  - Pain management
  - Prevention of constipation
  - Resumption of sexual activity

Perineal care and hygiene

- Women should be encouraged to start washing the perineum soon after birth. They should be educated that tap water will not cause any infection or delay healing. There is no indication for the use of any liquid antiseptic solutions.

- A Sitz bath is a warm, shallow bath that bathes the perineum and buttocks. A wide plastic basin, which can be kept on the floor, is used for this purpose. It helps to keep the perineum clean while also reducing pain and swelling. The vaginal and rectal areas, including any sutures, are fully immersed in the warm water. There is no evidence to support recommending the addition of antiseptic solution to the water.

Pain management

- NSAIDs are the first choice for perineal pain relief. A systematic review of the Cochrane Database showed that NSAIDs provided 50 per cent more relief than paracetamol (Wuytack et al., 2016). Ibuprofen 400 mg orally every 6–8 hours as needed provides good relief in the first postpartum week.

 Women with normal renal function can receive up to 1600–2000 mg per day of ibuprofen in divided doses. They should be encouraged to drink plenty of oral fluids to prevent renal damage (as with any NSAID).

- Local application of ice packs has also been reported to provide pain relief.
- Topical anesthetic agents like lidocaine and benzocaine may be a safe and effective treatment for perineal pain. However, there is no compelling evidence of the effectiveness of topically applied local anesthetics for treating perineal pain (Hedayati et al., 2005).

Prevention and management of constipation

- The new mother must be educated on maintaining soft bowel movements, which can be passed without straining. This helps in avoiding pain while passing motion. This is especially important in women with third- and fourth-degree tears to prevent disruption of the sutures.
- A high-fibre diet along with the intake of plenty of fluids helps in alleviating constipation.
- Additional treatment options include fibre supplements, stool softeners, and/or laxatives.
- Stool softeners must be routinely prescribed for women who have had repair of third- and fourth-degree tears.

Resuming sexual activity

- There are no evidence-based guidelines regarding the timing of resuming sexual activity following delivery.
- Good clinical practice suggests that sexual activity can be resumed 6–8 weeks after delivery if the following conditions are met:

 Since the first postpartum review visit is usually 4–6 weeks after delivery, it is a good opportunity to confirm that the perineum has healed well. Contraception must be discussed and prescribed since lactational amenorrhea is not reliable in preventing a pregnancy.

  - The perineum is fully healed
  - The mother is emotionally ready
  - The couple uses appropriate contraception

Breakdown or dehiscence of a repaired perineal laceration or episiotomy is discussed in **Chapter 16**, *Prevention and repair of perineal trauma occurring in childbirth.*

References

1. American College of Obstetricians and Gynecologists. 2018. ACOG Practice Bulletin No. 198. Prevention and management of obstetric lacerations at vaginal delivery. *Obstet Gynecol.* 132:e87–102.

2. Bonet M, Ota E, Chibueze CE, Oladapo OT. 2017. Antibiotic prophylaxis for episiotomy repair following vaginal birth. *Cochrane Database Syst Rev.* Issue 11. Art. no.: CD012136.

3. Hedayati H, Parsons J, Crowther CA. 2005. Topically applied anaesthetics for treating perineal pain after childbirth. *Cochrane Database Syst Rev.* Issue 2. Art. no.: CD004223.

4. Jiang H, Qian X, Carroli G, Garner P. 2017. Selective versus routine use of episiotomy for vaginal birth. *Cochrane Database Syst Rev.* Issue 2. Art. no.: CD000081.

5. Kettle C, Dowswell T, Ismail KM. 2012. Continuous and interrupted suturing techniques for repair of episiotomy or second-degree tears. *Cochrane Database Syst Rev.* Issue 11. Art. no.: CD000947.

6. Lund NS, Persson LK, Jangö H, Gommesen D, Westergaard HB. 2016. Episiotomy in vacuum-assisted delivery affects the risk of obstetric anal sphincter injury: A systematic review and meta-analysis. *Eur J Obstet Gynecol Reprod Biol.* 207:193-199.

7. Rodis JF. 2018. Shoulder dystocia: Intrapartum diagnosis, management, and outcome. Lockwood CW (Ed). *UpToDate.* Waltham, MA.

8. Sagi-Dain L, Sagi S. 2015. The role of episiotomy in prevention and management of shoulder dystocia: A systematic review. *Obstet Gynecol Surv.* 70:354.

9. Sathiyasekaran BWC, Palani G, Iyer RH, Edward S, Dharmappal CD, Rani A et al. 2007. Population-based study of episiotomy. *Sri Ramachandra J Med.* 9–14.

10. Singh S, Thakur T, Chandhiok N, Dhillon BS. 2016. Pattern of episiotomy use & its immediate complications among vaginal deliveries in 18 tertiary care hospitals in India. *Indian J Med Res.* 143(4):474–480.

11. World Health Organization. 2015. WHO recommendation against routine antibiotic prophylaxis for women with episiotomy. WHO, Geneva.

12. World Health Organization. 2018. WHO Recommendations: Intrapartum care for a positive childbirth experience. WHO, Geneva.

13. World Health Organization: Division of Family Health Maternal Health and Safe Motherhood. 1996. Care in normal birth: A practical guide. Report of a technical working group. WHO, Geneva.

14. Wuytack F, Smith V, Cleary BJ. 2016. Oral non-steroidal anti-inflammatory drugs (single dose) for perineal pain in the early postpartum period. *Cochrane Database Syst Rev.* Issue 7. Art. no.: CD011352.

Chapter 16

Prevention and Repair of Perineal Trauma Occurring in Childbirth

INTRODUCTION

- 50–80 per cent of women will sustain some type of perineal trauma at vaginal delivery, the majority being first- and second-degree tears or lacerations (Smith et al., 2013).
- After a vaginal delivery, it is mandatory to inspect the vagina, perineum, and anorectum to identify and repair significant tears and lacerations.
- An unrecognised injury to the anal sphincter complex sustained during an otherwise uncomplicated delivery can contribute to distressing symptoms—perineal pain in the short term and fecal incontinence in the long term.
- Even after a third- or fourth-degree tear is recognised and repaired, there may be residual anal sphincter dysfunction.

PREVENTION OF SIGNIFICANT PERINEAL TRAUMA

Perineal support

- Obstetric anal sphincter injuries (OASIS) or third- and fourth-degree perineal tears represent a serious complication of vaginal birth.
- Perineal support and the use of the Ritgen manoeuvre (Figure 16.1) have been traditionally used to reduce the occurrence of significant perineal trauma during childbirth.
- Perineal support has been found to be particularly protective against OASIS. Two interventional studies in Norway, undertaken to reduce the incidence of OASIS, showed

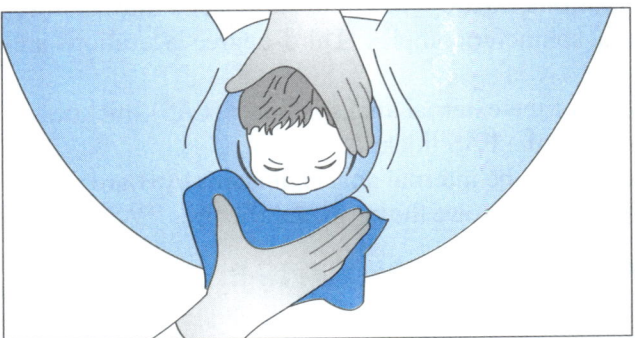

Figure 16.1   Ritgen manoeuvre: One hand of the obstetrician supports the perineum while the other hand gently flexes the fetal head to control the speed of birth. As the head crowns, delivery of the head is controlled to allow gradual delivery and not an abrupt expulsion.

that with perineal support, the occurrence of OASIS reduced by 50–70 per cent (Hals et al., 2010; Laine et al., 2012). These results were replicated in a recent study conducted in the United Kingdom (Naidu et al., 2017), which reported a 23 per cent reduction of OASIS and a 71 per cent reduction of major OASIS.

Perineal massage

- Perineal massage and gentle stretching of the introitus during the second stage of labour reduces the incidence of third- and fourth-degree tears.
- Perineal massage is performed with two fingers of the lubricated gloved hand moving from side to side over the fourchette with mild, downward pressure.
- This intervention is supported by a systematic review of the Cochrane Database for perineal techniques during the second stage of labour for reducing perineal trauma (Aasheim et al., 2011).

Avoiding episiotomy

- Episiotomy has been shown to result in more perineal trauma than spontaneous delivery without an episiotomy (Thacker and Banta, 1983).
- A meta-analysis showed that reducing the incidence of episiotomy decreased the rates of serious perineal trauma (Carroli and Mignini, 2009). However, anterior perineal tears are more common with the restrictive use of episiotomy.

CLASSIFICATION OF PERINEAL TRAUMA OCCURRING IN CHILDBIRTH

The following is the accepted classification of perineal lacerations that may occur during vaginal birth (ACOG, 2018):

- **First-degree lacerations** involve injury to the perineal skin only. The perineal muscles remain intact.
- **Second-degree lacerations** extend into the fascia and musculature of the perineal body, which includes the deep and superficial transverse perineal muscles and fibres of the pubococcygeus and bulbocavernosus muscles. The anal sphincter muscles remain intact.
- **Third-degree lacerations** extend through the fascia and musculature of the perineal body and involve the anal sphincter complex. Third-degree lacerations are further classified as follows:
  - 3a: <50 per cent of the external anal sphincter (EAS) thickness is torn
  - 3b: >50 per cent of the EAS thickness is torn
  - 3c: Both the EAS and the internal anal sphincter (IAS) are torn
- **Fourth-degree lacerations** involve the perineal structures, EAS, IAS, and the rectal mucosa.

REPAIR OF PERINEAL TRAUMA OCCURRING IN CHILDBIRTH

Optimising repair

- Lighting should be provided by a focused lamp (preferably with LED bulbs), for proper visualisation. It should be adjustable and flexible so that light can be directed into the vagina.

- Visualisation should be facilitated with the use of a speculum or narrow vaginal retractors.
- Positioning of the woman in a dorsolithotomy position is essential, especially when third- or fourth-degree lacerations are present.
- The labour bed should have the facility to fold down or remove the distal half of the bed so that the perineum can be accessed easily.
- The obstetrician should sit on a stool and have direct access to the perineum. If such an arrangement is not available, the woman should be moved into the operation theatre, especially for the repair of major lacerations and third- and fourth-degree tears.

> Third- and fourth-degree lacerations may be repaired in the operation theatre, if facilities are available. This makes it easier to position the woman, have adequate lighting, and provide anesthesia while carrying out the repair in aseptic conditions.

- Suturing should preferably be started after placental expulsion to avoid disruption of sutures, which may occur if manual removal becomes necessary with a retained placenta.

Inspection and assessment of vaginal, cervical, and perineal lacerations

- It is mandatory to inspect and identify lacerations that may have occurred during vaginal birth.
- The periurethral, periclitoral, and labial regions should be inspected for tears. Only tears that are bleeding profusely need suturing. The majority will stop bleeding with pressure applied with a gauze pad.

> Before starting the process of identification and repair of lacerations, the obstetrician should explain the procedure to the mother. It should be borne in mind that she has just gone through an extremely painful process and will still be deeply apprehensive. It is also of utmost importance to ensure that the mother receives adequate and effective analgesia and is pain-free during the procedure.

- Thorough visual inspection of the distal vagina, perineum, and anorectum should be performed.
- It is important to identify the apex of the vaginal laceration. The posterior vagina is gently displaced downwards by placing four fingers on the fourchette. A speculum can also be gently introduced to improve visualisation of the apex of the laceration if it has extended upwards or into the fornices. The author has found that a second speculum, inserted gently into the anterior vaginal fornix (with the handle of the speculum facing upwards), is very useful in visualising the fornices.
- The cervix is inspected for tears. A sponge-holding forceps is applied at the 12 o'clock position. Another one is then applied at the 2 o'clock position. The sponge-holding forceps are then alternatively removed and reapplied around the circumference of the cervix until the entire cervix has been visualised.
- With a deep second-degree tear, the anal sphincter should be identified to confirm that it is intact (Figure 16.2).
- If the anal sphincter cannot be visually identified, a rectal examination may be performed to exclude injury to the anal sphincter. The rectovaginal examination is accomplished by gently placing the well-lubricated index finger in the rectum and the thumb over the anal

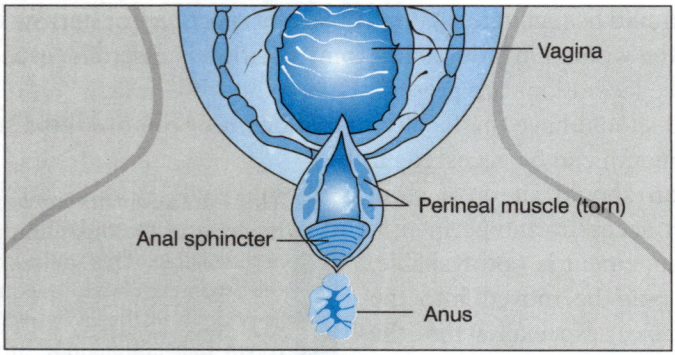

Figure 16.2   Second-degree tear: the anal sphincter is visualised and seen to be intact.

sphincter and using a pill-rolling motion to assess the sphincter. It is important to remember that the anal sphincter may be disrupted even in women with an otherwise intact perineum.

Routine endoanal ultrasonography immediately postpartum for the identification of occult OASIS is not recommended (ACOG, 2018).

- During the examination of the anal sphincter, the anorectal mucosa must also be examined with the index finger that is inside the rectum. An effort must be made to look for a 'buttonhole' laceration of the rectal mucosa that may occur proximal to an intact sphincter. If missed, this may result in fecal incontinence immediately after delivery.

Analgesia and anesthesia

- It is essential to keep the mother comfortable and as pain-free as possible during the repair.
- Adequate local anesthesia must be provided for the repair of second-degree tears. For third- or fourth-degree tears, ideally spinal analgesia, or even general anesthesia, may be required.

Repair of significant tears and lacerations can be very painful for the mother. It is absolutely essential that adequate and effective analgesia is provided. Failure to do so is tantamount to abuse. Compassionate and respectful care in the labour room includes this important aspect of maternity services.

- If the patient has already received epidural analgesia for delivery, it may be adequate for the repair. However, a top-up may be required if the analgesia is wearing off.

Antibiotics

- Antibiotics are not required for the repair of first- and second-degree tears.
- Though the evidence is not strong and is based on a single study (Duggal et al., 2008), it is currently recommended that a single dose of antibiotic (cefazolin or cefuroxime) at the time of repair is a reasonable choice in the setting of obstetric anal sphincter injuries (ACOG, 2018a).

Choice of suture and needle

- Chromic catgut (2–0) has been traditionally used for the repair of episiotomies and lacerations. However, this has been largely replaced by rapidly-absorbable polyglactin 910.

 If the cost of suture is a constraint, 2–0 chromic catgut can still be used since there is no difference between the long-term pain or dyspareunia associated with chromic catgut and synthetic suture (Kettle et al., 2010).

- A systematic review of the Cochrane Database (Kettle et al., 2010) compared catgut and synthetic materials. Synthetic absorbable suture material (2–0 polyglactin 910) is associated with the following:
  - Less short-term pain
  - A reduction in the use of analgesia
  - Lesser wound dehiscence
- The need for suture removal may arise if standard synthetic sutures are used instead of rapidly absorbable synthetic suture, so they are better avoided.
- A round-bodied needle is used for the suture of all layers except for the subcuticular skin layer, for which a reverse cutting needle is useful.

Periclitoral, periurethral, and labial lacerations

- Following vaginal delivery, it is common to see small tears in the anterior vaginal wall. Most of these stop bleeding when pressure is applied with a gauze pad and do not require repair.
- Periclitoral suturing can be extremely painful because of the rich nerve supply and should be avoided.
- Repair of periclitoral, periurethral, and labial lacerations should be carried out only if there is bleeding or distortion of anatomy (Cunningham et al., 2014).

Cervical lacerations

- The cervix must always be inspected for tears (see section above on *Inspection and assessment of vaginal, cervical, and perineal lacerations*).
- Commonly, cervical lacerations occur at the 9 o'clock and 3 o'clock positions. Hemorrhage from cervical lacerations usually arises from the apex and edges of the laceration.
- The repair of a cervical laceration is performed in the following manner:
  - Two sponge-holding forceps are applied on the lips of the cervix, one on either side of the laceration (Figure 16.3).
  - The first suture, using absorbable material (2–0 chromic or polyglactin), is placed above the apex of the laceration. Subsequently, continuous locking sutures are placed through the raw edges of the laceration up to the external os. Care must be taken to incorporate the entire thickness of the cervix.

Spontaneous first- and second-degree lacerations

- No randomised controlled studies are available to categorically establish that first- and second-degree tears need to be repaired.

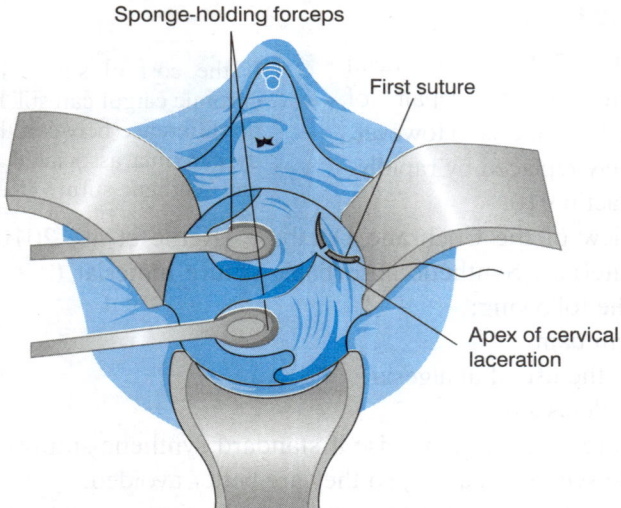

Figure 16.3   Suturing of cervical laceration at 3 o'clock position. The first suture is placed above the apex. This ensures that a bleeding vessel at the apex is not missed.

- Common clinical practice suggests that first-degree tears do not require suturing, unless bleeding is not controlled by simple pressure with a gauze.
- Second-degree tears may be sutured based on clinical judgement and the possibility of discomfort to the mother if left unsutured. A gaping tear may be painful and may burn during urination or washing. Approximation of the wound edges may avoid these problems.
- A small study (Leeman et al., 2007) showed that there was no difference between the sutured and unsutured group at 6 and 12 weeks with regard to urinary and anal incontinence, sexual activity, and sexual function.
- Suturing of a second-degree laceration is done using the same technique as that for an episiotomy (See **Chapter 15**, *Evidence-based approach to episiotomy*).

Third- and fourth-degree lacerations or obstetric anal sphincter injuries (OASIS)

- Though developed countries report a rate of 4–5 per cent of OASIS identifiable at delivery, developing countries tend to either under- or over-report the occurrence of significant third- and fourth-degree lacerations.
- An analysis of the WHO Global Survey (Hirayama et al., 2012) found a reported incidence of 0.1 per cent of OASIS in India and China. The WHO recommends training medical personnel to facilitate the early detection and treatment of postpartum women with third- and fourth-degree perineal lacerations to reduce sequelae.
- Repair of third- and fourth-degree tears involves the following steps:

1. Repair of the anorectal mucosa

- The rectal mucosa is repaired using a continuous (non-locking) 3–0 or 4–0 polyglactin 910 suture on a tapered needle (Figure 16.4). The sutures are continued till the squamo-cutaneous junction of the anus.

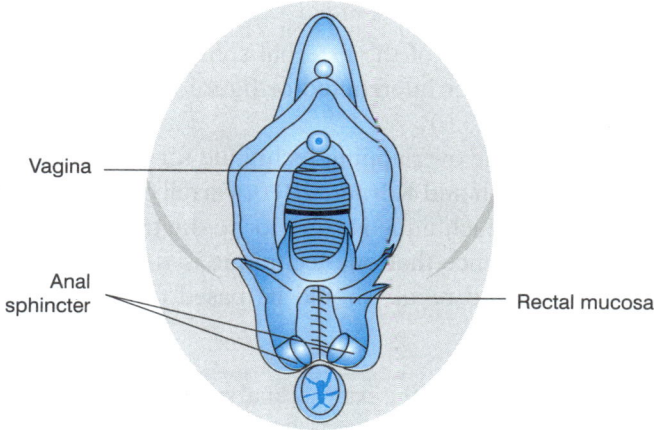

Figure 16.4   The torn rectal mucosa is repaired using a running stitch. Though interrupted stitches are also acceptable, they involve leaving more foreign material behind because of the number of knots.

2. Repair of the anal sphincters

Internal anal sphincter

- The internal anal sphincter should be properly identified and repaired as a separate layer. It appears as thickened, pale pink, shiny tissue just above the anal mucosa and is often referred to as perirectal fascia.
- Reapproximation of this layer is important for the strength and integrity of the repair and for achieving anal continence (Figure 16.5). A continuous 3–0 polyglactin 910 suture on a tapered needle is recommended for this repair.

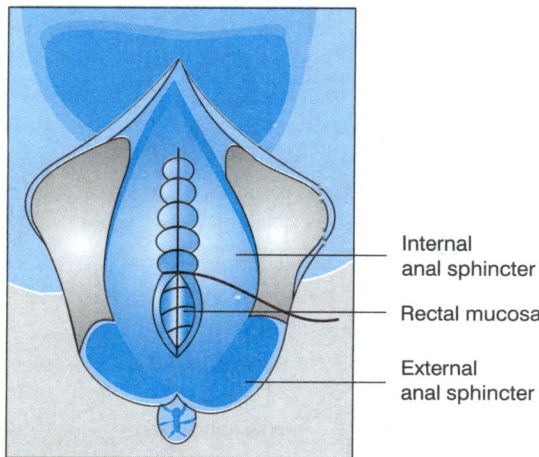

Figure 16.5   The internal rectal sphincter (also referred to as the perirectal fascia) is approximated using a continuous (non-locking) suture.

External anal sphincter

- The most common type of repair of the external sphincter (including the capsule) is an end-to-end repair, wherein either interrupted or figure-of-eight sutures are inserted into the sphincter muscle (Figure 16.6).
- In 1999, Sultan introduced the overlapping technique for sphincter repair at delivery.
- Two randomised studies (Rygh and Körner, 2010; Farrell et al., 2012) found no evidence to show that the overlapping technique is superior to the traditional end-to-end repair.
- Since there is no strong evidence that one technique is superior to the other, the choice between overlap or end-to-end repair should be based on the obstetrician's preference and experience.

> Immediate primary overlap repair of the external anal sphincter, when compared to immediate primary end-to-end repair, appears to be associated with lower risks of developing fecal urgency and anal incontinence symptoms. However, a review of the Cochrane Database (Fernando et al., 2013) found no difference between the two techniques at the end of 24 and 36 months in flatus or fecal incontinence.

- The cut ends of the external sphincter tend to retract. Allis forceps should be used to grasp each end of the sphincter and approximate them. It may be necessary to push the Allis clamp deep into the surrounding connective tissue to locate the sphincter.
- It is also important to identify the capsule of the external sphincter. It is a whitish layer surrounding the muscle. This should be included in the suture, otherwise the suture will tear through the sphincter muscle.

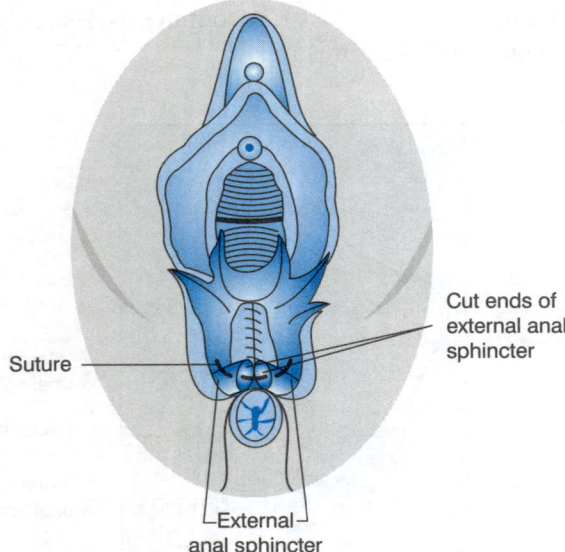

Figure 16.6   The external sphincter is identified and repaired. The repair consists of either end-to-end or overlapping plication of the disrupted external anal sphincter and capsule, using interrupted or figure-of-eight sutures. It is important to take the suture through the capsule of the sphincter.

- The anus should easily admit one finger after the repair.
- At the end of the repair, the skin next to the anus should be stroked with a blunt instrument. If the sphincter has been properly approximated, the anus will pucker in its entirety. This confirms that the sphincter has been restored anatomically.

MANAGEMENT OF BREAKDOWN OF PERINEAL WOUND

- An episiotomy or a second-degree laceration may break down occasionally. Though not common, it can be of great concern to the woman and her family. Repairs of third- and fourth-degree lacerations appear to be at increased risk of infection and breakdown compared to repairs of first- and second-degree lacerations.
- Current clinical practice favours early re-repair (Dudley et al., 2013). This is usually done in the first two weeks postpartum. Early repair decreases perineal pain during healing and reduces dyspareunia.
- Delayed repair after 6–8 weeks does not seem to have any advantages and also causes the mother pain and discomfort for a longer period of time.

Antibiotics and pre-op preparation

- A single prophylactic dose of a second-generation cephalosporin (cefuroxime) is recommended at the beginning of the secondary repair of an episiotomy or second-degree laceration.
- For the repair of a third- or fourth-degree laceration breakdown, antibiotic prophylaxis with aerobic and anaerobic coverage, such as a second-generation cephalosporin plus metronidazole is recommended.
- To reduce the risk of fecal contamination perioperatively, an enema the night before the surgery is considered good clinical practice.

References

1. Aasheim V, Nilsen AB, Lukasse M, Reinar LM. 2011. Perineal techniques during the second stage of labour for reducing perineal trauma. *Cochrane Database Syst Rev.* Issue 12. Art. no.: CD006672.
2. American College of Obstetricians and Gynecologists. 2018. ACOG Practice Bulletin No. 198. Prevention and management of obstetric lacerations at vaginal delivery. *Obstet Gynecol.* 132:87–102.
3. American College of Obstetricians and Gynecologists. 2018a. ACOG Practice Bulletin No. 199. Use of prophylactic antibiotics in labor and delivery. *Obstet Gynecol.* Volume 132. Issue 3.
4. Cunningham FG, Leveno KJ, Bloom SL, Spong CY et al. 2014. *Williams Obstetrics.* 24th ed. New York (NY): McGraw-Hill Medical.
5. Carroli G, Mignini L. 2009. Episiotomy for vaginal birth. *Cochrane Database Syst Rev.* Issue 1. Art. no.: CD000081.
6. Dudley LM, Kettle C, Ismail KM. 2013. Secondary suturing compared to non-suturing for broken down perineal wounds following childbirth. *Cochrane Database Syst Rev.* Issue 9. Art. no.: CD008977.

7. Duggal N, Mercado C, Daniels K, Bujor A et al. 2008. Antibiotic prophylaxis for the prevention of postpartum perineal wound complications: A randomized controlled trial. *Obstet Gynecol.* 111:1268–73.

8. Farrell SA, Flowerdew G, Gilmour D et al. 2012. Overlapping compared with end-to-end repair of complete third-degree or fourth-degree obstetric tears: Three-year follow-up of a randomized controlled trial. *Obstet Gynecol.* 120:803.

9. Fernando RJ, Sultan AH, Kettle C, Thakar R. 2013. Methods of repair for obstetric anal sphincter injury. *Cochrane Database Syst Rev.* Issue 12. Art. no.: CD002866.

10. Hals E, Øian P, Pirhonen T, Gissler M et al. 2010. A multicenter interventional program to reduce the incidence of anal sphincter tears. Obstet Gynecol. 116:901–908.

11. Hirayama F, Koyanagi A, Mori R, Zhang J, Souza J, Gulmezoglu A. 2012. Prevalence and risk factors for third- and fourth-degree perineal lacerations during vaginal delivery: A multi-country study. *BJOG.* 119:340–347.

12. Kettle C, Dowswell T, Ismail KMK. 2010. Absorbable suture materials for primary repair of episiotomy and second-degree tears. *Cochrane Database Syst Rev.* Issue 6. Art. no.: CD000006.

13. Laine K, Skjeldestad F E, Sandvik L et al. 2012. Incidence of obstetric anal sphincter injuries after training to protect the perineum: Cohort study. *BMJ Open.* 2(5), 001649.

14. Leeman LM, Rogers RG, Greulich B, Albers LL. 2007. Do unsutured second-degree perineal lacerations affect postpartum functional outcomes? *J Am Board Fam Med.* 20:451–7.

15. Naidu M, Sultan AH, Thakar R. 2017. Reducing obstetric anal sphincter injuries using perineal support: Our preliminary experience. *Int Urogynecol J.* 28: 381.

16. Sultan AH, Monga AK, Kumar D, Stanton SL. 1999. Primary repair of obstetric anal sphincter rupture using the overlap technique. *Br J Obstet Gynaecol.* 106(4):318–23.

17. Rygh AB, Körner H. 2010. The overlap technique versus end-to-end approximation technique for primary repair of obstetric anal sphincter rupture: A randomized controlled study. *Acta Obstet Gynecol Scand.* 89:1256.

18. Smith LA, Price N, Simonite V, Burns EE. 2013. Incidence of and risk factors for perineal trauma: A prospective observational study. *BMC Pregnancy Childbirth.* 13:59.

19. Thacker SB, Banta HD. 1983. Benefits and risks of episiotomy: An interpretative view of the English language literature, 1860–1980. *Obstet Gynecol Survey.* 38: 322–338.

Chapter 17

Pain Relief in Labour

INTRODUCTION

- The process of labour and childbirth is the only physiological function that is associated with pain. Labour pain has been reported to be the most severe pain that a woman experiences in her lifetime.
- Shockingly, this is also the only situation where a woman under the care of a physician or nurse is expected to tolerate severe pain with either no treatment or only partial treatment.
- The maximum amount of abuse faced by labouring women is in response to their desperate cry for pain relief: globally, women are ignored, scolded, and physically and emotionally abused when they request for help and alleviation of the pain they are experiencing.
- Pain during labour is due to multiple factors and involves complex physiological and psychosocial issues. The perception of labour pain intensity varies from mild discomfort to severe, excruciating pain.
- Neither the mother nor her physician can predict her reaction to pain. It is therefore imperative that all women be offered optimum relief of pain in labour.
- All mothers must be educated about labour pain (without frightening them unnecessarily) and also be informed about the choices available for pain relief prior to the onset of labour. Once the mother is in the throes of labour contractions, she loses her objectivity and the ability to make safe decisions. Every woman in labour wants to be involved in the decisions made about her labour and to be asked for her opinion on the same; it is imperative that she be offered such autonomy.

 Most women are aware that labour is painful and are frightened and anxious even before labour begins. However, they believe and hope that they will be given pain relief. In the majority of cases, there is a mismatch between women's expectations and their actual experience (Lally et al., 2008).

CAUSES AND CHARACTERISTICS OF PAIN DURING LABOUR

First stage of labour

- The pain during the first stage is caused by the following:
  - Distention of uterine and cervical mechanoreceptors
  - Ischemia of uterine and cervical tissues
- It coincides with the contraction and increases in intensity as labour progresses.
- The pain is referred to the abdominal wall, lumbosacral region, gluteal areas, and the inner thighs.

Second stage of labour

- In the second stage of labour, the intensity of pain increases further.
- It is caused by the following:
  - Uterine contractions and cervical stretching leading to visceral pain
  - Distension of vaginal and perineal tissues leading to somatic pain
- The pain originates in the pelvic floor, perineum, vaginal tissues, and pelvic ligaments.

ADVERSE EFFECTS OF LABOUR PAIN

- Unrelieved pain during labour is emotionally traumatic for most women. It has also been linked to postpartum depression (Suhitharan et al., 2016).
- The pain and stress of labour cause the release of adrenocorticotropic hormones, cortisol, catecholamines, and beta-endorphins, which induce changes in maternal blood pressure, decrease placental perfusion, and lead to alterations in fetal acid-base status.
- Maternal hyperventilation in response to labour pain may lead to alkalosis.

METHODS OF PAIN RELIEF IN LABOUR

A wide range of pharmacological and non-pharmacological methods of pain relief is available for women in labour (see box).

Labour analgesia
- Non-pharmacological
  - Childbirth education
  - Supportive birth environment
    - Mobility
    - Touch and massage
    - Hot and cold packs
  - Rhythmic breathing techniques
  - Continuous emotional and physical support by partner or a person of woman's choice
  - Other therapies
    - Music
    - Birthing ball
    - Hypnosis
    - Acupuncture and acupressure
    - Transcutaneous electrical nerve stimulation (TENS)
- Pharmacological
  - Systemic analgesia
  - Inhalational analgesia (Entonox)
  - Neuraxial analgesia
    - Epidural
  - Local analgesia
    - Pudendal block
    - Paracervical block
    - Perineal infiltration

Anesthesia
- Without loss of consciousness
  - Spinal
  - Epidural
  - Combined spinal–epidural
- With loss of consciousness
  - General

Non-pharmacological methods of pain relief

- In India, where systemic analgesics and epidural analgesia are not available to all women, non-pharmacological methods of pain relief help women cope with labour.
- None of the non-pharmacologic techniques currently available have been found to adversely affect the woman, the fetus, or the progress of labour (ACOG, 2017).
- On the other hand, some basic processes put in place to help the woman cope with the pain go a long way in making childbirth a more positive experience (WHO, 2018).

Childbirth education

- One of the biggest shocks that a woman faces in labour is the intensity of the pain. Nothing ever prepares her for it, and some women find it very difficult to cope with it.
- Educating women and their families during the late third trimester about what to expect in labour and the techniques available to cope with the pain helps them make an informed choice in the labour room.
- Childbirth education can be in the form of group classes or graphic brochures. The birth companion should also be encouraged to attend the educational classes. The most important aim of such education is to provide the woman with a realistic understanding of the quality of pain and to assure her that labour pain can be managed in both non-pharmacological and pharmacological ways.
- Breathing techniques to induce relaxation should be taught in these classes.

Supportive birth environment

- All facilities that provide care for birthing mothers should implement measures to provide a supportive birth environment. This has been shown to improve a woman's ability to cope with pain.
- Studies have shown that women would opt not to go to a facility if they feel that they are not supported during their labour and childbirth (WHO, 2018).
- A supportive environment allows the woman to have:
  - A comfortable labouring table
  - The ability to be mobile for as long as possible
  - Massage and counter-pressure provided by a birth companion
  - Hot or cold packs

 A systematic review of the Cochrane Database (Lawrence et al., 2013) showed clear and important evidence that walking and assuming upright positions in the first stage of labour reduce the need for epidural analgesia. In addition, such meaures decrease the duration of labour and the risk of cesarean birth.

Rhythmic breathing techniques

Rhythmic, controlled breathing allows the woman to divert her mind from the pain. This contributes to her ability to cope with labour pain. Women express high satisfaction with breathing techniques; hence these should be taught during antenatal classes or even during labour.

Continuous support during labour

- Labour can be very isolating. In most centres, the mother is moved into a labour room where she is largely in the midst of strangers and separated from the people she is closest to and whom she trusts.
- There is mounting evidence that continuous one-to-one emotional support provided by a midwife or the woman's partner, mother or female friend is associated with improved outcomes for the woman in labour (Bohren et al., 2017). This is quite logical since a woman who feels comforted and supported will feel more in control of the birth process.
- A systematic review of the Cochrane Database by Bohren et al. (2017) showed that a woman who received continuous support had a greater chance of having a vaginal delivery, and a reduced risk of a cesarean birth or a newborn with a low 5-minute Apgar score.
- One of the most important benefits of such a measure is the decreased need for analgesia. Bohren et al. (2016) showed the value of the non-pharmacological pain relief measures that companions help to facilitate with the following:
    - Soothing touch (holding hands, massage, and applying counter pressure)
    - Breathing and relaxation techniques
    - Adopting alternative positions to ease pain such as:
        - Squatting
        - Sitting
        - Walking
    - Spiritual support (when their companions read holy texts or pray)
- The author has allowed husbands/partners in the labour room since 1981 and has a deep personal conviction that it brings enormous comfort and allows the woman to make more rational choices regarding analgesia.

Other non-pharmacological methods of pain relief

- Music
- Acupuncture and acupressure
- Birthing ball
- Transcutaneous electrical nerve stimulation (TENS)
- Hypnosis

Pharmacological methods of pain relief

Systemic analgesics (opioid and non-opioid)

- Systemic analgesics are the most commonly available form of analgesia in low-resource countries like India. Even in high-resource facilities, they are useful as first-line drugs. They are useful for patients who choose not to use epidural, or in cases where these techniques are contraindicated.
- The most commonly used systemic agents are opioids (e.g., pethidine) or mixed opioid agonist–antagonists (e.g., tramadol).

- Opioids are most commonly administered as intramuscular (IM) or intravenous (IV) injections. However, they may also be administered with a pump (patient-controlled analgesia [PCA]).

Pethidine

- Pethidine is an opioid and a recommended option for healthy pregnant women requesting pain relief during labour (WHO, 2018a).

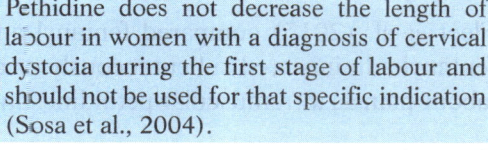 Pethidine does not decrease the length of labour in women with a diagnosis of cervical dystocia during the first stage of labour and should not be used for that specific indication (Sosa et al., 2004).

- Compared to epidural analgesia, opioids like pethidine have the following advantages:
  - Ease of administration
  - Availability
  - Low cost
  - Non-invasive
- The recommended dose of pethidine is 50–100 mg IM every 4–6 hours. The IM route is most commonly used.
- It can also be used IV as a dose of 25 mg every two hours.
- The onset of action is within 45 minutes of IM administration and almost immediately after IV administration.
- Pethidine takes the edge off the pain by inducing drowsiness. A 2018 systematic review of the Cochrane Database by Smith et al. found that parenteral opioids (IM or IV, including patient-controlled analgesia) during labour provided some pain relief and moderate satisfaction with analgesia. However, the pain relief tended to wear off one or two hours after administration in two-thirds of women who received opioids.
- Pethidine is associated with maternal nausea, vomiting, and drowsiness. Since nausea is one of the most common side effects of pethidine, an antiemetic is often administered along with it.

Timing of pethidine administration to prevent neonatal respiratory depression
- Pethidine crosses the placenta.
- The peak concentration of pethidine in the fetus is achieved 2–3 hours after administration.
- The risk of respiratory depression in the neonate is maximum from 1–4 hours after the administration of pethidine.
- The best timing of delivery is within one hour of, or >4 hours after a dose of pethidine, as pethidine reaches a maximal concentration in the fetus 2–3 hours after maternal dosing.
- Delivering the infant within 2–3 hours after the administration of pethidine may result in neonatal respiratory depression.
- The probability of when the mother will deliver should be kept in mind when administering a dose of pethidine.

Tramadol

- Tramadol (an opioid receptor agonist) is a systemic analgesic administered to women in labour. It is easily available and is not associated with the neonatal depression caused by pethidine. However, there are not enough high-quality studies regarding its efficacy.

- Tramadol is administered as a dose of 100 mg intramuscularly. The onset of action is within 10 minutes of IM administration, and the effect lasts for 2–3 hours. It is not as effective as pethidine.

Fentanyl

Fleet et al. (2015) compared fentanyl and pethidine for labour analgesia and found that fentanyl administered subcutaneously or as an intranasal spray is as efficacious in relieving labour pain as intramuscular pethidine, and resulted in greater satisfaction and less sedation.

Paracetamol

- In low-resource areas, where narcotics may not be freely available without a narcotics license, several recent studies (Kaur Makkar et al., 2015; Elbohoty et al., 2012; Aimakhu et al., 2017) have found that both IM and IV paracetamol provide moderate reduction in pain scores in labour.

 In low-resource areas, intramuscular paracetamol is proving to be useful in alleviating the pain of labour to a certain extent (Aimakhu et al., 2017).

- Compared to pethidine and tramadol, IV paracetamol has comparable reduction in pain scores with fewer side effects.
- Paracetamol may be given as a dose of 600 mg IM or as a 1 g IV infusion. The dose may be repeated after four hours.

Other non-opioid agents

- Various non-opioid agents like promethazine, phenothiazine, and benzodiazepine have been used as adjuncts with opioid analgesics to potentiate the analgesic effect and decrease the side effects.
- The evidence for their effectiveness is very poor and of low certainty (WHO, 2018a).

Inhalational analgesia

- A mixture of 50 per cent nitrous oxide and 50 per cent oxygen **(Entonox)** is the most commonly used inhalational agent for pain relief in labour.
- Its advantage is that it does not affect uterine contractility and does not cause neonatal depression (Klomp et al., 2012).
- The labouring woman self-administers the anesthetic gas, as required, by holding a handheld facemask over her nose and mouth.
- As the gas takes effect, the woman becomes drowsy and becomes unable to hold the facemask, which then falls off. This prevents overdosage.
- Due to the time lag for nitrous oxide to take effect, inhalation should begin approximately 30 seconds before the contraction is expected to begin and should cease as the contraction begins to recede.

Neuraxial techniques

- Neuraxial techniques (epidural, spinal, and combined epidural–spinal analgesia) have been shown to be most effective in providing pain relief in labour.

- Neuraxial techniques involve the injection of a local anesthetic with or without an opioid into the epidural or intrathecal space close to the spinal nerves that transmit sensory impulses from the contracting uterus and vagina.
- These agents provide analgesia without affecting the motor function and appreciation of pressure sensation. This helps in maternal expulsive efforts in the second stage. This also allows the mother to be ambulant in the first stage (ACOG, 2019).

Since epidural analgesia is the most popular and effective form of pain relief in labour, the next section will focus on this form of labour analgesia.

Epidural analgesia

- The availability of epidural analgesia depends on the resources available in the facility that the woman delivers in. The two major constraints are the cost of providing epidural analgesia and the non-availability of skilled anesthetists trained in administering epidurals.
- A woman's request for pain relief is the most important indication for providing epidural analgesia.
- Epidural analgesia must block T10 to L1 for the first stage of labour and extend from S2 to S4 during the late first stage and second stage of labour.

Contraindications

- There are very few contraindications for an epidural; they are as follows:
  - Existing coagulopathy
  - Thrombocytopenia with a platelet count <70,000/mL (ACOG, 2019)
  - A local infection on the back
  - Increased intracranial pressure

Epidural analgesia and anticoagulants

- If the mother is on a prophylactic dose of heparin, there is a specified time interval from the last dose to the placement/removal of the epidural catheter (Table 17.1). This is to prevent the risk of the woman developing a spinal epidural hematoma.
- If the mother is on low-dose aspirin or NSAIDs as the sole antithrombotic medication up until the day of the procedure, it will have no effect on the risk of epidural or spinal. In such cases, these analgesics may be given at any time in relation to the last dose.

 Neuraxial techniques must **not** be performed on women receiving two or more antithrombotic drugs simultaneously, e.g., heparin plus aspirin (Horlocker et al., 2018).

Drugs used for epidural analgesia

- The following drugs are used for epidural analgesia:
  - **Local anesthetics:** Bupivacaine and ropivacaine are the most commonly used long-acting local anesthetics for epidural analgesia. They inhibit nerve conduction by blocking sodium channels in the cell membrane of nerves. They exert a

Table 17.1   Timing of neuraxial techniques in women receiving anticoagulant prophylaxis

Anticoagulant	Interval from last dose to placement	Interval from placement/removal to next dose
Low-molecular-weight heparin (prophylactic dose)	≥12 hours	First postoperative dose ≥12 hours after neuraxial procedure; subsequent dose ≥24 hours after the first dose
Unfractionated heparin (prophylactic dose)	≥24 hours	6 hours

concentration-dependent blockade of various modalities of sensation. At low concentration, they selectively block the sensory component with minimal or no motor blockade. Adjuvant epinephrine may be added to enhance the analgesic effect of local anesthetics.

- **Opioids:** Fentanyl or sufentanil are the most commonly used lipophilic opioids for epidural analgesia. The addition of lipophilic opioids improves the quality of analgesia and reduces the dosage of the anesthetic drug used and also produces a more rapid onset of analgesia.

• A combination of local anesthetic and an opioid is given as a bolus via the epidural catheter.

Technique

• Epidural analgesia is performed with the mother either sitting or lying in the lateral position.
• The level at which neuraxial blockade is given is the L2–L3 intervertebral space.
• Epidural catheterisation is done using an 18–20 gauge catheter through an epidural Tuohy needle (16–18 gauge).
• A combination of a local anesthetic and an opioid is injected into the catheter.
• Epidural analgesia usually starts taking effect 5–10 minutes after injection. The maximal effect may not be achieved for 15–20 minutes.
• Blood pressure must be monitored every 15–30 minutes.
• Epidural analgesia can be maintained by the following:
  – Intermittent bolus dosage
  – Continuous infusion technique
  – Patient-controlled epidural analgesia (PCEA)

Intermittent epidural bolus technique

• This is the most cost-effective and standard technique used for pain relief in labour, especially when an infusion pump is not available.
• Regular 'top-ups' are given every 90 minutes to 2 hours, or less frequently, depending on the patient's requirement for analgesia.
• The limitations of the intermittent bolus technique are as follows:
  – Intermittent dosing requires frequent intervention by clinicians/skilled nurses
  – Waning of analgesic effect occurs between top-up doses
• A combination of bupivacaine and fentanyl is the most economical and effective.

Dosage of intermittent epidural bolus
- 10 mL of 0.0625% bupivacaine with 15 µg of fentanyl
- May be repeated every 1.5–2 hours

Continuous infusion technique

- Continuous infusion technique overcomes the disadvantages of the intermittent technique.
- It offers smooth analgesia throughout labour without peaks and valleys unlike the intermittent technique.
- The only notable disadvantage of the continuous technique is that motor block increases with prolonged infusion despite the low concentration and low dose of local anesthetics.
- Since a low dose is used, there may be breakthrough pain that may be managed by administering a bolus dose.

Dosage of continuous infusion
- Bupivacaine 0.04–0.125% with fentanyl 1–3 µg/mL OR
- Ropivacaine 0.08–0.2% with fentanyl 1–3 µg/mL

Patient-controlled epidural analgesia (PCEA)

- Patient-controlled epidural analgesia allows the mother to titrate the dose of the local anesthetic depending on the intensity of the perceived pain.
- This can be used along with continuous low-dose infusion.
- Advantages of PCEA
  - The total dose of local anesthetic used is less.
  - There is a lower incidence of motor blockade.
  - There is decreased need for intermittent additional top-ups.

Effects of epidural analgesia on labour

Timing of epidural

- The timing of epidural analgesia has no effect on labour progression; therefore, it is not necessary to wait until the active phase of labour to administer epidural analgesia. The mother's need for analgesia should guide timing.
- The first stage of labour can decrease by up to 90 minutes with the early administration of epidural (Wong et al., 2005).
- A systematic review of the Cochrane Database (Sng et al., 2014) compared early initiation (<4 cm cervical dilatation) with later initiation of epidural analgesia and found no difference in cesarean delivery rate, instrumental delivery, duration of the second stage of labour, and fetal outcomes.

Effect on the second stage of labour

- Due to the motor blockade induced by the analgesic, there is a small increase in duration of the second stage (an average of 7.66 minutes), but this does not affect outcome (Anim-Somuah et al., 2018).

- The practice of discontinuing epidural analgesia at the time of full cervical dilatation to help the mother feel the urge to push is not supported by any studies and is not recommended.

 A recent RCT supports pushing at the start of the second stage of labour for women receiving epidural analgesia (Cahill et al., 2018). This is contrary to earlier recommendations for delayed pushing with epidural.

- A systematic review of the Cochrane Database (Torvaldsen et al., 2004) has shown that the only effect achieved by halting epidural analgesia in the second stage is an increase in pain.

Effect on the need for instrumental delivery

- Earlier studies reported that the risk of instrumental vaginal delivery increased with the use of epidural analgesia.
- However, an analysis of trials conducted after 2005 failed to demonstrate a significant difference and may reflect a lower concentration of local anesthetics used in modern epidurals (ACOG, 2019).

Effect on cesarean section rates

Systematic reviews found no overall increase in cesarean section rates with the use of epidural analgesia (Anim-Somuah et al., 2018).

 There is no increase in instrumental delivery or cesarean section with epidural.

Effect on fetal heart rate changes

- In the absence of maternal hypotension prior to delivery, epidural analgesia does not negatively affect the neonate.
- A non-reassuring fetal heart rate pattern can occur after an epidural due to maternal hypotension (Abrão et al., 2009). These changes are transient and reversible.

Effect on residual back pain

- One of the most frequently voiced concerns that a mother has about epidural analgesia is residual back pain.
- In a randomised controlled study, Howell et al. (2002) found no increase in the risk of post-delivery back pain after epidural analgesia.

Combined spinal–epidural analgesia

- Combined spinal–epidural (CSE) analgesia is not a commonly practiced technique and is technically difficult.
- It combines a sequential spinal and epidural in the same intervertebral space through a special combined spinal–epidural needle.
- It is a needle-through-needle approach to deposit the opioid in the subarachnoid space followed by a catheter that is threaded into the epidural space to administer a local anesthetic.

- It is associated with a higher incidence of fetal heart rate abnormalities and a higher incidence of maternal pruritus.

Adverse effects of neuraxial techniques

Maternal hypotension

- Hypotension is the most common side effect of neuraxial techniques, be it spinal or epidural.
- This occurs due to sympathetic vasomotor blockade and may occur with epidural analgesia, and may be worse with spinal analgesia.
- In the event that hypotension occurs, phenylephrine can be used safely to treat it.

Preventing hypotension
Preloading the mother, prior to the epidural, with 500–1000 mL of normal saline IV helps prevent this problem as doing so expands the maternal vascular space. In women with severe preeclampsia, a lower volume of fluid may be administered as a preload.

Pruritus

- Pruritus is a common side effect of neuraxial analgesia.
- It occurs more commonly after spinal opioid administration than after epidural administration, with a reported incidence of close to 100 per cent for fentanyl, which is often used for combined spinal–epidural labour analgesia.
- The incidence of pruritus after neuraxial opioid administration is dose-dependent.

Postdural puncture headache

- Postdural puncture headache (PDPH) or spinal headache is caused by the leakage of cerebrospinal fluid through a dural puncture. This can happen after a spinal or due to inadvertent dural puncture during an epidural. The incidence is 1.5 per cent with an epidural and can be as high as 11 per cent with a spinal.
- The headache is positional and worsens when the mother sits or stands.
- Pencil-point needles are associated with significantly lower incidence of PDPH than with the cutting-needle design (Zorrilla-Vaca et al., 2018).
- Conservative management with complete bed rest, caffeine, NSAIDs and parenteral narcotics can be prescribed if the headache is not incapacitating. Intense, debilitating PDPH is treated with an epidural blood patch.

Epidural blood patch (EBP)
- Epidural blood patch is the treatment of choice for women with severe, debilitating headache and inability to nurse following epidural analgesia.
- The best means of controlling the leak of CSF from the dural puncture is to plug it with a blood clot. EBP has more than a 95 per cent chance of resolving the headache.
- An epidural needle is inserted into the epidural space above the previous epidural puncture, and 15–20 mL of autologous (maternal) blood is injected into the epidural space.
- EBP reduces the duration and intensity of postdural puncture headache and usually provides immediate relief (Boonmak and Boonmak, 2010).

Shivering and fever

- Central neuraxial blockade-related shivering is due to vasodilatation caused by sympathetic blockade, with redistribution of heat from the core to the periphery (Sessler, 2008).
- Several studies have reported an association between the use of epidural analgesia and rise in maternal temperature. The etiology of the temperature increase associated with epidural analgesia is not clear.

Rare complications

Rare complications that have been described with neuraxial analgesia are postpartum nephropathy, epidural abscess, and meningitis.

Perineal infiltration for episiotomy

- Perineal infiltration with a local anesthetic can be used if an episiotomy is to be performed (see **Chapter 15**, *Evidence-based approach to episiotomy*).
- Perineal infiltration acts on the terminal nerves in the posterior fourchette and perineum.
- The commonly used anesthetic agent is a 2 per cent solution of lidocaine.
- If inadvertently injected intravenously, lidocaine can cause hypotension, tachycardia, and central nervous system toxicity. Prior to injecting the anesthetic, the piston of the syringe should be withdrawn to ascertain that the needle is not in a blood vessel.
- If the infiltration is done during a contraction, the mother will experience less discomfort from the injection.

References

1. Abrão KC, Francisco RP, Miyadahira S, Cicarelli DD, Zugaib M. 2009. Elevation of uterine basal tone and fetal heart rate abnormalities after labor analgesia: A randomized controlled trial. *Obstet Gynecol.* 113(1):41.16.

2. Aimakhu C O, Saanu O O, Olayemi O. 2017. Pain relief in labor: A randomized controlled trial comparing intramuscular tramadol with intramuscular paracetamol at the University College Hospital, Ibadan, Nigeria. *Trop J Obstet Gynaecol.* 34:91-8.

3. American College of Obstetricians and Gynecologists. 2017. ACOG Committee Opinion No. 766. Approaches to limit intervention during labor and birth. *Obstet Gynecol.* 133(2):e164–e173.

4. American College of Obstetricians and Gynecologists. 2019. ACOG Practice Bulletin No. 209. Obstetric Analgesia and Anesthesia. *Obstetrics & Gynecology.* Volume 133. Issue 3. p 595–597.

5. Anim-Somuah M, Smyth RM, Cyna AM et al. 2018. Epidural versus non-epidural or no analgesia for pain management in labour. *Cochrane Database Syst Rev.* Issue 5. Art. no.: CD000331.

6. Bohren MA, Hofmeyr G, Sakala C, Fukuzawa RK, Cuthbert A. 2017. Continuous support for women during childbirth. *Cochrane Database Syst Rev.* Issue 7. Art. no.: CD003766.

7. Bohren MA, Munthe-Kaas H, Berger BO, Allanson EE, Tunçalp Ö. 2016. Perceptions and experiences of labour companionship: A qualitative evidence synthesis (protocol). *Cochrane Database Syst Rev.* Issue 12. Art. no.: CD012449.

8. Boonmak P, Boonmak S. 2010. Epidural blood patching for preventing and treating post-dural puncture headache. *Cochrane Database Syst Rev.* Issue 1. Art. no.: CD001791.

9. Cahill AG, Srinivas SK, Tita ATN, Caughey AB et al. 2018. Effect of immediate vs delayed pushing on rates of spontaneous vaginal delivery among nulliparous women receiving neuraxial analgesia: A randomized clinical trial. *JAMA.* 320:1444–54.

10. Elbohoty AE, Abd-Elrazek H, Abd-El-Gawad M et al. 2012. Intravenous infusion of paracetamol versus intravenous pethidine as an intrapartum analgesic in the first stage of labor. *Int J Gynaecol Obstet.* 118:7.

11. Fleet J, Belan I, Jones MJ, Ullah S, Cyna AM. 2015. A comparison of fentanyl with pethidine for pain relief during childbirth: A randomised controlled trial. *BJOG.* 122: 983–992.

12. Horlocker TT, Vandermeuelen E, Kopp SL et al. 2018. Regional anesthesia in the patient receiving antithrombotic or thrombolytic therapy: American Society of Regional Anesthesia and Pain Medicine Evidence-Based Guidelines (Fourth Edition). *Reg Anesth Pain Med.* 43:263.

13. Howell CJ, Dean T, Lucking L et al. 2002. Randomised study of long-term outcome after epidural versus non-epidural analgesia during labour. *BMJ.* 325:357.

14. Kaur Makkar J, Jain K, Bhatia N, Jain V, Mal Mithrawal S. 2015. Comparison of analgesic efficacy of paracetamol and tramadol for pain relief in active labcr. *J Clin Anesth.* 27(2):159–163.

15. Klomp T, van Poppel M, Jones L et al. 2012. Inhaled analgesia for pain management in labour. *Cochrane Database Syst Rev.* Issue 9. Art. no.: CD009351.

16. Lally JE, Murtagh MJ, Macphail S, Thomson R. 2008. More in hope than expectation: A systematic review of women's expectations and experience of pain relief in labour. *BMC Med.* 6:7.

17. Lawrence A, Lewis L, Hofmeyr GJ, Styles C. 2013. Maternal positions and mobility during first stage labour. *Cochrane Database Syst Rev.* Issue 8. Art. no.: CD003934.

18. Sessler DI. 2008. Temperature monitoring and perioperative thermoregulation. *Anesthesiology.* 109:318.

19. Sosa CG, Balaguer E, Alonso JG et al. 2004. Meperidine for dystocia during the first stage of labor: A randomized controlled trial. *American Journal of Obstetrics and Gynecology.* 191. 1212e8

20. Smith LA, Burns E, Cuthbert A. 2018. Parenteral opioids for maternal pain management in labour. *Cochrane Database Syst Rev.* Issue 6. Art. no.: CD007396.

21. Sng BL, Leong WL, Zeng Y et al. 2014. Early versus late initiation of epidural analgesia for labour. *Cochrane Database Syst Rev.* Issue 10. Art. no.: CD007238.

22. Suhitharan T, Pham TP, Chen H et al. 2016. Investigating analgesic and psychological factors associated with risk of postpartum depression development: A case-control study. *Neuropsychiatr Dis Treat.* 12:1333.

23. Torvaldsen S, Roberts CL, Bell JC, Raynes-Greenow CH. 2004. Discontinuation of epidural analgesia late in labour for reducing the adverse delivery outcomes associated with epidural analgesia. *Cochrane Database Syst Rev.* Issue 4. Art. no. CD004457.

24. World Health Organization. 2018. WHO recommendations: Intrapartum care for a positive childbirth experience. WHO, Geneva.

25. World Health Organization. 2018a. WHO recommendation: Opioid analgesia for pain relief during labour. WHO, Geneva.

26. Wong CA, Scavone BM, Peaceman AM, McCarthy RJ et al. 2005. The risk of cesarean delivery with neuraxial analgesia given early versus late in labor. *N Engl J Med.* 352:655–65.

27. Zorrilla-Vaca A, Mathur V, Wu CL, Grant MC. 2018. The impact of spinal needle selection on postdural puncture headache: A meta-analysis and metaregression of randomized studies. *Reg Anesth Pain Med.* 43:502.

Chapter 18

Fetal Health Surveillance in Labour

INTRODUCTION

- Modern obstetrics aims to minimise and prevent adverse fetal outcomes arising from fetal metabolic acidosis or cerebral hypoxia related to labour.
- Approximately half of all stillbirths and a quarter of neonatal deaths result from complications during labour and childbirth (Lawn et al., 2016).
- In low-resource countries like India, improving the quality of care in the intrapartum period has been identified as the most impactful strategy for reducing stillbirths and maternal and newborn deaths, even more than antenatal or postpartum care strategies (Bhutta et al., 2014).
- Every uterine contraction results in transient hypoxia. Healthy fetuses have the reserve to tolerate this. However, in fetuses that are already stressed, this hypoxia may cause alterations in fetal heart rate (FHR) patterns.
- FHR patterns are indirect markers of the fetal cardiac and medullary responses to blood volume changes, acidemia, and hypoxemia since the brain modulates the heart rate. Monitoring the fetal heart rate (FHR) is a vital part of the care of the fetus during labour.

 In conditions with chronic placental insufficiency (e.g., hypertension, diabetes, fetal growth restriction), the fetus may not tolerate the decrease in oxygenation during a contraction and may show signs of hypoxemia. The preterm fetus also tolerates hypoxia poorly.

AIM OF INTRAPARTUM FETAL SURVEILLANCE

- Intrapartum fetal surveillance aims to detect potential fetal harm due to decreased oxygenation. Timely detection allows for prompt and effective intervention to prevent perinatal/neonatal morbidity or mortality.
- Decreased oxygenation may result in brain injury. At present, no technology is available to directly assess brain injury during labour.
- Certain fetal heart rate changes occur prior to brain injury. The recognition of these heart rate changes is the basis of fetal monitoring in labour.

FETAL HYPOXIA

Causes of fetal hypoxia in labour

Fetal oxygenation in labour can be compromised when there is any interference with the uterine blood flow. This may result from maternal factors, placental dysfunction, or fetal factors (Table 18.1).

Table 18.1   Conditions that may lead to fetal hypoxia in labour

Maternal factors	Clinical condition
Chronic maternal conditions	Chronic hypertension Insulin-dependent diabetes Antiphospholipid antibody syndrome Significant nutritional anemia
Decreased uterine blood flow	Hypotension (e.g., acute blood loss) Regional anesthesia (epidural, spinal) Maternal positioning (supine hypotension)
Uteroplacental factors	
Excessive uterine activity	Hyperstimulation Placental abruption
Uteroplacental dysfunction	Fetal growth restriction Postterm pregnancy Oligohydramnios
Fetal factors	
Cord compression	Oligohydramnios Cord prolapse or entanglement
Decreased fetal oxygen-carrying capacity	Significant anemia due to: • Rh alloimmunsation • Maternal–fetal bleed

Effect of fetal hypoxia on the fetus

The fetus experiences three stages of deterioration when oxygen levels are depleted (Martin, 2008). These stages are as follows:

Transient hypoxia without metabolic acidosis
↓
Tissue hypoxia with a risk of metabolic acidosis
↓
Hypoxia with metabolic acidosis

Consequences of fetal hypoxia in labour

Hypoxic injury affects the fetus in several ways. Though it could result in multiorgan dysfunction, it is the fetal nervous system that is the most vulnerable to long-term injury. Hypoxic insult may manifest in the neonatal period as the following:

• **Hypoxic ischemic encephalopathy (HIE)**

HIE usually occurs due to **prolonged intrapartum hypoxia**. It may be mild, moderate, or severe. Severe HIE may be associated with neonatal death or disabilities in survivors.

• **Neonatal encephalopathy**

The majority of cases of neonatal encephalopathy are the result of **conditions that may exist even before labour starts,** like prenatal stroke, infection, cerebral malformation, and genetic disorders. It is important to remember that only 4 per cent of encephalopathy can be attributed directly to hypoxic events that occur during the process of labour (Hankins and Speer, 2003).

> **Cerebral palsy**
> 99.8 per cent of 'abnormal' FHR tracings are not associated with the later development of cerebral palsy (Nelson et al., 1996). The majority of cerebral palsies are not due to asphyxia during labour but due to **an insult that occurs in the antenatal period, or genetic and environmental factors**. Less than 0.5 per cent of cerebral palsy is the result of acute intrapartum hypoxia, which usually results in spastic quadriplegic cerebral palsy.

METHODS OF INTRAPARTUM FETAL SURVEILLANCE

The methods available for evaluating and assessing fetal response to labour include the following:

- Fetal heart rate monitoring
  - Intermittent auscultation (IA)
    - Pinard fetoscope
    - Stethoscope
    - Handheld Doppler device
  - Cardiotocography (CTG) or electronic fetal monitoring (EFM)
    - Intermittent (when required)
    - Continuous
- Fetal scalp blood sampling
  - Scalp pH
  - Fetal lactate concentration
- Fetal electrocardiography
- Pulse oximetry

Fetal heart rate monitoring

- Fetal heart rate (FHR) is affected by the brain's responses to peripheral and central stimulation of the fetus.
- The fetal heart rate changes significantly in response to prolonged hypoxia, making fetal heart rate monitoring a valuable and commonly used tool for assessing fetal oxygenation status in labour.
- Depending on the resources available, monitoring is done with **intermittent auscultation** or scaled up to **cardiotocography**.
- Intermittent auscultation (IA) of the FHR is recommended for low-risk women in established labour in any birth setting, including low-resource areas (NICE, 2014; WHO, 2018). If an FHR abnormality is detected using this method, then cardiotocography may be used to identify the nature of the abnormality.
- Cardiotocography (CTG), also known as electronic fetal monitoring (EFM), may be used (when available) where risk factors for fetal hypoxia exist (ACOG, 2009).
- In India, fetal heart rate monitors may not always be available in a facility.

- The World Health Organization does not recommend continuous cardiotocography for the assessment of fetal well-being in healthy pregnant women undergoing spontaneous labour (WHO, 2018a).
- Despite the frequency of its use, CTG has limitations, which include poor interobserver and intraobserver reliability, uncertain efficacy, and a high false positive rate (ACOG, 2009).

Does cardiotocography (CTG) improve perinatal outcomes?

CTG is utilised when available and is particularly useful in high-risk pregnancies where a normal heart rate tracing reassures us that the fetus is tolerating labour well. However, perinatal outcomes do not seem to improve with the use of CTG. A systematic review of the Cochrane Database (Alfirevic, 2017) showed that CTG during labour is associated with reduced rates of neonatal seizures, but with no clear differences in infant mortality or other standard measures of neonatal well-being. On the other hand, continuous CTG was associated with an increase in cesarean sections and instrumental vaginal births, though more contemporary trials demonstrate no significant difference in the rate of cesarean delivery between patients monitored continuously and those monitored by intermittent auscultation (Miller, 2018).

CTG has become a part of the protocol in labour rooms because there is no other technology available at present for intrapartum fetal surveillance.

Intermittent auscultation (IA)

- The World Health Organization recommends intermittent auscultation of the fetal heart rate with either a handheld Doppler device or a Pinard fetal stethoscope for healthy pregnant women in labour (WHO, 2018).

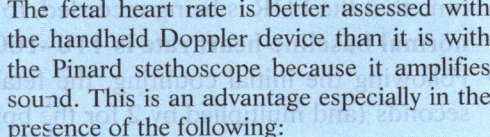

The fetal heart rate is better assessed with the handheld Doppler device than it is with the Pinard stethoscope because it amplifies sound. This is an advantage especially in the presence of the following:
- Obesity
- Polyhydramnios
- An actively moving fetus

- IA is quite often the only method available for fetal heart rate monitoring in many medical facilities in low- and middle-income countries like India.
- A strict protocol for intermittent auscultation has been recommended by the FIGO consensus guidelines on intrapartum fetal monitoring (Lewis and Downe, 2015). These guidelines must be followed to ensure that the maximum benefit is obtained from the fetal heart rate monitoring (Table 18.2).
- Although low nurse-to-patient ratios make it difficult to practice this protocol in busy labour and delivery suites, these guidelines should be adhered to as closely as possible to avoid missing fetal hypoxia.
- An important drawback of intermittent auscultation is *its inability to determine decreased beat-to-beat variability*, which is a very important feature of hypoxia.
- Fetuses with abnormal findings on auscultation (tachycardia or bradycardia) need to be shifted to cardiotocography (if available) to define the patterns, to identify non-reassuring fetal status, and determine the need for operative intervention (NICE, 2014).

Table 18.2 Recommended protocol for intermittent auscultation based on FIGO consensus guidelines on intrapartum fetal monitoring (Lewis and Downe, 2015)

Factors in intermittent auscultation	Recommendation
Interval between auscultation	1st stage of labour : Every 15–30 minutes 2nd stage of labour : Every 5 minutes During pushing : After each contraction
Duration	Each auscultation should last for at least 1 minute If an abnormality is noted, auscultate over at least 3 contractions
Timing	Auscultate during a uterine contraction and continue for at least 30 seconds after the contraction
Documentation	Record the baseline FHR (e.g., 130 beats per minute) and the presence or absence of accelerations or decelerations

 It is important to explain to the mother that the baby's heartbeat is being monitored and, if the FHR is normal, to tell her that the baby is doing well. This reassures the mother and helps her go through labour with confidence. In case of an abnormal finding, a clear explanation of the subsequent course of action should be given so that she is aware and involved.

Interpretation of fetal heart rate by auscultation

Baseline heart rate

- The fetal heartbeats are counted between contractions for 60 seconds, at least for the first time that the FHR is being recorded, to establish the baseline fetal heart rate (FHR). **The normal baseline heart rate is 110–160 beats per minute (bpm)**.
- Following the initial counting, the fetal heartbeat can be intermittently counted for 30 seconds (and multiplied by 2 for the bpm) to continue monitoring heart rate.

Fetal heart rate changes detected by auscultation

- **Accelerations** are a reassuring sign of fetal well-being. An acceleration is defined as an abrupt rise in the FHR above the baseline for 15–60 seconds.
- **Decelerations** are said to occur when the FHR abruptly drops below the baseline for 15–60 seconds or more.
- **Tachycardia** is defined as a fetal heart rate above 160 bpm for >10 minutes.
- **Bradycardia** is defined as FHR below 110 bpm for >10 minutes. If bradycardia is suspected, it is important to compare FHR to maternal pulse to ensure that the maternal heartbeat is not being confused for the fetal heartbeat.

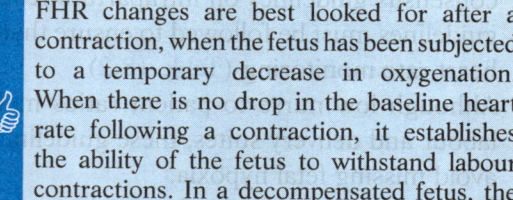 FHR changes are best looked for after a contraction, when the fetus has been subjected to a temporary decrease in oxygenation. When there is no drop in the baseline heart rate following a contraction, it establishes the ability of the fetus to withstand labour contractions. In a decompensated fetus, the FHR will drop following a contraction.

Management of abnormal FHR patterns identified by auscultation

The management of abnormal FHR patterns identified by intermittent auscultation is summarised in Table 18.3.

Table 18.3   Management of abnormal FHR patterns identified by intermittent auscultation based on recommendations of the FIGO Intrapartum Fetal Monitoring Expert Consensus Panel (Lewis and Downe, 2015)

FHR pattern	Possible causes	Management	Intervention
FHR <110 bpm for >5 minutes	Fetal hypoxia	Rule out cord prolapse, change maternal position, administer maternal oxygen	Immediate delivery by cesarean or instrumental vaginal delivery based on the obstetric condition and local resources
Tachycardia during at least 3 contractions	• Fetal hypoxia • Maternal fever • Intrauterine infection • Drugs (salbutamol, terbutaline, ritodrine)	Check and treat fever, intrauterine infection	Increased frequency of intermittent auscultation
Repetitive decelerations (common in 2nd stage of labour)	• Aortocaval compression • Cord compression • Head compression	Change maternal position	No intervention if decelerations disappear
Repetitive decelerations that start >20 seconds after the onset of a contraction and take >30 seconds to return to baseline values (late decelerations)	Fetal hypoxia/acidosis	Mother to stop pushing till decelerations disappear	If no rapid reversal, delivery by cesarean or instrumental vaginal delivery
Decelerations lasting >3 minutes (prolonged deceleration)	Fetal hypoxia/acidosis	Mother to stop pushing till decelerations disappear	If no rapid reversal, delivery by cesarean or instrumental vaginal delivery

Cardiotocography (CTG)

- Although continuous CTG is the accepted standard of care in most high-resource settings, the use of continuous CTG in low-resource settings is not feasible or recommended.
- The sensitivity of CTG for the presence of fetal acidosis or hypoxia has been shown to be poor.
- CTG is best used to increase the frequency of surveillance when an abnormality is noted on IA.
- Non-reassuring fetal heart rate patterns are observed in approximately 15 per cent of labours (East et al., 2015). Therefore, depending on this tool alone for identifying a decompensated, hypoxic fetus increases operative intervention rates.

> CTG is a better predictor of the absence of fetal hypoxia than the presence of hypoxia. In other words, when the fetal heart rate tracing is normal, the fetus is definitely normal. On the other hand, non-reassuring signs on the tracing do not necessarily equate with hypoxia or acidosis.

Indications for electronic fetal monitoring (ACOG, 2009; NICE, 2014)

- High-risk pregnancies (e.g., preeclampsia, suspected fetal growth restriction, maternal type 1 diabetes mellitus) should be monitored with continuous CTG, if available.

- In low-resource areas, it is quite acceptable to monitor the FHR with intermittent auscultation and then start CTG if an abnormal FHR is suspected.

> **Admission test**
> - The admission CTG is a screening test consisting of a short (usually 20 minutes) recording of the FHR and uterine activity, which is performed on the mother's admission to the labour ward.
> - For women at low risk of complications, there is insufficient evidence to determine whether cardiotocography as part of the initial assessment improves outcomes or if it results in harm for women and their babies as compared to intermittent auscultation alone (NICE, 2017).
> - A systematic review of the Cochrane Database (Devane et al., 2017) found no evidence of benefit from the performance of the admission CTG for low-risk women. On the contrary, the admission test has been shown to increase the cesarean section rate by 20 per cent.
> - However, the admission test may be of some benefit in women who are at high risk of labour complications, e.g., postterm pregnancy, growth-restricted fetus, oligohydramnios, and hypertensive disorders.
> - In a study by Akhavan et al. (2017), the admission test was found to be a useful screening tool in women with high-risk factors and was able to predict neonatal outcomes in terms of NICU admission and the need for cesarean birth.
> - In a high-risk pregnancy, a normal admission test, especially when combined with assessment of amniotic fluid volume, reassures the obstetrician and the mother that the fetus is likely to tolerate labour well.

Terms and definitions used with CTG

- Specific terms are used to describe the tracings generated by electronic fetal heart rate recording (ACOG, 2010).
- Since there is so much variability in inter- and intraobserver interpretation of FHR tracings, it is important that everybody uses the same terminology.

Baseline: This is the average FHR in increments of 5 beats per minute for a minimum of 2 minutes during a 10-minute segment.
- Normal FHR baseline : 110–160 beats per minute
- Tachycardia   : Baseline >160 beats per minute
- Bradycardia   : Baseline <110 beats per minute

Baseline variability: This refers to fluctuations in the baseline FHR that are irregular in amplitude and frequency.
- Absent   : Amplitude range undetectable
- Minimal   : Amplitude range detectable but ≤5 beats per minute
- Moderate (normal) : Amplitude range 6–25 beats per minute
- Marked   : Amplitude range >25 beats per minute

> - Good variability reflects a healthy nervous system, chemoreceptors, baroreceptors, and cardiac responsiveness.
> - The absence of baseline variability may be the result of cerebral hypoxemia and acidosis.
> - Non-hypoxic causes of decreased/absent variability include:
>   – Quiet fetal sleep   – Opiates
>   – Sepsis   – Complete heart block

Accelerations: These are abrupt increases (onset to peak in <30 seconds) in the FHR (Figure 18.1). In a mature fetus (after 32 weeks), an acceleration has a peak of 15 or more beats per minute above baseline, with a duration of ≥15 seconds but <2 minutes from onset to return.

Accelerations, along with moderate variability, clearly rule out the presence of fetal acidosis (Macones et al., 2008).

Decelerations: These are decreases in FHR which go at least 15 beats below the baseline and last at least 15 seconds.

- **Early deceleration:** Early decelerations are uniform, mirror the contractions, and decelerate only 10–20 beats per minute. They are caused by intrapartum compression of the fetal head during a uterine contraction and maternal expulsive efforts. Early decelerations are clinically benign and are not associated with fetal hypoxia.

- **Late deceleration:** Late decelerations commence after the start of the contraction and return to the baseline a few seconds after the contraction is over. The lowest point of the deceleration occurs after the peak of the contraction. They are caused by placental insufficiency.

 Recurrent **late decelerations** are indicative of fetal acidosis.

- **Variable deceleration:** This refers to abrupt drops in FHR which may or may not be related to contractions and vary in onset, depth, and duration. These are caused by cord compression (Figure 18.2).

 Persistent, deep, and recurrent **variable decelerations** are indicative of fetal acidosis.

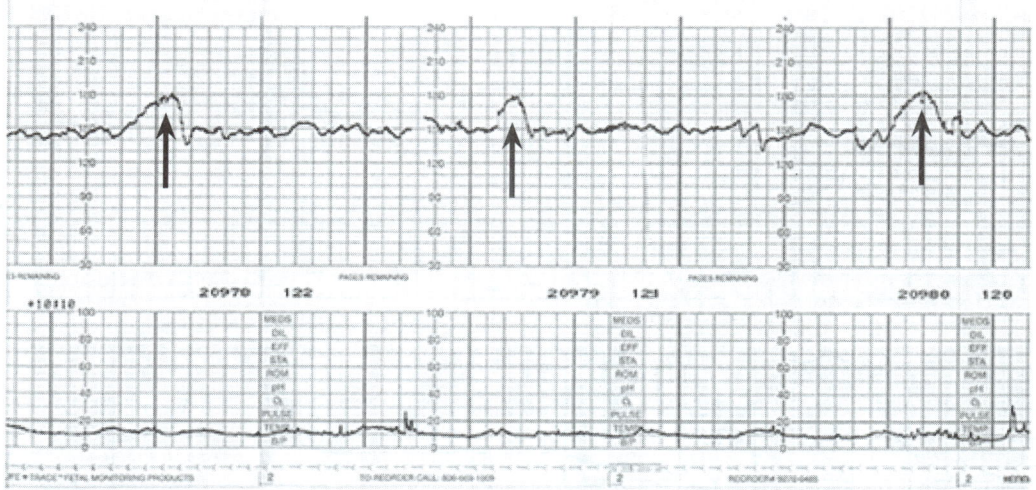

Figure 18.1 Category I or 'normal' (reassuring) fetal heart rate tracing. The basal heart rate is 145 bpm with good variability. Accelerations are present (arrows) and are a reassuring sign.

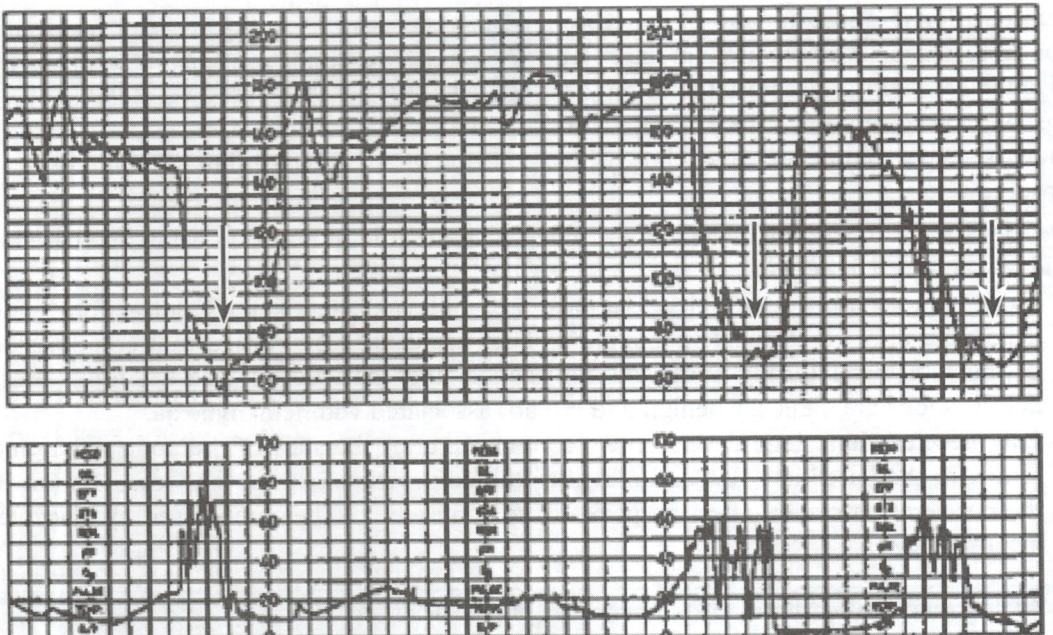

Figure 18.2 Recurrent variable decelerations (arrows) with poor variability are seen in the upper half of the graph.

Prolonged deceleration: This is a decrease in FHR from the baseline, that is ≥15 beats per minute, lasting ≥2 minutes but <10 minutes in duration (Figure 18.3).

Sinusoidal pattern: Usually associated with fetal anemia, this pattern is a smooth, sine wave-like undulating pattern in FHR baseline with a cyclic frequency of 3–5 per minute, which persists for ≥20 minutes (Figure 18.4).

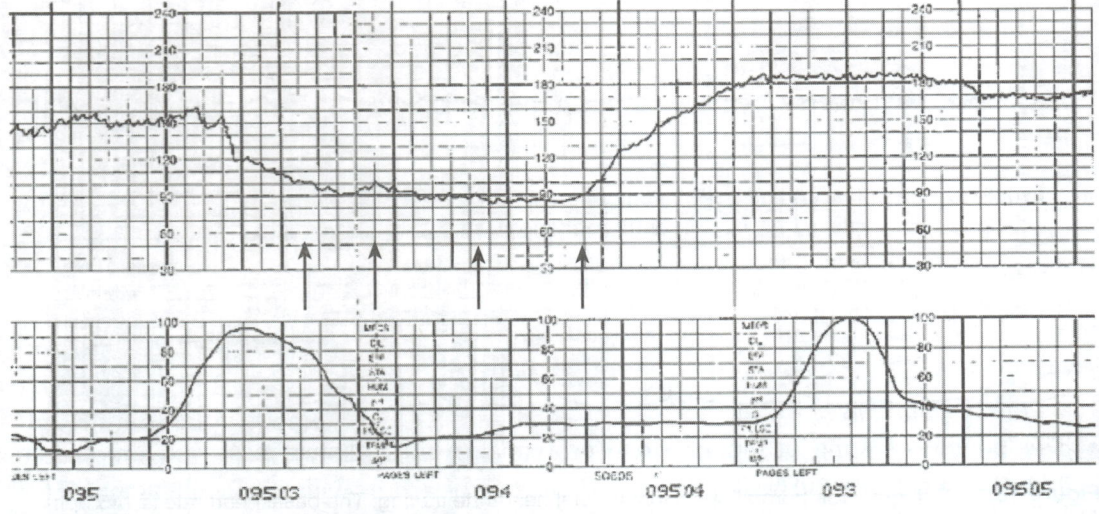

Figure 18.3 Prolonged bradycardia (arrows) with poor variability.

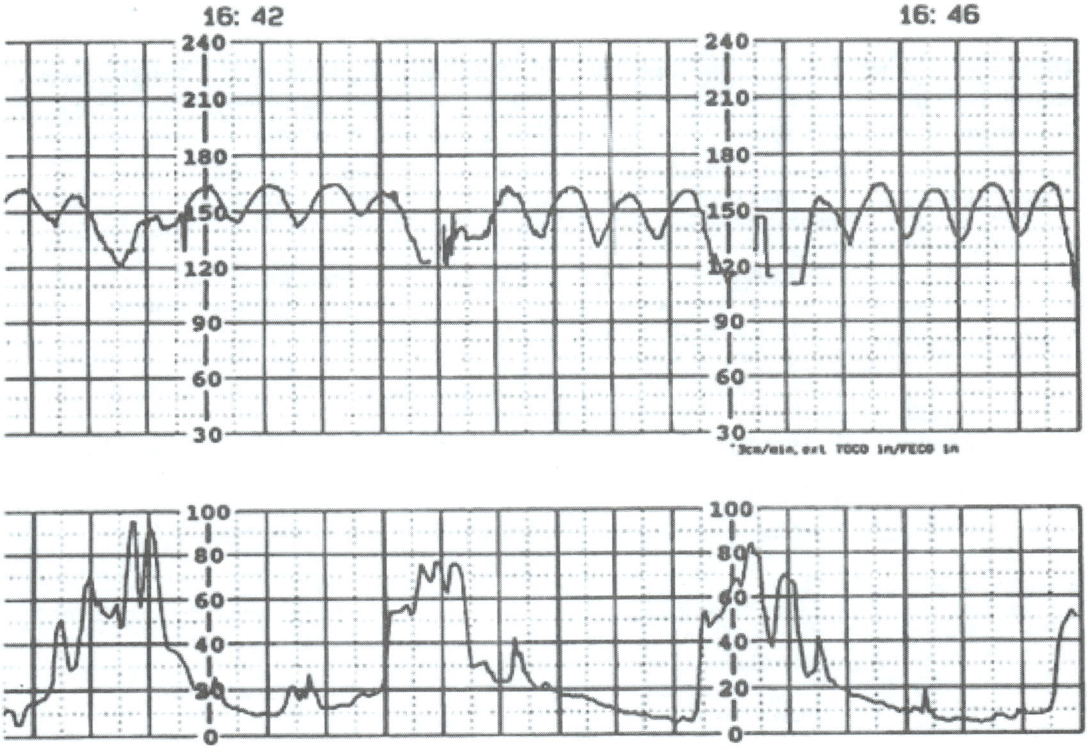

16: 42   16: 46

Figure 18.4   Sinusoidal fetal heart rate pattern is seen in the upper half of the graph.

Reassuring and non-reassuring FHR patterns

- The status of the fetus is assessed based on FHR patterns. These can either be *reassuring,* i.e., the fetal status is good, or *non-reassuring,* i.e., the fetal condition needs to be further evaluated immediately.

- The most commonly used classifications of FHR patterns come from the National Institute of Child Health and Human Development (NICHD; Macones et al.,

 The presence of a reassuring pattern indicates that **at the time of recording**, there is very little likelihood of acidemia.

2008) and The International Federation of Gynecology and Obstetrics (FIGO; Ayres-de-Campo et al., 2015). The classifications are compared in Table 18.4.

- A Category I or 'normal' FHR pattern is considered reassuring. A Category III or 'pathological' FHR pattern is considered non-reassuring.

Further evaluation of non-reassuring patterns on CTG

Fetal scalp stimulation test

- In the presence of a non-reassuring FHR pattern, the scalp stimulation test is a reassuring technique for determining fetal reserves and ruling out fetal hypoxia and acidemia. It was

Table 18.4   Comparison of NICHD and FIGO guidelines for the interpretation of fetal heart rate using continuous cardiotocography

NICHD three-tier fetal heart rate interpretation system (2008)		FIGO consensus guidelines on intrapartum fetal monitoring CTG tracing classifications (2015)	
FHR pattern	Description	FHR pattern	Description
Category I tracing (Figure 18.1)	*Baseline heart rate:* 110–160 bpm *Variability:* Moderate *Decelerations:* • No late decelerations • Early decelerations may be present or absent • Accelerations may be present or absent	Normal	*Baseline heart rate:* 110–160 bpm *Variability:* 5–25 bpm *Decelerations:* No repetitive decelerations
Category II tracing	FHR tracing does not meet criteria for category I or category III	Suspicious	Lacking at least one characteristic of normality, but with no pathologic features
Category III tracing (Figure 18.2, Figure 18.3, and Figure 18.4)	*Variability:* Absent FHR baseline variability AND any of the following: • Recurrent late decelerations • Recurrent variable decelerations • Bradycardia (FHR <110 bpm) OR Sinusoidal pattern	Pathological	*Baseline heart rate:* <100 bpm *Variability:* • Reduced variability for >15 min • Increased variability for >30 min OR • Sinusoidal pattern for >30 min *Decelerations:* Repetitive late or prolonged decelerations for >30 min (or >20 min if reduced variability) OR One prolonged deceleration >5 min

bpm, beats per minute; *FHR*, fetal heart rate

first proposed as a clinical alternative to fetal scalp blood sampling (Clark et al., 1984).

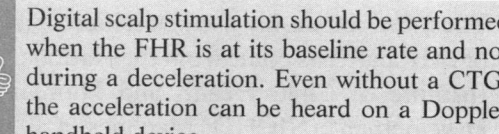

Digital scalp stimulation should be performed when the FHR is at its baseline rate and not during a deceleration. Even without a CTG, the acceleration can be heard on a Doppler handheld device.

- During a vaginal examination, the examiner strokes the fetal scalp with a finger, using firm pressure. This should elicit a fetal heart rate acceleration of ≥15 bpm above the baseline lasting for ≥15 seconds. Even without a CTG, the acceleration can be heard on a Doppler handheld device.

- When there are no spontaneous FHR accelerations, this test is easily performed and immediately reassuring, especially in a low-resource setting.

- A positive test (acceleration elicited) rules out fetal acidosis in 90 per cent of cases (Clark et al., 1984). Skupski et al. (2002) found that a negative test (acceleration not elicited) could be indicative of fetal acidemia in 50 per cent of fetuses and should be followed-up with careful fetal evaluation.

Fetal scalp blood sampling

- A difficult test to perform, both technically and in terms of laboratory support, fetal scalp blood sampling never became widely available in India.
- Its use has been questioned since it has not been shown to reduce emergency cesarean sections or operative vaginal births or improve long-term perinatal outcomes (Chandraharan, 2016; Carbonne et al., 2016). Fetal scalp blood sampling is now rarely performed, even in developed countries.

Other methods of fetal surveillance in labour

Fetal pulse oximetry

A systematic review of the Cochrane Database (East et al., 2014) found no evidence that assessment of fetal oxygen saturation by fetal pulse oximetry as an adjunct to electronic FHR monitoring improves neonatal outcome or reduces cesarean rates. It has not proved to be useful clinically.

Fetal electrocardiography

Fetal electrocardiography can be recorded by performing internal fetal monitoring with special equipment that processes fetal ECG, known as the STAN system. Fetal hypoxia causes ST segment and T-wave changes in the fetal ECG. Randomised trials and meta-analyses did not reveal improvement in neonatal or maternal outcomes with fetal electrocardiography.

Management of non-reassuring FHR patterns on CTG

Management of non-reassuring fetal heart rate patterns (Category II or suspicious, Category III or pathological) has three primary goals:

 If membranes are not ruptured yet, artificial rupture of membranes (AROM) could help assess the amniotic fluid. Thick meconium adds to the seriousness of the situation.

I. Increase fetal oxygenation and improve uteroplacental blood flow
II. Reduce uterine activity
III. Relieve umbilical cord compression

I. Increase fetal oxygenation and improve uteroplacental blood flow

- Decreased fetal oxygenation and acidemia could be associated with the following non-reassuring patterns:
  - Recurrent late decelerations
  - Prolonged decelerations or bradycardia
  - Minimal or absent fetal heart rate variability
- The interventions to improve fetal oxygenation include the following (ACOG, 2010, reaffirmed 2021):
  - Turning the mother to her left or right side (whichever improves the heart rate)
  - Administering oxygen (8–10 L/min of oxygen) to the mother with a facial mask or nasal prongs

– Administering an intravenous fluid bolus in the presence of maternal hypotension (e.g., for a mother who has received epidural analgesia)
– Discontinuing oxytocin (if it is being administered)

II. Reduce uterine activity

- Tachysystole (uterine hyperstimulation) may result in non-reassuring FHR patterns.
- The interventions to reduce uterine activity include the following:
  – Discontinuing oxytocin (if it is being administered)
  – Administering tocolytics, e.g., terbutaline 250 µg subcutaneously

III. Relieve umbilical cord compression

- Umbilical cord compression can result in:
  – Recurrent variable decelerations
  – Prolonged decelerations or bradycardia
- The interventions to relieve umbilical cord compression include the following:
  – Repositioning the mother to her left or right side (whichever improves the heart rate). If that does not help, the mother may be asked to assume the knee–chest position or get down on all fours.
  – Though amnioinfusion has been suggested as an intervention, there is limited evidence for improvements in short-term or long-term neonatal outcomes (ACOG, 2010).
  – In the presence of a prolapsed umbilical cord, the presenting fetal part is elevated, and preparations are made for cesarean delivery.

References

1. Akhavan S, Lak P, Rahimi-Sharbaf F, Mohammadi SR, Shirazi M. 2017. Admission test and pregnancy outcome. *Iranian J Med Sci.* 42(4):362–8.

2. Alfirevic Z, Devane D, Gyte GML, Cuthbert A. 2017. Continuous cardiotocography (CTG) as a form of electronic fetal monitoring (EFM) for fetal assessment during labour. *Cochrane Database Syst Rev.* Issue 2. Art. no.: CD006066.

3. American College of Obstetricians and Gynecologists. 2010 (reaffirmed 2021). ACOG practice bulletin no: 116. Management of intrapartum fetal heart rate tracings. *Obstet Gynecol.* 116(5):1232–40.

4. American College of Obstetricians and Gynecologists. 2009 (reaffirmed 2017). ACOG practice bulletin no: 106. 2009. Intrapartum fetal heart rate monitoring: Nomenclature, interpretation, and general management principles. *Obstet Gynecol.* 114(1):192–202.

5. Ayres-de-Campos D. Spong CY, Chandraharan E. 2015. FIGO consensus guidelines on intrapartum fetal monitoring: Cardiotocography. *International Journal of Gynecology & Obstetrics.* 131: 13–24.

6. Bhutta ZA, Das JK, Bahl R, Lawn JE, Salam RA, Paul VK et al. 2014. Can available interventions end preventable deaths in mothers, newborn babies, and stillbirths, and at what cost? *Lancet.* 384(9940):347–70.

7. Carbonne B, Pons K, Maisonneuve E. 2016. Foetal scalp blood sampling during labour for pH and lactate measurements. *Best Pract Res Clin Obstet Gynaecol.* 30:62.

8. Chandraharan E. 2016. Should national guidelines continue to recommend fetal scalp blood sampling during labor? *J Matern Fetal Neonatal Med.* 29:3682.

9. Clark SL, Gimovsky ML, Miller FC. 1984. The scalp stimulation test: A clinical alternative to fetal scalp blood sampling. *Am J Obstet Gynecol.* 148:274.

10. Devane D, Lalor JG, Daly S, McGuire W, Cuthbert A, Smith V. 2017. Cardiotocography versus intermittent auscultation of fetal heart on admission to labour ward for assessment of fetal wellbeing. *Cochrane Database Syst Rev.* Issue 1. Art. no.: CD005122.

11. East CE, Begg L, Colditz PB, Lau R. 2014. Fetal pulse oximetry for fetal assessment in labour. *Cochrane Database Syst Rev.* Issue 10. Art. no.: CD004075.

12. East CE, Leader LR, Sheehan P, Henshall NE, Colditz PB, Lau R. 2015. Intrapartum fetal scalp lactate sampling for fetal assessment in the presence of a non-reassuring fetal heart rate trace. *Cochrane Database Syst Rev.* Issue 5. Art. no.: CD006174.

13. Hankins GD, Speer M. 2003. Defining the pathogenesis and pathophysiology of neonatal encephalopathy and cerebral palsy. *Obstet Gynecol.* 102:628–36.

14. Lawn JE, Blencowe H, Waiswa P, Amouzou A, Mathers C, Hogan D et al. 2016. Stillbirths: Rates, risk factors, and acceleration towards 2030. *Lancet.* 387(10018):58–603.

15. Lewis D, Downe S. 2015. FIGO Intrapartum Fetal Monitoring Expert Consensus Panel. FIGO consensus guidelines on intrapartum fetal monitoring: Intermittent auscultation. *Int J Gynecol Obstet.* 131(1):9–12.

16. Macones GA, Hankins GD, Spong CY, Hauth J, Moore T. 2008. The 2008 National Institute of Child Health and Human Development workshop report on electronic fetal monitoring. Update on definitions, interpretation, and research guidelines. *Obstet Gynecol.* 112:661–6.

17. Martin CB Jr. 2008. Normal fetal physiology and behavior, and adaptive responses with hypoxemia. *Semin Perinatol.* 32(4):239–42.

18. Miller DA. 2018. Prenatal care: Intrapartum fetal heart rate assessment. Berghella V (Ed). *UpToDate.* Waltham, MA.

19. National Institute for Health and Clinical Excellence. NICE Clinical Guideline 190. 2017. Intrapartum Care. London: National Institute for Health and Care Excellence. pp. 10–13.

20. National Institute for Health and Clinical Excellence. 2014. NICE clinical guideline 190. Intrapartum care for healthy women and babies. London: National Institute for Health and Care Excellence.

21. Nelson KB, Dambrosia JM, Ting TY, Grether JK. 1996. Uncertain value of electronic fetal monitoring in predicting cerebral palsy. *N Engl J Med.* 334:613.

22. Skupski DW, Rosenberg CR, Eglinton GS. 2002. Intrapartum fetal stimulation tests: a meta-analysis. *Obstet Gynecol.* 99:129.

23. World Health Organization. 2018. WHO recommendation on intermittent fetal heart rate auscultation during labour. 2018. WHO, Geneva.

24. World Health Organization. 2018a. WHO recommendation on continuous cardiotocography during labour. 2018a. WHO, Geneva.

Chapter 19

Induction of Labour

INTRODUCTION

- Induction of labour is defined as the process of artificially stimulating uterine contractions before the onset of spontaneous labour. This is a therapeutic option offered in cases where the benefits of delivery outweigh the risks of continuing the pregnancy. It aims to achieve a vaginal delivery. It commonly involves the administration of oxytocin or prostaglandins and may also include amniotomy.
- The cervical status at the start of labour induction has a definite impact on the rate of successful vaginal delivery. Induction with a favourable or ripened cervix will decrease the duration of labour.
- If the cervical status is unfavourable, techniques to ripen the cervix should be used before starting formal induction.
- While it is a safe process in modern obstetrics, induction is not without risks to the mother and the baby. It is therefore imperative that the decision to intervene be based on clear indications and that the process be undertaken with strict adherence to protocols. Its clinical relevance lies in the fact that induction of labour is responsible for a major share of the obstetric workload, requiring several man-hours of work.
- Traditionally, obstetricians have believed that induction of labour increases the risk of cesarean section. Though observational studies have shown an increase in cesarean section rates following induction of labour, the risk of cesarean actually decreases in women with post-dates and term prelabour rupture of membrane (Wood et al., 2014).

Does induction increase the rate of cesarean section?
When performed with strict adherence to clear medical indications and with proper ripening protocols in place, induction of labour between 34 and 39 weeks does not increase the incidence of cesarean sections (Danilack et al., 2016).
Grobman et al. (the ARRIVE trial, 2018) found that induction of labour at 39 weeks in low-risk nulliparous women resulted in a significantly lower frequency of cesarean delivery.

- However, it must not be forgotten that induction is a medical intervention and has contributed to the medicalisation of labour and delivery. If done electively, it should be planned after the evaluation of the cervical status.

Rate of induction
- Though the induction rate varies depending on various factors, it has been estimated that approximately 20 per cent of women worldwide undergo induction of labour.
- Induction of labour (indicated and elective) is generally less common in lower-income countries than it is in higher-income one. However, Vogel et al. (2013), in an analysis of the World Health Organization's Global Survey on Maternal and Neonatal Health, found a higher incidence of induction of labour in India and Sri Lanka as compared to other Asian countries.

This chapter will address the following:
- Ripening of an unfavourable cervix
- Induction of labour at term
- Induction of labour in special situations
- Induction of labour in the second trimester
- Cervical ripening and induction of labour in women with a previous cesarean scar

INDICATIONS FOR INDUCTION OF LABOUR

- Induction can only be offered when there are no contraindications to labour and vaginal birth.
- Induction of labour is indicated when the maternal/fetal risks associated with continuing the pregnancy are thought to be greater than the maternal/fetal risks associated with early delivery.
- The decision to induce labour is influenced by the following factors:
  - Gestational age
  - Severity of the maternal/fetal condition
- Though it is difficult to be precise, induction is chosen when the gestational age is appropriate for neonatal survival. However, this has to be balanced against any possible harm from severe maternal or fetal conditions that might jeopardise the mother or child if the pregnancy is continued.
- The indications for the induction of labour periodically change and new ones evolve. While in some pregnancies there is clear benefit to the mother or fetus from intervention and delivery, in certain other situations, the benefit is less specific. The indication and benefit of induction must be clearly delineated before initiating the process.
- There is considerable overlap between maternal and fetal indications for induction and therefore, they can be combined as follows:
  - Postterm pregnancy
  - Preeclampsia/hypertension/HELLP syndrome
  - Maternal diabetes
  - Premature rupture of membranes
  - Multifetal pregnancy
  - Rh alloimmunisation
  - Fetal growth restriction
  - Fetal demise
  - Psychosocial and logistical reasons

The indications are discussed in greater detail in the respective chapters.

ELECTIVE INDUCTION OF LABOUR

- Induction of labour without a medical indication is termed elective induction of labour.
- Sometimes, this is done for reasons like a previous history of precipitate labour, distance from the hospital, or for psychosocial reasons.

- It is also being done more frequently now to ensure that the delivery occurs at a time when the hospital has an optimum number of staff, and essential services (e.g., blood bank) are accessible.

Elective induction

- ACOG (2013) and NICE (2018) guidelines have suggested that when elective induction is undertaken for the above-mentioned reasons, it should be at 39 completed weeks and not earlier.
- Just as preterm birth before 37 weeks is associated with neonatal morbidity, it is now emerging that early-term birth (37^{+0} to 38^{+6} weeks) is also associated with greater neonatal morbidity (Dietz et al., 2012).
- However, it is important to remember that Indian babies are born earlier and mature earlier in utero than Caucasian babies. **In the Indian scenario, it may be prudent to schedule planned delivery at 38 completed weeks.**

> **Is optimal gestational age for elective induction different in Indian women?**
> It is important to remember that the median gestational age at delivery in Indian women is <39 weeks.
> - The WHO Multinational Longitudinal Study to establish growth charts for developing countries (Kiserud et al., 2017) found the median gestational age at birth was 38^{+4} weeks in India.
> - A large study (122,000 women) conducted in a mixed-population hospital in London (Patel et al., 2004) reported the following findings:
>   - Normal gestational length is shorter in Indian, Pakistani, and Bangladeshi women.
>   - Meconium-stained amniotic fluid, which is a sign of fetal maturity, was significantly more frequent in preterm South Asian infants than it was in white European infants.

Elective induction at 39 weeks for low-risk nulliparous women

- Traditionally, in a low-risk pregnancy between 39 and 41 weeks of gestation, obstetricians would wait expectantly for the spontaneous onset of labour.
- In the multicentre ARRIVE trial, which evaluated the perinatal and maternal consequences of planned induction of labour at 39 weeks of gestation versus expectant management in low-risk nulliparous women, Grobman et al. (2018) found that induction reduced the chances of cesarean delivery, hypertensive disorders of pregnancy, and the need for neonatal respiratory support.
- Offering elective induction of labour to low-risk nulliparous women at 39 weeks of gestation is a reasonable option (SMFM, 2018; ACOG, 2018) because it provides an opportunity to choose a time that is most optimal for the presence of an adequate number of staff, the presence of senior/experienced obstetricians, and access to essential services.

CONTRAINDICATIONS TO INDUCTION OF LABOUR

- The contraindications to labour induction are generally the conditions that contraindicate labour and vaginal delivery.

- Some of these are as follows:
  - Increased risk of uterine rupture
    - Prior classical or other high-risk cesarean incision
    - Prior uterine rupture
    - Prior transmural uterine incision entering the uterine cavity (as in previous myomectomy)
  - Suspected cephalopelvic disproportion
  - Placenta previa or vasa previa
  - Umbilical cord prolapse
  - Abnormal fetal presentation like transverse lie, breech, brow, or face presentation
  - Category III fetal heart rate tracing indicating fetal distress (see **Chapter 18**, *Fetal health surveillance in labour*)
  - Active genital herpes infection

PREDICTION OF SUCCESS OF INDUCTION

Maternal characteristics

The success of induction of labour can be predicted by maternal characteristics. The following are associated with an increased chance of successful induction:

- Gestational age close to term
- Favourable pelvic configuration
- Multiparity
- Fetal weight <3.5 kg
- Tall stature
- Normal body mass index
- High Bishop score

Bishop score

- The readiness of the cervix for spontaneous labour is a crucial factor in determining response to induction of labour. In other words, the process of induction is faster and more successful if the cervix is already soft, short, and has started to dilate and when the presenting part is sufficiently low in the pelvis.

- The success of induction can be indirectly predicted by the modified Bishop score. This system uses a score based on the station of the presenting part and four characteristics of the cervix: dilatation (in cm), effacement (in length of cervix), consistency, and position (Table 19.1).

Checklist for the induction of labour
- Review indication
- Assess and discuss
  - Indication
  - Probability of failed induction
- Confirm gestational age
  - LMP
  - Ultrasound scan before 20 weeks
- Document fetal weight estimate
- Evaluate fetal well-being
  - Cardiotocography (CTG)
  - Biophysical profile/Doppler if required
- Abdominal examination
  - Fetal size
  - Presentation
  - Descent of presenting part
- Pelvic examination
  - Favourability of cervix
  - Station of presenting part
  - Adequacy of pelvis

Table 19.1   Modified Bishop score

Parameters	Bishop score			
	0	1	2	3
Cervical dilatation	<1 cm	1–2 cm	2–4 cm	>4 cm
Length of cervix/effacement	>4 cm/0–30%	2–4 cm/40–50%	1–2 cm/ 60–70%	<1 cm/80%
Station (cm from ischial spines)	–3	–2	–1/0	+1/+2
Consistency	Firm	Average	Soft	–
Position	Posterior	Mid-position	Anterior	–

- Cervical dilatation is considered to be the most important predictive element of the Bishop score.
- Laughon et al. (2011) have shown that a simplified Bishop score using only cervical dilatation, effacement, and station is quite effective in predicting a successful delivery.

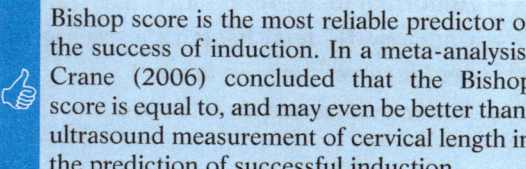

Bishop score is the most reliable predictor of the success of induction. In a meta-analysis, Crane (2006) concluded that the Bishop score is equal to, and may even be better than, ultrasound measurement of cervical length in the prediction of successful induction.

- **A high Bishop score (≥8) before induction is associated with a vaginal delivery rate comparable to that with spontaneous onset of labour. A low Bishop score (≤6) predicts an increased rate of failed induction, resulting in cesarean section.**
- When the Bishop score is low, cervical ripening is performed to improve the score before proceeding with induction.

PRE-INDUCTION CERVICAL RIPENING

- Cervical ripening typically begins prior to the onset of labour contractions and is necessary for cervical dilatation and the passage of the fetus. It is the term used to denote the process of cervical softening, thinning, and dilatation. A favourable cervix is one that has softened, thinned, and dilated to a certain extent prior to labour.
- Cervical ripening results from a series of complex biochemical processes that ends with the rearrangement and realignment of collagen molecules in the cervix.
- Several techniques are available to initiate cervical ripening in an unfavourable cervix, with the goal of reducing the rate of failed induction and the induction-to-delivery time.
- A Bishop score of <6 is an indication for initiating cervical ripening to increase the chances of successful induction.
- The commonly used methods of cervical ripening are as follows:
  - Sweeping of membranes
  - Mechanical agents
    - Balloon catheters
    - Hygroscopic dilators
  - Pharmacological agents
    - Prostaglandin E$_1$ (intracervical, intravaginal)
    - Prostaglandin E$_2$ (vaginal, oral)

- Both mechanical agents and prostaglandins have similar success in achieving cervical ripening. Chen et al. (2016) compared Foley catheters, misoprostol, and dinoprostone for cervical ripening in the induction of labour and concluded that no method of cervical ripening demonstrated superiority over the others. Each method has its advantages and disadvantages (Table 19.2).

The following methods are not recommended for cervical ripening or induction of labour because of the lack of robust data regarding their safety and efficacy:
- Nipple stimulation
- Sexual intercourse
- Castor oil
- Acupuncture
- Hot baths
- Enema
- Isosorbide mononitrate

Table 19.2 Advantages and disadvantages of cervical ripening agents

Ripening agent	Advantages	Disadvantages
Intravaginal misoprostol or dinoprostone	Best chance of achieving vaginal delivery within 24 hours	• Increased risk of uterine hyperstimulation with adverse FHR changes • Contraindicated in a scarred uterus
Intracervical dinoprostone	Less expensive than intravaginal dinoprostone	• Risk of uterine hyperstimulation but less than with intravaginal dinoprostone • Contraindicated in a scarred uterus
Foley catheter	• Inexpensive • Universally available • Very low risk of hyperstimulation • Safe in a scarred uterus	Higher rate of requirement of augmentation with oxytocin
Oral misoprostol	• Inexpensive • Easy to administer • Lowest risk of cesarean delivery	Contraindicated in a scarred uterus

Sweeping of membranes

- Sweeping of fetal membranes, also called *stripping* of membranes, is a simple outpatient technique that does

 Sweeping of membranes is known to reduce the need for formal induction of labour.

not require admission to hospital. It involves stripping the amniotic membrane off the lower uterine segment.
- The sweeping is done by gently inserting a finger through the external os into the space between the membranes and the lower uterine segment and rotating through 360 degrees, keeping the finger close to the uterine wall. In order to sweep the membranes, the cervix should be dilated enough to allow the insertion of a finger.
- The procedure works due to increased local production and release of prostaglandin $F_2\alpha$ ($PGF_2\alpha$) from the decidua and adjacent membrane, which lead to the onset of labour.
- A systematic review of the Cochrane Database (Boulvain et al., 2005) showed that sweeping of membranes reduced the need for more formal forms of labour induction.

- Sweeping of the membranes, performed as a routine policy in women at term, is associated with reduced duration of pregnancy and reduced the frequency of pregnancy continuing beyond 41 weeks.
- Nulliparous women at 40 and 41 weeks and parous women at 41 weeks may be offered membrane sweeping (NICE Guidelines, 2008).
- The response to membrane sweeping is unpredictable and slow. Therefore, it should be used only if the indication for induction is non-urgent.
- The potential serious complications of sweeping are bleeding from an undiagnosed previa or vasa previa, and the rupture of membranes.
- Women should be counselled about bleeding, discomfort, and contractions that may not lead to labour in 24 hours.

Mechanical methods of cervical ripening

Balloon catheters

- Both single-balloon (Foley) and double-balloon catheters have been subjected to randomised controlled trials and have been found to be equally effective (Yang et al., 2018).
- The action of the balloon catheter is a mechanical one. It leads to the stripping of the membranes from the lower uterine segment, thus releasing prostaglandins. This leads to cervical ripening and an increase in myometrial contractility.
- The advantages of a Foley catheter are its low cost and lower rate of excessive uterine stimulation (tachysystole), with or without FHR changes.
- The World Health Organization (2011) recommends combining a balloon catheter for cervical ripening with oxytocin for subsequent induction as an alternative method when prostaglandins are not available or contraindicated, such as in a scarred uterus.
- In a multicentre and randomised controlled study (INFORM trial) conducted in India, the two available inexpensive options for cervical ripening were compared. Oral misoprostol was found to be more effective than transcervical Foley catheter placement for the induction of labour in women with preeclampsia or hypertension (Mundle et al., 2017).

Foley catheter vs. double-balloon catheter
When the Foley catheter was compared with a double-balloon catheter, no clinically important differences were found in outcomes (Salim et al., 2018). However, the Foley catheter is less expensive and more readily available in developing countries like India.

Oxytocin concurrently with or after Foley placement?
A recent study (Schoen et al., 2017) showed that induction with intravenous oxytocin infusion started **concurrently** with Foley placement significantly increased the rate of delivery within 24 hours, compared with Foley placement **followed by** oxytocin infusion. 64% of nulliparous women delivered within 24 hours in the concurrent group as compared to 43% in the group that received oxytocin either after 12 hours of Foley placement or after the expulsion of the catheter. In multiparous women, the percentages were 87% and 72% respectively.

Role of amniotomy

- Early amniotomy is recommended after cervical ripening with a Foley catheter.
- Battarbee et al. (2016) found that in women undergoing labour induction after cervical ripening with a balloon catheter, amniotomy within one hour of catheter removal was more likely to result in a vaginal delivery within 24 hours of catheter placement (42.9 vs. 33.0 per cent) and was associated with a shorter interval to delivery.

> **Procedure for the placement of a transcervical balloon catheter**
> - Under strict aseptic conditions, a 16F Foley catheter with a 30 mL bulb is inserted into the cervix, past the internal os and into the extra-amniotic space.
> - This is usually possible even if the cervix is not dilated since the pregnant cervix is usually soft and allows the passage of the catheter.
> - The bulb is then filled with 30 mL of saline and the Foley is pulled back gently so that the bulb rests against the internal os.
> - The catheter is taped with tension to the medial aspect of the woman's thigh.
> - The catheter is left in place until it is extruded or it is removed after 12 hours.
> - If a double-balloon catheter is used, it is placed with one balloon below and the other, above the internal os.
> - Cervical ripening is usually achieved with a balloon catheter and may also result in the onset of labour.
> - Sufficient time should be allowed for effacement before formal agents of induction are used subsequently.

Extra-amniotic saline infusion (EASI)

- Extra-amniotic saline infusion is a modification of the use of a Foley catheter for cervical ripening.
- Room temperature sterile saline is infused through the catheter port at the rate of 30–40 mL/hour using an infusion pump.
- There is no clear advantage of this method over other methods of cervical ripening (NICE, 2008; Lin et al., 2007). It is not used commonly.

Hygroscopic dilators

- There are two types of hygroscopic dilators. *Laminaria tents* are made from natural seaweed and are currently being replaced by a more commonly available *synthetic product*.
- Hygroscopic dilators absorb moisture and thus gradually expand within the cervical canal. They disrupt the chorioamniotic decidual interface, causing lysosomal destruction and leading to prostaglandin release. The passive mechanical stretching provided by the dilator triggers changes in cervical tissue, resulting in ripening.
- Though they continue to be used more commonly for medical termination of pregnancy (MTP), hygroscopic dilators are proving to be as safe and effective as other cervical ripening agents in term pregnancies. A recent study (Saad et al., 2019) showed that the synthetic hygroscopic dilator was not inferior to the Foley catheter in bringing about cervical ripening. Women were also more satisfied with the hygroscopic dilator because, unlike the catheter, it does not protrude from the introitus and is therefore more comfortable.

- Oxytocin, with or without amniotomy, is usually administered following ripening with hygroscopic dilators.

> **Procedure for hygroscopic dilator placement**
> - Under aseptic conditions, the anterior lip of the cervix is held with a non-traumatic clamp.
> - The tip of the dilator is dipped into sterile lubricant to make the insertion easier.
> - As many dilators as possible are gently inserted into the endocervical canal. The number of dilators inserted must be documented.
> - Care must be taken not to exert undue force. Women may complain of cramping during the procedure.
> - A moistened roller gauze is then gently placed in the vagina to keep the dilators in place.
> - Synthetic dilators are removed after 6–8 hours. Laminaria tents are removed 12–24 hours after placement.

Pharmacological methods of cervical ripening

Prostaglandins

- In an **unscarred uterus**, prostaglandins are most effective for cervical ripening.
- The commonly used prostaglandins are prostaglandin E_1 (PGE$_1$) and prostaglandin E_2 (PGE$_2$).
- If prostaglandin E_1 or E_2 is administered for cervical ripening, 50 per cent of women will go into labour and may not require oxytocin (Thomas et al., 2014).

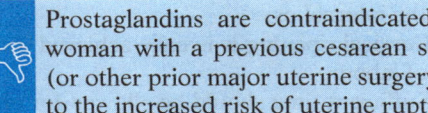

> Prostaglandins are contraindicated in a woman with a previous cesarean section (or other prior major uterine surgery) due to the increased risk of uterine rupture.

Prostaglandin E₁ (misoprostol)

- Misoprostol, a synthetic PGE$_1$ analogue, is an effective drug for the induction of labour.
- It is cheap and stable at room temperature and very useful in developing countries. The World Health Organization (2011) recommends it for pre-induction cervical ripening.
- Misoprostol is available as a 25 µg or 100 µg tablet. The 100 µg tablet can be broken into four equal-sized pieces for cervical ripening.
- The tablets can be administered both vaginally and orally.

Vaginal misoprostol
- A 25 µg dose of misoprostol is placed high in the vagina.
- The dose can be repeated every 3–6 hours (Table 19.3) for a maximum of six doses.

> **Oxytocin after misoprostol**
> If oxytocin is required for augmentation, it may be administered four hours after the final dose of vaginal or oral misoprostol.

Oral misoprostol
- Oral misoprostol is both convenient and effective for cervical ripening and labour induction.
- It is more effective than placebo, as effective as vaginal misoprostol, and results in fewer cesarean sections than vaginal dinoprostone or oxytocin (Alfirevic et al., 2014).

- Either a dose of 50 μg every four hours (Ten Eikelder et al., 2016) or 25 μg every two hours, as recommended by the WHO and others (Tang et al., 2013; Weeks et al., 2017) may be used for a maximum of six doses (Table 19.3). If oxytocin is required for augmentation, it may be administered four hours after the final dose of misoprostol.

Prostaglandin E$_1$ (misoprostol)
- Route
  - Vaginal
  - Oral
- Induces cervical ripening
- More effective than PGE$_2$
- Associated with
  - Tachysystole (>5 contractions in 10 minutes during a 30-minute period)
  - Fetal heart rate abnormalities
  - Meconium staining
- Can cause uterine rupture in a scarred uterus
- No increase in cesarean section rate
- Effects are dose-related
- If oxytocin is required for augmentation, it may be administered **four hours** after the final dose of misoprostol

---

Prostaglandin E$_2$ (dinoprostone)

- There are two prostaglandin E$_2$ preparations available.
- One is in the form of a pre-loaded intracervical gel which contains 0.5 mg of dinoprostone in 2.5 mL of gel. PGE$_2$ gel should be refrigerated to remain active and is more expensive than oxytocin and misoprostol.
- The other PGE$_2$ preparation is an intravaginal insert which contains 10 mg of dinoprostone in a timed-release formulation.

PGE$_2$ intracervical gel

- 0.5 mg of the intracervical gel is administered into the cervical canal every six hours up to a maximum of three doses in a 24-hour period (Table 19.3).
- If oxytocin is required for augmentation, it may be administered six hours after the final dose of PGE$_2$ gel.

Procedure for intracervical gel placement
- The mother is placed in the dorsolithotomy position.
- Under aseptic conditions, a speculum is used to visualise the cervical os.
- The anterior lip of the cervix is held with a sponge-holding forceps.
- The plastic inserter of the pre-loaded syringe is placed into the cervical canal, taking care not to go beyond the internal os.

PGE$_2$ intravaginal insert

- This contains 10 mg of dinoprostone in a small white polymer mesh sac and has an attached tape for removal.
- It is left in the vagina until active labour starts or for 12 hours (Table 19.3).

Prostaglandin E$_2$
- Route
  - Intracervical
  - Intravaginal
- Induces cervical ripening
- Reduces failed induction rate
- Reduces need for oxytocin
- Shortens induction–delivery interval
- If oxytocin is required for augmentation, it may be administered **six hours** after the final dose of PGE$_2$ gel

Table 19.3 Prostaglandin regimens for cervical ripening (in an unscarred uterus)

Drug	Route/dose	Caution
Misoprostol (PGE$_1$)	• Vaginal: 25 μg tablet every 3–6 hours • Oral: 50 μg every 4 hours OR 25 μg every 2 hours for a maximum of 6 doses	• Tachysystole common with vaginal dose of >25 μg • Interval of 4 hours before oxytocin is started for augmentation
Dinoprostone gel (PGE$_2$) intracervical	0.5 mg intracervically every 6 hours for a maximum of 3 doses	Oxytocin may be started 6 hours after final dose of PGE$_2$ (to avoid hyperstimulation)
Dinoprostone (PGE$_2$) intravaginal insert 10 mg	• Placed high in posterior fornix for a maximum of 12 hours • Easy to remove in case of tachysystole	Uterine tachysystole (hyperstimulation) most common with PGE$_2$ vaginal insert

Side effects of prostaglandins

Prostaglandins are associated with both systemic and uterine side effects in 1–5 per cent of women. The main criticisms against prostaglandins are that they are associated with a higher risk of uterine tachysystole, fetal distress, and uterine rupture (Alfirevic et al., 2014; ACOG, 2009). These complications are directly related to the dose and the frequency of administration.

Prostaglandin E$_2$
- Systemic side effects
  - Vomiting and nausea
  - Transient fever
  - Diarrhea
  - Headache
  - Chills
  - Transient decrease of >20 mmHg in diastolic blood pressure
- Tachysystole (>5 contractions in 10 minutes during a 30-minute period)

Misoprostol (prostaglandin E$_1$)
- Systemic side effects as above
- Hyperstimulation (tachysystole leading to non-reassuring fetal heart rate pattern)
- Risk of uterine rupture (contraindicated in case of previous cesarean section)

INDUCTION OF LABOUR AT TERM

- For successful induction of labour, the cervix needs to be favourable. Methods of ripening an unfavourable cervix have been described in the preceding section. Prostaglandins used for ripening the cervix may also stimulate uterine contraction, which may result in the onset of labour.
- Once the cervix becomes favourable, labour is induced, usually with oxytocin, with or without amniotomy.
- Amniotomy in itself may be ineffective without the use of oxytocin. In any case, it cannot be done unless the cervix is dilated enough to allow the passage of an instrument.
- Oxytocin is most effective when the cervix is already favourable or when the membranes have ruptured.

> **Terminology used to describe contractions during labour induction**
> The best way to monitor the efficacy of oxytocin is to monitor contractions. It is important to quantify uterine contractions with the use of the following terms:
> - *Frequency:* Desired frequency is 3–5 contractions in 10 minutes
> - *Duration:* Effective duration is 30–60 seconds
> - *Intensity:* Desired intensity – the uterus cannot be indented by palpating fingers at the peak of the contraction
> - *Relaxation time between contractions:* Optimal relaxation time between contractions is ≥3 minutes
> - *Tachysystole:* >5 contractions in 10 minutes
> - *Uterine hypertonus:* Single contraction lasting >2 minutes
> - *Hyperstimulation:* Tachysystole or hypertonus associated with non-reassuring fetal heart rate pattern

Induction of labour with oxytocin

- A systematic review of the Cochrane Database (Alfirevic et al., 2016), which looked at the best and most cost-effective method for induction of labour, found that oxytocin infusion along with amniotomy, and vaginal misoprostol were the most effective in achieving a vaginal delivery within 24 hours.
- Synthetic oxytocin is among the most potent uterotonic agents known and is administered as an intravenous infusion. The uterus responds to oxytocin with increasing sensitivity with advancing gestational age due to increase in myometrial oxytocin-binding sites.
- Each obstetric unit should adopt an evidence-based protocol for oxytocin administration, and the protocol should be readily available in the labour ward.
- An infusion pump should be used to control the rate of infusion precisely. In the absence of an infusion pump, the rate of drops-per-minute has to be titrated and monitored accurately.
- The maximum dose of oxytocin has not been established. The end point is usually the achievement of at least three uterine contractions in 10 minutes, each lasting for 40 seconds.
- The strength of uterine contractions should be monitored by palpation, and their frequency, duration, and intensity (strength) should be documented. It should also be noted whether the uterus relaxes between contractions and for how long.

> **Labour progression with oxytocin-induced labour**
> - Latent phase is prolonged.
> - Once active phase is reached, there is no difference in labour progression between induced and spontaneous labour.

Dosage of oxytocin

Two regimens are described for the administration of intravenous oxytocin: low-dose and high-dose regimens (Table 19.4).

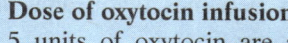

> **Dose of oxytocin infusion**
> 5 units of oxytocin are added to 500 mL of normal saline solution. The infusion is preferably given through an infusion pump. If an infusion pump is not available, a regular intravenous set may be used with close monitoring.

- **Low-dose regimens:** A low dose of oxytocin and less frequent increases in dose have the advantage of a lower risk of the occurrence of uterine tachysystole and associated FHR changes.

- **High-dose regimens:** A high dose of oxytocin and more frequent dose increases are associated with shorter labour and lower rates of cesarean delivery for dystocia. The disadvantage of this regimen is increased rates of uterine tachysystole with associated FHR changes.

Table 19.4   Low- and high-dose regimens for oxytocin administration

Regimen	Starting dose (mU/min)	Incremental dose	Dosage interval
Low-dose	0.5–2	1–2 (mU/min)	15–40 (minutes)
High-dose	6	3–6 (mU/min)	15–40 (minutes)

Incremental administration of oxytocin

- When 5 units of oxytocin are added to 500 mL of Ringer's lactate or normal saline, the concentration achieved is 10 mU/mL.
- A flow rate of 15 mL/hour will deliver the drug at the rate of 2 mU/min (Table 19.5). The maximum rate for oxytocin ranges from 32–40 mU/min, but it is rarely required.
- Optimal interval for dose increase:
  - Low-dose regimens and less frequent increases in dose are associated with a lower risk of uterine tachysystole with associated FHR changes.
  - Though increasing the dose of oxytocin at 20-minute intervals may be associated with tachysystole, it results in a significant reduction of cesarean sections for dystocia.
  - Increasing the dose at 40-minute intervals seems to offer no clear advantage over the 20-minute intervals.

The oxytocin dosage in mU, drops/per minute, and mL/hour (using 5 units of oxytocin in 500 mL of normal saline) is presented in Table 19.5.

> **Latent phase in induction**
> The latent phase is said to begin once cervical ripening has ended, oxytocin is initiated, and rupture of membranes has occurred. It is determined as having ended once a dilatation of 5 cm is achieved.

Table 19.5 Dosage of oxytocin for induction of labour

mU of oxytocin	Drops/minute (manual)	mL/hour (infusion pump)
0.5	1	3.75
2	4	15
4	8	30
6	12	45
8	16	60
10	20	75
14	24	90
16	28	105
18	32	120
20	36	135
24	40	150
28	44	165
30	48	180
32	52	195

Role of amniotomy

- Early amniotomy is recommended to increase the success of induction with oxytocin.
- The combination of early amniotomy and oxytocin administration during induction appears to shorten the time to vaginal delivery.
- In a randomised trial of nulliparous women undergoing labour induction, Macones et al. (2012) found that routine early amniotomy (**defined as being performed at a cervical dilatation ≤4 cm**) shortened the time to delivery by approximately two hours and increased the proportion of deliveries within 24 hours.
- Early amniotomy also provides the opportunity to assess the amniotic fluid for the presence of meconium.

Complications of induction with oxytocin

Uterine hyperstimulation

- Hyperstimulation may present as tachysystole (>5 contractions in 10 minutes) or hypertonus (single contraction lasting >2 minutes) and is associated with a non-reassuring fetal heart rate pattern.
- Excessive uterine activity leads to increased perinatal morbidity only when associated with abnormal fetal heart rate changes, particularly changes such as the absence of baseline variability, recurrent variable or late decelerations, and prolonged bradycardia.
- The incidence of uterine tachysystole is 5 per cent with oxytocin but may be as high as 15 per cent if dinoprostone and oxytocin are used concurrently.

Management of hyperstimulation (ACOG, 2009)
- Discontinue intravenous oxytocin infusion
- Turn the patient to the left lateral position
- Administer oxygen by face mask (at 10 L/min)
- Increase intravenous hydration if not contraindicated by the maternal condition (a bolus of 500 mL of Ringer's solution)
- Assess blood pressure
- Perform a pelvic examination to assess cervical dilatation and to rule out cord prolapse
- Administer a tocolytic if the hypertonus does not respond to the discontinuation of the drug; subcutaneous or intravenous terbutaline (250 µg) is recommended
- Proceed with cesarean section if the abnormal FHR pattern does not improve with these measures

Restarting oxytocin after tachysystole

- Oxytocin should be restarted carefully after an episode of tachysystole.
- If there are no persistent abnormal changes in the fetal heart rate, the oxytocin is restarted at a lower dosage.
- The incremental increase should be reduced to 3. mU/minute if hyperstimulation is present, and to 1 mU/minute if there is recurrent hyperstimulation.

Uterine rupture

- Uterine rupture is very rare with induction of labour in an unscarred uterus, even in parous women.
- It is more likely to occur in a grand multipara (a woman who has given birth five or more times) or in neglected cases of obstructed labour.

Hyponatremia ('water intoxication')

- Water intoxication is a very rare complication in modern obstetrics.
- It may occur when high concentrations of oxytocin are infused in large quantities of hypotonic solutions, and is very unusual in the doses used for labour induction.

Chorioamnionitis

- If the interval between the onset of induction and delivery is prolonged, the risk of chorioamnionitis increases. Once the membranes are ruptured, the risk of chorioamnionitis increases with increase in the duration between amniotomy and delivery.

Failed induction

- Though the criteria for failed induction are not uniform, it can be defined as failure to progress from the latent phase to the active phase of labour. A failed induction will necessitate a cesarean section.
- Enough time should be given before the induction is considered to have failed. Grobman et al. (2018) suggest that cesarean delivery should not be undertaken during the latent phase unless at least 15 hours have passed after initiating oxytocin, and rupture of membranes has occurred.

Risk of cesarean section with induction of labour

- Any increase in the risk of cesarean delivery related to induction appears to be associated primarily with an unfavourable cervix at admission.

- Though obstetricians have long believed that the induction of labour increases the risk of cesarean section, recent data have challenged this belief. Systematic reviews and meta-analyses have concluded that when performed with strict adherence to clear medical indications and with proper ripening protocols in place, *induction of labour between 34 and 39 weeks does not increase the incidence of cesarean sections* (Danilack et al., 2016; Wood et al., 2014).

INDUCTION OF LABOUR IN SPECIAL SITUATIONS

Postterm pregnancy

- The chief goals in the management of postterm pregnancies are reduction in perinatal mortality rate and choosing the ideal time for intervention to achieve this goal without increasing the cesarean section rate.
- A systematic review of the Cochrane Database (Middleton et al., 2018) has concluded that elective labour induction at 40 or 41 weeks' gestation is associated with fewer perinatal deaths and fewer cesarean sections as compared to expectant management.

Routine induction at 40–41 weeks (Middleton et al., 2018)
- 70% reduction in stillbirth
- 70% reduction in perinatal mortality
- 8% reduction in cesarean
- 28% reduction in macrosomia
- 23% reduction in meconium aspiration syndrome

Preterm prelabour rupture of membranes (PPROM)

- In PPROM, expectant management up to 34 weeks is recommended to attain fetal maturity. Expectant management can be followed in the absence of maternal or fetal infection (see **Chapter 33**, *Preterm labour and preterm prelabour rupture of membranes*).
- In the presence of a favourable cervix, labour can be induced at 34 weeks with oxytocin. Either vaginal PGE_2 or misoprostol can be used if the cervix is unfavourable (Zhang et al., 2015).

Prelabour rupture of membranes (PROM) at term

- Women with term PROM should be induced promptly.
- A systematic review of the Cochrane Database (Middleton et al., 2018) comparing induction and expectant

Prompt induction of labour is recommended for women with prelabour rupture of membranes at term. Oxytocin is the first choice.

management showed that induction resulted in a shorter time to delivery with no increase in cesarean delivery. A decrease in maternal infection was also noted with early induction.
- Oxytocin is regarded as the first option, though prostaglandins may be considered if the Bishop score is low.

INDUCTION OF LABOUR IN THE SECOND TRIMESTER

- Intrauterine fetal demise (IUFD) in the late second trimester is the commonest indication for induction of labour in the second trimester.
- Immediate delivery, as soon as the diagnosis is made, is indicated in conditions that jeopardise maternal well-being such *as severe preeclampsia/eclampsia, placental abruption, ruptured membranes*, and *chorioamnionitis*.
- If the fetus is not salvageable, induction might be a better option than a cesarean, which would scar the uterus.
- Though the majority of women spontaneously go into labour within three weeks of intrauterine fetal demise, most women and their families opt for delivery within 24–48 hours. Approximately 90 per cent deliver within 24 hours of induction with minimal complications.
- Maternal coagulopathy associated with fetal death is uncommon up to four weeks after the event. However, blood tests should be done to rule out this complication, especially if expectant management is chosen.
- The choice of the method of induction depends on the following:
  - Gestational age
  - Presence or absence of a previous scar (see section below on *Cervical ripening and induction of labour in women with a previous cesarean scar*)

> The following options have been recommended by the ACOG (2013) for the use of a combined regimen with mifepristone and vaginal misoprostol in second trimester induction of labour for termination of pregnancy:
> 1. **Mifepristone** 200 mg, administered orally, followed by:
>   - **Misoprostol** 800 μg administered vaginally, followed by 400 μg administered vaginally or sublingually every three hours for up to a maximum of five doses **or**
>   - **Misoprostol** 400 μg administered buccally every three hours for up to a maximum of five doses
> 2. **If mifepristone is not available, the following is recommended**:
>   - Misoprostol 400 μg administered vaginally or sublingually every three hours for up to five doses; vaginal placement is superior to sublingual placement for nulliparous women **or**
>   - A vaginal loading dose of 600–800 μg of misoprostol followed by 400 μg administered vaginally or sublingually every three hours may be more effective
> 3. **If misoprostol is not available**, the following is recommended:
>   - Oxytocin 20–100 units infused intravenously over three hours followed by one hour without oxytocin to allow diuresis; oxytocin dose may be slowly increased to a maximum of 300 units over three hours
> **If the termination is not complete after five doses, the woman may be allowed to rest for 12 hours before starting the cycle again.**

- A combination of mifepristone followed by vaginal misoprostol is the most effective regimen in the second trimester (Chaudhuri and Datta, 2015; Panda et al., 2013). This combination may be used safely up to 34 weeks of gestation. Compared to misoprostol alone, this combination has the following advantages:
  - It results in a significantly high rate of successful delivery.
  - It shortens the induction–delivery interval in women who have experienced fetal death as compared to the use of misoprostol alone (see box above).
  - It significantly reduces the need for oxytocin augmentation.

CERVICAL RIPENING AND INDUCTION OF LABOUR IN WOMEN WITH A PREVIOUS CESAREAN SCAR

- Compared to spontaneous labour, induction of labour is associated with higher rates of uterine rupture in women with a previous scar. Though the absolute

 The use of prostaglandins is contraindicated in a woman who has had a previous cesarean section.

risk of uterine rupture in labour following a previous cesarean is low, a trial of labour after prior cesarean delivery is associated with a greater risk of uterine rupture as compared to elective repeat cesarean delivery without labour (Landon et al., 2004).
- Jozwiak and Dodd (2013), in a systematic review of the Cochrane Database, were unable to come to a conclusion regarding the optimal method of inducing labour in women with a prior cesarean birth.
- Each case has to be individualised and if induced, the increased risks of the need for emergency cesarean section and the risk of uterine rupture should be discussed with the couple (Table 19.6).
- In women who opt for trial of labour after cesarean (TOLAC), the following would be the options available:
  - Woman with a favourable cervix:
    - Amniotomy followed by oxytocin infusion
  - Woman with an unfavourable cervix:
    - Cervical ripening with a Foley catheter followed by oxytocin infusion
- The risk of uterine rupture is higher in the presence of a previous cesarean scar (or a deep transmyometrial uterine scar following a myomectomy where the uterine cavity was entered).

 Induction of labour in women attempting vaginal birth after cesarean (VBAC) is associated with less success of vaginal delivery as compared to those with spontaneous onset of labour. It is also associated with an increased risk of serious maternal morbidity (Sims et al., 2001).

- Because of the risk of uterine rupture (Table 19.6), induction of labour for trial of labour following a previous cesarean must be done in a tertiary centre with immediate access to an operation theatre, anesthetist, and blood bank.

Table 19.6   Risk of uterine rupture depending on labour status

Labour status	Risk of rupture
Planned repeat cesarean section	0
Spontaneous labour	4 ruptures per 1000 spontaneously labouring women
Augmented labour	9 ruptures per 1000 augmented labours
Induced labour (with oxytocin alone)	11 ruptures per 1000 women induced
Induced labour (mechanical dilatation with or without oxytocin)	9 ruptures per 1000 women induced
Induced labour (prostaglandin with or without oxytocin)	14 ruptures per 1000 women induced

MONITORING INDUCTION OF LABOUR

- Wherever induction is carried out, facilities for close monitoring of the fetus should be available, preferably with an electronic fetal monitor (cardiotocograph). However, a good one-to-one monitoring by trained staff is equally safe.
- A normal fetal heart rate pattern should be confirmed before induction is started and as soon as the contractions are established.
- Further monitoring will depend upon the condition of the fetus and the indication for which induction is being carried out. Intermittent auscultation may be used if the pregnancy is low-risk and if the initial assessment is normal.

PAIN RELIEF DURING INDUCTION OF LABOUR

Women in whom labour is induced have greater analgesic requirement than those with spontaneous labour, particularly those induced with oxytocin (see **Chapter 17**, *Pain relief in labour*).

References

1. Alfirevic Z, Aflaifel N, Weeks A. 2014. Oral misoprostol for induction of labour. *Cochrane Database Syst Rev.* Issue 6. Article no.: CD001338.
2. Alfirevic Z, Keeney E, Dowswell T et al. 2016. Which method is best for the induction of labour? A systematic review, network meta-analysis and cost-effectiveness analysis. *Health Technol Assess.* 20(65):1–584.
3. American College of Obstetricians and Gynecologists. 2009 (reaffirmed 2020). ACOG Practice Bulletin Number 107. Induction of labor.
4. American College of Obstetricians and Gynecologists. 2013 (reaffirmed 2017). ACOG Practice Bulletin No. 135: Second-trimester abortion. *Obstet Gynecol.* 121:1394.
5. American College of Obstetricians and Gynecologists. 2018. ACOG Practice Advisory: Clinical guidance for integration of the findings of The ARRIVE Trial: Labor Induction versus Expectant Management in Low-Risk Nulliparous Women.
6. Battarbee AN, Palatnik A, Peress DA, Grobman WA. 2016. Association of early amniotomy after foley balloon catheter ripening and duration of nulliparous labor induction. *Obstet Gynecol.* 128(3):592–597.
7. Boulvain M, Stan C, Irion O. 2005. Membrane sweeping for induction of labor. *Cochrane Database Syst Rev.* Issue 1. Article no.: CD000451.
8. Chaudhuri P, Datta S. 2015. Mifepristone and misoprostol compared with misoprostol alone for induction of labor in intrauterine fetal death: A randomized trial. *J Obstet Gynaecol Res.* 41:1884.
9. Chen W, Xue J, Peprah MK et al. 2016. A systematic review and network meta-analysis comparing the use of Foley catheters, misoprostol, and dinoprostone for cervical ripening in the induction of labour. *BJOG.* 123:346.
10. Crane JM. 2006. Factors predicting labor induction success: A critical analysis. *Clin Obstet Gynecol.* 49:573.
11. Danilack VA, Dore DD, Triche EW et al. 2016. The effect of labour induction on the risk of caesarean delivery: Using propensity scores to control confounding by indication. *BJOG.* 123: 1521–1529.

12. Dietz PM, Rizzo JH, England LJ et al. 2012. Early term delivery and health care utilization in the first year of life. *J Pediatr.* 161:234.

13. Grobman WA, Rice MM, Reddy UM et al. 2018. Labor induction versus expectant management in low-risk nulliparous women. *N Engl J Med.* 379:513–523.

14. Jozwiak M, Dodd JM. 2013. Methods of term labour induction for women with a previous caesarean section. *Cochrane Database of Syst Rev.* Issue 3. Art No.: CD009792.

15. Kiserud T, Piaggio G, Carroli G et al. 2017. The World Health Organization fetal growth charts: A multinational longitudinal study of ultrasound biometric measurements and estimated fetal weight. *PLoS Med.* 14: e1002220.

16. Landon MB, Hauth JC, Leveno KJ et al. 2004. Maternal and perinatal outcomes associated with a trial of labor after prior cesarean delivery. *N Engl J Med.* 351:2581.

17. Laughon SK, Zhang J, Troendle J et al. 2011. Using a simplified Bishop score to predict vaginal delivery. *Obstet Gynecol.* 117:805.

18. Lin MG, Reid KJ, Treaster MR et al. 2007. Transcervical Foley catheter with and without extraamniotic saline infusion for labor induction: A randomized controlled trial. *Obstet Gynecol.* 110:558.

19. Macones GA, Cahill A, Stamilio DM, Odibo AO. 2012. The efficacy of early amniotomy in nulliparous labor induction: A randomized controlled trial. *Am J Obstet Gynecol.* 207:403.e1.

20. Middleton P, Shepherd E, Crowther CA. 2018. Induction of labour for improving birth outcomes for women at or beyond term. *Cochrane Database Syst Rev.* Issue 7. Art. no.: CD004945.

21. Mundle S, Bracken H, Khedikar V et al. 2017. Foley catheterisation versus oral misoprostol for induction of labour in hypertensive women in India (INFORM): A multicentre, open-label, randomised controlled trial. *Lancet.* 12;390 (10095):669–680.

22. NICE clinical guideline 70. Induction of labour. 2008. National Institute for Health and Clinical Excellence.

23. Panda S, Jha V, Singh S. 2013. Role of combination of mifepristone and misoprostol verses misoprostol alone in induction of labour in late intrauterine fetal death: A prospective study. *J Family Reprod Health.* 7:177.

24. Patel RR, Steer P, Doyle P et al. 2004. Does gestation vary by ethnic group? A London-based study of over 122 000 pregnancies with spontaneous onset of labour. *International Journal of Epidemiology.* Volume 33, Issue 1 Pages 107–113.

25. Saad AF, Villarreal J, Eid J et al. 2019. A randomized controlled trial of Dilapan-S vs Foley balloon for pre-induction cervical ripening (DILAFOL trial). *American journal of obstetrics and gynecology.* 220(3):275-e1.

26. Salim R, Schwartz N, Zafran N et al. 2018. Comparison of single- and double-balloon catheters for labor induction: A systematic review and meta-analysis of randomized controlled trials. *J Perinatol.* 38:217.

27. Schoen, CN, Grant G, Berghella V et al. 2017. Intracervical foley catheter with and without oxytocin for labor induction: A randomized controlled trial. *Obstetrics & Gynecology.* 129(6):1046–1053.

28. Sims EJ, Newman RB, Hulsey TC. 2001. Vaginal birth after cesarean: To induce or not to induce. *Am J Obstet Gynecol.* 184:1122–4.

29. Society for Maternal-Fetal Medicine (SMFM) Publications Committee. 2018. Statement on Elective Induction of Labor in Low-Risk Nulliparous Women at Term: The ARRIVE Trial. *American Journal of Obstetrics and Gynecology.*

30. Tang J, Kapp N, Dragoman M, de Souza JP. 2013. WHO recommendations for misoprostol use for obstetric and gynecologic indications. *Int J Gynaecol Obstet.* 121:186.

31. Ten Eikelder ML, Oude Rengerink K, Jozwiak M et al. 2016. Induction of labour at term with oral misoprostol versus a Foley catheter (PROBAAT-II): A multicentre randomised controlled non-inferiority trial. *Lancet*. 387:1619.

32. Thomas J, Fairclough A, Kavanagh J, Kelly AJ. 2014. Vaginal prostaglandin (PGE2 and PGF2a) for induction of labour at term. *Cochrane Database Syst Rev*. Issue 6. Art. No.: CD003101.

33. Vogel JP, Souza JP, Gülmezoglu AM. 2013. Patterns and Outcomes of Induction of Labour in Africa and Asia: A secondary analysis of the WHO Global Survey on Maternal and Neonatal Health. *PLoS One*. 8(6):e65612.

34. Weeks AD, Navaratnam K, Alfirevic Z. 2017. Simplifying oral misoprostol protocols for the induction of labour. *BJOG*. 124:1642.

35. Wood S, Cooper S, Ross S. 2014. Does induction of labour increase the risk of cesarean section? A systematic review and meta-analysis of trials in women with intact membranes. *BJOG*. 121(6): 674–85.

36. World Health Organization. 2011. WHO recommendations for induction of labour. WHO, Geneva.

37. Yang F, Huang S, Long Y, Huang L. 2018. Double-balloon versus single-balloon catheter for cervical ripening and labor induction: A systematic review and meta-analysis. *J Obstet Gynaecol Res*. 44:27.

38. Zhang Y, Wang J, Yu Y et al. 2015. Misoprostol versus prostaglandin E2 gel for labor induction in premature rupture of membranes after 34 weeks of pregnancy. *Int J Gynaecol Obstet*. 130:214.

Chapter 20

Abnormal Progression of Labour

INTRODUCTION

- Once the diagnosis of labour has been established, normal labour usually progresses in a predictable fashion. However, in some women, labour may be prolonged or may even end in complete cessation of progress.
- When the labour pattern diverges from that observed in the majority of women who have spontaneous vaginal deliveries, ill-defined terms like 'abnormal labour', 'dystocia', and 'failure to progress' are used. The risk of dystocia is highest in *nulliparous women with term pregnancies* (Kjaergaard, 2009).
- It is important to understand normal and abnormal progression of labour so that timely management may help avoid unnecessary interventions like cesarean sections.

NORMAL PROGRESSION OF LABOUR

- For more than 50 years, the progress of labour was measured based on data derived by Friedman (1954). The Friedman curve (Figure 20.1) has long been accepted as the standard for the assessment of labour progression. Friedman defined normal cervical dilatation during the active phase as 1.2 cm/hour for nulliparous women and 1.5 cm/hour for multiparous women. If cervical dilatation was slower than 1 cm/hour, labour was considered to be protracted or prolonged.
- Recent studies have questioned the Friedman curve. Contemporary data (Zhang et al., 2010) have led to the plotting of a smoother curve (Figure 20.2) with the acceleration of cervical dilatation in the active stage starting at 5–6 cm.
- A recent systematic review (Oladapo et al., 2018) concluded that an expectation of a minimum cervical dilatation threshold of 1 cm/hour throughout the first stage of labour is unrealistic for most healthy nulliparous and parous women. Labour progresses at a slower rate until cervical dilatation of 5–6 cms is reached.

ABNORMAL PROGRESSION OF LABOUR

- Abnormal progression of labour is not uncommon. Approximately 20 per cent of all labours ending in a live birth involve a protraction and/or arrest disorder (Zhu et al., 2006). In nulliparous women, this may occur in up to 37 per cent (Kjaergaard, 2009).

Non-progress of labour is the commonest reason for primary cesarean delivery. In one study, the indication was the lack of progress in labour in 68 per cent of the cesarean deliveries (Kjaergaard, 2009).

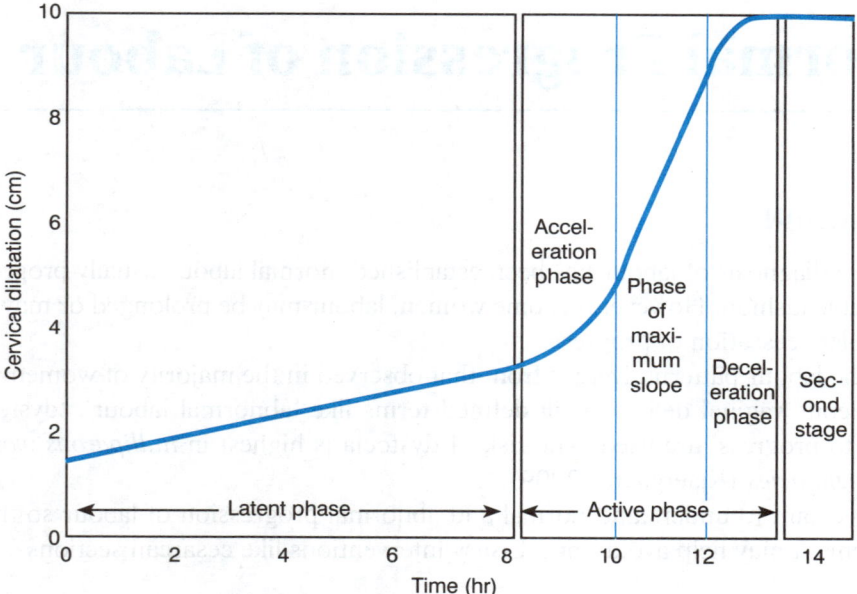

Figure 20.1 Friedman curve: The transition from the latent phase to active phase occurs at 3–4 cm cervical dilatation. The normal cervical dilatation during the active phase is considered to be 1.2 cm/hour for nulliparous women and 1.5 cm/hour for multiparous women. The active phase of the first stage is divided into acceleration phase, phase of maximum slope, and deceleration phase.

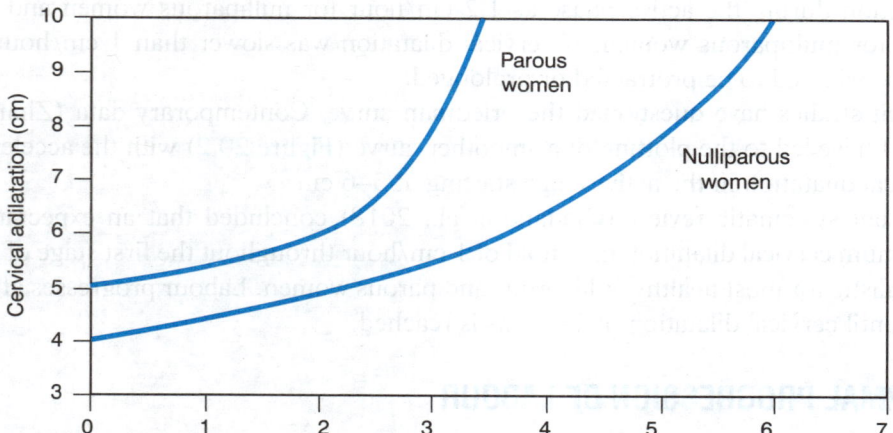

Figure 20.2 Contemporary patterns of spontaneous labour (Zhang et al., 2010). The acceleration of cervical dilatation starts at about 6 cm for multiparous women. There is no clear point where cervical dilatation accelerates for nulliparous women. There is no deceleration phase.

Risk factors

- Risk factors for abnormal progression of labour include:
  - Inadequate contractions

- ◆ Not strong on palpation and/or
- ◆ Infrequent (<3 or 4 contractions/10 minutes) and/or
- ◆ Short duration (<50 seconds)
- Cephalopelvic disproportion (CPD)
- Occiput posterior or occiput transverse position
- Macrosomia
- Maternal obesity
- Epidural analgesia

> In nulliparous women in active labour, a persistently floating head at 7 cm dilatation (indicative of CPD) was predictive of cesarean delivery in 100 per cent of the studied cases (Debby et al., 2003).

LABOUR DISORDERS

I. Prolongation disorders:
- Prolonged latent phase
- Prolonged second stage

II. Protracted active phase: Slower than expected progress of labour in the active phase

III. Arrest of labour: Complete cessation of dilatation or descent

MANAGEMENT OF LABOUR DISORDERS IN THE LATENT PHASE

Prolonged latent phase

- The diagnosis of latent phase is difficult since it may mimic false labour. The definition of latent phase based on contemporary data is the period **from the beginning of painful contractions to a cervical dilatation of 6 cm**.

> The duration of latent labour being highly variable, supportive and expectant management is most appropriate in the management of a prolonged latent phase.

- Prolonged latent phase is associated with increased perinatal mortality and is the harbinger of other labour abnormalities (Simon and Grobman, 2005).

Management

- If the mother is extremely uncomfortable and exhausted and the cervical dilatation is <6 cm, the following therapeutic option may be employed:
  - **Rest:** The mother is given an IM injection of pethidine (50–100 mg). Around 60–85 per cent of these women will wake up in the active phase of labour (Koontz and Bishop, 1982; Mackeen et al., 2014). 5 per cent will continue to have dysfunctional labour and may require a cesarean section.
- In women who are well rested and have a prolonged latent phase, the following are good options:
  - **Augmentation with oxytocin:** Early augmentation with oxytocin at 4 cm dilatation will help the labour to progress to the active phase (Bräne et al., 2014).

– **Amniotomy**: By itself, amniotomy will not help in the progression of labour, but in combination with oxytocin, it helps cut short the latent phase.

MANAGEMENT OF LABOUR DISORDERS IN THE FIRST STAGE

Protracted active phase of labour

- According to Friedman, the minimum rate of acceptable cervical dilatation during the active phase of labour is:
  - 1.2 cm/hour for nulliparous women
  - 1.5 cm/hour for multiparous women
- The **current definition** of protracted active phase is dilatation <1–2 cm/hour in women who have reached ≥6 cm dilatation (Zhang et al., 2010).
- The **diagnosis** of protracted active phase is made in mothers (nulliparous or multiparous) in the active phase (cervix ≥6 cm) who dilate ≤1 cm over two hours.

 With protracted active phase dilatation, the risk for subsequent arrest of dilatation or descent may be increased 2.5-fold to 8-fold, regardless of parity.

Management of protracted active phase

- There is significant evidence that augmentation with oxytocin is an effective and safe approach to the management of protracted active phase dilatation, especially in nulliparous women (see **Chapter 19**, *Induction of labour*).
- A systematic review of the Cochrane Database (Wei et al., 2013) concluded that early intervention with oxytocin and amniotomy appears to be associated with an increase in spontaneous vaginal delivery and a modest reduction in the rate of cesarean section over expectant care.

Arrest of active phase of labour

- Traditionally, secondary arrest of dilatation was diagnosed when there had been no change in cervical dilatation for at least two hours after the cervix had dilated to 4 cms or more.
- A workshop convened by the United States National Institute of Child Health and Human Development, Society for Maternal–Fetal Medicine, and American College of Obstetricians and Gynecologists (Spong et al., 2012) concluded that arrest of active phase of labour is diagnosed if cervical dilatation is ≥6 cm in a woman with ruptured membranes but there is:
  - No cervical change for **≥4 hours despite adequate contractions**
  - No cervical change for **≥6 hours with inadequate contractions**
- Arrest in the first stage is associated with:
  - Inadequate uterine contractions
  - Cephalopelvic disproportion

– Malpositions like persistent occiput posterior and persistent occiput transverse positions; however, it is difficult to say whether the associated malposition is a result or cause of the arrest disorder

- If there has been protracted active-phase dilatation, the risk of secondary arrest of dilatation increases 5-fold in nulliparas and 8-fold in multiparas.

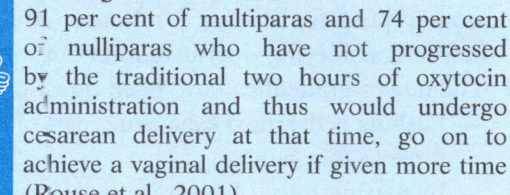

Why the change from 2 hours to 4 hours in the diagnosis of arrest?
91 per cent of multiparas and 74 per cent of nulliparas who have not progressed by the traditional two hours of oxytocin administration and thus would undergo cesarean delivery at that time, go on to achieve a vaginal delivery if given more time (Rouse et al., 2001).

Management of arrest of active-phase dilatation

- Oxytocin augmentation should be used to promote adequate contractions. It is important to give the woman enough time to achieve a vaginal delivery. If no cervical change is achieved even after augmentation, then a cesarean section is the only option.

- Despite the use of oxytocin, arrest in the active phase can result in cesarean section rates as high as 60 per cent (Handa and Laros, 1993).

- The maternal status must be monitored continuously while waiting for vaginal delivery. The diagnosis of arrest in the active phase should be followed-up with stringent monitoring because, if ignored, it might result in a ruptured uterus.

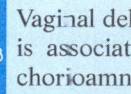

Vaginal delivery following active-phase arrest is associated with a significant increase in chorioamnionitis and shoulder dystocia (Henry et al., 2008).

- Fetal status must also be monitored carefully.

MANAGEMENT OF LABOUR DISORDERS IN THE SECOND STAGE

Prolongation of second stage of labour

After complete cervical dilatation, if the fetal head descends at a rate slower than 1 cm per hour, it is called prolonged second stage.

Arrest of second stage of labour

After complete cervical dilatation, if the fetal head does not descend despite good maternal efforts, it is called arrest of the second stage.

 If the arrest of descent has been preceded by protracted active-phase labour, the chances of cesarean section rise exponentially (Sokol and Blackwell, 2003).

Duration of second stage

- Traditionally, the second stage is considered prolonged if it lasts more than two hours in a nullipara or one hour in a multipara. If epidural analgesia is used, the time limits could be extended for one more hour.

- Newer guidelines (ACOG-SMFM, 2014) are suggesting that nulliparous women push for at least three hours (and up to four hours with epidural analgesia) and multiparous women push for at least two hours (and up to three hours with epidural analgesia) prior before considering operative intervention.
- The newer guidelines have been questioned for the following reasons:
  - Pushing is the most exhausting part of labour. It is unfair to expect the woman to push for three to four hours.
  - Increasing rates of cesarean delivery, operative vaginal delivery, and perineal trauma are associated with the second stage getting prolonged beyond the first hour (Cheng et al., 2004).
  - A prolonged second stage is often associated with persistent malposition or macrosomia. Vaginal delivery in these situations is associated with neonatal morbidity (Cheng et al., 2007).
  - Increased duration of the second stage is associated significantly with admission to a neonatal intensive care unit (Rouse et al., 2009).
  - Rate of birth asphyxia-related complications gradually increase with the duration of the second stage (Sandström, 2017).
  - If a cesarean delivery is necessary, a prolonged second stage may result in the fetal head being trapped deep in the pelvis, which increases the difficulty of delivering the fetus. A prolonged second stage may also further thin the lower uterine segment, increasing intraoperative morbidity.
  - Prolonging the second stage appears to increase the risk of postpartum hemorrhage (Miller et al., 2017).

Factors that favour successful vaginal delivery

- A previous vaginal delivery
- Mother is not exhausted and is pushing effectively
- Fetal status is normal
- Pelvis appears adequate on physical examination
- Mother is not short and/or obese
- Fetus in occiput anterior position with minimal caput and moulding
- Absence of macrosomia by clinical estimation or estimated fetal weight (EFW) by ultrasound

Management of arrest of second stage disorders

- The mother is encouraged to increase her expulsive forces or she is taught how to push more effectively (see **Chapter 14**, *Normal labour and delivery – evidence-based management*).
- Augmentation with oxytocin is initiated or its dose is judiciously increased if oxytocin is already being administered and contractions are ineffectual.
- If the head is low down in the pelvis (+2 station or below), instrumental vaginal delivery can be carried out (with forceps or ventouse), provided all the conditions for instrumental delivery are met with (see **Chapter 21**, *Operative vaginal delivery*).

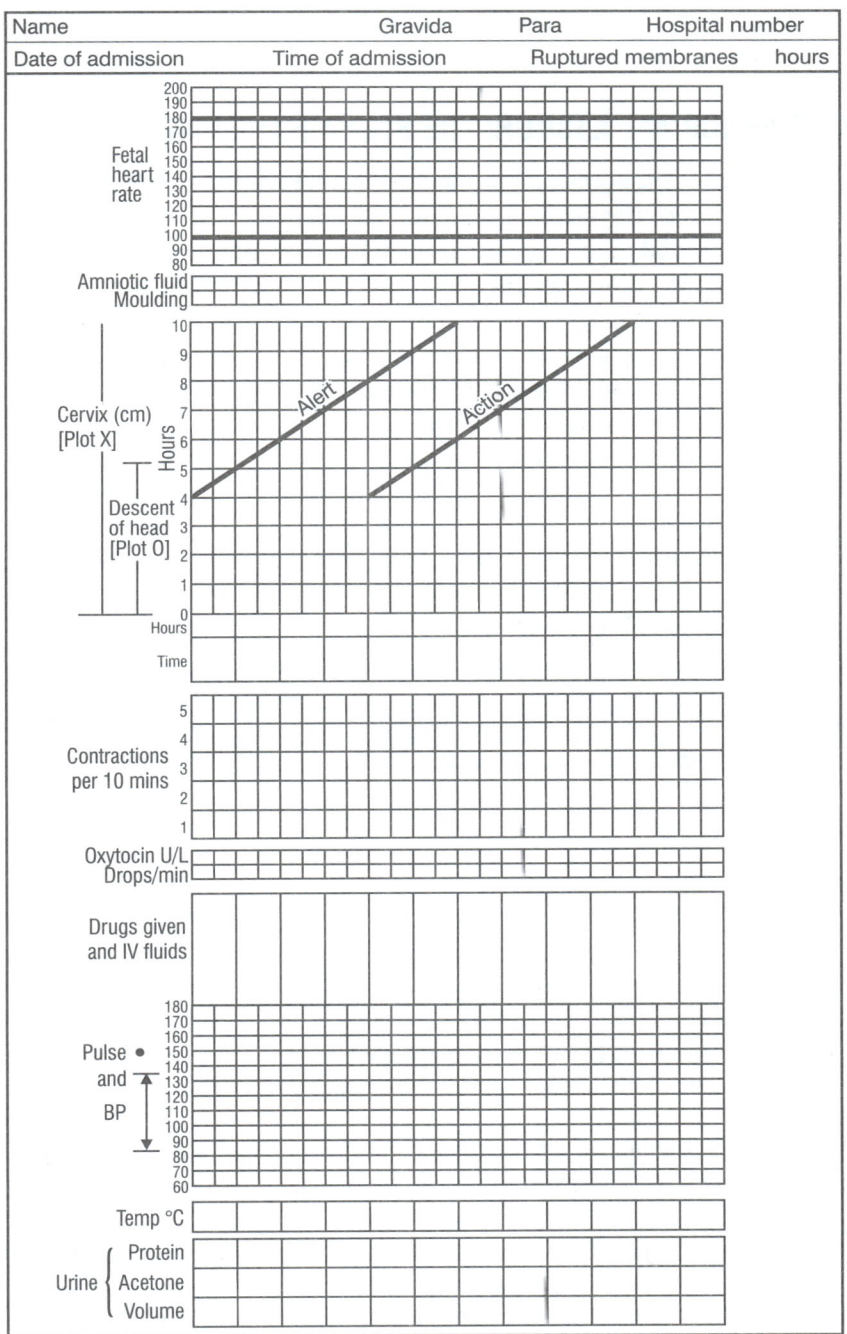

Figure 20.3 World Health Organization partograph showing the alert line and action line that are recorded when the woman is in the active phase of labour. When the cervical dilatation falls to the right of the alert line, it indicates that labour is slower than 1 cm/hour. Augmentation with oxytocin is indicated at this point. The WHO partograph does not differentiate between nulliparous or multiparous women.

- Cesarean section would be the next logical option if the conditions for a safe instrumental delivery are not met with.

DIAGNOSING ABNORMAL LABOUR: THE ROLE OF THE PARTOGRAPH

- It is imperative that some sort of labour record be maintained so that progress in cervical dilatation and station of the vertex are recorded systematically and meticulously. As long as all the people involved in taking care of the labouring mother have a standard protocol they can follow for recording cervical dilatation and descent of the fetal vertex, abnormal progress of labour can be diagnosed and managed.
- The partograph (or partogram) was introduced nearly 40 years ago and is a visual record of the progress of labour. The World Health Organization partographs are the best-known partographs in low-resource settings (Figure 20.3).
- The partograph is a record of all the observations made on a woman in labour, and most importantly, the graphic recording of the dilatation of the cervix as assessed by vaginal examination.
- Clinicians often resist using partographs, usually because of their busy schedules. Globally, there is evidence that partographs are not being used as anticipated in practice, often being filled in after the delivery is over.

 A systematic review of the Cochrane Database (Lavender et al., 2018) could not prove that the routine use of partographs significantly improves obstetric outcome. Further, no single partograph has been proven to be superior to others.

References

1. American College of Obstetricians and Gynecologists, Society for Maternal-Fetal Medicine. 2014. ACOG-SMFM Obstetric care consensus no. 1: Safe prevention of the primary cesarean delivery. *Obstet Gynecol.* 123:693.

2. Bräne E, Olsson A, Andolf E. 2014. A randomized controlled trial on early induction compared to expectant management of nulliparous women with prolonged latent phases. *Acta Obstet Gynecol Scand.* 93:1042.

3. Cheng YW, Hopkins LM, Caughey AB. 2004. How long is too long: Does a prolonged second stage of labor in nulliparous women affect maternal and neonatal outcomes? *Am J Obstet Gynecol.* 91(3):933–938.

4. Cheng YW, Hopkins LM, Laros RK Jr, Caughey AB. 2007. Duration of the second stage of labor in multiparous women: Maternal and neonatal outcomes. *Am J Obstet Gynecol.* 196(6):585.e1–585.e5856.

5. Debby A, Rotmensch S, Girtler O et al. 2003. Clinical significance of the floating fetal head in nulliparous women in labor. *J Reprod Med.* 48:37.

6. Friedman EA. 1954. The graphic analysis of labor. *Am J Obstet Gynecol.* 68:1568.

7. Handa VL, Laros RK. 1993. Active phase arrest in labor: Predictors of cesarean in nulliparous population. *Obstet Gynecol.* 81:758.

8. Henry DE, Cheng YW, Shaffer BL, Kaimal AJ, Bianco K, Caughey AB. 2008. Perinatal outcomes in the setting of active phase arrest of labor. *Obstet Gynecol.* 112(5):1109-15.

9. Kjaergaard H, Olsen J, Ottesen B, Dykes AK. 2009. Incidence and outcomes of dystocia in the active phase of labor in term nulliparous women with spontaneous labor onset. *Acta Obstet Gynecol Scand.* 88:402.

10. Koontz WL, Bishop EH. 1982. Management of the latent phase of labor. *Clin Obstet Gynecol.* 25:111.

11. Lavender T, Cuthbert A, Smyth RM. 2018. Effect of partograph use on outcomes for women in spontaneous labour at term and their babies. *Cochrane Database Syst Rev.* Issue 8. Art. no.: CD005461.

12. Mackeen AD, Fehnel E, Berghella V, Klein T. 2014. Morphine sleep in pregnancy. *Am J Perinatol.* 31:85.

13. Miller CM, Cohn S, Akdagli S et al. 2017. Postpartum hemorrhage following vaginal delivery: Risk factors and maternal outcomes. *J Perinatol.* 37:243.

14. Oladapo OT, Diaz V, Bonet M et al. 2018. Cervical dilatation patterns of 'low-risk' women with spontaneous labour and normal perinatal outcomes: A systematic review. *BJOG.* 125:944.

15. Rouse DJ, Owen J, Savage KG, Hauth JC. 2001. Active phase labor arrest: Revisiting the 2-hour minimum. *Obstet Gynecol.* 98:550–4.

16. Rouse DJ, Weiner SJ, Bloom SL et al. 2009. Second-stage labor duration in nulliparous women: Relationship to maternal and perinatal outcomes. *Am J Obstet Gynecol.* 201:357.e1.

17. Sandström A, Altman M, Cnattingius S et al. 2017. Durations of second stage of labor and pushing, and adverse neonatal outcomes: A population-based cohort study. *J Perinatol.* 37:236.

18. Simon CE, Grobman WA. 2005. When has an induction failed? *Obstet Gynecol.* 105: 705-709.

19. Sokol RJ and Blackwell SC. 2003. Abnormal labor: Diagnosis and management. *Gynecology and Obstetrics* on CD-ROM. Lippincott Williams & Wilkins.

20. Spong CY, Berghella V, Wenstrom KD et al. 2012. Preventing the first cesarean delivery: Summary of a joint Eunice Kennedy Shriver National Institute of Child Health and Human Development, Society for Maternal-Fetal Medicine, and American College of Obstetricians and Gynecologists Workshop. *Obstet Gynecol.* 120:1181.

21. Wei S, Wo BL, Qi HP et al. 2013. Early amniotomy and early oxytocin for prevention of, or therapy for, delay in first stage spontaneous labour compared with routine care. *Cochrane Database Syst Rev.* Issue 8. Art. no.: CD006794.

22. Zhang J, Landy HJ, Branch DW et al. 2010. Contemporary patterns of spontaneous labor with normal neonatal outcomes. *Obstet Gynecol.* 116:1281.

23. Zhu BP, Grigorescu V, Le T et al. 2006. Labor dystocia and its association with interpregnancy interval. *Am J Obstet Gynecol.* 195:121.

Chapter 21

Operative Vaginal Delivery

INTRODUCTION

- Operative vaginal delivery, with a vacuum device (ventouse) or forceps, is an important aspect of obstetric care. It assists in accomplishing or expediting safe vaginal delivery for maternal or fetal indications.

> The goal of operative vaginal delivery is to mimic spontaneous vaginal birth, thereby expediting delivery with minimum maternal or neonatal morbidity.

- The ability to perform a vacuum- or forceps-assisted delivery is an essential skill for those who provide maternity care (Bailey, 2005). However, over the past three decades, there has been a global decline in instrumental delivery rates while cesarean rates have increased. This may be attributed to the inadequate teaching of instrumental delivery, which results in obstetricians not receiving sufficient hands-on experience during their training.

- A five-year retrospective study conducted on trends of instrumental deliveries at a tertiary teaching hospital in Puducherry, India, showed a 7.7 per cent rate of instrumental vaginal deliveries (Dhodapkar and Chauhan, 2015). During the study period, a decline in the trend of instrumental deliveries was observed.

- The decrease in instrumental deliveries may be ascribed to concerns over neonatal and maternal safety as well as a declining number of obstetricians skilled in instrumental delivery. Unfortunately, this decrease is reflected in the rising rates of cesarean section.

INDICATIONS FOR OPERATIVE VAGINAL DELIVERY

- The indications for both vacuum- and forceps- assisted deliveries are the same (see box).
- The commonest indication is to cut short the second stage of labour (ACOG, 2015).

> **Indications for vacuum extraction or forceps delivery**
> **Maternal**
> - Prolonged second stage of labour
> - Maternal exhaustion
> - Epidural block with diminished urge to push
> - Shortening of second stage for maternal medical conditions that preclude pushing (cardiac disease class III/IV, severe preeclampsia/hypertension)
>
> **Fetal**
> - Suspicion of immediate or potential fetal compromise
> - Rotational instrumental delivery for malpositioned fetus
> - Delivery of the head at assisted breech delivery (singleton or twin)

CONTRAINDICATIONS

Contraindications to operative delivery include the following:

- Unengaged head
- Incompletely dilated cervix
- Suspected cephalopelvic disproportion/macrosomia
- Fetal malpresentation (brow or face presentation)
- Rotation >45° from occiput anterior or occiput posterior
- Fetal prematurity <34 weeks
- Fetal bleeding disorders, e.g., hemophilia and thrombocytopenia
- Fetal demineralising disease, e.g., osteogenesis imperfecta

CLASSIFICATION OF OPERATIVE VAGINAL DELIVERY

- A standard classification of operative vaginal delivery should be used.
- The American College of Obstetricians and Gynecologists (ACOG, 2020) and the RCOG Green-top Guidelines (2011) define the delivery by station and position (see box).
- Midforceps delivery should be performed only by an experienced obstetrician after cephalopelvic disproportion is excluded and the fetal station is reassessed. High forceps delivery is not performed in modern obstetrics.

Classification of forceps delivery

Outlet forceps
- Scalp is visible at the introitus without separating labia
- Fetal skull has reached pelvic floor
- Sagittal suture is in the anteroposterior diameter or right or left occiput anterior or posterior position
- Fetal head is at or on the perineum
- Rotation does not exceed 45°

Low forceps
- Leading point of fetal skull (not caput) is at station ≥+2 cm and not on the pelvic floor
- Rotation
  - 45° or less from the occipito-anterior position
  - More than 45°, including the occipito-posterior position

Midforceps
- Fetal head is no more than 1/5th palpable per abdomen
- Leading point of the skull is above +2 cm but not above the ischial spines (engaged)
- Rotation
  - 45° or less from the occipito-anterior position
  - More than 45°, including the occipito-posterior position

PREREQUISITES FOR OPERATIVE VAGINAL DELIVERY

Forceps should only be applied after an abdominal and vaginal examination confirm the following:

- The fetal head is ≤1/5th palpable per abdomen

- It is a vertex presentation
- The cervix is fully dilated and the membranes are absent

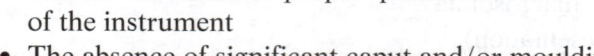 Safe operative vaginal delivery requires careful assessment of the clinical situation, clear communication with the mother, and expertise in the chosen procedure.

- The exact position of the head is known—to achieve proper placement of the instrument
- The absence of significant caput and/or moulding
- Adequacy of pelvis

Preparation of mother

- A clear explanation should be given to the mother and her informed consent obtained.
- Appropriate and adequate analgesia should be given for mid-cavity rotational deliveries. An epidural may be appropriate.
- The mother should be in the dorsolithotomy position with her legs in stirrups. The lower end of the labour table should be dropped and the operator should be seated on a stool.
- The maternal bladder should be emptied. An in-dwelling catheter, if present, should be removed or the balloon deflated.
- The entire procedure should be performed using aseptic precautions.

Preparation of staff

- The obstetrician must have the necessary knowledge, experience, and skill. A senior obstetrician competent in performing mid-cavity deliveries should

 An experienced obstetrician should be present from the outset for all attempts at rotational or mid-cavity operative vaginal delivery.

  be present if a junior trainee is performing the delivery.
- Adequate facilities should be available (appropriate equipment, bed, lighting, etc.).
- A back-up plan should be in place in case of failure to deliver. When conducting mid-cavity deliveries, theatre staff should be informed and should be immediately available to allow a cesarean section to be performed without delay (ideally, <30 minutes).
- Complications that may arise (e.g., shoulder dystocia, postpartum hemorrhage, etc.) must be anticipated and prepared for.
- Personnel who are trained in neonatal resuscitation should be available.

Informed consent

- For deliveries in the delivery room, verbal consent should be obtained before an operative vaginal delivery and the discussion documented in the labour room notes.
- If circumstances allow and institutional protocols are in place, written consent may also be obtained.
- Written consent should be obtained for the trial of operative vaginal delivery in the operating theatre.

Antibiotics

- The role of prophylactic antibiotics in operative delivery remains controversial.

- A systematic review of the Cochrane Database (Liabsuetrakul et al., 2020) concluded that prophylactic intravenous antibiotics are effective in reducing infectious puerperal morbidities in terms of superficial and deep perineal wound infections or serious infectious complications in women undergoing operative vaginal deliveries. This was based on the findings of a large study in the UK (Knight et al., 2019) in which almost 90 per cent of the women had a mediolateral episiotomy.
- A single dose of 1.2 g of intravenous amoxicillin and clavulanic acid is recommended within six hours of instrumental vaginal delivery.
- However, ACOG (2020) does not recommend the use of routine prophylactic antibiotics before operative delivery. They recommend considering the use of antibiotics if a third- or fourth-degree laceration occurs.

CHOICE OF INSTRUMENT: FORCEPS VS. VACUUM

- There have been no randomised controlled trials comparing different types of forceps; it is recognised that the choice is often subjective (Wegner and Bernstein, 2019). However, there has been a marked shift to vacuum deliveries in the past decades, probably due to less training available in forceps delivery.
- The operator should choose the instrument most appropriate to the clinical circumstances and his/her level of skill.
- In a systematic review of the Cochrane Database, O'Mahony and colleagues (2010) evaluated the relative merits of vacuum-assisted delivery and forceps (Table 21.1). They found that forceps cause more maternal trauma, whereas vacuum devices cause more neonatal trauma. The risk of failed delivery was found to be least with forceps and most with soft-cup vacuum, with metal-cup and handheld vacuum devices in the middle.

Table 21.1 Comparison of forceps and vacuum devices (O'Mahony et al., 2010)

Forceps	Vacuum devices
Need more expertise to apply	Easier to apply
More likely to succeed in delivery	More likely to fail
Rotation has to be done actively	Fetal head rotation may occur passively during fetal extraction
Increased risk of maternal and fetal trauma	Less maternal tissue trauma
Increased need for regional anesthesia	Less need for regional anesthesia
Lower risk of scalp injury and cephalohematoma compared to vacuum devices	Increased risk of neonatal cephalohematoma and fetal retinal hemorrhages

TRIAL OF INSTRUMENTAL DELIVERY

- Instrumental delivery should be attempted when the possibility of successful delivery is high and all the prerequisites are met.
- However, when difficulty in vaginal delivery is anticipated, a **trial of forceps** is attempted, with the intention of abandoning the procedure if fetal descent meets with resistance or if excessive force is required.

- Trial of instrumental delivery should be conducted by an experienced operator and in a facility where immediate recourse to cesarean section is possible. Most often, it is performed in the operating room.
- It is important to remember that failed forceps- or vacuum-assisted deliveries are associated with greater maternal and neonatal morbidity.
- Walsh et al. (2013) found that the rate of serious neonatal complications associated with operative vaginal delivery is similar to that associated with cesarean delivery at full dilatation. They also found no significant differences between adverse neonatal outcomes of vacuum-assisted and forceps-assisted deliveries.
- It is good clinical practice to reappraise the situation if there is no descent with the first three pulls.

There are no evidence-based guidelines for the number of forceps pulls or vacuum detachments that are permissible before considering the procedure a failure. Clinical consensus advises abandoning the procedure if more than three pulls are required.

FAILED INSTRUMENTAL DELIVERY

- Occasionally, in spite of no anticipated difficulty, an attempted forceps procedure fails to deliver the baby. This is known as **failed forceps**.
- The risk of neonatal morbidity and maternal injury is higher with a failed forceps.
- The procedure should be abandoned if the following occur:
  - There is difficulty in the application or approximation of the blades.
  - There is no progressive descent with moderate traction.
  - Delivery is not imminent after three pulls.

Higher rates of failure are associated with the following factors:
- Fetal macrosomia
- Occipito-posterior positions
- A higher station of the presenting part
- Higher maternal BMI
- Protracted second stage of labour
- Excessive moulding of the fetal head

FORCEPS

- All obstetric forceps share the same basic design (Figure 21.1). They consist of two crossing halves with a locking mechanism in the centre. Each half of the forceps consists of a handle, shank, lock, and blade.
- The blades usually have a pelvic curve and a cephalic curve.
- Various versions differ from each other in features like blade length, fenestration, type of lock, and presence or absence of a pelvic curve.
- Forceps used for non-rotational deliveries have a more pronounced pelvic curve and a fixed (English) lock (Figure 21.2).
- Rotational forceps like the Kielland's forceps have a less pronounced pelvic curve and a sliding (French) lock to correct asynclitism (Figure 21.3).

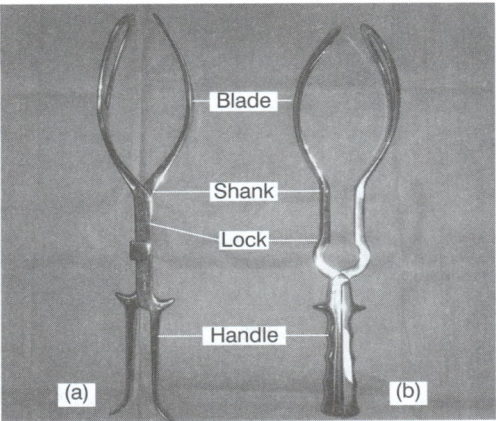

Figure 21.1   Parts of (a) rotational and (b) non-rotational forceps.

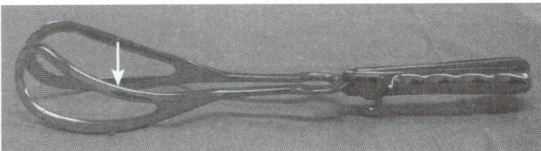

Figure 21.2   Side view of non-rotational forceps showing prominent pelvic curve (arrow).

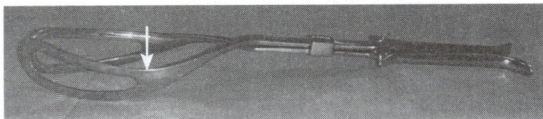

Figure 21.3   Side view of Kielland's forceps showing a ess pronounced pelvic curve (arrow).

The use of rotational forceps

Modern obstetric guidelines advise the use of rotational forceps with caution. Their use has declined due to reports of adverse outcomes. However, data from contemporary large studies suggest that they are associated with a low neonatal complication rate (Stock et al., 2013). Bahl and colleagues (2013) compared Kielland forceps to vacuum extraction, and manual rotation, and found that maternal and perinatal outcomes were the same, with few adverse effects. The present consensus is that Kielland forceps may be safe and effective in trained hands and significantly more successful at achieving operative vaginal delivery than either rotational ventouse or manual rotation (Nash et al., 2015).

VACUUM DEVICES

- Vacuum devices (Figure 21.4) consist of a soft or rigid plastic cup, a vacuum pump to provide suction between the cup and fetal scalp, and a traction system.
- The original vacuum device was the Malmström disc-shaped metal cup (Figure 21.4a).
- The soft cups were introduced in the 1980s. The *soft cup* is a pliable funnel- or bell-shaped cup made of silicone (Figure 21.4b) and is available in 3 sizes (40 mm, 50 mm, and 60 mm). The commonly used size for a term fetus is 50 mm.
- The Kiwi™ hand-held device (Figure 21.4c) is a disposable device that has a simple hand-operated pump. While it is less successful than conventional ventouse in achieving vaginal delivery, its safety profile is comparable (Groom et al., 2006).

Soft cups

- A systematic review of the Cochrane Database (O'Mahony et al., 2010), compared soft and rigid vacuum extractor cups. They found that soft cups:
  - Were more likely to fail to achieve a vaginal delivery because of more frequent detachments (pop-offs).
  - Were associated with fewer scalp injuries.

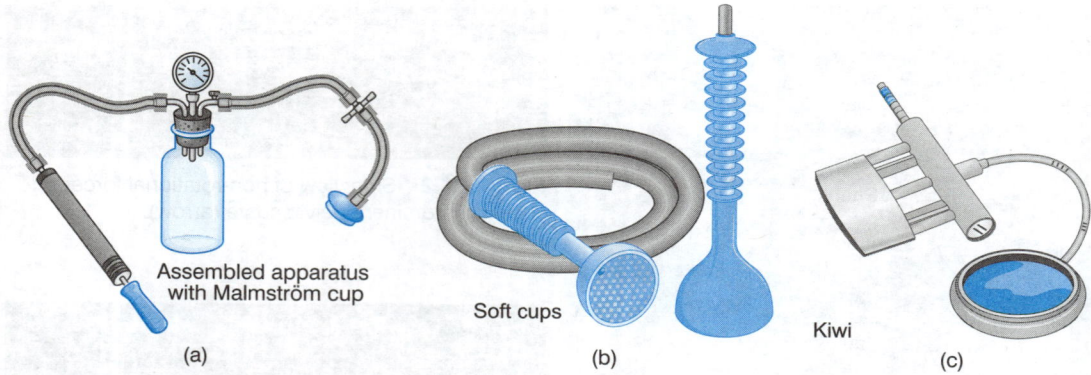

Figure 21.4   Different types of vacuum devices. The three main types of handheld disposable vacuum devices are: (a) the firm and mushroom-shaped rigid cup, (b) the pliable and funnel-/bell-shaped soft cup and (c) the Kiwi disposable handheld device.

- Studies have demonstrated no significant differences between the handheld (Kiwi™) and the standard vacuum in achieving a successful delivery.
- Soft cups should be considered for more straightforward occiput anterior deliveries.

> Soft cups should be considered for more straightforward occiput anterior deliveries and rigid cups should be reserved for more complicated deliveries.

Rigid cups

- The rigid cup is able to generate more traction force than the soft cup and is better at achieving a successful delivery. It is, however, associated with more risk of injury to the baby (O'Mahony et al., 2010).
- The rigid cup is a better choice for more complicated deliveries such as occiput posterior, occiput transverse, and difficult occiput anterior deliveries because it is less likely to get detached from the fetal head.

TECHNIQUE OF FORCEPS DELIVERY

The technique of forceps delivery consists of application, traction, and delivery of the fetal head.

Application of forceps

The application of forceps can be by one of two methods—cephalic and pelvic.

Cephalic application

- The optimum cephalic application is with the fetal head in the occiput anterior position.
- The blades of the forceps are applied along the sides of the head, grasping the biparietal diameter in-between the widest part of the blades (Figure 21.5).

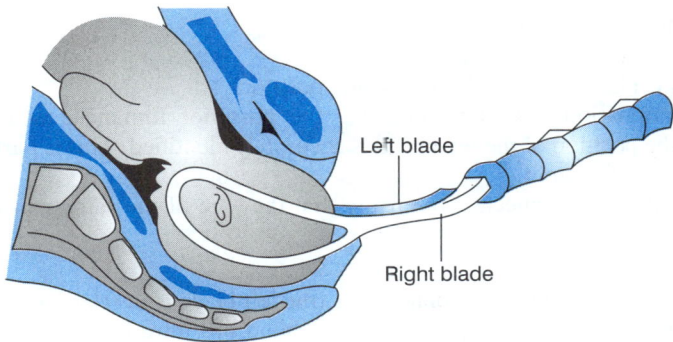

Figure 21.5 Correct cephalic application of forceps. The blades are applied along the sides of the fetal head, grasping the biparietal diameter in-between the widest part of the blades. The tips of the blades lie over the cheeks.

- The long axis of the blades corresponds to the occipito-mental plane.
- The tips of the blades lie over the cheeks. In the occipito-anterior position, the major part of the blade is on the fetal face.
- The blades should lie symmetrically on either side of the head.
- The sagittal suture of the fetal head should be in the middle, and the blades should be equidistant from the sagittal and occipital sutures.
- At no time should any part of the forceps cover any midline structure.
- The forceps should lock easily without any force and the handles should be parallel to the plane of the floor.
- The correctness of application should be confirmed before applying traction.

Identifying the right and left blades
With the patient in the lithotomy position, the blades of the forceps need to be applied with the pelvic curve directed anteriorly and the cephalic curve directed medially.
    To facilitate the identification of the right and left blades, the forceps can be articulated and held in front of the perineum in the position that the blades will be applied. This makes it easy to identify the left blade and the right (here, right and left refer to the mother's right and left).

Pelvic application

- The term pelvic application is used when the left blade is applied on the left side of the maternal pelvis and the right blade is applied on the right side of the pelvis, regardless of the fetal position.

> Serious compression effects can occur on the fetal cranium with an improper pelvic application, so it should be used with caution.

- Pelvic application may be appropriate in some instances, as in a direct occiput posterior presentation.
- Pelvic application should never be used as a substitute for exact knowledge of the fetal position because inappropriate pelvic application may cause significant harm.
- Pelvic application is only justified in low forceps operations.

Technique of forceps application
- Aseptic precautions must be taken.
- The woman is placed in the dorsolithotomy position.
- A pelvic examination is done, and using the posterior fontanelle and sagittal suture as guidelines, the position of the fetal head is accurately identified. This is particularly important in the presence of a caput.
- The forceps blades are checked to ensure that they are of the same pair and that they lock easily.

Left blade
- By convention, the left blade is applied first (the left blade is in relation to the maternal left).
- Two or more fingers of the operator's right hand are introduced inside the left posterior portion of the vagina, sliding in between the fetal head and the vaginal wall.
- The left blade is grasped between the thumb and two fingers of the left hand. The shank and handle of the blade are held vertical with the tip pointing towards the floor.
- The tip of the blade is then gently passed into the vagina between the fetal head and the palmar surface of the right hand and smoothly guided into the posterior aspect of the vagina.
- A good clinical tip is to move the handle through a wide arc while slipping the blade behind the fetal head.
- Care should be taken not to exert unnecessary pressure or to force the blade into the vagina.

Right blade
- For the application of the right blade, two or more fingers of the operator's left hand are introduced into the right and posterior part of the vagina to guard the maternal soft tissues and serve as guides for the right blade.
- The blade is held by the operator's right hand.
- With proper application, the sagittal suture of the fetal skull lies in the midline of the blades, the blades are symmetrical, and the application and locking are smooth.
- Difficulty with locking signifies asymmetrical application on the fetal head and can cause fetal injuries.

Removal of blades
- The right blade should be removed first, followed by the left.

Traction with forceps

- During a forceps delivery, traction should be applied during contractions.
- Minimal traction can be used to maintain the station of the fetal head between contractions.
- Traction is applied along the axis of the birth canal, along the curve of Carus. From the level of the ischial spines, the maternal pelvis is 'J'-shaped. Hence the direction of traction depends on the station of the fetal head in the birth canal.
- After confirming proper forceps application, traction starts horizontally until the head crowns and the perineum bulges (Figure 21.6a). It then follows It is important to support the perineum while applying traction to the forceps to prevent lacerations or extension of the episiotomy.

the curve of the birth canal (Figure 21.6b). Finally, the forceps are elevated to an almost vertical position as the fetal head extends (Figure 21.6c).
- The amount of traction should be the least necessary to accomplish safe fetal head descent.

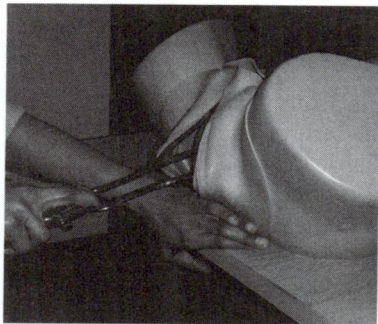

Figure 21.6 (a) First, traction is applied horizontally until the head crowns and the perineum bulges. The perineum should be supported.

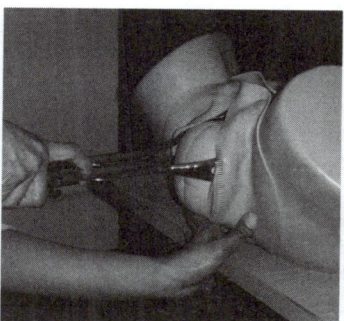

Figure 21.6 (b) As the fetal head descends, traction follows the curve of the pelvis (the curve of Carus).

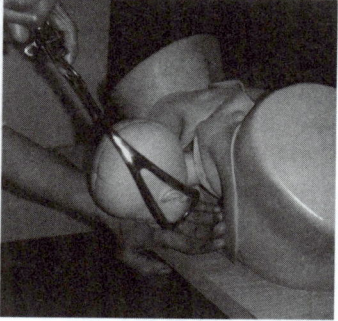

Figure 21.6 (c) As the fetal head is delivered, the handles are elevated almost to a vertical position (*Images 21.6 a-c courtesy:* Cruz Winston Justin and Tulika Singh).

- The angle of traction is as important as the force applied in effecting delivery.
- Assuming that everything has been done according to proper protocols and no progress is observable in three reasonable traction attempts, operative vaginal delivery should be discontinued and preparation for abdominal delivery should be initiated as soon as possible.
- **Delivery in the occipito-posterior position:** For a fetus in the occipito-posterior position, traction is applied in the horizontal plane until the root of the nose is under the pubic symphysis. Then, upward traction is applied until the occiput emerges over the perineum. Finally, the blades are pulled downwards.

> **Use of episiotomy at the time of instrumental delivery**
> There is no consensus on whether episiotomy is indicated with operative vaginal delivery. It is probably better to avoid episiotomy as in a spontaneous vaginal delivery. However, episiotomy may facilitate the placement of the forceps or vacuum extractor in women with a narrow vaginal outlet (see **Chapter 15**, *Evidence-based approach to episiotomy*).
>
> An episiotomy may prevent anal sphincter damage in women with a short perineum who require operative vaginal delivery. A systematic review (Lund et al., 2016) showed that mediolateral or lateral episiotomy significantly reduced the risk of obstetric anal sphincter injury (OASIS) in vacuum-assisted deliveries in primiparous women. An observational study from the Netherlands (de Leeuw et al., 2008) concluded that mediolateral episiotomy is protective against obstetric anal sphincter injury in both vacuum extraction and forceps delivery.

TECHNIQUE OF VACUUM-ASSISTED DELIVERY

Patient preparation

- The woman is placed in the dorsolithotomy position.
- The maternal bladder is emptied (by catheterisation if necessary).
- A vaginal examination is done to determine the position and station of the fetal head.

Determining the flexion point

- In the normally moulded fetal head, the flexion point is in the midline, over the sagittal suture, approximately 6 cm from the anterior fontanelle and 3 cm from the posterior fontanelle.
- Outward traction on this point will bring about natural flexion of the fetal neck.

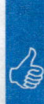 Correct placement of the cup over the flexion point will facilitate flexion, descent, and rotation of the vertex when traction is applied and will minimise injury to both the fetus and maternal soft tissues.

Positioning of the cup

- The labia are spread and the soft cup is introduced by compressing and inserting it into the vagina while angling the device towards the occiput.
- If a rigid cup is used, the device is inserted sideways into the vagina while angling it posteriorly.
- When the cup makes contact with the fetal head, the centre of the cup is placed over the flexion point and symmetrically across the sagittal suture (Figure 21.7a).
- The entire circumference of the cup must then be digitally palpated to ensure that no vaginal, cervical, or vulvar tissues are trapped between the cup and the fetal surface.

 Care must be taken not to cover either fontanelle with the ventouse cup.

Application of suction

- After the correct placement of the cup is confirmed, the negative pressure is rapidly raised to maintain the cup's position. The edges of the cup should again be swept with a finger to ensure that no maternal tissues are entrapped.

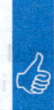 The traction should be applied in concert with uterine contractions and maternal expulsive efforts. The safe limits for vacuum duration and number of pulls are still unknown (Åberg et al., 2019).

- The thumb and index finger of one hand are kept on the edges of the cup to apply counter pressure while the other hand applies traction (Figure 21.7b).
- With application of vacuum suction, part of the scalp is sucked into the cup, creating an artificial caput succedaneum (known as a **chignon**).

Application of traction

- The exact traction force required to safely deliver the baby is unknown.
- The dominant hand exerts traction while the non-dominant hand monitors the progress of descent and prevents cup detachment by applying counter pressure directly to the vacuum cup.
- Sustained downward traction should be applied along the pelvic curve while supporting the perineum (Figure 21.7c and d). Traction is applied gradually as the contraction builds

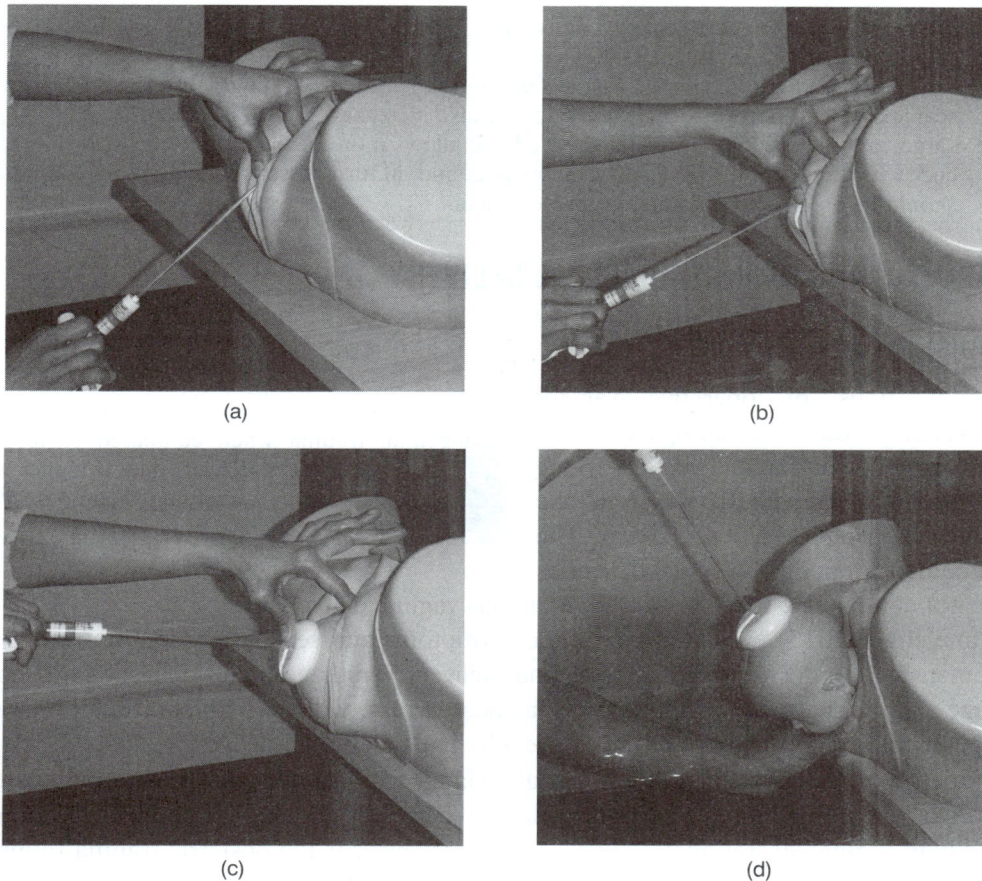

(a)   (b)

(c)   (d)

Figure 21.7   Steps of a vacuum-assisted delivery. (a) Positioning the cup; (b) The thumb and index finger of one hand are kept on the edges of the cup to apply counter pressure while the other hand applies traction; (c) Sustained downward traction applied along the pelvic curve; (d) Supporting the perineum, while the head is delivered (*Image credits for Figures 21.7a-d:* Cruz Winston Justin and Tulika Singh).

and is maintained as long as the contraction lasts, in conjunction with the mother's expulsive efforts.

- In an observational study, Murphy and colleagues (2003) found that 82 per cent of successful deliveries were achieved within one to three pulls, and that more than three pulls was associated with a 45 per cent risk of neonatal trauma.
- Åberg et al. (2019) investigated the impact of protracted vacuum extraction on the risk of neonatal intracranial hemorrhage in term infants and found that the safe limits for vacuum duration and number of pulls are still unknown and that intracranial hemorrhage may occur even when performed in accordance with safety recommendations.
- Cephalohematoma is more likely to occur as the duration of vacuum application increases (ACOG, 2015).

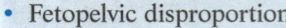

Reasons for failed vacuum-assisted delivery
- Fetopelvic disproportion
- Incorrect technique: Upwards traction before the head is crowning will release the vacuum seal and lead to pop-offs. Incorrect cup size also increases the risk of failure.
- Large caput succedaneum: Fetal scalp edema allows more of the scalp to be drawn into the cup, which reduces the available vacuum area, and, in turn, lessens total traction. A rigid cup should be used for better success in such cases.

COMPLICATIONS OF INSTRUMENTAL DELIVERY

Maternal complications

- Complications of operative vaginal deliveries should be compared with outcomes of cesarean section done for second-stage arrest, which is the clinical alternative (ACOG, 2015). The outcomes of operative vaginal deliveries are not comparable to those of a spontaneous vaginal delivery.

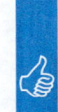 Vacuum delivery causes less maternal genital trauma when compared to forceps delivery. Forceps delivery has a higher risk of anal sphincter injury than vacuum delivery (O'Mahony et al., 2010).

- Crane et al. (2013) evaluated pelvic floor symptoms and sexual function in primiparous women who underwent operative vaginal delivery versus cesarean delivery for second-stage arrest. They found that at one year postpartum, women with successful operative vaginal delivery did not differ from those who had a cesarean delivery.
- Midpelvic operative vaginal delivery is associated with a high rate of maternal obstetric trauma (including third- and fourth-degree perineal lacerations, cervical lacerations, and high vaginal lacerations), which significantly exceeds the obstetric trauma (injury to pelvic organ/joint, pelvic hematoma, and extension of uterine incision) with second-stage cesarean delivery (Muraca et al., 2017).

Fetal complications

Forceps delivery

- Injuries with forceps are more common if the blades are not placed properly or if they are forcibly locked. This can lead to facial palsies, other facial injuries, and depressed skull fractures. Fortunately, persistent disabilities are rare (Dupuis et al., 2005).
- In a systematic review of the Cochrane Database, O'Mohony et al. (2010) found that facial injury was five times more likely with forceps than it was with a vacuum device.

Vacuum delivery

- Fetal scalp abrasions and lacerations, cephalohematoma, retinal hemorrhage, and brachial plexus injury may occur with vacuum delivery. The retinal hemorrhages typically resolve without sequelae within four weeks of birth. The majority of cephalohematomas resolve spontaneously over the course of a few weeks without any intervention.

- Intracranial hemorrhage (epidural, subdural, intraparenchymal, and subarachnoid), intraventricular hemorrhage, and subgaleal hemorrhage are more common with vacuum delivery and may occasionally be life-threatening.

SEQUENTIAL ATTEMPTS WITH DIFFERENT INSTRUMENTS

- When the first attempt at delivering the head is unsuccessful with either a vacuum or a pair of forceps, another instrument is sometimes applied to try to deliver the head—this is called **sequential use of instruments**. In other words, a vacuum device is followed by the use of a pair of forceps or vice versa. If proper placement of forceps cannot be achieved or a vacuum device fails to achieve suction and traction has not yet been applied, switching to another device should not be considered a sequential attempt.
- In some situations, a vacuum device is used to achieve rotation and then forceps are used to deliver the head. When planned as a sequential use of devices, morbidity is not increased. Ezenagu and colleagues (1999) found that the prudent use of sequential instruments at operative vaginal delivery did not engender higher rates of maternal or neonatal morbidity.
- However, problems arise when an instrumental delivery fails and an alternative device is used in the hope of somehow achieving a delivery. In this situation, the sequential use of instruments

 The sequential use of vacuum extractors and forceps has been associated with increased rates of neonatal complications and therefore, should not routinely be performed (ACOG, 2020).

is associated with an increase in neonatal morbidity, trauma, intracranial hemorrhage, and asphyxia. Cesarean delivery is a safer alternative and should be resorted to in this clinical scenario.

TRAINING IN OPERATIVE VAGINAL DELIVERY

- The morbidity associated with instrumental deliveries depends more on the operator's skills than on the instrument itself.
- Training must ensure that obstetricians can identify indications and contraindications, choose the appropriate instrument and use it correctly, and that they know the principles applied to operative vaginal delivery.
- The training programme must include simultaneous training in both forceps use as well as vacuum extraction. The knowledge of obstetric mechanics should be imparted.
- Clinical hands-on training may be reinforced with simulations using mannequins.

References

1. Åberg K, Norman M, Pettersson K et al. 2019. Protracted vacuum extraction and neonatal intracranial hemorrhage among infants born at term: A nationwide case-control study. *Acta Obstet Gynecol Scand.* 98:523.

2. American College of Obstetricians and Gynecologists. 2020. ACOG Practice Bulletin No. 219. Operative vaginal birth. *Obstet Gynecol.* 135:e149–59.

3. Bahl R, Van de Venne M, Macleod M, Strachan B, Murphy DJ. 2013. Maternal and neonatal morbidity in relation to the instrument used for mid-cavity rotational operative vaginal delivery: A prospective cohort study. *BJOG.* 120: 1526–33.

4. Bailey PE. 2005. The disappearing art of instrumental delivery: Time to reverse the trend. *Int J Gynaecol Obstet.* 91(1):89-96.

5. Crane AK, Geller EJ, Bane H, Ju R, Myers E, Matthews CA. 2013. Evaluation of pelvic floor symptoms and sexual function in primiparous women who underwent operative vaginal delivery versus cesarean delivery for second-stage arrest. *Female Pelvic Med Reconstr Surg.* 19:13–6.

6. De Leeuw JW, de Wit C, Kuijken JP, Bruinse HW. 2008. Mediolateralepisiotomy reduces the risk for anal sphincter injury during operative vaginal delivery. *BJOG.* 115:104–8.

7. Dhodapkar SB, Chauhan RC. 2015. Trends of instrumental deliveries at a tertiary care teaching hospital in Puducherry. *Indian Journal of Applied Research.* Vol.5.

8. Dupuis O, Silveira R, Dupont C et al. 2005. Comparison of "instrument-associated" and "spontaneous" obstetric depressed skull fractures in a cohort of 68 neonates. *Am J Obstet Gynecol.* 192:165.

9. Ezenagu LC, Kakaria R, Bofill JA. 1999. Sequential use of instruments at operative vaginal delivery: Is it safe? *Am J Obstet Gynecol.* 180:1446.

10. Groom K, Jones B, Miller N, Paterson-Brown S. 2006. A prospective randomised controlled trial of the Kiwi Omnicup versus conventional ventouse cups for vacuum-assisted vaginal delivery. *BJOG.* 113: 183–189.

11. Knight M, Chiocchia V, Partlett C, Rivero-Arias O, Hua X, Hinshaw K et al. 2019. Prophylactic antibiotics in the prevention of infection after operative vaginal delivery (ANODE): A multicentre randomised controlled trial. ANODE collaborative group. *Lancet.* 393: 2395–403.

12. Liabsuetrakul T, Choobun T, Peeyananjarassri K, Islam QM. 2020. Antibiotic prophylaxis for operative vaginal delivery. *Cochrane Database Syst Rev.* Issue 3. Art. no.: CD004455.

13. Lund NS, Persson LK, Jangö H, Gommesen D, Westergaard HB. 2016. Episiotomy in vacuum-assisted delivery affects the risk of obstetric anal sphincter injury: A systematic review and meta-analysis. *Eur J Obstet Gynecol Reprod Biol.*

14. Muraca GM, Sabr Y, Lisonkova S et al. 2017. Perinatal and maternal morbidity and mortality after attempted operative vaginal delivery at mid-pelvic station. *CMAJ.* 189:e764.

15. Murphy DJ, Liebling RE, Patel R, Verity L, Swingler R. 2003. Cohort study of operative delivery in the second stage of labour and standard of obstetric care. *BJOG.* 110(6):610–5.

16. Nash Z, Nathan B, Mascarenhas L. 2015. Kielland's forceps: From controversy to consensus? *Acta Obstet Gynecol Scand.* 94: 8–12.

17. O'Mahony F, Hofmeyr GJ, Menon V. 2010. Choice of instruments for assisted vaginal delivery. *Cochrane Database Syst Rev.* Issue 11. Art. no.: CD005455.

18. RCOG Green-top Guideline No. 26. *Operative vaginal delivery.* 2011.

19. Stock S, Josephs K, Farquharson S et al. 2013. Maternal and neonatal outcomes of successful Kielland's rotational forceps delivery. *Obstet Gynecol.* 121: 1032–9.

20. Walsh CA, Robson M, McAuliffe FM. 2013. Mode of delivery at term and adverse neonatal outcomes. *Obstet Gynecol.* 121:122–8.

21. Wegner EK, Bernstein IM. 2019. Operative vaginal delivery. Berghella V (Ed). *UpToDate.* Waltham, MA.

Chapter 22

Breech Delivery

INTRODUCTION

- Breech presentation is seen in 3–4 per cent of all pregnancies at term. A fetus with no anatomical defects will adopt the cephalic presentation near term as long as it has normal activity and the amniotic fluid volume and placental location are normal. Cephalic presentation is the best fit for the normal uterine shape at term.
- Up to 25 per cent of fetuses are in breech position before 28 weeks; this percentage drops as pregnancy progresses. At 34 weeks, 10 per cent of fetuses could be in breech presentation (Hickock et al., 1992).
- Vaginal breech delivery is associated with increased neonatal morbidity and mortality as compared to the vaginal delivery of a cephalic presentation (Hofmeyr, 2019).

> Though the absolute risks of perinatal mortality, fetal neurologic morbidity, birth trauma, 5-minute Apgar score <7, and neonatal asphyxia with vaginal breech delivery are low, the relative risks are 2- to 5-fold higher than they are with elective cesarean delivery for breech (Berhan and Haileamlak, 2016).

RISK FACTORS FOR BREECH PRESENTATION

There are certain maternal and fetal factors that increase the risk of breech presentation. These are as follows:

Maternal factors

- Preterm gestation
- Previous breech presentation
- Primiparity
- Older mother
- Uterine abnormality (e.g., bicornuate or septate uterus, fibroid distorting the lower segment)
- Multiparity resulting in a lax abdominal wall and more rounded intrauterine space
- Contracted maternal pelvis

> The following conditions must be ruled out when a breech presentation is diagnosed:
> - Prematurity
> - Congenital anomalies (e.g., hydrocephalus and anencephaly)
> - Placenta previa

Fetal factors

- Fetal anomaly (e.g., anencephaly, hydrocephaly, sacrococcygeal teratoma)
- Placental location (e.g., placenta previa, cornual placenta)
- Amniotic fluid volume abnormalities (polyhydramnios, oligohydramnios)
- Fetal growth restriction

- Crowding from multiple gestation
- Extended fetal legs
- Fetal neurologic impairment (affecting movement)
- Short umbilical cord

CLASSIFICATION

Classification of breech presentation is important clinically because of the different outcomes with each type of breech. It is important to establish the type of breech with a detailed ultrasound examination.

There are three types of breech presentation, which are as follows:

Frank breech
- Both the hips and knees of the fetus are extended.

> 👍 A frank breech is the most amenable for a trial of vaginal delivery.

- The compact breech fits snugly in the lower uterine segment; therefore, labour progresses well and cord prolapse is less common.
- This is the most common type of breech presentation.

Complete breech
- Both the hips and knees of the fetus are flexed.
- The irregular, bulky breech does not fit well in the lower uterine segment.
- Labour does not progress well and cord prolapse is common.
- This is the least common type of breech presentation.

Incomplete breech
- One or both hips are extended.
- A foot or knee is below the level of the breech.
- The breech may escape through the incompletely dilated cervix, and head entrapment is common.

DIAGNOSIS OF BREECH

- The diagnosis of breech presentation is made by clinical examination and confirmed by ultrasonography.
- Abdominal palpation reveals the head near the uterine fundus and the broad, irregular, soft breech in the lower pole.
- On vaginal examination, the sacrum and ischial tuberosities of the fetus are felt. One or both feet can be felt in incomplete breech presentation.
- Ultrasonographic examination assists in the following:
  - Identifying the type of breech
  - Estimating fetal weight
  - Defining the attitude of the fetal head (flexed/extended)
  - Locating the placenta
  - Assessing liquor volume
  - Assigning gestational age

– Identifying fetal anomalies
– Identifying uterine anomalies

COMPLICATIONS OF BREECH PRESENTATION

Maternal morbidity

Maternal morbidity is increased in breech presentation and delivery. Complications depend on the mode of delivery.

- Vaginal breech delivery involves vaginal and occasionally intrauterine manipulations. These can result in the following complications:
  - Vaginal/cervical lacerations
  - Extension of episiotomy
  - Perineal tears
  - Uterine rupture (resulting from intrauterine manipulations)
- When a breech is delivered by cesarean section, it carries with it the morbidity associated with surgery: increased blood loss, longer hospitalisation, anesthetic complications, sepsis, and thromboembolic phenomena.

Perinatal morbidity and mortality

- The perinatal mortality and morbidity are higher with vaginal delivery of a breech presentation as compared to an elective cesarean birth.
- A recent study from Sweden (Ekéus et al., 2019) found that infants in breech presentation who were delivered vaginally had significantly higher risk of brachial plexus injury, Apgar score <7 at 5 minutes, intracranial hemorrhage (ICH), or convulsions. They also had a higher risk of perinatal mortality than those delivered by elective cesarean. This was in spite of the fact that these deliveries occurred in pre-selected women who were considered to be good candidates for vaginal breech delivery.

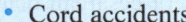

Perinatal complications of breech delivery
- Cord accidents
- Cord prolapse
- Short cord
- Cord entanglement
- Birth asphyxia
- Entrapment of aftercoming head
- Birth trauma

- The increased risk to the fetus is not only due to inherent problems in the fetus presenting as breech but also from complications of breech delivery.

EXTERNAL CEPHALIC VERSION (ECV)

- Breech presentation is delivered by cesarean section in >90 per cent of cases, and this contributes to the overall cesarean rate, which is high globally. Converting a breech presentation to a cephalic presentation can reduce the cesarean rate for this indication.

External cephalic version at term reduces the chance of non-cephalic presentation at birth and cesarean section. Studies suggest that complications are rare with ECV (Hofmeyr et al., 2015; Melo et al., 2019).

- External cephalic version is the manipulation of the fetus through the mother's abdomen to convert a non-cephalic to a cephalic presentation. A short video of the procedure is available on WHO's Reproductive Health Library (RHL) website (https://extranet.who.int/rhl/resources/videos/external-cephalic-version-why-and-how).

 Factors that increase the chances of success of ECV:
- Posterior placental location
- Complete breech position
- Normal amniotic fluid volume (≥3 cm single deepest vertical pocket)

External cephalic version is recommended at 36 weeks in a primigravida and at 37 weeks in a multigravida.

- A systematic review of the Cochrane Database (Hofmeyr, 2015) demonstrated that ECV led to a 60 per cent reduction in the incidence of breech delivery and a 40 per cent reduction in cesarean section at term.
- The success rate of ECV is high if the version is performed at 34 weeks. However, since spontaneous version is also likely up to 36 weeks, external version is recommended at 36 weeks in a primigravida and at 37 weeks in a multigravida.
- Melo et al. (2019) published a study of their experience with ECV over 18 years. Their success rate was 40 per cent in nulliparous women and 64 per cent in parous women. After successful ECV, 97 per cent of fetuses remained cephalic at birth, of whom 86 per cent were delivered vaginally.

 Although the frequency of cesarean deliveries with ECV is lesser than that without it, the cesarean delivery rate even after successful ECV remains higher than that in women with cephalic presentation. The cesarean delivery rate after successful ECV is approximately twice as high as the rate in women with cephalic-presenting fetuses who had no ECV. Both dystocia and non-reassuring fetal heart rate patterns contribute to the higher risk of cesarean delivery (Hofmeyr, 2019a).

Contraindications for ECV

ECV is contraindicated in the following situations:
- Multifetal pregnancy
- Antepartum hemorrhage
- Placenta previa
- Severe hypertension
- Oligohydramnios
- Hyperextended fetal head
- Fetal growth restriction
- Fetal macrosomia
- Previous cesarean section (relative contraindication)

Preparation for ECV

- The procedure is explained clearly to the mother. Informed consent should then be obtained from her. It should be explained that if the procedure is successful, she may avoid the risk of cesarean section. She should also be informed about the chances of the procedure not being sucessful.
- Ultrasonography is performed and contraindications ruled out. Knowing the placental location and the side of the fetal spine helps in deciding how to proceed with the manoeuvre.
- Cardiotocography is performed and a baseline fetal heart rate (FHR) tracing recorded.
- The mother is positioned on a narrow, firm examination table with the fetal back towards the operator. The author uses the examination table in the ultrasound room so that ultrasound can be used periodically during the procedure to assess the fetal position.
- The woman is asked to keep her knees flexed since this helps in relaxing the abdominal wall muscles.

 Anesthesia or sedation should not be used for performing ECV since it permits the use of undue force.

- Anesthesia is not needed and should not be used.

Tocolysis: Near term, manipulation of the uterus can cause painless myometrial contractions, as a result of which, ECV may become difficult. A tocolytic agent administered before the procedure keeps the uterus relaxed during the procedure.

- Nifedipine 10 mg orally may be given 30 minutes before the procedure and has been shown to be an effective tocolytic for the procedure (Salim et al., 2008).
- Terbutaline (0.25 mg) is administered subcutaneously as a tocolytic 15–30 minutes prior to ECV. Injectable terbutaline is sporadically unavailable in India.

Steps of ECV

- The breech is disengaged from the pelvis (Figure 22.1a).
- The fetal head is manipulated towards the pelvis in the direction in which the fetus is facing ('forward roll') (Figure 22.1b). At the end of a successful ECV, the fetal head is felt in the lower pole (Figure 22.1c).
- Lifting the breech and manipulating it gently is easier than trying to put excessive pressure on the head.

 Though complications resulting from ECV are relatively uncommon, it should only be performed in a centre where an emergency cesarean section can be carried out.

- If this manoeuvre is unsuccessful, the fetus can be turned in the other direction ('backward flip'); however, this has less chances of success.
- Once the fetal head is in the lower pole, it is held in place gently for a few minutes. The woman is now asked to extend her legs. The tightening of the abdominal muscles caused by this helps keep the fetus in position.
- During the procedure, the fetal position and fetal heart motion are periodically checked with ultrasound examination.
- At the end of the procedure, the fetal heart rate is checked. The cardiotocograph is repeated. A short run of fetal bradycardia is not uncommon immediately after the completion of

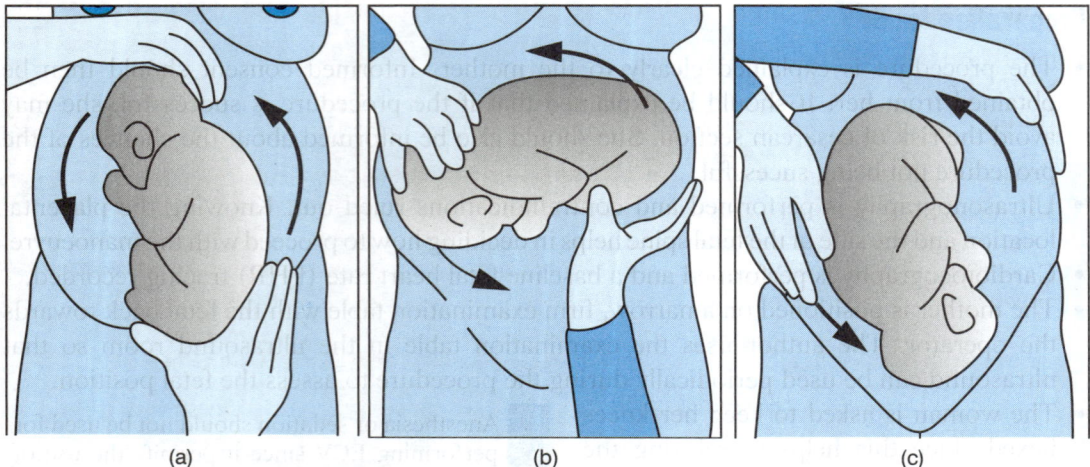

(a)	(b)	(c)

Figure 22.1   (a) The breech is disengaged from the pelvis by gently lifting it cephalad; (b) the fetal head is gently turned towards the pelvis in the direction in which the fetus is facing ('forward-roll'); (c) at the end of the procedure, the fetal head is felt in the lower pole.

ECV, but persistent fetal heart rate abnormality should be acted upon without delay as it may indicate cord entanglement.

MODE OF DELIVERY OF TERM SINGLETON BREECH

The mode of delivery of term breech is a topic of debate and controversy.
- A recent ACOG Committee Opinion (2018), states that 'planned vaginal delivery of a singleton breech fetus may be reasonable under hospital-specific protocol guidelines for eligibility and labour management'. However, if the criteria for vaginal delivery are not met or if experience in vaginal breech delivery is lacking, cesarean section is recommended for persistent singleton breech presentation at term.
- Hannah and colleagues, in the Term Breech Trial (2000), showed that vaginal breech delivery is associated with a higher risk of perinatal mortality than cesarean section (5 per cent vs. 1.6 per cent).
- Though subsequent trials have questioned this view (Goffinet et al., 2006), the two decades following the Term Breech Trial have seen a global switch to cesarean sections for term singleton fetuses in breech presentation.

 A relatively recent systematic review of the Cochrane Database (Hofmeyr et al., 2015a) showed that an elective cesarean section reduced perinatal or neonatal death and serious neonatal morbidity in comparison with planned vaginal birth for a term breech.

- In developed countries, almost 90–95 per cent of breech presentations are delivered by cesarean section. Even in India, the number of practitioners with the skills and experience to perform vaginal breech delivery has decreased. Hence training in vaginal breech delivery is also on the decline.

- With rising rates of litigation, obstetricians are reluctant to attempt vaginal breech delivery. Therefore, except in the setting of a teaching institution, cesarean section seems to have become the preferred mode of delivery for breech presentation, even in India.

> Even if vaginal breech deliveries are becoming rarer, all obstetricians should be trained in the art of breech delivery since the same manoeuvres are applied during cesarean section for a breech presentation. Moreover, the need for vaginal breech delivery may arise when a woman presents in an advanced stage of labour. Vaginal breech delivery may also be required for the second of twins (see **Chapter 35**, *Multiple pregnancy*) and for a dead or malformed fetus.

Elective cesarean section

If a cesarean section has been decided upon, it should be a planned one, performed prior to the onset of labour (38–39 completed weeks). This has a better outcome than an emergency cesarean section in the second stage of labour (Su et al., 2004).

Planned vaginal breech delivery

- Vaginal delivery can be undertaken for a multigravida with a previous vaginal delivery if the following criteria are satisfied:
  - Gestational age >37 weeks
  - Adequate maternal pelvis
  - Ultrasound documentation of the following:
    - Frank or complete breech presentation
    - No fetal anomalies
    - Estimated fetal weight between 2.5 kg and 3.5 kg
    - Fetal head flexion
    - Adequate amniotic fluid volume (defined as ≥3 cm single deepest vertical pocket)
- Most vaginal breech deliveries are assisted breech deliveries, i.e., the fetus is delivered spontaneously up to the umbilicus and then the obstetrician uses various manoeuvres to deliver the rest of the body.
- Neither oxytocin induction nor augmentation should be offered.
- Strict criteria should be followed to assess whether labour is progressing normally.

Procedure for assisted breech delivery

- When in the second stage, the mother should be placed in the dorsolithotomy position with her buttocks just over the edge of the delivery table.
- There is no data available for routine *episiotomy* for vaginal breech delivery. If it is required to facilitate delivery, it should only be done after the fetal anus is visible at the vulva (Hofmeyr, 2019).
- The fetus is allowed to deliver spontaneously till the umbilicus. The baby is wrapped in a towel to make it easier to hold. This also helps avoid cutaneous stimulation, which might initiate fetal breathing. Meconium passage is common.

- The fetus should be held by placing the thumbs on the sacrum and the index fingers on the iliac crests – this is known as the *femoro-pelvic grip*. The back of the fetus should face the obstetrician throughout the procedure.

 Rotation of the trunk and extraction of limbs is acceptable. However, traction on the trunk should be avoided as it may lead to the extension of the neck and arms, and nuchal arms, which may complicate the delivery.

- At this point, the assistant applies suprapubic pressure to promote neck/head flexion and descent.
- The mother continues expulsive efforts until the feet, legs, and buttocks have been delivered and the trunk is visible to the level of the scapulae.
- The feet may be hooked out if required. If the legs are extended, the obstetrician may use the fingers to exert pressure on the back of the fetus' knee (**Pinard manoeuvre**). This causes the knee to flex and allows the extraction of the foot and the leg.
- After the legs are delivered, a small loop of cord is pulled down and kept to one side to prevent compression and traction.
- The mother continues to push until the shoulders are delivered along with the arms. If the arms do not deliver spontaneously, the fetus is rotated through 180° to deliver the first shoulder and arm, then in the opposite direction so that the other shoulder and arm are delivered under the symphysis pubis (**Lovset manoeuvre**).
- The duration between the delivery of the fetus up to the umbilicus and the delivery of the mouth is crucial as prolongation may result in asphyxia. This usually takes 2–3 minutes but should not exceed 5 minutes.
- The mother is encouraged to push, suprapubic pressure is applied and traction is avoided until the head is delivered.
- The aftercoming head may also be delivered by forceps.

MODE OF DELIVERY FOR PRETERM BREECH

- The fetal head is larger than the body in preterm fetuses, and the risk of entrapment of the head in a partially dilated cervix is high.
- A cesarean section is the preferred mode of delivery for a preterm breech. Vaginal delivery of the preterm breech fetus (gestational age 25^{+0} to 36^{+6} weeks) results in a neonatal mortality almost four times more than that with cesarean birth (Bergenhenegouwen, 2013).

References

1. American College of Obstetricians and Gynecologists. 2018. ACOG Committee Opinion No. 745. Mode of term singleton breech delivery. *Obstet Gynecol.* 132:e60–3.
2. Bergenhenegouwen LA, Meertens LJ, Schaaf J et al. 2014. Vaginal delivery versus caesarean section in preterm breech delivery: A systematic review. *Eur J Obstet Gynecol Reprod Biol.* 172:1.
3. Berhan Y, Haileamlak A. 2016. The risks of planned vaginal breech delivery versus planned caesarean section for term breech birth: A meta-analysis including observational studies. *BJOG.* 123

4. Ekéus C, Norman M, Åberg K, Winberg S, Stolt K, Arcnsson A. 2019. Vaginal breech delivery at term and neonatal morbidity and mortality – a population-based cohort study in Sweden. *The Journal of Maternal-Fetal & Neonatal Medicine.* 32:2. 265–270.

5. Goffinet F, Carayol M, Foidart JM et al. 2006. Is planned vaginal delivery for breech presentation at term still an option? Results of an observational prospective survey in France and Belgium. *Am J Obstet Gynecol.* 39:385.

6. Hannah ME, Hannah WJ, Hewson SA, Hodnett ED, Saigal S, Willan AR et al. 2000. Planned caesarean section versus planned vaginal birth for breech presentation at term: A randomized multicentre trial. *Lancet Term breech trial collaborative group.* 356: 1375.

7. Hickock DE, Gordon DC, Milberg JA et al. 1992. The frequency of breech presentation by gestational age at birth: A large population-based study. *Am J Obstet Gynecol.* 166:851.

8. Hofmeyr GJ. 2019. Delivery of the singleton fetus in breech presentation. Lockwood CJ (Ed). *UpToDate.* Waltham, MA.

9. Hofmeyr GJ, Kulier R, West HM. 2015. External cephalic version for breech presentation at term. *Cochrane Database Syst Rev.* Issue 4. Art. no.: CD000033

10. Hofmeyr GJ. 2019a. External cephalic version. Lockwood CJ (Ed). *UpToDate.* Waltham, MA.

11. Hofmeyr GJ, Hannah M, Lawrie TA. 2015a. Planned caesarean section for term breech delivery. *Cochrane Database Syst Rev.* Issue 7. Art. no.: CD0001E6.

12. Melo P, Georgiou EX, Hedditch A et al. 2019. External cephalic version at term: A cohort study of 18 years' experience. *BJOG.* 126:493.

13. Salim R, Zafran N, Nachum Z et al. 2008. Employing nifedipine as a tocolytic agent prior to external cephalic version. *Acta Obstet Gynecol Scand.* 87(4):434-7.

14. Su M, Hannah WJ, Willian A et al. 2004. Planned cesarean section decreases the risk of adverse perinatal outcome due to both labor and delivery complications in the Term Breech Trial. *BJOG.* 111:1065.

Chapter 23

Cesarean Section: Procedure and Technique

INTRODUCTION

- Cesarean section rates have increased dramatically over the past three decades. This is a global phenomenon. The latest available data show that almost 1 in 5 women in the world gives birth by cesarean section (Betrán, 2016).
- Cesarean sections are life-saving procedures that are firmly ensconced in obstetric practice. Though advances in anesthetic services and improved surgical techniques have reduced the morbidity and mortality of this procedure, there is evidence that there are short- and long-term risks for the mother and infant (see **Chapter 24**, *Reducing cesarean section rates*).
- Cesarean section being the most common surgical procedure performed by an obstetrician, it is important for a practitioner to be up-to-date with evidence-based procedures and surgical techniques involved in a cesarean.

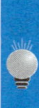 In India, as in other developing countries, the probability of cesarean delivery increases with improved socio-economic status, higher education, lower birth order, higher age, and with more number of antenatal check-ups. In other words, delivering in a private facility increases the risk of having a cesarean. On the other hand, the economically disadvantaged strata of society do not receive the optimal rate of cesareans.

TYPES OF CESAREAN SECTION

- **Primary cesarean section:** When a cesarean section is performed for the first time on a pregnant woman, it is called a primary cesarean section. In India, approximately 70 per cent of cesareans are primary cesarean sections (Mittal et al., 2014).
- **Repeat cesarean section:** When a woman has had one or more previous cesarean sections, it is known as a repeat cesarean. With the rising rate of primary cesareans, repeat cesareans are adding to the total cesarean section rate.
- **Lower segment cesarean section (LSCS):** In modern obstetrics, the uterine incision is made in the lower uterine segment.
- **Classical cesarean section:** In rare cases, a vertical incision is made in the upper uterine segment. This is called a classical cesarean section. It is not routinely used in modern obstetrics because of the increased risk of uterine rupture in a subsequent pregnancy.
- **Cesarean hysterectomy:** This procedure is uncommon but may be life-saving. The most common indications are intractable hemorrhage due to uterine atony, placenta percreta or increta, or uterine rupture.

CLASSIFICATION OF CESAREAN SECTIONS

- **Emergency cesarean section:** A cesarean section done in a labouring woman (intrapartum) is known as an **emergency** cesarean section.
- **Elective cesarean section:** A cesarean section done in a woman who has not gone into labour is known as an **elective** cesarean section. 'Cesarean on-demand' is an elective cesarean section done on the woman's request and without a medical indication.

Cesarean on-demand

If a woman does not want to undergo a vaginal delivery and wants an elective cesarean section in the absence of a medical indication, the procedure is known as a *cesarean on-demand or cesarean on maternal request.*

In 2016, the World Health Organization issued a statement (Betrán et al., 2016a) that cesareans should only be performed for a medical indication.

The American College of Obstetricians, in a Committee Opinion (ACOG, 2019a), recommended that in the absence of maternal or fetal indications for cesarean delivery, **vaginal delivery should be recommended as being the safest and most appropriate option.**

If after offering counselling (that includes information on pain relief and continuous support during labour), the mother still wants a planned cesarean, then the following is recommended:

- Explain to the mother the short- and long-term risks of cesarean
- Schedule the cesarean at or after 38–39 completed weeks of gestation

For Indian women, an elective cesarean should be performed at or after 38 completed weeks of gestation (see below in section on *Scheduling an elective cesarean section*).

If an obstetrician is not comfortable with performing a cesarean on-demand, they can refer the woman to a colleague (NICE, 2011; updated 2019).

EMERGENCY CESAREAN SECTION (INTRAPARTUM)

Indications for emergency cesarean section

The majority of primary cesarean sections are performed as an emergency procedure due to problems that arise in labour.

Maternal indications

- **Dystocia** or **failure to progress** is the most common indication for an emergency cesarean section done for a labouring woman (see **Chapter 20,** *Abnormal progression of labour*). Failure to progress in labour may occur due to the following:
  - *Dysfunctional labour,* resulting from abnormal uterine action, protraction, and arrest disorders may require a cesarean section if other treatment modalities fail.
  - *Cephalopelvic disproportion (CPD)* is one of the reasons for failure to progress in labour. This may be due to an inadequate maternal pelvis resulting in CPD. Although it may be suspected prior to labour, it is usually diagnosed during labour.
  - *Failed induction* is the term used when labour has been induced but does not progress to a vaginal delivery. A cesarean section is indicated in this situation.

- **Primary genital herpes** with visible lesions at the onset of labour is an indication for an immediate cesarean section. This reduces exposure of the fetus to HSV, which may be present in maternal genital secretions. Though the risk of neonatal infection increases if membranes have been ruptured for more than four hours, cesarean is still recommended in these cases.

The commonest indications for 85 per cent of cesareans performed globally are as follows:
- Failure to progress
- Previous cesarean delivery
- Non-reassuring fetal status
- Breech presentation

Fetal indications

- *Non-reassuring fetal status (fetal distress)* is the second commonest indication for cesarean sections. Non-reassuring fetal status is diagnosed by the following:
  - The presence of abnormal fetal heart rate on auscultation (persistent tachycardia or bradycardia)
  - Abnormal fetal heart tracing on cardiotocograph—absent baseline variability, recurrent variable decelerations, recurrent late decelerations, or bradycardia (see **Chapter 18**, *Fetal health surveillance in labour*)
- *Placental abruption* occurring during labour, and leading to fetal hypoxia, can be an acute indication for a cesarean section (see **Chapter 31**, *Antepartum hemorrhage*).
- *Fetal macrosomia* leading to CPD and prolonged labour is an indication for a cesarean section.
- Difficulty in delivery of the *second twin* may also necessitate a cesarean section.

Timing of emergency cesarean section

- Once a decision has been made to proceed with a cesarean, it is recommended that the decision-to-surgery interval be 30 minutes or less.
- However, all indications are not the same. The time to delivery varies depending on the situation, which may be as follows:
  - It is a life-threatening situation for the mother or fetus
  - Maternal or fetal compromise is present but there is no immediate danger to either life
  - Indication for delivery is present but there is no evidence of maternal or fetal compromise
- The time to cesarean also depends on the infrastructure of the facility and the availability of theatre facilities, staff and anesthetist, and access to blood products.

ELECTIVE CESAREAN SECTION

Indications for elective cesarean section

Maternal indications

- *Previous cesarean section* is a leading indication for elective cesarean sections. A previous classical cesarean section (though rare) is an absolute indication for an elective cesarean section.
- *Placenta previa* partially or completely covering the internal os is an indication for an elective cesarean section.

- *Maternal HIV* is an indication for a cesarean section. This helps minimise transmission to the baby.
- *Primary genital herpes* within six weeks of the expected date of delivery is an indication for an elective cesarean section.
- An *elderly primigravida* who has conceived after extensive infertility treatment may be offered an elective cesarean delivery. She may also have associated complications such as gestational and pre-gestational diabetes, hypertension, and fetal growth restriction/macrosomia.
- *Soft tissue dystocia* resulting from uterine fibroids or ovarian tumours obstructing labour is an indication for cesarean section.
- *Anomalies of the lower genital tract* such as vaginal septum and scarring of the vagina or cervix are also indications for planned cesarean section.
- *Previous vaginal surgery* for pelvic organ prolapse is an indication; this approach avoids the recurrence of the problem.
- *Extensive vaginal lacerations* after a previous vaginal delivery may be an indication for an elective cesarean section.
- *Cervical cancer* necessitates a cesarean section because a vaginal delivery can pose a risk of hemorrhage and dissemination of disease.

Fetal indications

- *Fetal growth restriction* with oligohydramnios/abnormal Doppler findings requires a cesarean delivery to prevent fetal compromise in labour.
- *Twin pregnancy with the first baby in a non-cephalic presentation* is an indication for a planned cesarean section.
- *Malpresentations*
  - Term singleton breech, if external cephalic version is contraindicated or has failed, is considered an indication for an elective cesarean section; however, each obstetric unit needs to work out its policy for allowing a vaginal delivery in selected cases of breech presentation (see **Chapter 22**, *Breech delivery*).
  - Transverse lie
- *Suspected macrosomia* (estimated fetal weight >3500–4000 g), especially in diabetic mothers, is an indication for elective cesarean section.
- *Fetal anomalies* such as severe hydrocephalus are also an indication for cesarean section.
- *A previous adverse perinatal event*, for example, stillbirth or a difficult vaginal delivery resulting in a severely asphyxiated infant, may be considered an indication for an elective cesarean section.

Scheduling an elective/planned cesarean section

- An elective cesarean prior to the onset of labour for a medical or obstetric indication may need to be done:
  - Immediately, regardless of gestational age because of worsening maternal or fetal condition **or**
  - At the best gestational age for the mother and fetus.

- If there is no urgency for the cesarean, it is best scheduled at 38 completed weeks to reduce the risk of respiratory distress syndrome (RDS). Though ACOG (2013) and NICE (2011) guidelines have suggested 39 completed weeks, it is important to remember that Indian babies are born earlier and mature earlier in-utero than Caucasian babies.

> **The median gestational age at birth in Indians**
> The median gestational age at delivery is <39 weeks in Indian women.
> - The WHO's Multinational Longitudinal Study to establish growth charts for developing countries (Kiserud et al., 2017) found that the median gestational age at birth was 38 weeks + 4 days in India.
> - A large study (122,000 women) done in a mixed-population hospital in London (Patel et al., 2004), reported the following findings:
>   - The normal gestational length is shorter in Indian, Pakistani, and Bangladeshi women
>   - Meconium-stained amniotic fluid, which is a sign of fetal maturity, was significantly more frequent in preterm South Asian infants than it was in white European infants.

PREOPERATIVE PREPARATION

Patient safety checklist

- As for any surgery, a woman undergoing a cesarean should have a safety checklist (Figure 23.1) that is filled by a nurse or physician before taking the woman to the operation theatre. The checklist is completed at the end of surgery by documenting the surgical count.

Figure 23.1 A sample patient safety checklist for cesarean section

PATIENT SAFETY CHECKLIST		
Patient data		
Name: _____ Age/DOB: _____		
Doctor: _____ Gravida: _____ Para: _____ Live: _____		
Allergies: _____ Blood group: _____ Rh type: _____		
Indication: _____		

	Yes	No
1. Consent form signed	☐	☐
2. Lab reports (Hgb/Hct, blood sugar) checked	☐	☐
3. Jewellery removed and handed to attendant	☐	☐
4. Glasses/contacts/dentures removed	☐	☐
5. Anesthetist and neonatologist/pediatrician informed	☐	☐
6. Blood reserved	☐	☐
7. Skin prep done	☐	☐
8. Intravenous line started	☐	☐
9. Pre-medication given	☐	☐
10. Prophylactic antibiotic given	☐	☐
11. Presence of fetal heart tones documented before incision	☐	☐
12. Surgical (instrument and pad) counts done before and after surgery	☐	☐

- A checklist ensures that important patient data is not overlooked. This decreases mishaps due to simple errors of omission.

Oral intake and intravenous access

Practice Guidelines for Obstetric Anesthesia (2016) and the ACOG (2019) recommend the following:
- The uncomplicated mother undergoing elective cesarean delivery may have moderate amounts of clear liquids up to two hours before the induction of anesthesia.
- The woman undergoing elective cesarean delivery should not consume solids for 6–8 hours prior to surgery.
- Intravenous access should be established with an 18-gauge intravenous (IV) catheter. 5% dextrose in normal saline, 0.45% saline, or lactated Ringer's solution may be administered.

 If a labouring woman requires an emergency cesarean section, she may be given H_2-receptor antagonists (e.g., ranitidine 50 mg IV) and/or metoclopramide to prevent complications in the rare case of anesthetic aspiration.

Hair removal at surgical site

- If there is hair that will interfere with the operative area, it is shaved/clipped on the day of surgery. Pubic hair need not be shaved routinely.
- Shaving on the night before surgery increases the risk of wound infection and is not recommended.

Bathing on the day of surgery

In elective surgery, bathing on the day of surgery has been shown to decrease surgical site infection. However, there is no clear evidence that using antiseptic solutions like chlorhexidine is better than regular soap (Webster and Osborne, 2015).

Prophylactic antibiotics

- Prophylactic antibiotics are strongly recommended for a cesarean section as they reduce the risk of surgical site infection, endometritis, and postoperative urinary tract infection (Smaill and Grivell, 2014).
- Antibiotics used for prophylaxis for cesarean delivery should be effective against gram-positive, gram-negative, and some anaerobic bacteria.
- Only a single dose of antibiotic should be given within 60 minutes before making

 A single dose of cefazolin 2g IV or cefuroxime 1.5 g IV should be given at the start of surgery, just before induction of anesthesia. Cefazolin (a first-generation cephalosporin) is the most inexpensive. Cefuroxime is a second-generation cephalosporin and is almost 10 times as expensive as cefazolin.

 Co-amoxiclav (amoxicillin and clavulanic acid) should not be used because of the increased risk of neonatal necrotising enterocolitis if it is given as prophylaxis before skin incision or cord-clamping (NICE, 2011).

the incision. Intravenous antibiotic can be given at the start of surgery, just before the induction of anesthesia.

- The antibiotic regimens that have been recommended and are the gold standard globally (Bratzler et al., 2013; Kawakita et al., 2018) are listed in the box below.

> **Recommended antibiotic regimens for cesarean section**
>
> *No penicillin allergy:*
> - Cefazolin 2 g IV **or**
> - Cefuroxime 1.5 g IV (if cefazolin is not available)
>
> *Penicillin allergy:*
> - Clindamycin 900 mg intravenously PLUS gentamicin 5 mg/kg IV
>
> In the case of ruptured membranes >12 hours prior to cesarean, 1 or 2 more doses of antibiotics may be given at 8 hourly intervals following surgery.

Prophylactic anticoagulation

- Anticoagulation to prevent venous thromboembolism (VTE) is not recommended for cesarean sections in low-risk pregnancies. It may be used in women at high risk of VTE. This includes women with previous VTE, high-risk thrombophilia (inherited or acquired), or body mass index (BMI) >40 kg/m^2.
- Anticoagulation is begun 6–12 hours postoperatively, after the risk of hemorrhage has decreased and is continued until ambulation. *Unfractionated heparin*, 5000 units every 12 hours, or *low-molecular-weight heparin* (enoxaparin) 40 mg daily can be used.

ANESTHESIA

Regional anesthesia

- **Spinal anesthesia** is the most common type of anesthesia used for a cesarean delivery (see **Chapter 17**, *Pain relief in labour*). It has the advantage of quick placement and rapid onset of anesthesia.
- **Epidural analgesia** is used when an epidural catheter is already in place for labour analgesia or when the cesarean section is not an emergency.
- **Combined spinal–epidural** is preferred by some anesthetists.

General anesthesia

- The indications for general anesthesia are as follows:
  - Urgency of delivery of the baby
  - Inadequate or failed regional anesthesia
  - Coagulation disorders
  - Spinal abnormalities (preventing spinal anesthesia)
- General anesthesia is induced with propofol and succinylcholine. After endotracheal intubation, anesthesia is maintained by an inhalational agent such as sevoflurane.

TECHNIQUE OF CESAREAN DELIVERY

The steps of a cesarean section have been standardised over the years since it is the most common surgical procedure in obstetrics. The common steps are presented here based on current evidence.

Positioning of the woman

The gravid uterus may cause aortocaval compression and cardiovascular compromise. Therefore, the woman should be positioned supine with a 15° left lateral tilt. Alternatively, a wedge may be placed under her right hip. However, there is limited evidence to support or refute this recommendation.

Bladder drainage

An indwelling bladder catheter is placed and is usually removed 12–24 hours after surgery. A deflated bladder helps in better visualisation of the lower uterine segment.

Documenting fetal presentation and placental location

- To anticipate and plan for problems that may complicate safe delivery, it is important to know the following about the fetal presentation before starting the procedure:
  > It is good clinical practice to document fetal heart tones prior to surgery.
  - Whether the fetus is in cephalic, breech, or transverse presentation
  - Whether the fetal head is engaged or floating
- The placental location should be documented by ultrasound examination, especially in women with a previous cesarean section since the risk of placenta previa and morbidly adherent placenta is increased in such cases.

Skin cleansing techniques

- A systematic review of the Cochrane Database (Hadiati et al., 2018) found insufficient evidence to recommend one agent over the other.
- Either 10% povidone-iodine solution or chlorhexidine (as soap or in an alcohol base) can be used to prep the skin.

Opening the abdomen

Skin incision

The commonly used skin incisions for a cesarean delivery are as follows:

- Transverse incisions (Pfannenstiel, Joel-Cohen)
- Vertical (midline) incision

> If a prominent scar or keloid is present from a previous cesarean, the incision may be made above or below it, and the scar excised after the cesarean section is completed.

The type of incision is usually dictated by the clinical situation and the preferences of the operator.

Transverse skin incisions

- A low transverse skin incision is the preferred option for a cesarean delivery.
- It is associated with less postoperative pain, greater wound strength, less risk of incisional hernia, and better cosmetic results than vertical midline incisions (Bickenbach et al., 2013).

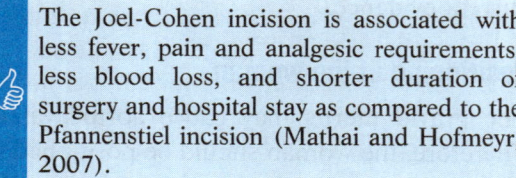 The Joel-Cohen incision is associated with less fever, pain and analgesic requirements, less blood loss, and shorter duration of surgery and hospital stay as compared to the Pfannenstiel incision (Mathai and Hofmeyr, 2007).

- The Pfannenstiel and the Joel-Cohen incisions are commonly used. The Pfannenstiel incision is usually 2–3 cm above the pubic symphysis and placed in a natural fold of skin (the 'smile' or 'bikini' incision). The Joel-Cohen type of incision is straight, 3 cm below the line that joins the anterior superior iliac spines, and slightly more cephalad than the Pfannenstiel.

Vertical skin incisions

- Though vertical incisions generally allow faster abdominal entry, are associated with less bleeding and nerve injury, and can be easily extended cephalad if more space is required for access, they do not improve neonatal outcomes.

 A midline incision is the preferred vertical incision.

 Paramedian incisions are not advised as they have a greater risk of incisional hernia.

- Vertical midline incisions are associated with a greater risk of postoperative wound dehiscence and development of incisional hernia than transverse skin incisions.
- The scar is cosmetically less pleasing.

Length of skin incision

A skin incision measuring at least 15 cm in length (the length of a standard Allis clamp) is deemed sufficient and avoids difficulty in delivering the fetus.

Subcutaneous tissue

The subcutaneous tissue is dissected sharply until the glistening fascia is seen.

Rectus fascia

One of two methods can be used with no difference between the two regarding postoperative pain. These are as follows:
- In the Pfannenstiel incision, the fascia is cut with a transverse incision and raised as flaps.
- In the Joel-Cohen incision, the fascia is nicked in the midline and opened transversely with blunt finger dissection or by pushing laterally with slightly opened scissor tips.
- Care must be taken to avoid cutting the superficial and deep epigastric vessels.

Rectus muscles

- In the Pfannenstiel technique, the rectus muscles are separated in the midline with blunt finger dissection. Then, the rectus fascia is dissected from the muscle. This appears to be unnecessary and is less physiological.
- In the Joel-Cohen technique, the rectus muscles are separated by applying traction with the fingers.
- In the Maylard muscle-cutting technique, after incising the fascia transversely, the rectus muscles are undermined from the midline or the lateral edge with a finger. The muscle is then completely transected with sharp dissection or electrocautery, approximately 2 cm above the insertion into the pubic bone. This technique provides much greater exposure.

Opening the peritoneum

The peritoneum is nicked open in the midline. The opening in the peritoneum is then widened sharply with fine scissors or widened bluntly using fingers. The CORONIS trial found no short- or long-term differences when the two techniques were compared (Abalos et al., 2016).

Dextrorotation of the uterus
Once the peritoneal cavity is entered and the lower part of the uterus exposed, it is important to bear in mind that the uterus is often dextrorotated, with the left round ligament lying more anterior and closer to the midline than the right round ligament. This dextrorotation can be quickly corrected by inserting a hand between the uterus and the right pelvic sidewall and lifting the uterus gently upwards and to the left.

Opening the uterus (hysterotomy)

Raising the bladder flap

- There is no strong evidence to either support or oppose the creation of a bladder flap.

 The location of the bladder is best delineated by palpating the bulb of the Foley catheter.

- In women who are not in labour, the lower uterine segment may be better approached after creating a bladder flap. Similarly, creating a bladder flap may be useful in women who have had a previous cesarean and in whom the bladder is attached well above the lower uterine segment. Pushing the bladder out of harm's way may decrease the risk of inadvertent bladder injury.
- The uterovesical fold of the peritoneum is grasped with toothed forceps, just above the upper margin of the bladder, and a small nick is made in the midline with fine scissors. The blades of the scissors are then inserted under the loose fold of peritoneum and intermittently opened and closed to separate the peritoneum from the underlying tissue. This strip is then cut sharply to both sides, taking care to cut so that the incision forms a curve, with the lateral ends curving upwards.
- The lower edge of the peritoneal flap is then grasped with a toothed forceps or artery clamp, and the bladder is separated gently by blunt dissection. In the presence of a previous cesarean scar, sharp dissection may be required to release the adherent bladder.

Uterine incision

- A transverse uterine incision is made in the lower segment. Rarely, a vertical uterine incision is used. The low vertical incision has not found much favour in practice because of the possibility of extension upward into the uterine fundus or downwards into the bladder.

 It is important to be aware of the placental position at the time of making the uterine incision, especially if an ultrasound scan has indicated a low-lying placenta or placenta previa. This helps in avoiding going through the placenta and prevents significant hemorrhage.

- The type of uterine incision used is dictated by the fetal size, presentation, placental location, and the presence of large fibroids.
- The uterine incision must be large enough to allow atraumatic delivery of the fetal head and trunk without either tearing into or having to cut the uterine vessels at the lateral margins of the uterus.

 A 'J' or inverted 'T' extension is often required if a larger incision is needed to deliver the infant, particularly with a breech or a transverse lie. The 'J' or 'T' incision may result in problems in future pregnancies because of the potential for uterine scar rupture. **If such an incision is made, it should be documented in the woman's medical records for future reference.**

Technique

- A small incision is made in the midline with the scalpel, 1 cm below the upper margin of the peritoneal reflection.
- If possible, membranes are left intact until complete extension of the incision.
- When entry into the uterine cavity is achieved, the hysterotomy incision can be extended using blunt side-to-side expansion with the index fingers. Blunt expansion is fast and has less risk of inadvertent trauma to the fetus as compared to the use of scissors. It also

 The risk of nicking the baby's skin is increased if:
- The lower uterine segment is thinned out
- The fetus is in breech presentation

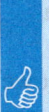 In women who have been in labour and may have undergone significant cervical effacement and dilatation, it is prudent to place the incision relatively higher. This will not only prevent lateral extension into the uterine vessels but will also avoid opening into the vagina.

reduces the lateral extension of the incision and decreases blood loss (Saad et al., 2014).

Classical cesarean

- A vertical incision that extends into the upper uterine segment/fundus is termed a 'classical' incision and is very rare in modern obstetrics because of the higher frequency of catastrophic uterine rupture in future pregnancies associated with such an incision.
- The only indication for a classical cesarean incision may be the need for a quick delivery in a woman who will also be undergoing tubal ligation.

Delivering the fetus

- After the uterine incision is made, the membranes (if still intact) are ruptured. The obstetrician inserts a hand into the uterine cavity and quickly assesses the presentation (if not known earlier).
- When the fetus is in a cephalic presentation, the hand is used to scoop the head up and bring it to the level of the uterine incision. The head is then extracted through the uterine incision. To facilitate delivery of the head through the uterine incision, the surgical assistant usually applies transabdominal fundal pressure.
- The shoulders are then delivered by gentle traction; the rest of the body will readily follow. The mouth and nostrils of the infant are immediately aspirated with a bulb syringe.
- Once the infant's cord is clamped and cut, it is handed over to an appropriately trained clinician who takes over the care of the infant.

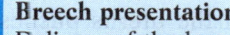

> **Breech presentation**
> Delivery of the breech fetus may require the same manoeuvres as are used for vaginal breech delivery.
> **Transverse lie**
> The fetus is turned to either a vertex or breech presentation and then delivered.

Special situations

Instrumental delivery at cesarean

A systematic review of the Cochrane Database (Waterfall et al., 2016) found insufficient information available from randomised trials to support or refute the routine or selective use of forceps or vacuum devices to facilitate infant birth at the time of a difficult cesarean section.

Delivering the deeply impacted head

- A deeply impacted fetal head may be encountered during a cesarean delivery following prolonged labour. The head may be wedged deep in the pelvis, making it hard to disengage and deliver it.

> Delivery of a deeply impacted head could also be facilitated by extending the uterine incision into an inverted 'T' shape.

- In such cases, the fingers of one hand are insinuated between the fetal head and the cervix and vagina and then wiggled gently. This releases the suction with which the fetal head is stuck in the pelvis. A sucking sound is produced as air rushes into the space between the head and the pelvis, and then the head can be extracted.
- However, with prolonged labour, the tissues may become very edematous and friable and this could lead to the extension of the incision laterally into the broad ligament and uterine vessels.
- If this procedure fails, upward pressure applied by the assistant's hand in the vagina can push the head back through the vagina and out of the pelvis.

Delivering the floating head

When the head is floating above the hysterotomy incision (found more often in pre-labour cesarean section), it is difficult to grasp the head and bring it out through the hysterotomy. In such cases, there are two options, which are as follows:

 A recent study (Elshwaikh et al., 2019) found internal podalic version to be a safe and rapid technique as compared to forceps or vacuum extraction in the presence of a floating head at cesarean.

- **Internal podalic version:** Both the feet of the fetus are identified and are grasped by the obstetrician. With gentle traction, the feet are guided out through the hysterotomy. External pressure on the uterus pushes the head towards the fundus, and the infant is delivered as a footling breech.
- **Instrumental delivery:** Some obstetricians use forceps or a vacuum device to deliver the floating head.

Delivering the placenta

- Spontaneous delivery of the placenta is encouraged with gentle traction on the cord and the use of oxytocin to enhance uterine expulsive forces.
- A systematic review of the Cochrane Database (Anorlu et al., 2008) showed that manual extraction results in more postoperative endometritis, greater blood loss, and lower postpartum hematocrit.

 After placental extraction, it is important to ensure that the entire placenta, along with the membranes, has been removed. The uterine cavity is explored with the hand or the uterine cavity is wiped with one hand holding a gauze sponge. The fundus of the uterus is stabilised with the other hand during this procedure.

Prophylaxis against postpartum hemorrhage (PPH)

- The uterus is massaged immediately after the delivery of the placenta to promote uterine contraction.
- The commonest uterotonic used is oxytocin. This is usually given intravenously in a dose of 10–20 units in 500 mL of normal saline.

 Oxytocin given IV in a dose of 10–20 units in 500 mL of normal saline is recommended as a uterotonic after a cesarean section.

- The next three bottles of postoperative intravenous solutions also contain the same dosage, and the fluid is run in at 125 mL/hour.
- Oxytocin has fewer side effects than ergot alkaloids, especially in hypertensive women.

Closure of hysterotomy

Exteriorisation of the uterus

- Closure of the uterine incision may be aided by the exteriorisation of the uterus. This involves the temporary removal of the uterus from the abdominal cavity to facilitate the repair of the uterine incision.

- Exteriorisation is particularly valuable when exposure of the uterine incision is difficult or there is need for immediate hemostasis due to excessive bleeding.

 Since exteriorisation helps in easy visualisation of the adnexae, it is good clinical practice to rapidly rule out ovarian or tubal pathology.

- Exteriorisation allows easy access to the tubes for tubal ligation.
- Exteriorisation also allows for the direct massage of a non-contracted, flabby uterus.

 In a meta-analysis comparing uterine exteriorisation with in-situ repair for cesarean, Zaphiratos et al. (2015) found that exteriorisation may reduce blood loss, but not significantly. There was no statistically significant difference between the two repair techniques for intraoperative nausea, vomiting, or pain.

Choice of suture

- In India, the choice of suture is heavily influenced by the cost to the patient.
- Both chromic catgut and delayed absorbable synthetic sutures, e.g., polyglactin 910 (Vicryl) are used to close the uterine incision.

 Chromic catgut can be used for uterine repair, especially since it is a cheaper option. The CORONIS trial compared it with polyglactin 910 and found no short- or long-term adverse effects.

- The CORONIS trial (Abalos et al., 2013 and 2016) clearly showed that in the short- and long-term, there was no difference between the results obtained with the use of chromic catgut and polyglactin 910.

Single-layer versus double-layer closure

- Traditionally, the uterine incision is closed by a two-layer repair. The first layer is closed with a continuous locking suture which ensures hemostasis. This is followed by a continuous non-locking imbricating layer.
- A single-layer closure was introduced by Lal (1988) and Hauth (1992), which considerably reduced operating time.
- However, the long-term risk of uterine rupture in a subsequent pregnancy following a single-layer closure has been a matter of debate. Earlier reports (Bujold et al., 2002; Bujold et al., 2010) stated that the risk of uterine rupture in vaginal deliveries after single-layer closures increased two- to four-fold when compared with pregnancies after a double-layer closure.
- A recent meta-analysis (di Spiezio Sardo et al., 2017) reported that single- and double-layer closure of the uterine incision following cesarean delivery are associated with a similar incidence of cesarean scar defects as well as uterine dehiscence and rupture in a subsequent pregnancy.
- The CORONIS trial (Abalos et al., 2016) also found no evidence of difference in maternal death or complications when comparing the long-term effects of single- and double-layer closure.
- With conflicting data, some of which is of poor-quality, it would be prudent to restrict single-layer closure to women undergoing tubal ligation.

 A single-layer closure can be used in women undergoing tubal sterilisation.

A double- (or even triple-) layer closure may be necessary when the myometrium is thick, such as with a classical cesarean, low vertical incisions, or a 'T' extension.

Extension of incision

Extension of the incision to the vagina, upper segment, or to the lateral angles (involving the uterine vessels) must be managed by careful suturing and ligation of the uterine vessels.

Inspection of adnexae

It is good clinical practice to inspect the ovaries and tubes at the time of a cesarean section. This ensures that a cyst or mass is not missed (see below in section on *Incidental surgery during cesarean section*).

Abdominal closure

Closure of peritoneum

There is currently no evidence to justify the time taken to close the visceral or peritoneal peritoneum. There is no difference in the adhesion rate whether the peritoneum is reapproximated or not (Berghella, 2021).

Fascial closure

- This is probably the most important step in the closure of the abdomen. A properly done fascial closure is essential in preventing incisional hernia.
- It is important to place the sutures with the appropriate tension—the aim is to reapproximate, not strangulate.
- The suture material used for fascial closure is a delayed absorbable suture like monofilament polydioxanone or polyglactin 910.
- A permanent suture like 1–0 nylon has

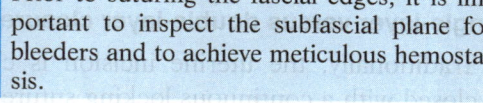 Prior to suturing the fascial edges, it is important to inspect the subfascial plane for bleeders and to achieve meticulous hemostasis.

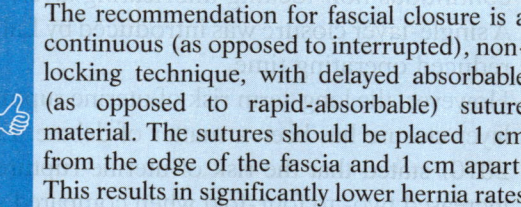 The recommendation for fascial closure is a continuous (as opposed to interrupted), non-locking technique, with delayed absorbable (as opposed to rapid-absorbable) suture material. The sutures should be placed 1 cm from the edge of the fascia and 1 cm apart. This results in significantly lower hernia rates (Diener et al., 2010).

also been recommended. In developing countries, nylon is a cost-effective permanent suture, which is associated with a lower incidence of suture sinus formation than polypropylene.

Closure of the subcutaneous tissue

- When the depth of the subcutaneous tissue is <2 cm, routine closure cannot be recommended. However, when the subcutaneous tissue is >2 cm in depth, closure with an interrupted delayed absorbable suture prevents the formation of seroma and subsequent wound breakdown.

- Placing a drain in the subcutaneous tissue is unnecessary and may lead to infection.
- If adhesive paper strips are being used to close the skin, a few sutures may be placed in the subcutaneous tissue to reduce the tendency of the skin to gape.

Closure of skin

- Better cosmesis and patient satisfaction can be achieved with subcuticular sutures using delayed absorbable suture.
- The skin can be closed with vertical mattress sutures using fine nylon.
- Adhesive paper strips are the least painful and have excellent cosmetic results. The skin edges are cleaned with saline and dried. An adhesive skin prep like tincture benzoin can be used on the edges to help the strips stick better. The edges are held together with forceps and the adhesive strips are applied by placing each strip on one edge and then pulling gently across to the other skin edge (Figure 23.2).

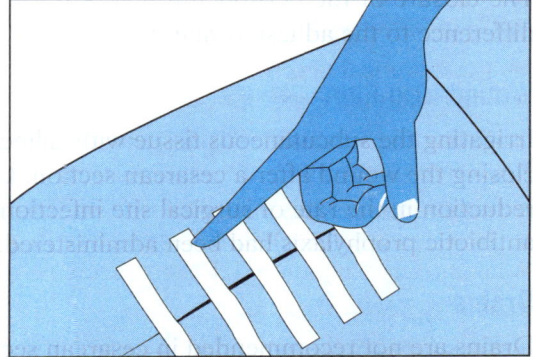

Figure 23.2 Closure of skin incision with adhesive skin tape.

Wound dressing

A light protective gauze dressing is recommended. One or two narrow strips of tape can be used to hold the dressing in place. An occlusive dressing is not necessary. The dressing can be removed after 24 to 48 hours.

UNNECESSARY INTERVENTIONS DURING CESAREAN SECTION

Abdominal irrigation

Other than suctioning out excessive amniotic fluid and blood which may have collected in the peritoneal cavity, there is no necessity for intra-abdominal irrigation (Harrigill et al., 2003).

Uterine irrigation with antibiotic solution

Uterine irrigation with an antibiotic solution is not recommended. A systematic review of the Cochrane Database (Nabhan et al., 2016) showed no strong evidence that this intervention was more effective in preventing infection than pre-incision parenteral antibiotic prophylaxis.

Adhesion barriers

Following cesarean section, the chances of intra-abdominal adhesions with and without the use of adhesion barriers are the same (11–70 per cent). Adhesion barriers are therefore not recommended. Proper surgical technique is crucial to reducing adhesion formation.

Suturing of rectus muscles

There is no necessity to reapproximate the rectus muscles. When the fascial edges are approximated, the muscles come together naturally. Suturing the rectus muscles only results in increased postoperative pain (Dahlke et al., 2013)

Closure of peritoneum

The closure of the peritoneum makes no difference to the adhesion rate.

 There is currently no evidence to justify the time taken and cost of peritoneal closure.

Wound irrigation

Irrigating the subcutaneous tissue with saline or povidone iodine is not recommended while closing the wound after a cesarean section. Güngordük et al. (2010) did not demonstrate a reduction in the rate of surgical site infection by this intervention when routine intravenous antibiotic prophylaxis had been administered.

Drains

Drains are not recommended in cesarean sections because the routine use of drains has not been shown to reduce the risk of seroma, hematoma, infection, or wound disruption (Gates and Anderson, 2013). Drains are not useful in obese women either.

Manual cervical dilatation

Postoperative manual cervical dilatation has no benefits, and there is no evidence to support this procedure (Dahlke et al., 2013).

INCIDENTAL SURGERY DURING CESAREAN SECTION

The two common incidental findings at cesarean section are adnexal masses and fibroids.

Ovarian mass

- Dede et al., (2007) suggest that an ovarian cyst or mass identified incidentally at the time of cesarean section should be removed. Excision of the mass is preferred, without which, malignancy could be missed. If malignancy is suspected and facilities for frozen section are available, then an oophorectomy is performed if the frozen section confirms the presence of malignancy. A staging laparotomy should be done at a later date.
- In most developing countries, facilities for frozen section may not be readily available. In that case, the mass may be excised in toto and if proven to be malignant by histopathology, an oophorectomy may be performed at a later date, along with a staging laparotomy.

Fibroids

- The term uterus receives 17 per cent of the cardiac output. Therefore, attempting a myomectomy at cesarean section can lead to significant hemorrhage. Myomectomy is generally contraindicated for this reason.

- Retrospective studies on women undergoing myomectomy during cesarean show a more marked decrease in hemoglobin levels and approximately 40 per cent increase in the use of blood transfusion.
- It is advisable to avoid a concomitant *intramyometrial* myomectomy during a cesarean because of the risk of severe hemorrhage. However, the excision of a *pedunculated fibroid* is acceptable.

POSTOPERATIVE CARE

Intravenous fluids

- Intravenous fluids are continued for the first 24–48 hours after cesarean and until the patient is able to tolerate and retain oral feeding.
- Typically, lactated Ringer solution or a similar crystalloid solution containing 5% dextrose is used.
- The usual amount administered is 500 mL every 4 hours. Urine output is recorded, and input and output are charted.

Feeding after cesarean section

Early oral intake after cesarean delivery (clear liquids or solids according to the mother's preference) can be resumed within six hours of surgery. This improves the return of gastrointestinal function without increasing the occurrence of gastrointestinal complications (Hsu et al., 2013).

> Early intake of oral fluids or food is associated with the following:
> - Reduced time to first food intake
> - Reduced time to return of bowel sounds
> - Reduced postoperative hospital stay

Pain relief

Pain relief after cesarean requires a multimodal approach.
- **Paracetamol** (1 g in 100 mL vial) is infused intravenously over 15 minutes as the surgery is coming to an end. This is repeated every 6–8 hours for the first 24 hours (Mitra et al., 2012).
- **Opioid:** Tramadol is most commonly used in India for postoperative analgesia. It can be given intravenously or orally. It is associated with nausea.
- **NSAIDs:**
  - Diclofenac 100 mg suppository can be used at the end of surgery and may be repeated every 8 hours for the first 24 hours.
  - After 24 hours, oral ibuprofen 400 mg along with 500 mg/650 mg of paracetamol provide good pain relief.
  - Ketorolac may also be given orally after the first 24 hours.
- **Transversus abdominis plane (TAP) block:** Using ultrasound guidance, a local anesthetic is injected into the neurovascular plane between the transversus abdominis (TA)

and internal oblique (IO) muscles. TAP block is now becoming part of the multimodal approach to postoperative pain relief.

Urinary catheter

The urinary catheter may be removed after 12–24 hours. Routine urine culture after catheterisation is not recommended.

Postoperative complications after cesarean section

- Postoperative complications following a cesarean section include wound infection, endometritis, and hemorrhage.
- Long-term complications of a cesarean section include the following:
  - Abnormal placentation in the subsequent pregnancy
  - Scar dehiscence or rupture in the next pregnancy
  - Subfertility
  - Complications related to the uterine and abdominal scar include ectopic pregnancy in the hysterotomy scar, pain and numbness over the abdominal scar, and scar endometriosis
- Neonatal complications include transient tachypnea of the newborn or respiratory distress syndrome (due to unexpected prematurity).

References

1. American College of Obstetricians and Gynecologists. 2013 (reaffirmed 2017). ACOG Committee Opinion No. 561. Non-medically indicated early-term deliveries. *Obstet Gynecol.* 121:911.

2. American College of Obstetricians and Gynecologists. 2019a. ACOG Committee Opinion No. 761. Cesarean delivery on maternal request. *Obstet Gynecol.* 133:e73–7.

3. American College of Obstetricians and Gynecologists. 2019. ACOG Committee Opinion No. 766. Approaches to limit intervention during labor and birth. *Obstet Gynecol.*

4. Anorlu RI, Maholwana B, Hofmeyr GJ. 2008. Methods of delivering the placenta at caesarean section. *Cochrane Database of Syst Rev.* Issue 3. Art. no.: CD004737.

5. Berghella V. Cesarean delivery: Surgical technique. 2021. Lockwood CJ (Ed). *UpToDate.* Waltham, MA.

6. Betrán AP, Ye J, Moller AB, Zhang J, Gülmezoglu AM, Torloni MR. 2016. The increasing trend in caesarean section rates: Global, regional and national estimates: 1990–2014. *PLoS One.* 11(2):e-0148343.

7. Betrán AP, Torloni MR, Zhang JJ, Gülmezoglu AM. 2016a. WHO Working Group on Caesarean Section. WHO Statement on Caesarean Section Rates. *BJOG.* 23(5):667–670.

8. Bickenbach KA, Karanicolas PJ, Ammori JB et al. 2013. Up and down or side to side? A systematic review and meta-analysis examining the impact of incision on outcomes after abdominal surgery. *Am J Surg.* 206:400.

9. Bujold E, Bujold C, Hamilton EF et al. 2002. The impact of a single-layer or double-layer closure on uterine rupture. *Am J Obstet Gynecol.* 186:1326.

10. Bujold E, Goyet M, Marcoux S, Brassard N et al. 2010. The role of uterine closure in the risk of uterine rupture. *Obstet Gynecol.* 116(1):43-50.

11. Bratzler DW, Dellinger EP, Olsen KM et al. 2013. Clinical practice guidelines for antimicrobial prophylaxis in surgery. *American Journal of Health-System Pharmacy.* Volume 70, Issue 3. 195–283.

12. CORONIS Collaborative Group, Abalos E, Addo V et al. 2013. Caesarean section surgical techniques (CORONIS): A fractional, factorial, unmasked, randomised controlled trial. *Lancet.* 382:234.

13. CORONIS Collaborative Group, Abalos E, Addo V et al. 2016. Caesarean section surgical techniques: 3-year follow-up of the CORONIS fractional, factorial, unmasked, randomised controlled trial. *Lancet.* 388:62.

14. Di Spiezio Sardo A, Saccone G, McCurdy R et al. 2017. Risk of cesarean scar defect following single- vs double-layer uterine closure: Systematic review and meta-analysis of randomized controlled trials. *Ultrasound Obstet Gynecol.* 50:578.

15. Dahlke JD, Mendez-Figueroa H, Rouse DJ et al. 2013. Evidence-based surgery for cesarean delivery: An updated systematic review. *Am J Obstet Gynecol.* 209:294.

16. Dede M, Yenen MC, Yilmaz A et al. 2007. Treatment of incidental adnexal masses at cesarean section: A retrospective study. *Int J Gynecol Cancer.* 17:339.

17. Diener MK, Voss S, Jensen K et al. 2010. Elective midline laparotomy closure: The INLINE systematic review and meta-analysis. *Ann Surg.* 251(5):843–56.

18. Elshwaikh SL, Elsokary AA, Abuhamama AM. 2019. Internal podalic version for delivery of high floating head during cesarean section and neonatal outcome. *J Obstet Gynaecol Res.*

19. Güngördük K, Asicioglu O, Celikkol O et al. 2010. Does saline irrigation reduce the wound infection in caesarean delivery? *J Obstet Gynaeco.* 30:662.

20. Gates S, Anderson ER. 2013. Wound drainage for caesarean section. *Cochrane Database Syst Rev.* Issue 12. Art. no.: CD004549.

21. Hsu YY, Hung HY, Chang SC, Chang YJ. 2013. Early oral intake and gastrointestinal function after cesarean delivery: A systematic review and meta-analysis. *Obstet Gynecol.* 121:1327.

22. Harrigill KM, Miller HS, Haynes DE. 2003. The effect of intraabdominal irrigation at cesarean delivery on maternal morbidity: A randomized trial. *Obstet Gynecol.* 101:80.

23. Hadiati DR, Hakimi M, Nurdiati DS et al. 2018. Skin preparation for preventing infection following caesarean section. *Cochrane Database Syst Rev.* Issue 10. Art. no.: CD007462.

24. Kapustian V, Anteby EY, Gdalevich M et al. 2012. Effect of closure versus nonclosure of peritoneum at cesarean section on adhesions: A prospective randomized study. *Am J Obstet Gynecol.* 206:56.e1.

25. Kawakita T, Huang CC, Landy HJ. 2018. Choice of prophylactic antibiotics and surgical site infections after cesarean delivery. *Obstet Gynecol.* 132(4):948-955.

26. Kiserud T, Piaggio G, Carroli G et al. 2017. The World Health Organization fetal growth charts: A multinational longitudinal study of ultrasound biometric measurements and estimated fetal weight. *PLoS Med.*14: e1002220.

27. Mitra S, Khandelwal P, Sehgal A. 2012. Diclofenac-tramadol vs. diclofenac-acetaminophen combinations for pain relief after caesarean section. *Acta Anaesthesiol Scand.* 56(6):706-11.

28. Mittal S, Pardeshi S, Mayadeo N, Mane J. 2014. Trends in cesarean delivery: rate and indications. *J Obstet Gynaecol India.* 64(4):251-4.

29. Mathai M, Hofmeyr GJ. 2007. Abdominal surgical incisions for caesarean section. *Cochrane Database of Syst Rev.* Issue 1. Art. no.: CD004453.

30. Nabhan AF, Allam NE, Hamed Abdel-Aziz Salama M. 2016. Routes of administration of antibiotic prophylaxis for preventing infection after caesarean section. *Cochrane Database Syst Rev.* Issue 6. Art. no.: CD011876.

31. National Institute for Health and Clinical Excellence. 2011 (Updated 2019). Caesarean section (update) (Clinical guideline 132). http://guidance.nice.org.uk/CG132.

32. Patel RR, Steer P, Doyle P et al. 2004. Does gestation vary by ethnic group? A London-based study of over 1,22,000 pregnancies with spontaneous onset of labour. *Int Journal of Epidemiology.* Volume 33, Issue 1. 107–113.

33. Practice Guidelines for Obstetric Anesthesia: An Updated Report by the American Society of Anesthesiologists Task Force on Obstetric Anesthesia and the Society for Obstetric Anesthesia and Perinatology. 2016. *Anesthesiology.* 124(2):270-300.

34. Saad AF, Rahman M, Costantine MM, Saade GR. 2014. Blunt versus sharp uterine incision expansion during low transverse cesarean delivery: A meta-analysis. *Am J Obstet Gynecol.* 211:684.e1.

35. Smaill FM, Grivell RM. 2014. Antibiotic prophylaxis versus no prophylaxis for preventing infection after cesarean section. *Cochrane Database Syst Rev.* Issue 10. Art. no.: CD007482.

36. Waterfall H, Grivell RM, Dodd JM. 2016. Techniques for assisting difficult delivery at caesarean section. *Cochrane Database of Syst Rev.* Issue 1. Art. no.: CD004944.

37. Webster J, Osborne S. 2015. Preoperative bathing or showering with skin antiseptics to prevent surgical site infection. *Cochrane Database of Syst Rev.* Issue 2. Art. no.: CD004985.

38. Zaphiratos V, George RB, Boyd JC, Habib AS. 2015. Uterine exteriorization compared with in situ repair for cesarean delivery: A systematic review and meta-analysis. *Can J Anaesth.* 62:1209.

Chapter 24

Reducing Cesarean Section Rates

INTRODUCTION

- There is no doubt that a cesarean section is a life-saving procedure when it is done for an acceptable medical indication. It should be universally accessible to save mothers and their children.
- However, this surgical intervention is also associated with short- and long-term health effects on women and their children (Sandall et al., 2018).

 The latest available data show that almost 1 in 5 women in the world gives birth by cesarean section (Betrán, 2016). On the other hand, in low-resource areas, mothers and their babies are dying because of lack of access to facilities where they can have a safe cesarean section.

- Cesarean section is well-recognised as a maternal healthcare indicator. Lack of facilities for cesarean can increase maternal and perinatal mortality. The World Health Organization issued a statement (Betrán et al., WHO Statement on Cesarean Section Rates, 2016a) that when cesarean section rates rise towards 10–15 per cent across a population, maternal and newborn deaths decrease. When the cesarean rate is less than 10 per cent, it usually means that women and their babies are receiving less than optimum care.
- Globally, the cesarean section rate has been increasing alarmingly. Current rates of cesarean section, except in the least developed countries, are consistently higher than what is considered medically justifiable. This has received enormous attention from women, governmental agencies, public authorities, and the media.
- A high rate of cesarean section is a major public health concern and contributes to the healthcare cost burden of a country, particularly in emerging economies.
- The obstetric community has to take ownership of the problem and make sweeping changes to keep the cesarean section rate at a level that is beneficial to mothers and their children. Efforts must be made to reduce the number of

 Reducing the **primary** cesarean section rate should be the main focus of all efforts. Once the uterus is scarred, the possibility of having a vaginal delivery in a subsequent pregnancy decreases exponentially.

unnecessary cesarean sections and at the same time, make sure that women in need of a cesarean have access to it.

SHORT- AND LONG-TERM HEALTH EFFECTS OF CESAREAN SECTION

Maternal risks

Short–term risks

- As with any surgery, a cesarean can be associated with infection, hemorrhage, injury to other organs, and anesthetic risks.

- The risk of maternal mortality is higher after a cesarean than after a vaginal birth.

Long–term risks

In the subsequent pregnancy, a cesarean leads to an increased risk of the following:
- Uterine rupture
- Abnormal placentation
- Ectopic pregnancy
- Stillbirth
- Preterm birth

Risk for the baby

- Emerging evidence shows that not passing through the vaginal canal prevents the baby from being exposed to maternal vaginal bacteria (Sandall et al., 2018). This could preclude proper colonisation of the fetal gut and lead to reduced neonatal intestinal gut microbiome diversity, which is now being linked to the following:
  - Altered immune development
  - Increased likelihood of allergy, atopy, and asthma

'Vaginal seeding'
This refers to the practice of applying a cotton swab with vaginal fluids to the mouth, nose, or skin of an infant delivered by cesarean. This is done in an effort to transfer the maternal vaginal bacteria to the newborn. This practice is **unproven and not recommended** (ACOG, 2017).

- Babies who have cesarean birth are also exposed to different hormonal, physical, and medical factors (such as intrapartum antibiotics and uterotonic drugs) which can subtly alter neonatal physiology.
- Long-term risks have been less well investigated, but there seems to an association between cesarean birth and the following:
  - Late childhood obesity
  - Asthma

OPTIMUM CESAREAN SECTION RATE

- So far, the optimum rate of cesarean deliveries has not been defined, though recommendations certainly exist.
- In 1985, the WHO released a statement that 'there is no justification for any region to have a cesarean section rate higher than 10–15 per cent'. This was based on 'populations' and was not specific to the obstetric demographic that is served by the varied range of facilities around the world.
- This range of 10–15 per cent has been misinterpreted, questioned, and criticised. Consequently, the WHO released the 'WHO Statement on Cesarean Section Rates' (Betrán et al., 2016a).
- In this statement, Betrán et al., emphasised that cesarean should be undertaken when medically necessary, and rather than attempting to achieve a specific rate, efforts should focus on providing cesarean section to all women in need.

> **How to define the woman 'in need' of a cesarean?** This can only be determined by the healthcare providers caring for the woman on a case-by-case basis and should be based on strong medical indications.

- The greatest challenge in determining the optimal cesarean rate is the lack of a reliable and internationally accepted classification system to produce standardised data.
- The WHO strongly recommends the Robson classification (see section below on *Auditing to reduce cesarean section rates*), and expects that it will help healthcare facilities to:
  - Optimise the use of cesarean section by identifying, analysing, and focusing interventions on specific groups of particular relevance for each healthcare facility
  - Assess the effectiveness of strategies or interventions targeted at optimising the use of cesarean section

CESAREAN SECTION RATES IN INDIA

- The National Family Health Survey (2015–2016) charted several healthcare indicators that included cesarean section.
- The survey found that the disparity between private and public facilities is very marked (Table 24.1). In several states, there are private facilities where 1 of 2 pregnant women is having a cesarean birth. On the other hand, the public facilities in several states have cesarean rates well below 10 per cent, resulting in unacceptable and preventable maternal and perinatal mortality. The unfortunate fact is that private facilities in those same states have high cesarean birth rates that are medically unjustified.

Table 24.1 Percentage of women who deliver by cesarean section in India (data from National Family Health Survey, 2015–2016)

State	Private facility: C-section rate (in %)	Public facility: C-section rate (in %)
Andhra Pradesh	57	25.5
Chhatisgarh	46.6	5.7
Gujarat	26.6	10.8
Karnataka	40.3	16.9
Kerala	38.6	31.4
Madhya Pradesh	40.8	5.8
Maharashtra	33.1	13.1
Odisha	53.7	11.5
Punjab	39.7	17.8
Rajasthan	23.2	6.1
Tamil Nadu	51.3	26.3
Telangana	74.9	40.6
Uttar Pradesh	31.3	4.7
West Bengal	70.9	18.8

- The inequity in healthcare delivery in India needs to be monitored. Guidelines need to be laid down by professional bodies to ensure that one segment is not receiving cesareans at a rate that is **too little** and **too late** while another segment is having surgical intervention **too early** and **too frequently**.

 In India, segments of marginalised populations have almost no access to potentially life-saving cesareans. On the other hand, more than half the urban and wealthier population has cesarean rates in excess of the medical need.

FACTORS CONTRIBUTING TO INCREASED CESAREAN RATES

Maternal perception

- There is a misconception among women and their families that a cesarean is safer for them and their babies. This perception is sometimes fueled by healthcare professionals and the media.
- Some women are terrified of the pain of labour, as a result of which, they are unwilling to undergo a vaginal delivery. Empathetic counselling, and offering continuous support and pain relief during labour usually convince such women to attempt a vaginal delivery.
- There is also a concern among women and their partners that vaginal delivery will lead to vaginal laxity, sexual dysfunction, and urinary/fecal incontinence.

Social factors

- Cesarean birth is considered to be a more 'modern' approach to delivery and hence wealthier sections of society tend to opt for it.
- Choosing the date of the baby's delivery on the basis of good luck and 'controlling' the baby's horoscope, and thereby the future of the baby, is one of the cultural pressures leading to the scheduling of a cesarean.
- Some families choose a cesarean for the convenience of a scheduled delivery to allow the husband and other family members to be present at the time of the delivery.

Healthcare professionals

- Globally, there is evidence that some healthcare professionals opt for cesarean section due to the convenience of a scheduled delivery.
- Fear of medical litigation is becoming a driving force for the increasing rate of cesareans. Women and their families have a much lower tolerance to any complications or outcomes that do not result in the 'perfect baby'. A neonatal complication is much better accepted after a cesarean than with a vaginal delivery.

AUDITING TO REDUCE CESAREAN SECTION RATES

- It is difficult to have the same cesarean section rate across all obstetric units and populations, i.e., teaching hospitals, private hospitals, public hospitals, and hospitals catering to high-risk pregnancies. Auditing helps an obstetric unit understand what changes can be introduced to bring down their cesarean rates.

- To understand the cesarean rates in specific groups across different populations, the Robson Ten-Group Classification of Cesarean Sections (Figure 24.1) should be introduced into every unit providing maternity care. This allows the audit of cesareans across all types of hospitals and populations. It has proved useful in reducing cesarean rates in units that have implemented it (Tanaka and Mahomed, 2017).

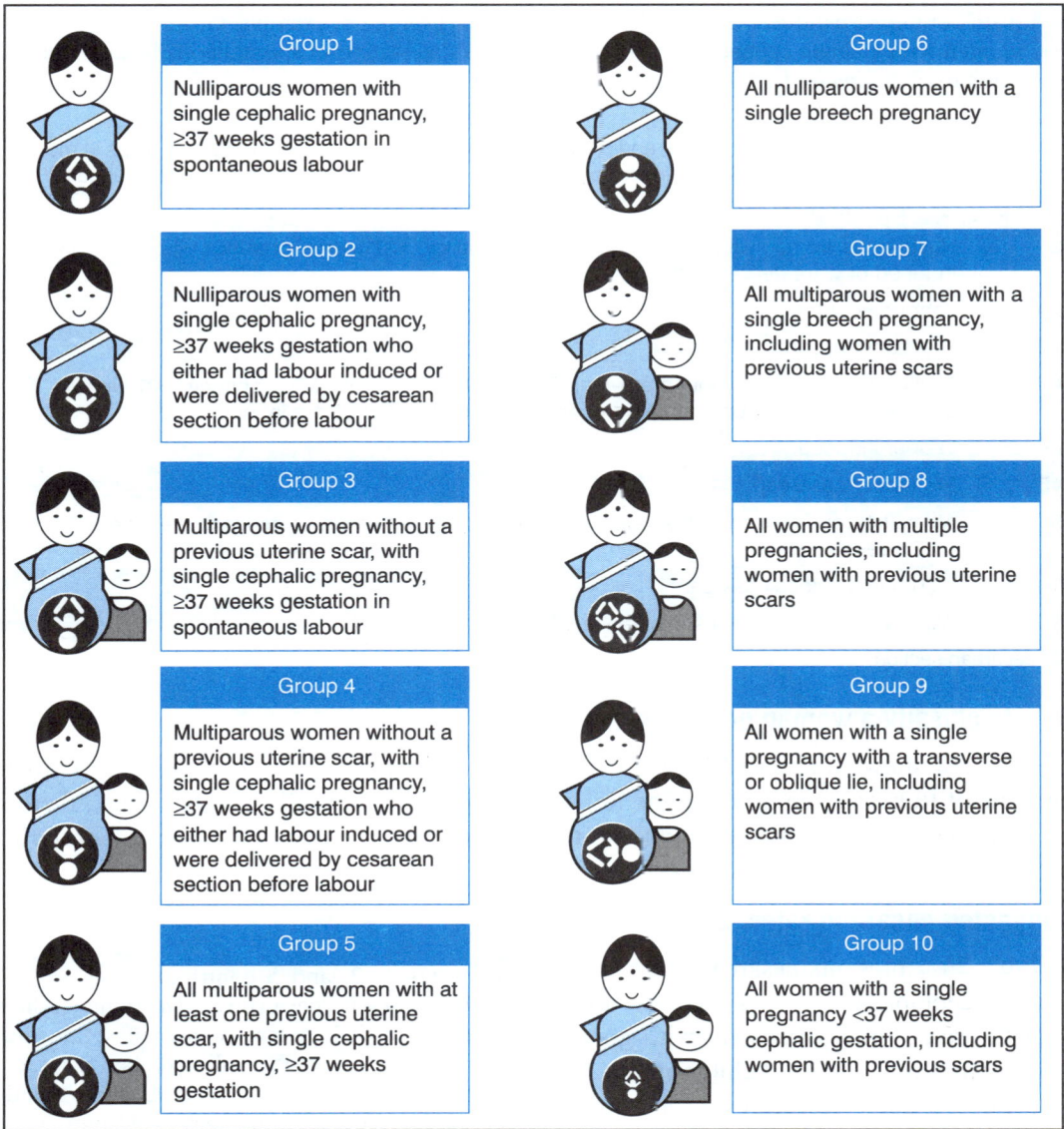

Figure 24.1 The Robson Ten-Group Classification of Cesarean Sections (adapted from the WHO Implementation Manual, 2017).

- The Robson Ten-Group Classification is easy to implement because of its simplicity, robustness, reproducibility, and flexibility (WHO: Robson Classification–Implementation Manual, 2017).
- To get better uniformity and homogeneity among the groups, certain subdivisions have been introduced in some of the groups (Table 24.2) by stratifying women within those groups according to certain relevant characteristics.

> Classifying an obstetric population using the Robson's classification allows practitioners to justify or improve the cesarean rate for each individual group. For example, Group 1 (nulliparous women with a single cephalic pregnancy, ≥37 weeks' gestation in spontaneous labour) should not have a cesarean rate exceeding 10 per cent.

Table 24.2   Subdivisions for groups 2, 4, and 5, to improve uniformity and homogeneity; this helps in more accurate reporting and auditing (Adapted from the WHO: Robson Classification: Implementation Manual, 2017)

Group	Obstetric population
2	Nulliparous women with a single cephalic pregnancy, ≥37 weeks gestation who had labour induced or were delivered by CS before labour
2A	Labour induced
2B	Pre-labour cesarean
4	Multiparous women without a previous CS, with a single cephalic pregnancy, ≥37 weeks' gestation who had labour induced or were delivered by CS before labour
4A	Labour induced
4B	Pre-labour cesarean
5	All multiparous women with at least one previous CS, with a single cephalic pregnancy, ≥37 weeks' gestation
5.1	With one previous cesarean
5.2	With two or more previous cesareans

CS, cesarean section

How to classify a woman on admission

Figure 24.2 shows a simple flow chart to guide heathcare workers in classifying mothers into one of Robson's ten groups. The Robson's groups are **mutually exclusive** (i.e., there is no overlap between any two groups) and **totally inclusive** (i.e., every category of labouring women is covered in this classification).

Suggested cesarean rates for Robson's groups

- Table 24.3 presents cesarean rates that are acceptable and to be aimed for, and at the same time, consistent with good outcomes of labour and childbirth.
- Groups 6 and 7 (breech presentation) have a cesarean rate of >90 per cent globally.

> Groups 1, 2, and 5 contribute to 2/3rd of all cesareans performed. In units trying to reduce their cesarean rate, these are the groups where effort should be focused. Avoiding cesarean section in Groups 1 and 2 will reduce the numbers in Group 5 in subsequent years and thereby bring down the overall rate.

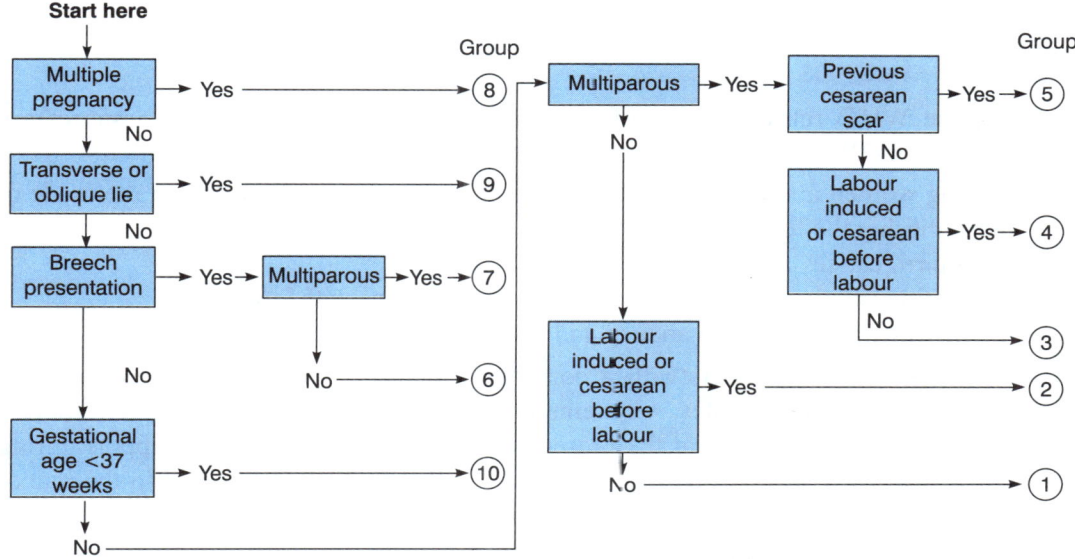

Figure 24.2   A simple flowchart that can be followed by any healthcare worker to place the woman in a Robson's group (adapted from the WHO Robson Classification: Implementation Manual, 2017).

Table 24.3   Guidelines for acceptable cesarean section rates in different Robson's groups

Group	Robson's guideline for acceptable CS rate	Remarks
Group 1 (Nullipara, single cephalic, ≥37 weeks)	10% or less	This group should be the main focus of efforts to reduce the overall CS rate.
Group 2 (Nullipara, single cephalic, ≥37 weeks + induced labour **or** pre-labour CS)	20–35%	If inductions of labour are resulting in high CS rates, better selection of candidates for induction may bring down the rate.
Group 3 (Multipara, single cephalic, ≥37 weeks, no CS scar)	No higher than 3.0%	A woman who has had a successful vaginal delivery with a previous pregnancy should be given every chance to have another vaginal delivery.
Group 4 (Multipara, single cephalic, ≥37 weeks, no CS scar + induced labour **or** pre-labour CS)	15%	A woman with a previous traumatic or prolonged labour may request a CS for the current pregnancy.
Group 5 (Multipara, single cephalic, ≥37 weeks, with CS scar)	50–60%	The CS rate could be higher if the hospital does not allow VBAC.
Group 8 (Multiple pregnancy, including women with previous CS scar)	60%	Rates will depend on type of twin pregnancy, being lowest when the first twin is in cephalic presentation.

CS, cesarean section; *VBAC*, vaginal birth after cesarean

STRATEGIES TO REDUCE CESAREAN SECTION RATES

Non-clinical strategies

In 2018, the WHO released a list of non-clinical interventions to reduce unnecessary cesarean sections (WHO, 2018). Their main suggestions include the following:

- **Educating women** and **their families** to help informed decision-making on the mode of delivery utilising the following:
  - Childbirth classes
  - Relaxation training programmes to help a woman cope with labour pain
  - Counselling for those with anxiety and extreme fear of labour pain
- **Continuous labour support** (with a companion of the woman's choosing) has been shown to reduce cesarean rates. A systematic review of the Cochrane Database (Hodnett et al., 2013) demonstrated that the presence of continuous one-on-one support during labour and delivery was associated with a statistically significant reduction in the rate of cesarean delivery
- **Utilising clinical guidelines, audits of cesarean sections**, and **timely feedback** to healthcare professionals about cesarean practices; the Robson's classification contributes greatly to this process
- **Implementation** of evidence-based clinical practice guidelines
- **Policy changes**—individuals, hospitals, and professional bodies should work to create a culture where policy changes regarding cesarean delivery are incorporated voluntarily. The safe lowering of the primary cesarean rate should be encouraged
- **Validation of indication**—a second opinion should be required for cesarean section indication at point-of-care in settings with adequate resources. Peer review after the cesarean (as an educational exercise and not as a 'blame game') will also contribute to reduction in cesarean rates
- **Introducing midwife-led obstetric units** because there is strong evidence of lower cesarean sections in such units than in obstetrician-led units
- **Financial incentives** seem to be a strong driver for cesarean sections as shown by the much higher cesarean rates in private facilities; equalising physician fees for vaginal births and cesarean sections might drive down the incidence of cesareans

Clinical strategies

In 2014, the ACOG released an Obstetric Care Consensus that addressed safe prevention of the primary cesarean delivery. Recommendations include the followeing:

- *Reducing surgical intervention in the first stage:*   Slow but progressive labour in the first stage should not be an indication for cesarean delivery.
- *Defining active phase:*   Cervical dilatation of 6 cm has been shown to be the beginning of the active phase for most women in labour. Thus, standards of active phase progress should not be applied before 6 cm of dilatation is achieved (see **Chapter 20**, *Abnormal progression of labour*).

- *Operative vaginal delivery:*   When performed in the second stage of labour by experienced and well-trained physicians, operative vaginal delivery is a safe, acceptable alternative to cesarean delivery. Training in operative vaginal delivery should be emphasised (see **Chapter 21**, *Operative vaginal delivery*).

- *Manual rotation of the fetal occiput*:   In the setting of fetal malposition in the second stage of labour, manual rotation of the fetal head is a reasonable intervention to consider before moving to operative vaginal delivery or cesarean delivery (see **Chapter 14**, *Normal labour and delivery – evidence-based management*). Assessing the fetal position in the second stage of labour, particularly when there is abnormal fetal descent, and then correcting malposition, will reduce cesarean rates.

- *Induction for postterm pregnancy*:   When induction for postterm pregnancy is scheduled at at 41^{+0} weeks of gestation and not earlier, the risk of cesarean delivery is reduced. Cervical ripening methods should be used when labour is induced in women with an unfavourable cervix.

- *External cephalic version (ECV):*   Fetal presentation should be assessed and documented beginning at 36^{+0} weeks of gestation to allow for ECV to be offered in the case of breech presentation (see **Chapter 22**, *Breech delivery*).

- *Twin pregnancy:*   Perinatal outcomes for twin gestations in which the first twin is in cephalic presentation are not improved by cesarean delivery. Women with either cephalic/cephalic-presenting twins or cephalic/non-cephalic presenting twins should be counselled to attempt vaginal delivery.

References

1. American College of Obstetricians and Gynecologists. 2017. ACOG Committee Opinion No. 725. Vaginal seeding. *Obstet Gynecol.* 130:e274–8.

2. American College of Obstetricians and Gynecologists. 2014. Obstetric Care Consensus No. 1. Safe prevention of the primary cesarean delivery. *Obstet Gynecol.* 123:693–711

3. Betrán AP, Ye J, Moller AB, Zhang J, Gülmezoglu AM, Torloni MR. 2016. The increasing trend in cesarean section rates: Global, regional and national estimates: 1990–2014. *PLoS One.* 11(2):e0148343.

4. Betrán AP, Torloni MR, Zhang JJ, Gülmezoglu AM. 2016a. WHO Working Group on Caesarean Section. WHO Statement on Caesarean Section Rates. *BJOG.* 123(5):667–670.

5. Hodnett ED, Gates S, Hofmeyr GJ, Sakala C. 2013. Continuous support for women during childbirth. *Cochrane Database Syst Rev.* Issue 7. Art. no.: CD003766.

6. Sandall J, Tribe RM, Avery L, Mola G, Visser GH, Homer CS et al. 2018. Short-term and long-term effects of caesarean section on the health of women and children. *Lancet.* 392(10155):1349–57.

7. Tanaka K, Mahomed K. 2017. The Ten-Group Robson Classification: A single centre approach identifying strategies to optimise caesarean section rates. *Obstetrics and Gynecology International.* Article ID: 5648938.

8. World Health Organization. 2017. WHO: Robson Classification: Implementation manual. WHO, Geneva.

9. World Health Organization. 2018. WHO recommendations: Non-clinical interventions to reduce unnecessary caesarean sections. WHO, Geneva.

Chapter 25

Vaginal Birth After a Previous Cesarean Delivery

INTRODUCTION

- A woman who has had a cesarean delivery can have one of two possible routes of delivery in the subsequent pregnancy: a *trial of labour* aiming for a vaginal delivery or an *elective repeat cesarean delivery* (ERCD).
- The term *trial of labour after cesarean* (TOLAC) refers to a trial of labour in women who have had a previous cesarean delivery, regardless of the outcome. The term *vaginal birth after cesarean delivery* (VBAC) is used to denote a successful vaginal birth following a trial of labour.

> **TOLAC:** A trial of labour in a woman who has had a previous cesarean delivery, regardless of the outcome
> **VBAC:** A vaginal birth after a trial of labour
> **ERCD:** Elective repeat cesarean delivery

- Attempting a vaginal birth after cesarean is a safe and appropriate choice that should be offered to select women who have had a prior cesarean delivery and who fulfil the criteria for the possibility of a successful VBAC (ACOG, 2019). This chapter will focus on practical guidelines for selecting women who have a high chance of a successful vaginal birth after a previous cesarean birth.
- All women who have had a prior cesarean delivery should be counselled about the maternal and perinatal risks and benefits of both planned vaginal birth and elective repeat cesarean section.
- A systematic review of the Cochrane Database (Dodd et al., 2013) found no large randomised controlled trials that have compared outcomes of VBAC with those of elective repeat cesarean delivery. Both forms of care have benefits and risks associated with them.
- Some of the complications of trial of labour with a scar are sudden and catastrophic, and the maternal/fetal morbidity is maximum when a trial of labour fails. Studies showing an association between TOLAC and uterine rupture discourage many patients and practitioners from attempting vaginal birth after cesarean delivery (Guise, 2004).
- Repeat cesarean sections account for almost one-third of cesareans, and contribute greatly to the overall cesarean section rates. Metz et al. (2013) estimated that if all women who were good candidates for VBAC underwent TOLAC, the repeat cesarean rate in women with a prior cesarean would be reduced from 70 per cent to 25 per cent.

- A large number of women choose an elective repeat cesarean section even though they are eligible candidates for TOLAC. This is generally because of the following:
  - Poor patient education
  - Reluctance on the part of obstetricians to face the following:
    - The consequences of a failed TOLAC
    - The recriminations from patients and their families when TOLAC fails
  - Lack of facilities for an emergency intrapartum cesarean in smaller hospitals

 VBAC is associated with less morbidity and mortality than elective repeat cesarean delivery, whereas a failed TOLAC is associated with more complications.

TRIAL OF LABOUR VERSUS ELECTIVE CESAREAN SECTION AFTER A PREVIOUS CESAREAN BIRTH

- In a woman who has had one previous low transverse uterine incision, the chances of a successful vaginal delivery in a subsequent pregnancy are approximately

 The term **trial of scar** is occasionally used instead of TOLAC. It is not a term that is used globally, and is best avoided.

50–60 per cent. However, a careful selection of the ideal candidate for TOLAC increases success rates.
- A TOLAC that ends in a successful vaginal birth is associated with fewer complications than a failed TOLAC.
- Guise et al. (2010) analysed available data on vaginal birth after cesarean and found that the rates of maternal hysterectomy, hemorrhage, and transfusions did not differ significantly between TOLAC and ERCD.
- A trial of labour after prior cesarean delivery is associated with a greater perinatal risk than ERCD without labour, although absolute risks are low (Landon et al., 2004).

 The ACOG (2019) recommends that most women with one previous cesarean delivery with a low transverse incision should be offered TOLAC after appropriate counselling.
In low-resource areas, the decision to offer TOLAC depends on the facilities available for emergency cesarean section.

Benefits of a successful TOLAC

- A successful trial of labour after a previous cesarean delivery results in VBAC.
- A VBAC is associated with much less morbidity and mortality as compared to both elective repeat cesarean delivery and failed TOLAC.
- The benefits of a VBAC are (ACOG, 2019) as follows:
  - Avoidance of major abdominal surgery
  - Reduced risks of hemorrhage and infection
  - Reduced risk of blood transfusion
  - Shorter recovery period
  - Reduced cost

- Less febrile morbidity
- Reduced risks resulting from multiple cesarean deliveries such as bladder/bowel injury and hysterectomy
- Reduced risk of placenta previa/accreta in future pregnancies
- Lower risk of neonatal respiratory distress syndrome (RDS)

Who can offer TOLAC?

Given the increased risk of uterine rupture with TOLAC, hospitals that offer TOLAC should have the ability to perform an emergency cesarean delivery within 30 minutes.

The hospital should have the following facilities:

- Experienced obstetrician/s capable of monitoring labour and performing an emergency cesarean delivery
- Anaesthetic service coverage for emergency cesarean delivery
- Theatre personnel to assist with emergency cesarean delivery
- Pediatrician/neonatologist to provide neonatal resuscitation
- Access to blood bank

The risks of a failed TOLAC

- When a trial of labour after a previous cesarean delivery does not succeed and results in an emergency cesarean delivery, all the risks of an operative delivery are exponentially increased.
- The risks with a failed TOLAC include operative injury, hemorrhage, infection, thrombo-embolism, hysterectomy and rarely, death. However, it is important to remember that the absolute risk of these complications is low.

Maternal risks

Uterine dehiscence and uterine rupture

- Uterine dehiscence and uterine rupture are significant complications associated with TOLAC. Uterine rupture may occur in 0.7 per cent of women attempting vaginal delivery following LSCS. The risk increases to 1.9 per cent with J-shaped or lower segment vertical incisions, and may be much higher in upper segment or high fundal incisions (classical section).
- **Uterine dehiscence** is an incomplete uterine scar separation where the visceral peritoneum remains intact. It may go unrecognised if the uterine scar is not explored after the vaginal delivery. The risk of hemorrhage or adverse maternal or perinatal outcomes is low.
- **Uterine rupture** is defined as the complete disruption of the uterine scar, including the visceral peritoneum. It is a catastrophic event, jeopardising the life of the mother and fetus. It may be associated with severe hemorrhage and bladder laceration, and may often necessitate hysterectomy. Perinatal morbidity and mortality may result from intrauterine hypoxia.
- Most studies describing uterine rupture following TOLAC do not differentiate between complete (rupture) or partial separation (dehiscence). However, catastrophic rupture is most commonly associated with maternal morbidity and mortality.

- For practical purposes, it has been hypothesised that approximately 1 in 200 TOLACs will lead to uterine rupture. With ERCD, the risk of uterine rupture is much lower—26 per 100,000 cases (Metz, 2019).
- The risk of rupture is maximum with the first VBAC and decreases with subsequent pregnancies.
- The risk of rupture is much lower in women who have had a prior vaginal delivery as compared to those who have not had a prior vaginal delivery (Smith et al., 2004).
- Women undergoing TOLAC after two prior cesareans are at a significantly higher risk of rupture than those with one prior cesarean (Tahseen and Griffiths, 2010).
- Risk of rupture is also higher in women whose labour is induced with prostaglandins (Lydon-Rochelle et al., 2001).

Factors associated with increased risk of rupture in TOLAC (Landon and Frey, 2020)
- Classical or low vertical uterine scars
- Increased number of prior cesareans
- Interpregnancy interval <18 months
- Induction of labour, more with prostaglandins than with oxytocin
- Previous uterine rupture
- Single layer uterine closure, especially with locked sutures
- Obesity
- Infant birth weight >4000 g

Can ultrasound imaging predict the risk of uterine rupture in TOLAC?
- In an attempt to predict whether a previous cesarean scar would rupture during TOLAC, ultrasound imaging has been used to assess the uterine scar in pregnancy. However, a systematic review that included 21 studies (Kok et al., 2013) found that **this was not useful in clinical practice**. No myometrial thickness threshold value was accurate enough in predicting whether a hysterotomy scar would rupture during labour or remain intact. A thinned uterine scar (3.5 mm) has a very low positive predictive value (Rozenberg et al., 1996) for rupture. There have been reports of uterine rupture in labour even with normal lower uterine segment thickness (Cheung, 2008).
- **Routine ultrasound imaging to assess the lower uterine segment thickness in women with a prior cesarean is not recommended** (Landon and Frey, 2020).

Hemorrhage and transfusion

- The risk of hemorrhage, infection, hysterectomy, and perinatal asphyxia is higher in women undergoing TOLAC if the attempt is unsuccessful and scar dehiscence or rupture results.
- However, there does not seem to be an increase in the risk of hemorrhage or transfusion when TOLAC is compared to elective repeat cesarean section (Table 25.1).

Fetal and perinatal risks

- Though the perinatal mortality and neonatal mortality are higher with trial of labour as compared to elective cesarean, the absolute risk associated with TOLAC is low (Cunningham et al., 2010).
- Neonatal respiratory morbidities such as transient tachypnea of newborn are more common in elective repeat cesareans as compared to trial of labour.

Table 25.1 Composite maternal risks in elective repeat cesarean delivery (ERCD) and trial of labour following cesarean (TOLAC) in term patients (Guise et al., 2010)

Maternal risks	ERCD after 1 previous cesarean (%)	TOLAC (%)
Infectious morbidity	3.2	4.6
Surgical injury	0.30–0.60	0.37–1.3
Blood transfusion	0.46	0.66
Hysterectomy	0.16	0.14
Uterine rupture	0.02	0.71
Maternal death	0.0096	0.0019

- There seems to be an increased risk of neonatal depression and NICU admission with TOLAC as compared to ERCD (Studsgaard et al., 2013).

Probability of success of a TOLAC

- Selecting the appropriate cases will ensure that 65–75 per cent of women attempting TOLAC achieve a successful vaginal delivery.
- Prediction of success in trial of labour may be crucial in reducing maternal and fetal morbidity and mortality in pregnancies with a previous scar.
- The maternal and fetal risks are integrally related to a woman's likelihood of achieving a vaginal delivery; several studies have attempted to estimate this probability of success. The factors associated with the decreased or increased possibility of success with TOLAC are listed in the box below.
- Calculators and predictive models have been developed to calculate the likely success rate of TOLAC. However, most of these have not been validated and are not useful during antenatal counselling as they take intrapartum factors into consideration.

Factors associated with an increased probability of success with TOLAC
- History of a prior vaginal delivery (before or after the cesarean section)
- History of a prior successful VBAC
- Onset of active spontaneous labour at ≤40 weeks' gestation
- Fetal weight not suggestive of macrosomia
- Non-recurrent indication for a previous cesarean section, for example, fetal malpresentation or fetal distress

Factors associated with a decreased probability of success with TOLAC
- Advanced maternal age
- BMI >35 kg/m^2
- Induced labour
- No previous vaginal birth
- Previous cesarean section for dystocia
- Postterm pregnancy
- Estimated fetal weight >3500–4000 g
- Occipito-posterior position and deflexion
- Inter-delivery interval <18 months
- Inter-pregnancy interval <12 months
- Cervical dilatation <4 cm on admission in labour

Contraindications to TOLAC
- Previous classical or inverted 'T' uterine scar
- Previous hysterotomy or myomectomy entering the uterine cavity
- Previous uterine rupture
- The presence of a contraindication to labour such as placenta previa or malpresentation
- Request from the mother for an elective repeat cesarean section
- Limited availability of the following:
  - Surgical, anesthetic, nursing, and pediatric staff
  - Blood and blood products

Planning a TOLAC

- The chances of a successful TOLAC are probably highest in a singleton pregnancy with cephalic presentation of an average-sized baby with one previous cesarean.

> The best chance of a successful TOLAC is in a pregnancy with the following characteristics:
> - Singleton pregnancy
> - Cephalic presentation
> - Average-sized baby
> - One previous cesarean

- The risks and benefits of TOLAC should be discussed with the mother and her partner. The possibility of a successful vaginal delivery should be estimated and contraindications excluded.

- Ultrasonography should be performed to estimate the weight of the baby and the placental location.

- Trial of labour should be undertaken in facilities where resources for emergency cesarean are immediately available (see section above on *Who should offer TOLAC?*). It should take no longer than 30 minutes to set up and proceed with an emergency cesarean.

- If such facilities are not available, the patient should be counselled, and alternate options such as referral to a suitable centre early in the course of antenatal care or an elective cesarean section should be offered.

- In smaller settings where additional staff can be mobilised should the need arise, all the concerned staff should be alerted and asked to be available.

- The patient's chance of having a VBAC and the risk of uterine rupture should be evaluated and clearly documented. A delivery plan should be drawn at 36 weeks and documented in the woman's case sheet.

- The hospital should have a plan for managing uterine rupture; drills may be useful in preparing for these emergencies.

INTRAPARTUM MANAGEMENT

- Women attempting TOLAC should be monitored on a one-on-one basis to keep track of the progress of labour and to look out for any signs of uterine rupture.

> The mother should be monitored during labour with the following tests:
> - Half-hourly pulse
> - Hourly BP
> - Cardiotocography, if available

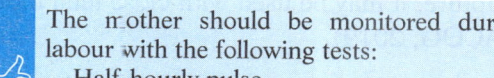

- Pelvic examination helps assess the pelvic configuration, cervical effacement, and dilatation.

- Continuous fetal monitoring with cardiotocography is preferable to intermittent monitoring as fetal heart rate abnormalities are often the earliest signs of rupture.
- The need for **augmentation** is associated with a decrease in successful VBAC. The decision to augment needs to be taken by a senior obstetrician and should be accompanied by careful surveillance. There should be a lower threshold to intervene with a cesarean section if labour does not progress normally.

> **Intrapartum signs of uterine rupture**
> - Non-reassuring fetal heart rate tracing (baseline bradycardia, tachycardia, variable and late decelerations)
> - Maternal tachycardia is an early sign of scar dehiscence.
> - Maternal hypotension is a late sign and indicates rupture with internal hemorrhage.
> - Increased maternal pain/or sudden cessation of pain
> - Loss of fetal station

Postpartum exploration of uterine cavity

Following a successful VBAC, exploration of the uterine cavity is practised by many obstetricians to check scar integrity. The benefits of this procedure are not clear. Moreover, surgical intervention is not required for asymptomatic dehiscence. For this reason, currently, there is no recommendation regarding routine scar exploration. However, it may be prudent to explore the scar in the presence of any of the following:

- Persistent vaginal bleeding
- Hemodynamic instability
- After an operative vaginal delivery

Requisites for TOLAC

- Intravenous access is absolutely essential and must be started at the beginning of labour.
- Continuous fetal heart rate and uterine activity monitoring with cardiotocography must be done, especially to identify uterine rupture.
- The anesthetist, theatre personnel and pediatrician/neonatologist must be informed and should be available.
- Blood should be reserved and available.

Epidural analgesia

- The option of adequate pain relief may encourage women to choose a trial of labour.
- Though theoretically, epidural analgesia may mask the signs and symptoms of uterine rupture, it may be used with close fetal monitoring and is not contraindicated in TOLAC (ACOG, 2019).

Induction and augmentation of labour

- Induction of labour in women attempting TOLAC is associated with an increased risk of uterine rupture (Ravasia et al., 2000) as compared to spontaneous onset of labour and hence should be avoided.

- A mechanical method of cervical ripening such as the use of a transcervical Foley catheter is preferable to other methods of induction in a scarred uterus as it is less likely to be associated with uterine hyperstimulation and scar dehiscence.
- Misoprostol is contraindicated for cervical ripening or labour induction in patients at term who have had a cesarean delivery or major uterine surgery (Aslan et al., 2004;

 Misoprostol is contraindicated for cervical ripening or induction of labour with a previous uterine scar.

ACOG, 2019). Most units will not use any prostaglandins with a previous cesarean scar. The use of prostaglandins followed by oxytocin is not recommended.

SPECIAL SITUATIONS

External cephalic version (ECV)

External cephalic version is not contraindicated in a candidate for TOLAC with a breech presentation (Sela et al., 2009). The chance of successful external version in a previous cesarean section has been reported to be similar to the chance of success in women without a scar.

More than one previous cesarean

- Data is limited regarding the risk for women attempting TOLAC with more than two previous cesarean deliveries.
- Tahseen and Griffiths (2010) found that women undergoing TOLAC after two prior cesareans were at a significantly higher risk of rupture than those who had undergone only one prior cesarean.

Postdated pregnancy

The chances of TOLAC resulting in a successful vaginal delivery decrease in gestations beyond 40 weeks (Coassolo et al., 2005).

Macrosomia

- Macrosomia is a relative contraindication to attempting TOLAC.
- Both the risk of rupture as well as failed TOLAC (Elkousy et al., 2003; Zelop et al., 2001) increase in the presence of macrosomia.

Unknown type of uterine incision

- Some women may not have any record of the type of uterine incision performed in the prior cesarean section.
- However, the majority of cesareans in modern obstetrics use a low transverse uterine incision. Therefore, women with one previous cesarean delivery with an unknown uterine scar type may be offered TOLAC (ACOG, 2019).

Twin gestation

Women with twin gestation have a similar chance of achieving a successful vaginal birth as a singleton pregnancy and do not incur an increased risk of rupture (Cahill et al., 2005; Varner et al., 2007).

Second trimester delivery

- Some women with a previous uterine scar may require delivery in the second trimester due to the following developments:
  - Preterm labour
  - Intrauterine fetal demise
- In women with preterm labour, TOLAC should be encouraged and is an appropriate option (ACOG, 2019).
- In a case of intrauterine fetal demise in the second trimester in a woman who has a prior scar, labour induction with prostaglandins (including misoprostol) has been shown to have outcomes that are similar to those in women with an unscarred uterus.

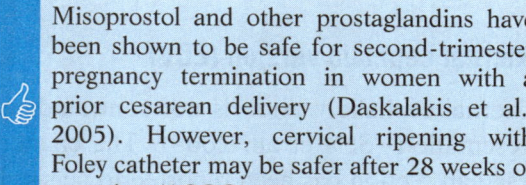

Misoprostol and other prostaglandins have been shown to be safe for second-trimester pregnancy termination in women with a prior cesarean delivery (Daskalakis et al., 2005). However, cervical ripening with Foley catheter may be safer after 28 weeks of gestation (ACOG, 2019).

- Most studies show that the frequency of uterine rupture with labour induction in this situation is less than 1 per cent (Daskalakis et al., 2005; Marinoni et al., 2007).
- In a case of intrauterine fetal demise after 28 weeks, cervical ripening with a transcervical Foley catheter is recommended.

References

1. American College of Obstetricians and Gynecologists. 2019. ACOG Practice Bulletin No. 205. Vaginal Birth After Previous Vaginal Delivery.

2. Aslan H, Unlu E, Agar M, Ceylan Y. 2004. Uterine rupture associated with misoprostol labor induction in women with previous cesarean delivery. *Eur J Obstet Gynecol Reprod Biol.* 113:45–8.

3. Cahill A, Stamilio DM, Pare E, Peipert JP, Stevens EJ, Nelson DB et al. 2005. Vaginal birth after cesarean (VBAC) attempt in twin pregnancies: Is it safe? *Am J Obstet Gynecol.*193:1050–5.

4. Cheung VY. 2008. Sonographic measurement of the lower uterine segment thickness: Is it truly predictive of uterine rupture? *J Obstet Gynaecol Can.* 30:148.

5. Coassolo KM, Stamilio DM, Pare E, Peipert JF, Stevens E, Nelson DB et al. 2005. Safety and efficacy of vaginal birth after cesarean attempts at or beyond 40 weeks of gestation. *Obstet Gynecol.* 106:700–6.

6. Cunningham FG, Bangdiwala S, Brown SS, Dean TM et al. 2010. National Institutes of Health Consensus Development Conference Statement. Vaginal Birth After Cesarean: New Insights. *Obstetrics & Gynecology.* 115(6):1279–1295.

7. Daskalakis GJ, Mesogitis SA, Papantoniou NE, Moulopoulos GG et al. 2005. Misoprostol for second trimester pregnancy termination in women with prior caesarean section. *BJOG.* 112:97–9.

8. Dodd JM, Crowther CA, Huertas E, Guise J, Horey D. 2013. Planned elective repeat caesarean section versus planned vaginal birth for women with a prev ous caesarean birth. *Cochrane Database Syst Rev*. Issue 12. Art. no.: CD004224.

9. Eden KB, McDonagh M, Denman MA et al. 2010. New insights on vaginal birth after cesarean: can it be predicted? *Obstet Gynecol*. 116:967–981.

10. Elkousy MA, Sammel M, Stevens E, Peipert JF, Macones G. 2003. The effect of birthweight on vaginal birth after cesarean delivery success rates. *Am J obstet Gyneco*. 188:824–30.

11. Guise JM, McDonagh MS, Osterweil P, Nygren P, Chan BK, Helfand M. 2004. Systematic review of the incidence and consequences of uterine rupture in women with previous caesarean section. *BMJ*. 329:19–25.

12. Guise JM, Eden K, Emeis C et al. 2010. Vaginal birth after cesarean: New insights. *Evid Rep Technol Assess* (Full Rep).

13. Kok N, Wiersma IC, Opmeer BC et al. 2013. Sonographic measurement of lower uterine segment thickness to predict uterine rupture during a trial of labor in women with previous cesarean section: A meta-analysis. *Ultrasound Obstet Gynecol*. 42:132.

14. Landon MB, Frey H. 2020. TD. Uterine rupture: After previous cesarean delivery. Berghella V (Ed). *UpToDate*. 2020. Waltham, MA.

15. Landon MB, Hauth JC, Leveno KJ, Spong CY, Leindecker S, Varner MW et al. 2004. Maternal and perinatal outcomes associated with trial of labour after prior cesarean delivery. National Institute of Child Health and Human Development Maternal-Fetal Medicine Units Networks. *N Eng J Med*. 351:2581–9.

16. Lydon-Rochelle M, Holt VL, Easterling TR, Martin DP. 2001. Risk of uterine rupture during labor among women with a prior cesarean delivery. *N Engl J Med*. 345:3–8.

17. Marinoni E, Santoro M, Vitagliano MP, Patella A, Cosmi EV, Di Iorio R. 2007. Intravaginal gemeprost and second-trimester pregnancy termination in the scarred uterus. *Int J Gynaecol Obstet*. 97:35–9.

18. Metz TD. 2019. Choosing the route of delivery after cesarean birth, Berghella V (Ed), *UpToDate*. Waltham, MA.

19. Metz TD, Stoddard GJ, Henry E et al. 2013. How do good candidates for trial of labor after cesarean (TOLAC) who undergo elective repeat cesarean differ from those who choose TOLAC? *Am J Obstet Gynecol*. 208:458.e1.

20. Ravasia DJ, Wood SL, Pollard JK. 2000. Uterine rupture during induced trial of labor among women with previous cesarean delivery. *Am J Obstet Gynecol*.183:1176–9.

21. Rozenberg P, Goffinet F, Phillippe HJ, Nisand I. 1996. Ultrasonographic measurement of lower uterine segment to assess risk of defects of scarred uterus. *Lancet*. 347:281.

22. Sela HY, Fiegenberg T, Ben-Meir A, Elchalal U, Ezra Y. 2009. Safety and efficacy of external cephalic version for women with a previous cesarean delivery. *Eur J Obstet Gynecol Reprod Biol*.142:111–4.

23. Smith GC, Pell JP, Pasupathy D, Dobbie R. 2004. Factors predisposing to perinatal death related to uterine rupture during attempted vaginal birth after caesarean section: Retrospective cohort study. *BMJ*. 329: 375–7.

24. Studsgaard A, Skorstengaard M, Glavind J et al. 2013. Trial of labor compared to repeat cesarean section in women with no other risk factors than a prior cesarean delivery. *Acta Obstet Gynecol Scand*. 92:1256.

25. Tahseen S, Griffiths M. 2010. Vaginal birth after two caesarean sections (VBAC-2): A systematic review with meta-analysis of success rate and adverse outcomes of VBAC-2 versus VBAC-1 and repeat (third) caesarean sections. *BJOG*. 117(1):5–19.

26. Varner MW, Thom E, Spong CY, Landon MB, Leveno KJ, Rouse DJ et al. 2007. Trial of labor after one previous cesarean delivery for multifetal gestation. National Institute of Child Health and Human Development (NICHD) Maternal–Fetal Medicine Units Network (MFMU). *Obstet Gynecol.* 110:814–9.

27. Zelop CM, Shipp TD, Repke JT, Cohen A, Liebermann E. 2001. Outcomes of labour following previous cesarean delivery among women with fetuses weighing more than 4000 g. *Am J Obstet Gynecol.* 185:903–5.

Chapter 26

Prophylactic Antibiotics in Obstetrics

THE CONCEPT OF ANTIBIOTIC PROPHYLAXIS

- The principles underlying the use of prophylactic antibiotics must be clearly distinguished from those governing the administration of therapeutic antibiotics in the presence of established infection (ACOG, 2018).
- Prophylactic antibiotics do not completely sterilise the tissues; instead, they reduce the colony count of microorganisms introduced to the surgical site. This lowers the level of contamination enough to allow the patient's immune system to handle it.
- Prophylaxis is administered:
  - Before exposure to the contaminating bacteria.
  - Only for a limited duration (usually 24 hours).
- Prophylaxis is intended for both elective procedures and emergency surgeries.

 Prophylactic antibiotics *prevent* infection. Therapeutic antibiotics *treat* established infections.

CHARACTERISTICS OF A PROPHYLACTIC ANTIBIOTIC

The ideal prophylactic antibiotic should:
- Reduce postoperative infection (including surgical site infection)
- Be inexpensive
- Have few side effects
- Be long-acting
- Be effective against organisms likely to be encountered during the surgical procedure

TIMING OF ANTIBIOTIC PROPHYLAXIS

- To be effective, the antibiotic should be administered within 60 minutes before the skin incision is made (Bratzler and Houck, 2005).
- The timing of the administration of the prophylactic antibiotic should ensure that serum and tissue levels are adequate before the incision is made and that therapeutic levels of the agent can be maintained in serum and tissue during surgery and for a few hours after the incision is closed (ACOG, 2018).
- A single dose is usually effective.

ANTIBIOTIC PROPHYLAXIS DURING LABOUR AND DELIVERY

In this section, antibiotic prophylaxis will be discussed for the following situations:
- Vaginal birth
- Operative vaginal delivery
- Third- and fourth-degree perineal tears during vaginal birth
- Cesarean delivery
- Obstetric complications
- Obstetric procedures
- Prophylaxis for bacterial endocarditis during delivery

Vaginal birth

- Spontaneous uncomplicated vaginal birth is not an indication for prophylactic antibiotics. Good standards of hygiene and aseptic techniques are recommended.

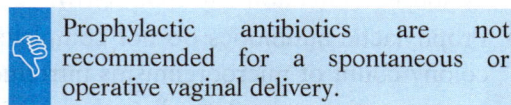 Prophylactic antibiotics are not recommended for a spontaneous or operative vaginal delivery.

- In a woman who has tested positive for human immunovirus (HIV-positive), treatment with antiretroviral medication can reduce perinatal transmission of the infection (see **Chapter 48**, *Infections in pregnancy*).

Operative vaginal delivery

A systematic review of the Cochrane Database (Liabsuetrakul et al., 2020) concluded that prophylactic intravenous antibiotics are effective in reducing infectious puerperal morbidities. However, ACOG (2020) does not recommend the use of routine prophylactic antibiotics before operative delivery. They recommend considering the use of antibiotics if a third- or fourth-degree laceration occurs (see **Chapter 21**, *Operative vaginal delivery*).

Third- or fourth-degree perineal laceration

- Antibiotics are not required for the repair of first- and second-degree tears.
- Though the evidence is not strong and is based on a single study (Duggal et al., 2008), the current recommendation is that a single dose of antibiotic (cefazolin or cefuroxime) at the time of repair is reasonable in the setting of obstetric anal sphincter injuries (ACOG, 2018).

Cesarean section

- Rates of infection after a cesarean section are significantly higher than they are with vaginal birth (Declercq et al., 2007). The risk of infection is 5- to 20-fold greater in women undergoing cesarean delivery than it is in women who give birth vaginally. The single most important risk factor for postpartum maternal infection is cesarean section (Smaill and Grivell, 2014). Studies have shown the incidence of wound infections to be as high as 30 per cent and that of endometritis to be as high as 60 per cent if prophylactic antibiotics have not been administered for a cesarean delivery.

Endomyometritis, urinary tract infection, wound infection, and sepsis may occur following cesarean section. The incidence is higher in an emergency cesarean section.

- A systematic review of the Cochrane Database (Smaill and Grivell, 2014) found strong evidence for the administration of prophylactic antibiotics in all women undergoing cesarean section, both elective and emergency.
- Though there is ample evidence to support the use of prophylactic antibiotics in cesarean delivery, it is not clear whether any one particular agent, dose or route of administration is superior.
- Antibiotics used for prophylaxis for cesarean delivery should be effective against gram-positive bacteria, gram-negative bacteria, and some anaerobic bacteria.
- The antibiotics that have demonstrated some efficacy either alone or in combination with another drug are:
  - Penicillins (ampicillin, ticarcillin, and piperacillin)
  - Cephalosporins (cefazolin, cefuroxime, cefoxitin, cefotetan, and cefotaxime)
  - Metronidazole in conjunction with gentamicin (activity against a very narrow range of potential pathogens)
- Gyte et al. (2014), in a systematic review of the Cochrane Database, found that based on current evidence, cephalosporins and penicillins have similar efficacy in preventing immediate postoperative infections when given as prophylaxis at cesarean section.

Recommended antibiotics

- The recommended regimens for cesareans that are accepted as the gold standard globally are listed in Table 26.1 (Bratzler et al., 2013; Kawakita et al., 2018).
- Co-amoxiclav (amoxicillin and clavulanic acid) **should not be used** because of the

 A single dose of cefazolin 2 g IV or cefuroxime 1.5 g IV should be given at the start of surgery, just before the induction of anesthesia. Cefazolin (a first-generation cephalosporin) is the most inexpensive. Cefuroxime, a second-generation cephalosporin, is almost ten times as expensive as cefazolin.

Table 26.1 Antibiotic regimen for cesarean section

Drug	Time of administration	Number of doses
No penicillin allergy Inj. cefazolin 2 g IV 6 hourly **or** Inj. cefuroxime 1.5 g IV (if cefazolin not available)	Within 60 minutes before skin incision **or** just before induction of anesthesia	Single dose
Penicillin allergy Clindamycin 900 mg IV **plus** gentamicin 5 mg/kg IV	Within 60 minutes before skin incision	Single dose
Emergency cesarean or membranes ruptured >4 hours before cesarean Azithromycin (500 mg IV, infused over 1 hour) in addition to routine antibiotic prophylaxis	Within 60 minutes before skin incision	Single dose

increased risk of neonatal necrotising enterocolitis if it is given as prophylaxis before skin incision or cord-clamping (NICE, 2011).

Dosage and timing

- It is recommended that a single dose of antibiotic be administered within 60 minutes before making the skin incision (NICE, 2011; ACOG, 2018). Intravenous antibiotic may be administered at the start of surgery, just before induction of anesthesia.
- Recent studies have suggested that the addition of a single dose of **azithromycin** (500 mg IV infused over 1 hour) to the routine single dose of prophylactic antibiotic in women who undergo a **cesarean in labour** (emergency cesarean section) or who have **ruptured membranes for >4 hours** prior to cesarean section significantly decreases the risk of wound infection and endometritis (Tita et al., 2016; Farmer et al., 2020). It is not recommended for elective cesarean sections (ACOG, 2018; Berghella, 2020).

Why a single dose?

The aim of prophylactic antibiotics is to get the most effective infection prevention with the least amount of exposure to both the mother and the fetus. Studies in general surgical populations have shown no benefit from postoperative antimicrobial prophylaxis; this has been applied to cesareans too.

Moreover, recent studies have focused attention on the ill-effects of early antibiotic exposure on the neonatal oral and gut microbiome. It is, therefore, essential to shorten fetal antibiotic exposure, which may have a negative impact on neonatal immune development.

Antibiotic prophylaxis for obstetric complications

Preterm premature rupture of membranes

- Mothers with preterm premature rupture of membranes (PPROM) at less than 34^{+0} weeks of gestation benefit from antibiotic prophylaxis, which helps

 In PPROM at $<34^{+0}$ weeks, antibiotic prophylaxis is indicated when delivery is not imminent.

in prolonging pregnancy and delaying delivery (Kenyon et al., ORACLE I study, 2001; ACOG, 2018).
- Mercer et al. (1997) were the first to establish that prophylactic antibiotics in this situation also reduce the incidence of respiratory distress syndrome, necrotising enterocolitis, intraventricular hemorrhage, and early-onset sepsis but do not significantly reduce perinatal mortality. A systematic review of the Cochrane Database confirmed this data (Kenyon et al., 2013).

Dosage and duration of antibiotic prophylaxis for PPROM

The recommendations for the antibiotic regimens for PPROM are based on the largest randomised controlled trial for this condition (Kenyon et al., 2001; SOGC, 2017; ACOG, 2018). The recommendations are summarised in Table 26.2.

 Amoxicillin/clavulanic acid should not be used because of the increased risk of necrotising enterocolitis in neonates exposed to this antibiotic.

Table 26.2 Antibiotic regimen for preterm premature rupture of membranes

Drug regimen	Duration
Inj. ampicillin 2 g IV 6 hourly **and** Inj. erythromycin 250 mg IV 6 hourly	48 hours
Followed by T. amoxicillin 250 mg orally every 8 hours **and** T. erythromycin 333 mg orally every 8 hours	5 days
Alternative regimen	
Azithromycin 1 g orally at admission **and** ampicillin 2 g IV at admission and every 6 hours	48 hours
Followed by Amoxicillin 500 mg orally every 8 hours	5 days

Preterm labour

A systematic review of the Cochrane Database (Flenady et al., 2013) showed that antibiotic prophylaxis is **not indicated** for pregnancy prolongation in women with preterm labour and intact membranes.

Antibiotic prophylaxis for obstetric procedures

Manual removal of placenta

- No data exists to support the administration of prophylactic antibiotics to mothers who gave birth vaginally and in whom a manual removal of the placenta has been performed.
- However, the WHO (2012) recommends a single dose of antibiotics (ampicillin or first-generation cephalosporin) if manual removal of the placenta has been performed. There is no good-quality evidence for this recommendation, which was reached by consensus.

Cerclage procedures

Elective (prophylactic) cervical cerclage

- The rate of complications (including infectious complications) after prophylactic cerclage is low (1–5 per cent) when it is performed before there is any evidence of cervical dilatation or shortening (Harger, 2002).

 Antibiotic prophylaxis is not indicated for prophylactic cervical cerclage.

- There is insufficient evidence to recommend antibiotic prophylaxis for elective cervical cerclage.

Emergency cervical cerclage

- Emergency cerclage performed when some degree of cervical dilatation and effacement has already occurred is associated with a high risk of chorioamnionitis and rupture of membranes. This risk increases further when the membranes are exposed significantly.
- Currently, there is insufficient evidence to recommend antibiotic prophylaxis for emergency cerclage (ACOG, 2018).

- However, if the membranes are exposed, a single dose of an IV cephalosporin (e.g., cefazolin or cefuroxime) may be given just before the beginning of the procedure.

Abdominal cerclage

- In accordance with recommendations for other gynecologic surgical procedures that do not involve entering the vagina, there is no indication for antibiotic prophylaxis for abdominal cerclage when done through a laparotomy.

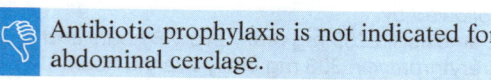 Antibiotic prophylaxis is not indicated for abdominal cerclage.

- Antibiotic prophylaxis is not recommended for patients undergoing operative laparoscopy in which entry of the bowel or vagina is not anticipated (ACOG, 2018a). Therefore, abdominal cerclage done laparoscopically does not require prophylactic antibiotics.

Prevention of bacterial endocarditis

- Infective endocarditis prophylaxis is not recommended for women with acquired or congenital structural heart disease for either vaginal or cesarean delivery according to the guidelines issued by the American Heart Association and the American College of Cardiology (Nishimura et al., 2017).
- The small subset of women who require prophylaxis for bacterial endocarditis are those who have either of the following:
  - Cyanotic cardiac disease
  - Prosthetic valves

Dangers of antibiotic overuse and abuse

As mentioned earlier, the aim of prophylactic antibiotics is to get the most effective infection prevention with the least amount of exposure to both the mother and the fetus. Recent studies have focused attention on the ill-effects of early antibiotic exposure on the neonatal oral and gut microbiome. It is, therefore, essential to shorten fetal antibiotic exposure, which may have a negative impact on neonatal immune development.

The inappropriate and irresponsible use of antibiotics has resulted in the emergence of pathogens that are multi-drug resistant. In obstetrics, this has reflected in increased neonatal infections and maternal infectious morbidity. What is more worrisome is that the bacterial spectrum causing sepsis is changing. Studies have shown that *Escherichia coli* is now the most common organism causing sepsis in neonates, particularly after maternal antibiotic administration (Bizzarro et al., 2008). Emerging strains of highly virulent methicillin-resistant *Staphylococcus aureus* (MRSA) in the community are posing concerns for populations at risk, including pregnant women and children.

Antimicrobial resistance in bacterial pathogens is a global emergency that is associated with high morbidity and mortality. Multi-drug resistance patterns in gram-positive and gram-negative bacteria are difficult to treat, and are proving to be resistant to conventional antibiotics. There is currently a shortage of effective therapies compounded by a lack of successful prevention measures (Frieri et al., 2017). Only a few new antibiotics are available currently since there has been a massive decline in the discovery of new drug molecules as far as antibiotics are concerned.

References

1. American College of Obstetricians and Gynecologists. 2018. ACOG Practice Bulletin No. 199. Use of prophylactic antibiotics in labor and delivery. *Obstet Gynecol*. 132: e103-19.

2. American College of Obstetricians and Gynecologists. 2018a. ACOG Practice Bulletin No. 195. Prevention of infection after gynecologic procedures. *Obstet and Gynecol*. 131: e172–189.

3. Berghella V. 2020. Cesarean delivery: Preoperative planning and patient preparation. Lockwood CJ (Ed). *UpToDate*. Waltham, MA.

4. Bizzarro MJ, Dembry LM, Baltimore RS, Gallagher PG. 2008. Changing patterns in neonatal *Escherichia coli* sepsis and ampicillin resistance in the era of intrapartum antibiotic prophylaxis. *Pediatrics*. 121:689–96.

5. Bratzler DW, Houck PM. 2005. Antimicrobial prophylaxis for surgery: An advisory statement from the National Surgical Infection Prevention Project. *Am J Surg*. 189(4):395–404.

6. Bratzler DW, Dellinger EP, Olsen KM et al. 2013. Clinical practice guidelines for antimicrobial prophylaxis in surgery. *American Journal of Health-System Pharmacy*. Volume 70, Issue 3. p195–283.

7. Declercq E, Barger M, Cabral HJ, Evans SR, Kotelchuck M, Simon C et al. 2007. Maternal outcomes associated with planned primary cesarean births compared with planned vaginal births. *Obstet Gynecol*. 109:669–77.

8. Farmer N, Hodgetts-Morton V, Morris RK. 2020. Are prophylactic adjunctive macrolides efficacious against caesarean section surgical site infection: A systematic review and meta-analysis. *Eur J Obstet Gynecol Reprod Biol*. 244:163-171.

9. Flenady V, Hawley G, Stock OM, Kenyon S, Badawi N. 2013. Prophylactic antibiotics for inhibiting preterm labour with intact membranes. *Cochrane Database Syst Rev*. Issue 12. Art. no.: CD000246.

10. Frieri M, Kumar K, Boutin A. 2017. Antibiotic resistance. *J Infect Public Health*. (4):369-378.

11. Gyte GML, Dou L, Vazquez JC. 2014. Different classes of antibiotics given to women routinely for preventing infection at caesarean section. *Cochrane Database Syst Rev*. Issue 11. Art. no.: CD008726.

12. Harger JH. 2002. Cerclage and cervical insufficiency: An evidence-based analysis. *Obstet Gynecol*. 100: 1313–27.

13. Kawakita T, Huang CC, Landy HJ. 2018. Choice of prophylactic antibiotics and surgical site infections after cesarean delivery. *Obstet Gynecol*. 132(4):948-955.

14. Kenyon SL, Taylor DJ, Tarnow-Mordi W. 2001. Broad-spectrum antibiotics for preterm rupture of the fetal membranes: The ORACLE I Randomised Trial. *Lancet*. 357:981-90.

15. Kenyon S, Boulvain M, Neilson J. 2013. Antibiotics for preterm rupture of membranes. *Cochrane Database Syst Rev*. Issue 12. Art. no.: CD001058.

16. Liabsuetrakul T, Choobun T, Peeyananjarassri K, Islam QM. 2017. Antibiotic prophylaxis for operative vaginal delivery. *Cochrane Database Syst Rev*. Issue 8. Art. no.: CD004455.

17. National Institute for Health and Clinical Excellence. 2011. Caesarean section (update). (Clinical guideline 132).

18. Nishimura RA, Otto CM, Bonow RO, Carabello BA et al. 2017. AHA/ACC focused update of the 2014 AHA/ACC guideline for the management of patients with valvular heart disease: A report of the American College of Cardiology/American Heart Association Task Force on Clinical Practice Guidelines. 135:e1159–195.

19. Smaill FM, Grivell R. 2014. Antibiotic prophylaxis versus no prophylaxis for preventing infection after cesarean section. *Cochrane Database Syst Rev.* Rev. Issue 10. Art. no.: CD007482.

20. Yudin MH, van Schalkwyk J, Eyk NV et al. SOGC Clinical Practice Guideline No. 233. 2017. Antibiotic therapy in preterm premature rupture of the membranes. *J Obstet Gynaecol.* Volume 39, Issue 9. e207–e212.

21. Tita AT, Szychowski JM, Boggess K et al. 2016. Adjunctive azithromycin prophylaxis for cesarean delivery. *N Engl J Med.* 375:1231.

22. World Health Organization. WHO Reproductive Health Library. 2012. WHO recommendation on the use of antibiotics for the manual removal of retained placenta. The WHO Reproductive Health Library. WHO, Geneva.

Chapter 27

Maternal Care in the Puerperium

INTRODUCTION

- The puerperium is the period starting from the delivery of the infant to the time when the physiological changes of pregnancy in different maternal systems have mostly returned to the pre-pregnant state.
- The puerperium is usually considered to last from six to eight weeks after delivery.
- This is an important time in the life of the woman as well as her newborn. Both the woman and her newborn require physical, emotional, and medical support during this period.
- After an uncomplicated vaginal birth in a health facility, healthy mothers and newborns should receive care in the facility for at least 24 hours after birth (WHO, 2014). After an uncomplicated cesarean delivery, the mother and her newborn should remain hospitalised for at least 48 to 72 hours after birth.

THE IMMEDIATE PUERPERAL PERIOD

- Immediately after an uncomplicated vaginal delivery, and for the first 24 hours, the woman must be monitored for the following:
  - Vaginal bleeding
  - Uterine contraction and fundal height—this is done confirm that the uterus has started involuting
  - Temperature
  - Pulse rate
  - Blood pressure—this should be measured shortly after birth; if normal, a second blood pressure measurement should be taken within six hours
  - Urine output—the first void should be documented within six hours
- **Postpartum shivering or chills:** 25–50 per cent of women develop shivering immediately after the birth of the baby. It is usually transient and usually settles down on its own. The mother should be reassured that it is a normal phenomenon. Warm blankets may be of use.

ROUTINE POSTPARTUM CARE

Perineal care

- The mother should be instructed to wash her perineum regularly to keep it clean. Lochia may drain for up to four weeks and hence she should be advised to change pads frequently. Reusable cloth pads are now available for maternity use. Disposable pads may be used, but are environmentally unsound.
- After urinating, the mother should be advised to wash and gently pat the perineum dry.

Bleeding and lochia

- After the placenta is extruded, the basal layer of the decidua is left behind. This is shed over the next few weeks. The normal shedding of blood and decidua appears reddish-brown for the first few days after delivery and is called **lochia rubra**. The vaginal discharge then becomes increasingly watery for the next two or three weeks (**lochia serosa**). Ultimately, the discharge turns yellowish-white (**lochia alba**). Microscopically, lochia consists of serous exudate, erythrocytes, leukocytes, decidua, epithelial cells, and bacteria.
- A foul-smelling lochia is a sign of infection. It may be accompanied by fever. The mother should be informed that she should seek medical help if this happens.

Voiding of urine and motion

- It is important to assess the bladder and make sure that the mother is voiding urine well. The first void should be within six hours of delivery. The bladder should be palpated to make sure that it is not overdistended. If the uterus is felt above the level of the umbilicus, it may be an indication of retention or partial voiding of urine.
- The mother will usually be concerned about the first motion after delivery. She may worry that defecation may be painful. Stool softeners or mild laxatives may be prescribed to avoid constipation.
- *Hemorrhoids* may become more prominent due to pushing during delivery. Painful hemorrhoids may be treated with a high-fibre diet, stool softeners and Sitz baths.

Pain management

Perineal pain

- Perineal pain can be managed with paracetamol (650–1000 mg 3–4 times a day) and/or ibuprofen (400 mg every 6–8 hours).

 Both paracetamol and ibuprofen are considered safe in breastfeeding women (Montgomery and Hale, 2012).

- Warm Sitz baths help relieve pain. Some women may prefer ice packs.
- Local anesthetic ointments may help relieve pain, particularly in the presence of an episiotomy.
- If the episiotomy is very painful and the mother finds it difficult to sit, she may be advised to use a ring cushion, which is normally used for hemorrhoids.

After pains

- Some women experience severe uterine contraction pains, especially during breastfeeding. These are called 'after pains' and usually last only for a week or two after delivery. Ibuprofen is usually effective for pain relief.
- After pains occur more often in multiparous women.

Lactation and breastfeeding

See **Chapter 29**, *Lactation and breastfeeding.*

Anti-D immunoglobulin

- Rh(D)-negative mothers of Rh(D)-positive infants should receive anti-D immune globulin as soon as possible after delivery and within 72 hours.
- If the facilities are available, Rh(D)-negative women should be tested for excessive fetomaternal bleeding at the time of delivery to ensure that they receive an adequate dose of anti-D immune globulin (see **Chapter 43**, *Management of Rh alloimmunisation in pregnancy* for further details).

Iron and vitamin supplements

- **Iron:** The WHO (2016) recommends oral iron supplementation, either alone or in combination with folic acid supplementation, to postpartum women for six to twelve weeks following delivery to reduce the risk of anemia. This is particularly important in India where anemia is a public health concern.
- **Calcium:** Lactating women require 1000 mg of calcium per day. Adolescent lactating girls require 1300 mg per day. Calcium supplementation is required if the mother's diet does not meet her daily calcium requirement, and should be continued for the duration of breastfeeding.

  See Chapter 23, *Cesarean section: procedure and technique* **for postpartum care specific to cesarean delivery.**

FIRST POSTPARTUM CHECK-UP

Following an uncomplicated birth, the first postpartum examination is usually offered at 4–6 weeks after the delivery.

Checklist for postpartum check-up

- The mother should be specifically asked about the following:
  - Abnormal vaginal bleeding/discharge
  - Difficulties in breastfeeding
- The physical examination should include the following:
  - Blood pressure recording to rule out persistent hypertension
  - Examination for signs of anemia
  - Breast examination to rule out
    - Cracked nipples
    - Mastitis/breast abscess
  - Abdominal examination to confirm uterine involution
  - Pelvic examination to confirm healing of episiotomy/lacerations
- The mother/couple should be advised on the following:
  - *Resumption of sexual activity:* Intercourse can be resumed when the mother is comfortable with it, usually at 4–6 weeks after birth.
  - *Contraception:* The couple should be advised on a contraceptive method ideal for them.

- *Postnatal exercises:* The importance of postnatal exercise must be stressed, and the mother should be advised to increase exercise gradually.
- *Weight reduction:* The initial weight loss after delivery should be recorded. The mother should be given dietary advice to reach her pre-pregnancy weight or her ideal weight.
- Women who were diabetic in pregnancy should undergo further testing after delivery (see **Chapter 40**, *Gestational and pre-gestational diabetes*).

References

1. Montgomery A, Hale TW. 2012. Academy Of Breastfeeding Medicine. ABM clinical protocol #15: Analgesia and anesthesia for the breastfeeding mother, revised 2012. *Breastfeed Med.* 7:547.
2. World Health Organization. 2014. WHO recommendations on postnatal care of the mother and newborn. WHO press, Geneva.
3. World Health Organization. 2016. World Health Organization Guideline: Iron supplementation in postpartum women. WHO, Geneva.

Chapter 28

Maternal Complications in the Puerperium

INTRODUCTION

The majority of women have an uneventful puerperium. However, some minor and major issues may arise. On rare occasions, potentially life-threatening complications may present themselves in the puerperium. The obstetrician should be aware of these and should be able to recognise and handle them. This chapter deals with some of the more common postpartum complications.

BREAKDOWN OR DISRUPTION OF THE EPISIOTOMY/ LACERATION FOLLOWING VAGINAL BIRTH

- An episiotomy or a second-degree laceration may break down occasionally. Though not common, it can be of great concern to the patient and her family. Repairs of third- and fourth-degree lacerations appear to be at increased risk of infection and breakdown as compared to repairs of first- and second-degree lacerations.
- Current clinical practice favours early re-repair (Dudley et al., 2013). This is usually done in the first two weeks postpartum. Early repair decreases perineal pain during healing and reduces dyspareunia.
- Delayed repair after 6–8 weeks does not seem to have any advantages and also causes the mother pain and discomfort for a longer period.

Antibiotics and pre-op preparation

- A single prophylactic dose of a second-generation cephalosporin (cefuroxime) is recommended at the beginning of the secondary repair of an episiotomy or second-degree laceration.
- For the repair of a third- or fourth-degree laceration breakdown, antibiotic prophylaxis with aerobic and anaerobic coverage, such as a second-generation cephalosporin plus metronidazole, is recommended.
- To reduce the risk of fecal contamination perioperatively, an enema administered the night before the surgery is considered good clinical practice.

HYPERTENSION AND/OR SEIZURES

- Hypertension and/or seizures related to preeclampsia/eclampsia may present for the first time in the postpartum period. Most of these cases present within 48 hours of the delivery.

- Acute severe hypertension (systolic blood pressure ≥160 mmHg and/or diastolic blood pressure ≥110 mmHg) should be treated immediately to reduce the risk of maternal stroke and other serious maternal complications.
- Magnesium sulphate is the medication recommended for the prevention of initial and recurrent eclamptic seizures (See **Chapter 39**, *Hypertensive disorders in pregnancy*).

INCOMPLETE VOIDING AND URINARY RETENTION

- Some women may be unable to void spontaneously within six hours of vaginal delivery or within six hours of the removal of the Foley catheter after a cesarean delivery. Voiding difficulty results from injury to the pudendal nerve during birth.
- Voiding difficulty or urinary retention should be suspected when the mother presents with the following:
  - No urge to void
  - Voiding small quantities of urine at a time
  - Urinary frequency or urgency
  - Bladder pain or discomfort
  - Urinary incontinence ('overflow incontinence')
- Clinically, bladder distension may be present, and may be recognised when either of these signs is present:
  - The uterus is difficult to palpate abdominally or
  - The uterus is felt above the umbilicus
- An incompletely emptying bladder can be confirmed by a post-void ultrasound.
- The risk factors associated with voiding difficulty are as follows (Mulder et al., 2014):
  - Primiparity
  - Instrument-assisted delivery
  - Episiotomy
  - Epidural analgesia

Treatment

- Intermittent catheterisation every 4–6 hours may help resolve the issue. The mother can be taught self-catheterisation. Catheterisation can be stopped when the residual urine is <150 mL.
- If the mother is reluctant to perform self-catheterisation, she can be sent home with a Foley catheter and a urine bag. She should be instructed to clamp the catheter for 2–4 hours at a time during the day. The clamp should be released and the bladder emptied every 2–4 hours. At night, the Foley should not be clamped and should be left attached to the urine bag. Usually, bladder function returns after 48–76 hours.

PROLAPSED OR THROMBOSED HEMORRHOIDS

- Symptomatic hemorrhoids are not uncommon after a delivery, especially if the mother already had hemorrhoids during pregnancy. Prolapsed hemorrhoids may result from pushing during a vaginal delivery.

- The mother usually presents with pain and discomfort. The pain may be acute with thrombosed hemorrhoids.

Treatment

- General treatment:
  - Sitz baths
  - High-fibre diet
  - Plenty of fluids
- Medications:
  - Stool softeners/bulk-forming laxatives
  - Topical corticosteroids
  - Local application of nitroglycerin ointment
- Thrombosed external hemorrhoids are best treated with hemorrhoid excision, rather than incision and simple evacuation of the clot. However, evacuation of the clot gives immediate relief.

PUBIC SYMPHYSIS DIASTASIS

- During pregnancy, the pubic symphysis relaxes by about 3–7 mm, starting in the first trimester of pregnancy. This is the result of both mechanical pressure and the influence of the hormones progesterone and relaxin.
- In some women, vaginal delivery results in the separation of the right and left pubic rami to a width of greater than 10 mm. This is known as diastasis, and its prevalence is reported to be 1 in 300 pregnancies to 1 in 30,000 pregnancies (Parker and Bhattacharjee, 2009).
- Diastasis results in severe pain in the midline, directly over the pubic symphysis. When severe, the woman may find it very painful to walk.
- Though the symptoms and signs are enough to make the diagnosis of diastasis, a plain X-ray can demonstrate the diastasis. An MRI is definitive but is an expensive test.

Treatment

- This condition is treated conservatively, using a brace or pelvic belt to stabilise the pelvis. Analgesics and anti-inflammatory medications are used to treat the pain as required.

FEVER AND INFECTIONS

- Fever (an oral temperature ≥38.0°C or ≥100.4°F) that occurs after the first 24 hours of delivery on any two of the first 10 days postpartum, is considered to be postpartum febrile morbidity.
- The common causes of postpartum fever are as follows:
  - Wound infection (episiotomy, laceration repair, or cesarean incision)
  - Endometritis
  - Urinary tract infection
  - Mastitis and breast abscess (see **Chapter 29**, *Lactation and breastfeeding*)

Wound infection

- Infection of the episiotomy is characterised by inflammation and edema around the area. There may or may not be purulent discharge and wound gaping.
- Infection of a cesarean incision is accompanied by fever, erythema, discharging sinuses, and possible wound dehiscence.
- Wound infection is treated with local care, debridement, opening of the wound, and culture-appropriate antibiotics. The wound is allowed to close by secondary intention. If required, reapproximation of the wound edges should only be carried out after the appearance of healthy granulation tissue.

Endometritis

- Postpartum fever associated with midline lower abdominal pain and uterine tenderness is indicative of endometritis.
- It may be associated with foul-smelling lochia.
- **Treatment:**
  - Treatment should include antibiotics to cover aerobic gram-positive, gram-negative, and anaerobic organisms.
  - Mild endometritis can be managed with **oral antibiotics**. In low-resource areas, the following regimens have been suggested (Meaney-Delman, 2015):
    - Amoxicillin-clavulanic acid 875 mg orally every 12 hours OR
    - Amoxicillin 500 mg plus metronidazole 500 mg orally every 8 hours OR
    - Clindamycin 600 mg orally every 6 hours plus gentamicin 5 mg/kg **intramuscularly** every 24 hours
  - Infection following cesarean sections, more severe infections with fever, chills, abdominal pain and purulent discharge should be treated with parenteral antibiotics. **A combination of clindamycin and gentamycin has a cure rate of 95 per cent and is the recommended first-line treatment** (Mackeen et al., 2015).

> Intravenous antibiotics for endometritis (with normal renal function):
> - Clindamycin 900 mg every 8 hours PLUS
> - Gentamicin 5 mg/kg every 24 hours (preferred) or 1.5 mg/kg every 8 hours

Urinary tract infection (UTI)

- The risk of UTI increases when the woman is catheterised during labour and delivery.
- The mother may present with symptoms of cystitis or an ascending UTI (pyelonephritis).
- Symptoms of cystitis include dysuria, frequency, urgency, suprapubic pain, and/or hematuria, usually without fever.
- Symptoms of pyelonephritis include all those associated with cystitis PLUS fever (>38°C), chills, flank pain, costovertebral angle tenderness, and nausea/vomiting.

Diagnosis

- UTI should be confirmed with a **urine culture**. $\geq 10^5$ (100,000) cfu/mL is considered significant and indicative of an infection. Some clinically symptomatic women with significant pyuria show a lower colony count on urine culture. In these women, $\geq 10^3$ cfu/mL may also be taken as indicative of significant infection.
- The determination of **antibiotic sensitivity** and resistance is very important. The final result of the test is the minimum inhibitory concentration (MIC) of commonly used antibiotics. This indicates which antibiotic may be used to treat the UTI successfully.

Treatment

- The treatment of UTI includes hydration with plenty of oral fluids.
- **Acute cystitis** is commonly treated with empiric antibiotic therapy, pending the report of the urine culture and sensitivity test.
- In low-resource settings, where facilities for culture are not available, the presence of more than two symptoms may be used as an indication for initiating therapy. In this situation, the UTI may also be confirmed by the dipstick test for nitrites.
  - The majority of infections are caused by *E. coli*. Hence empirical antibiotic therapy is started to treat this organism, since the culture results take 48 hours to be reported.
  - Oral antibiotics are the treatment of choice for acute cystitis. The commonly used antibiotics are nitrofurantoin, amoxicillin, amoxicillin-clavunate, cephalexin, cefuroxime, and fosfomycin.
  - The duration of treatment is 4–7 days; short-course treatments are associated with a higher rate of recurrence.
- **Acute pyelonephritis** requires hospitalisation and intravenous fluids.
  - Parenteral, broad-spectrum β-lactams are the preferred antibiotics for the initial empirical therapy of pyelonephritis. The commonly used antibiotics are third-generation cephalosporins such as cefepime or ceftriaxone, extended-spectrum penicillins, carbapenems, and aminoglycosides.

HEADACHE

Postpartum headache is of concern if accompanied by the following symptoms:
- Headache with altered mental status, seizures, papilledema, changes in vision, stiff neck, weakness, or focal neurological signs/symptoms
- Sudden onset of severe, unrelenting headache
- Change in headache characteristics (e.g., pain, pattern, severity) from usual headaches
- New-onset of migraine-type headache
- Headache that awakens the woman from sleep
- Headache unrelieved by pain medication

Postdural puncture headache

- Women who have received spinal or epidural anesthesia are at risk for developing a severe headache due to a dural puncture.

- The headache is characterised by postural increase in pain when the patient attempts to sit up.
- It is treated by asking the woman to lie flat, ensuring hydration with intravenous fluids and administering an autologous 'blood patch' (see **Chapter 17**, *Pain relief in labour*).

Cerebral venous sinus thrombosis

- Cerebral venous sinus thrombosis is a rare postpartum complication. In India, it has been reported to have an incidence of 450 per 100,000 deliveries (Srinivasan, 1983).
- The headache is intense and may be accompanied by vomiting. It is confirmed by imaging studies like MRI. The severity of symptoms correlates with the degree of thrombosis and the vessel involved.
- It is treated with anticoagulation.

POSTPARTUM MENTAL HEALTH ISSUES

- Postpartum mental health issues can be divided into three categories:
  - **Postpartum 'blues':** 300–750 per 1000 women experience postpartum 'blues' globally. It is characterised by mood swings, insomnia, anxiety, and crying spells that occur 2–3 days after delivery and peak by the 5th day. It usually resolves spontaneously in a few days or weeks with negligible negative sequelae. It only requires reassurance and support. If the postpartum 'blues' last for longer than two weeks, postpartum depression should be suspected.
  - **Postpartum depression:** Depressive episodes that first present in the first six weeks after birth are termed postpartum depression. Such a condition could also be a continuation of antenatal depression.
  - **Postpartum psychosis:** An uncommon disorder (0.89 to 2.6 per 1000 births), psychosis is a severe disorder that begins within four weeks postpartum and requires hospitalisation, antipsychotic therapy, and occasionally, electroconvulsive therapy (VanderKruik et al., 2017).

Postpartum depression

- **Incidence:** A systematic review and meta-analysis (Upadhyay et al., 2017) showed that the overall pooled estimate of the prevalence of postpartum depression in Indian mothers was 22 per cent, with the highest prevalence in the southern regions of the country.
- Postpartum depression may be precipitated by the following:
  - Genetic susceptibility
  - Hormonal changes
  - Stress and psychological pressures related to the early postnatal period
- **Signs and symptoms** of postpartum depression should not be ignored. They are similar to unipolar depression in adults.
  - Approximately 50 per cent of patients with postpartum depression may feel sad, cry for no reason, feel hopeless and discouraged, and may also exhibit intense irritability, anger, or hostility

- There may be sleep disturbances along with loss of appetite and intense fatigue
- Feelings of guilt may also be present, and this may be associated with suicidal ideation.
- **The consequences** of postpartum depression have adverse effects on both the mother and the infant, and include the following:
  - Poor nutrition and health in the offspring
  - Difficulties with breastfeeding
  - Interference with maternal–infant bonding
  - Poor care of the infant and other children
  - Breakdown in relationship with husband and other family members
- **Treatment** consists of psychotherapy and antidepressants. Selective serotonin re-uptake inhibitors are the drugs of choice. Exercise (e.g , walking for 30 minutes for three to five days per week) seems to improve the effects of the other two modalities (Daley et al., 2015).

References

1. Daley AJ, Blamey RV, Jolly K et al. 2015. A pragmatic randomized controlled trial to evaluate the effectiveness of a facilitated exercise intervention as a treatment for postnatal depression: The PAM-PeRS trial. *Psychol Med.* 45:2413.

2. Dudley LM, Kettle C, Ismail KM. 2013. Secondary suturing compared to non-suturing for broken down perineal wounds following childbirth. *Cochrane Database Syst Rev.* Issue 9. Art. no.: CD008977.

3. Mackeen AD, Packard RE, Ota E, Speer L. 2015. Antib otic regimens for postpartum endometritis. *Cochrane Database Syst Rev.* Issue 2. Art. no.: CD001067.

4. Meaney-Delman D, Bartlett LA, Gravett MG, Jamieson DJ. 2015. Oral and intramuscular treatment options for early postpartum endometritis in low-resource settings: A systematic review. *Obstet Gynecol.* 125:789.

5. Mulder FE, Hakvoort RA, Schoffelmeer MA et al. 2014. Postpartum urinary retention: A systematic review of adverse effects and management. *Int Urogynecol J.* 25:1605.

6. Parker JM, Bhattacharjee M. 2009. Images in clinical medicine. Peripartum diastasis of the symphysis pubis. *N Engl J Med.* 5;361(19).

7. Srinivasan K. 1983. Cerebral venous and arterial thrombosis in pregnancy and puerperium: A study of 135 patients. *Angiology.* 34:731–46.

8. Upadhyay RP, Chowdhury R, Salehi A et al. 2017. Postpartum depression in India: A systematic review and meta-analysis. Bulletin of the World Health Organization. 95:706-717C.

9. VanderKruik R, Barreix M, Chou D, Allen T, Say L, Cohen LS. 2017. Maternal Morbidity Working Group. The global prevalence of postpartum psychosis: A systematic review. *BMC Psychiatry.* 07 28;17(1):272.

Chapter 29

Lactation and Breastfeeding

INTRODUCTION

- Breastfeeding is beneficial for both the mother and her child.
- Breast milk is the best form of nutrition for neonates and infants because it has unique properties and is composed of a combination of nutrients essential to a child's health.

 In resource-poor countries like India, the overall morbidity and mortality is substantially lower in breastfed infants as compared to formula-fed infants (Sankar et al., 2015; Victora et al., 2016).

- While the infant's microbiome is largely determined by the mode of delivery, it is also influenced by the mother's milk. A mother's breast milk transmits elements of her own microbiome and immune response to the infant, and also provides specific prebiotics to support the growth of beneficial bacteria. A healthy microbiome influences both the immunity and cognitive function of the infant (Mayer et al., 2014). Therefore, breastfeeding sets the stage for protecting the infant against infectious and chronic diseases.
- Breastfeeding also provides short-term (during lactation) and long-term benefits to the mother.
- The World Health Organization and most professional bodies recommend that in the first six months, the baby should be nourished exclusively with breast milk. It is recommended that mothers breastfeed for at least the first year of their child's life.

BENEFITS OF BREASTFEEDING FOR THE INFANT

- Breast milk plays an important role in maintaining the infant's health and immunity.
- Breast milk improves gastrointestinal function.

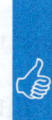 A meta-analysis by Victora et al. (2016) on breastfeeding in the 21st century demonstrated protection against childhood infections, increases in intelligence, and probable reductions in overweight and diabetes in the long-term.

- It also improves host defence by creating a favourable gut microbiome. Neonatal intestinal colonisation occurs with beneficial microbes of the *Bifidobacteria* and *Lactobacillus* species that prevent necrotising enterocolitis (Pannaraj et al., 2017).
- In both resource-rich and resource-poor nations, human milk, when compared with formula, has been found to decrease the risk of acute illnesses during the period in which the infant is fed. Bowatte et al. (2015) showed in a meta-analysis that breastfeeding protects against acute otitis media until two years of age, and the protection is greater with exclusive breastfeeding and breastfeeding of longer duration.

BENEFITS OF BREASTFEEDING FOR THE MOTHER

Breastfeeding has both short-term and long-term benefits for the mother.

Short-term benefits

- Uterine involution is promoted by the secretion of oxytocin during breastfeeding. This also decreases the risk of postpartum bleeding if breastfeeding is initiated soon after delivery.
- Lactational amenorrhea and anovulation have some advantages in providing a natural form of contraception. However, even among exclusively breastfeeding women, the return of ovulation varies and is not predictable. The couple should be advised regarding a more reliable form of contraception.

Long-term benefits

- Breastfeeding has been shown to reduce the risk of breast, ovarian, and endometrial cancers (Victora et al., 2016).
- Breastfeeding has been associated with cardiovascular health benefits (Nguyen et al., 2017).
- Lactation leads to improved glucose tolerance and insulin sensitivity. Breastfeeding significantly reduces the maternal risk of developing type 2 diabetes later in life (Martens et al., 2016).

COMPOSITION AND PROPERTIES OF HUMAN MILK

- Human milk is a unique, complex fluid with nutritional qualities, immunologic properties and growth-promoting characteristics essential for the healthy growth of the infant.
- Milk actually changes its composition to meet the changing needs of the baby during growth and maturation.
- Colostrum has lower concentrations of fat than mature milk but higher concentrations of protein and minerals. It also contains IgA, IgG, and IgM immunoglobulins. The IgA immunoglobulin represents over 90 per cent of milk antibodies. It protects the neonate against enteric infections. IgG antibodies from the mother provide passive immunisation to the infant in the first few months of life.

> **Passive immunity from mother to breastfed infant**
> - The mother's milk contains immunoglobulins which passively immunise the infant.
> - There is decreased risk of gastrointestinal infections by *E. coli* and rotavirus, dermatitis, allergies, and respiratory infections in breastfed infants, particularly during the first year of life.

- The composition of milk reverses as the infant matures. The quality of milk varies within a given breastfeeding session.
  - **Fore milk** is the milk first ingested by the infant and has a lower fat content than hind milk.
  - **Hind milk** is produced as the infant continues to breastfeed over the next several minutes. The fat content increases and facilitates satiety in the infant.

REGULATION OF MILK SYNTHESIS

- During pregnancy, changes occur in the breast (**mammogenesis**) which prepare it for the secretion of milk (**lactogenesis**) followed by the establishment and maintenance of milk secretion (**galactopoiesis** or **lactation**). The stage of galactopoiesis begins 4–6 days postpartum. Milk production continues at the established rate during this period until weaning is started. After breastfeeding has been stopped, involution occurs.
- The two hormones essential for the initiation and maintenance of lactation are **prolactin** and **oxytocin**. Prolactin and oxytocin act independently on different cellular receptors but their combined actions are critical for successful lactation.
- The regulation of milk synthesis is an efficient mechanism. The actual volume of milk secreted may be adjusted to the requirement of the infant by *feedback inhibitor of lactation*, a local factor secreted into the milk (Wilde et al., 1998). The rate of milk synthesis is related to the degree of breast emptiness or fullness.
- Increased suckling of the hungry infant, leading to increased emptying of the breast, is associated with an increased milk volume.
- If the breast remains full due to decreased inter-feeding intervals, breast milk production decreases.

> Milk production is affected by maternal stress and fatigue. Increased levels of dopamine, norepinephrine, or both, inhibit prolactin synthesis. The more anxious a mother is about her ability to feed the baby, the less milk she is able to produce. Relaxation and emotional support are essential for successful lactation.

INITIATING AND MAINTAINING BREASTFEEDING

Supporting the mother for successful breastfeeding

- Suckling and breastfeeding are areas that new mothers frequently struggle with. It is often taken for granted that the newborn infant will instinctively take to breastfeeding or that the mother will be able to successfully feed her baby right away.
- It is important to instruct all mothers on the proper techniques for breastfeeding to ensure a successful and uncomplicated breastfeeding experience.

> The baby should be given to the mother immediately after birth in the delivery room for the following reasons:
> - The infant is still alert soon after delivery.
> - Approximately 6–12 hours after birth, the baby enters a deep sleep period and will not be interested in feeding.
> - The mother's oxytocin levels are still high immediately postpartum, and this has been shown to help in:
>   – Milk letdown
>   – Bonding with the infant

- The World Health Organization (WHO, 2017) recommendations for promoting, protecting and supporting breastfeeding include the following:
  - **Early and uninterrupted skin-to-skin contact** between mothers and infants should be facilitated and encouraged as soon as possible after birth.

- Breastfeeding should be initiated as soon as possible after birth, **within the first hour** after delivery.
- Mothers should receive **practical support** to enable them to initiate and establish breastfeeding and manage common breastfeeding difficulties.
- In the event that the mother has to be separated temporarily from her infant, she should be taught how to **express breast milk** as a means of maintaining lactation. Breast pumps are the best option, but if not available, the mother should be coached on manual expression.

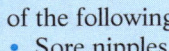

Unless a new mother receives support, she may stop breastfeeding within the first month because of the following:
- Sore nipples
- Perception of inadequate milk supply
- Concerns that the infant is not satisfied

- Mothers should be encouraged to stay with their infants and to practise rooming-in throughout the day and night. This does not apply in circumstances where infants need to be moved for specialised medical care.
- Mothers should be supported in practising responsive feeding (also called 'demand feeding') as part of nurturing care.
- If expressed breast milk or other feeds are medically indicated for term infants, feeding methods such as cups (traditional cups with spouts called *paladai*) and spoons may be used during their stay at the facility. Feeding bottles and teats are used only if absolutely essential.
- In preterm infants, if expressed breast milk or other feeds are medically indicated, feeding methods such as cups (*paladai*) or spoons are preferred over feeding bottles and teats.

MECHANICS OF BREASTFEEDING

Two factors that ensure successful breastfeeding are as follows:
- Positioning of the infant
- Latching-on

Positioning of the infant

- The mother must be in a comfortable position while breastfeeding her infant.
- The infant should be positioned to face the mother's body so that:
  - the infant's mouth is opposite the mother's nipple
  - the infant's neck is slightly extended
  - the infant's head, shoulders, and hips are in alignment

Latching-on

- Latching-on refers to the infant's lips forming a tight seal around the nipple and a sufficient portion of the surrounding areola. This facilitates efficient extraction of milk during suckling.

- It is a natural instinct for the baby to open its mouth wide when the nipple touches its upper or lower lip. The tongue extends under the nipple, and the nipple is drawn into the mouth, initiating the suckling reflex. While attempting to get the infant to latch on, the mother's nipple and areola should be manoeuvred into the infant's open mouth instead of pushing the infant's head toward the breast. This simple manoeuvre may seem difficult to an anxious first-time mother.
- When the latching-on is correct, the nipple and areola extend as far as the junction between the baby's hard and soft palates. The baby's jaw then moves the tongue toward the areola, compressing it. This process causes the milk to travel from the lactiferous sinuses into the infant's mouth.

ASSESSING ADEQUACY OF INFANT INTAKE

Adequacy of intake is assessed based on the following indicators:
- Frequency and duration of feeding
  - Average of 8–12 feeds in 24 hours for at least 10–15 minutes per feed
- Urine and stool output
  - Voiding of urine occurs 4–6 times during the third and fourth day, and 6–8 times on day five and after with adequate feeds
  - Meconium changes to transitional stools within approximately three days of birth; 3–4 stools per day after day four
- Weight of the infant
  - Weight loss is normal after delivery, and infants lose 5–7 per cent of birth weight in the first five days of life
  - Usually, infants stop losing weight by five days after birth and regain their birth weight by 1–2 weeks of age
  - If the breastfeeding is adequate, infants gain 15–40 g per day

Maternal nutrition during breastfeeding
The mother needs an additional 500–700 kCal/day during breastfeeding. Protein intake should be 25 g/day. Iron and calcium supplementation must be continued throughout the duration of breastfeeding. Vitamins and minerals should also be supplemented.

COMMON PROBLEMS DURING BREASTFEEDING

Retracted nipple

- This should be identified during antenatal checkups closer to term.
- The mother should be encouraged to draw out the nipple daily during her bath, with lubricant applied to her fingers.
- If the retracted nipple persists, the nipple should be pulled out by the *inverted syringe technique*. The nozzle of a 10 mL syringe is cut off and the piston introduced through the cut end. The smooth end is placed on the breast, around the nipple, and the piston withdrawn slowly. This procedure should be performed daily before each feed for a few days.

Engorgement

- Engorgement presents as swollen and painful breasts and can occur due to the following:
  - Interstitial edema and/or
  - Excessive milk
- Treatment focuses on frequent breastfeeding to ensure the adequate removal of the milk.
  - Positioning of the infant and proper latching-on will help
  - Initial pumping of milk may be required to soften the areola and allow better latching-on
  - Analgesics and firm support with well-fitting undergarments are recommended

Sore and cracked nipples

- This problem is commonly associated with improper latching-on. Hence it is crucial that the proper technique of getting the infant to latch on is taught.
- Placing a drop of milk on each nipple and allowing this to air dry after breastfeeding may help.

Mastitis

- Mastitis is a localised inflammation of the breast that is associated with fever, myalgia, breast pain, and redness. It is most common during the first six weeks postpartum and may follow a cracked or sore nipple.
- It is usually caused by *Staphylococcus aureus* transmitted to the breast from the infant's mouth.
- It is important to perform an ultrasound examination to differentiate mastitis from a breast abscess.

 Both community and hospital-acquired methicillin-resistant *S. aureus* (MRSA) are now being commonly implicated in lactational mastitis.

- **Treatment:**
  - NSAIDs, continued breastfeeding, and supportive undergarments help alleviate the pain.
  - Breastfeeding should be continued on the opposite breast. The mother should be encouraged to continue feeding from the affected breast.
  - Antibiotics are started after milk from the affected breast is sent for culture and sensitivity.
  - *S. aureus* can be treated with cephalexin (500 mg 4 times daily).
  - Methicillin-resistant *S. aureus* (MRSA) can be treated with trimethoprim-sulfamethoxazole (TMP-SMX; 1 double-strength tablet orally twice daily) or clindamycin (300 mg orally 3 times daily).

Breast abscess

- When mastitis does not respond to antibiotic treatment, it may progress to a breast abscess, which is a localised collection of pus in the breast tissue.
- Clinically, there is a fluctuant, tender, palpable mass. High, spiking fever is characteristic.

- Ultrasound features that help in confirming the diagnosis include a hypoechoic collection, mostly multiloculated, with no vascularity within the collection.
- **Treatment:**
  - Antibiotics are initiated after choosing one that will be effective against *S. aureus* or methicillin-resistant *S. aureus* based on culture and sensitivity (see management of mastitis above).
  - Ultrasound-guided aspiration of the pus is the current approach to the drainage of the abscess and ensure the complete removal of pus.
  - Surgical incision and drainage is indicated for a very large abscess or one that has not responded to needle aspiration.
- The mother should continue to breastfeed from the unaffected side and pump the affected side to relieve pressure and facilitate recovery.

INCREASING MILK PRODUCTION

Galactogogues

- Some women have a problem with the establishment of adequate lactation. If there is no improvement with proper techniques of breastfeeding, galactogogues may be considered.
- Galactagogues are drugs that facilitate milk production. The agents most commonly used are dopamine receptor antagonists–**metoclopramide** and **domperidone**. These are particularly useful for mothers of preterm infants.
- Either metoclopramide or domperidone is given in a dose of 10 mg three times a day for 10 days. Both drugs seem equally effective (Ingram et al., 2012).

SUPPRESSION OF LACTATION

- Suppression of lactation may be required in the following situations:
  - Stillbirth or perinatal death
  - The mother wishes to stop breastfeeding
  - There are contraindications to breastfeeding
    - HIV-positive mother
    - Active pulmonary tuberculosis
    - Maternal treatment with drugs that would be secreted in breast milk
    - Puerperal psychosis
- **Cabergoline** is the drug of choice for the suppression of lactation as it is well-tolerated. The dose is either one of the following:
  - 1 mg as a single dose OR
  - 2 doses of 0.5 mg given 12 hours apart.
- Bromocriptine is no longer recommended due to the high risk of vomiting, seizures, hypertension, and thromboembolism.
- There is currently no evidence that non-pharmacologic methods (for example, jasmine flowers or cabbage leaves tied to the breasts) are any better than placebo in lactation suppression.

References

1. Bowatte G, Tham R, Allen KJ et al. 2015. Breastfeeding and childhood acute otitis media: A systematic review and meta-analysis. *Acta Paediatr.* 104:85.

2. Ingram J, Taylor H, Churchill C et al. 2012. Metoclopramide or domperidone for increasing maternal breast milk output: A randomised controlled trial. *Arch Dis Child Fetal Neonatal Ed.* 97:F241.

3. Mayer EA, Knight R, Mazmanian SK et al. 2014. Gut microbes and the brain: Paradigm shift in neuroscience. *J Neurosci.* 34: 15490-15496.

4. Martens PJ, Shafer LA, Dean HJ et al. 2016. Breastfeeding Initiation Associated With Reduced Incidence of diabetes in mothers and offspring. *Obstet Gynecol.* 128:1095.

5. Nguyen B, Jin K, Ding D. 2017. Breastfeeding and maternal cardiovascular risk factors and outcomes: A systematic review. *PLoS One.* 12:e0187923.

6. Pannaraj PS, Li F, Cerini C et al. 2017. Association between breast milk bacterial communities and establishment and development of the infant gut microbiome. *JAMA Pediatr.* 171:647.

7. World Health Organization. 2017. Protecting, promoting and supporting breastfeeding in facilities providing maternity and newborn services. WHO, Geneva.

8. Sankar MJ, Sinha B, Chowdhury R et al. 2015. Optimal breastfeeding practices and infant and child mortality: A systematic review and meta-analysis. *Acta Paediatr.* 104:3.

9. Victora CG, Bahl R, Barros AJ et al. 2016. Breastfeeding in the 21st century: Epidemiology, mechanisms, and lifelong effect. *Lancet.* 387:475.

10. Wilde CJ, Addey CV, Bryson JM et al. 1998. Autocrine regulation of milk secretion. *Biochem Soc Symp.* 63:81.

Chapter 30

Obstetric Emergencies

This chapter will deal with the following obstetric emergencies:
- Shoulder dystocia
- Umbilical cord prolapse
- Uterine inversion
- Uterine rupture
- Amniotic fluid embolism

Postpartum hemorrhage (PPH) is discussed in **Chapter 32**, *Postpartum hemorrhage.* Eclampsia is discussed in **Chapter 39**, *Hypertensive disorders in pregnancy.*

SHOULDER DYSTOCIA

Introduction

- Shoulder dystocia is defined as a failure of the shoulders to deliver after the head has been delivered. A disproportion in size between the shoulders and the maternal pelvic dimensions results in obstruction occurring at the pelvic inlet.
- Gherman et al. (2006) characterised shoulder dystocia as 'the unpreventable obstetric emergency with empiric management guidelines'.
- Though shoulder dystocia occurs only in 0.2 to 3 per cent of all deliveries (Hoffman et al., 2011), it represents a major obstetric emergency.
- The incidence of shoulder dystocia is rising due to the increase in maternal obesity and diabetes. However, the majority of cases of shoulder dystocia occur in non-diabetic women with babies that are not macrosomic.
- Most shoulder dystocias cannot be predicted or prevented (ACOG, 2017).
- The aim of successful management of shoulder dystocia is to avoid neonatal complications like brachial plexus injury, fractures and asphyxia, while at the same time, minimising maternal morbidity.

 Though maternal diabetes and fetal macrosomia are associated with shoulder dystocia, the majority of cases occur in non-diabetic women with babies that are not macrosomic.

Why does shoulder dystocia occur?

- Shoulder dystocia is caused by a persistent anterior–posterior location of the fetal shoulders at the pelvic brim due to:
  - Obstruction of the descent of the anterior shoulder by the symphysis pubis or
  - Impaction of the posterior shoulder on the maternal sacral promontory.

 Obstruction of the anterior shoulder is more common than posterior shoulder obstruction.

- The factors that may lead to a persistent anterior–posterior location of the fetal shoulders at the pelvic brim are as follows:
  - Fetal macrosomia, which causes increased resistance between the fetus and the pelvic walls
  - Disproportion between the large fetal chest and the biparietal diameter with significantly large shoulders, as seen in fetuses of diabetic women
  - Precipitous labour when truncal rotation does not have time to occur

Can shoulder dystocia be predicted?

- Though antenatal risk factors or labour abnormalities may raise suspicion of shoulder dystocia, the occurrence of shoulder dystocia cannot be accurately predicted.
- Moreover, shoulder dystocia can occur without any of the classical risk factors. Therefore, obstetricians should be prepared to face this complication during any vaginal delivery.

Risk factors

While a number of factors are associated with an increased risk of shoulder dystocia (see box below), none have sufficient sensitivity or positive predictive value to allow their use clinically to reliably and accurately identify the occurrence of shoulder dystocia (ACOG, 2017).

> **Risk factors for shoulder dystocia (ACOG, 2017)**
> - Macrosomia
> - Maternal diabetes
> - Maternal obesity
> - Multiparity
> - Previous history of macrosomia
> - Previous history of shoulder dystocia
> - Instrumental delivery
> - Prolonged second stage of labour
> - Others
>   - Prolonged pregnancy
>   - Advanced maternal age

Can shoulder dystocia be prevented?

No preventive measures have proved to be effective for shoulder dystocia, though the following risk factors should alert the clinician to the possibility of this complication.

- **Macrosomia:**
  - *Induction of labour* at ≥38 weeks for suspected fetal macrosomia has been suggested as an intervention to reduce the risk of shoulder dystocia.
    - The available data is confusing. Though a meta-analysis by Magro-Malosso et al. (2017) suggested that the induction of labour at term was associated with a significant decrease in fetal fractures due to shoulder dystocia, a systematic review of the Cochrane Database (Boulvain et al., 2016) found that to prevent one fracture, it would be necessary to induce labour in 60 women.

❖ Currently, routine induction at <38 weeks is not recommended for macrosomia in non-diabetic women since there is insufficient evidence that the benefits of reducing shoulder dystocia risk would outweigh the harms of early delivery (ACOG, 2020).

❖ In diabetic mothers, a systematic review suggested a potential reduction in macrosomia and shoulder dystocia with labour induction at term (Witkop et al., 2009).

– Elective cesarean section:

✦ *In a non-diabetic mother:* Elective cesarean delivery for macrosomia diagnosed by ultrasonography is not routinely recommended for the sole purpose of avoiding shoulder dystocia (ACOG, 2020). Rouse et al. (1999) calculated that more than 1000 cesarean deliveries would be required to prevent one permanent injury in the presence of macrosomia of 4000–4500 g. In Indian mothers, a fetus weighing 3500 g or more may be considered an indication for a cesarean instead of opting for a difficult instrumental delivery in the presence of protracted active phase or prolonged second stage (see below in section on *Prolonged second stage*). In Indian women with a fetus suspected to weigh 3800–4000 g, serious consideration should be given to an elective cesarean section.

✦ *In a diabetic mother:* It has been estimated that 443 elective cesarean deliveries for a macrosomic fetus diagnosed by ultrasonography are required to prevent one permanent injury (Rouse et al., 1996). In Indian mothers with diabetes, a fetus weighing 3500 g or more may be considered an indication for an elective cesarean.

- **Previous shoulder dystocia:** If a woman has had a previous shoulder dystocia, the chance of recurrence in the next pregnancy is 10 per cent (Bingham et al., 2010). In such a case, the estimated fetal weight, gestational age, maternal diabetes status, and the severity of the prior neonatal injury should be taken into consideration. Though most women will not have a recurrent shoulder dystocia, counselling and informed consent are required for an attempt of vaginal delivery.

- **Prolonged second stage:** A large study involving 100,000 women (Laughon et al., 2014) found no correlation between a prolonged second stage and shoulder dystocia in nulliparous and multiparous women.

However, **in the presence of macrosomia**, a prolonged second stage may be a warning for the occurrence of shoulder dystocia. In this situation, if an operative delivery (forceps or vacuum) becomes necessary, the risk of shoulder dystocia increases. A cesarean may be a prudent decision in this clinical scenario.

 In the presence of macrosomia, a prolonged second stage may be a warning sign. If an operative delivery is required after a prolonged second stage, the risk of shoulder dystocia increases.

Recognition of shoulder dystocia

- A diagnosis of shoulder dystocia is usually made when there is failure of delivery of the fetal shoulder after the head has delivered, despite gentle traction being applied in conjunction with maternal pushing.

- **The 'turtle sign'**—this occurs when the fetal head retracts back against the mother's perineum after it emerges from the vagina. The baby's cheeks bulge out, resembling a turtle pulling its head back into its shell. This retraction of the fetal head is caused by the baby's anterior shoulder becoming impacted behind the pubic symphysis, preventing delivery of the rest of the baby.

Complications of shoulder dystocia

- The complications of shoulder dystocia are listed in Table 30.1.
- Though brachial plexus injury is the commonest neonatal complication of shoulder dystocia, its mere presence is not evidence that shoulder dystocia has occurred (ACOG, 2017).
- Cases of severe brachial plexus palsy have been documented in the absence of shoulder dystocia and without identifiable risk factors (Torki et al., 2012).

Table 30.1   Maternal and fetal complications of shoulder dystocia

Maternal	Fetal
Postpartum hemorrhage	Brachial plexus palsy
Third- or fourth-degree episiotomy or tear	Fracture of the humerus
Rectovaginal fistula	Clavicle fracture
Symphyseal separation or diathesis with or without transient femoral neuropathy	Fetal hypoxia with or without permanent neurologic damage
Uterine rupture	Fetal death

Brachial plexus injury
- Unilateral brachial plexus injury is one of the most common fetal complications of shoulder dystocia. The C5–C6 nerve roots are affected in 80 per cent of cases (**Erb-Duchenne palsy**).
- The right arm is usually affected (64.6 per cent) because of the fact that the left occiput anterior presentation leaves the right shoulder impacted against the symphysis pubis (Gherman et al., 1998).
- 88 per cent of brachial plexus injuries resolve within a year (Chauhan et al., 2005).
- The incidence of brachial plexus palsy also depends on the number of manoeuvres required to deliver the shoulders:
  - 7.7 per cent with 1–2 manoeuvres
  - 25 per cent with 3 or more manoeuvres
- Nocon et al. (1993) found that the number of injuries was the highest (37.9 per cent) with the delivery of the posterior arm.

Management of shoulder dystocia

- Regardless of the manoeuvres and management strategies employed, maternal and infant complications are unpredictable and may not always be avoidable.
- It is important to note the time at which the shoulder dystocia was diagnosed as well as the time at which complete delivery is achieved.

Time available to resolve shoulder dystocia

- Hypoxia due to shoulder dystocia results from the following:
  - Compression of the neck, leading to central venous congestion
  - Compression of the umbilical cord

– Reduced placental intervillous flow from prolonged increased intrauterine pressure and secondary fetal bradycardia
- Prolonged head-to-delivery intervals are associated with increasing hypoxia although the time required to resolve the shoulder dystocia without causing hypoxic injury is not yet clear.
- Stallings et al. (2001) concluded that a threshold interval of 7 or more minutes had 67 per cent sensitivity and 74 per cent specificity for predicting brain injury.

 A previously well-oxygenated term fetus will tolerate up to five minutes of head-to-body delivery interval before the risk of asphyxial injury increases (Leung et al., 2011).

The HELPERR mnemonic

The HELPERR mnemonic (Baxley and Gobbo, 2004) is a clinical tool that offers a structured process that deals with shoulder dystocia in a step-wise fashion (Table 30.2).

Table 30.2   The HELPERR mnemonic for the management of shoulder dystocia (adapted from Baxley and Gobbo, 2004)

H	Call for help	Activate the pre-arranged protocol and get more senior/trained staff into the labour room.
E	Evaluate for episiotomy	Episiotomy is necessary only to make more room if rotation manoeuvres are required. Since shoulder dystocia is a bony impaction, episiotomy alone will not release the shoulder.
L	Legs (the McRoberts' manoeuvre)	Flexion and abduction of the maternal hips and positioning the maternal thighs up onto the maternal abdomen straightens the sacrum, rotates the pubic symphysis anteriorly, and reduces the angle of inclination. The mother herself can be instructed to pull her legs upwards. Anyone in the labour room, including a family member, can provide assistance for this manoeuvre.
P	Suprapubic pressure	In combination with the McRoberts' manoeuvre, pressure is applied suprapubically by an assistant. The fetal anterior shoulder is dislodged from behind the symphysis pubis with a downward and lateral motion. This manoeuvre should be attempted while continuing downward traction.
E	Enter manoeuvres (internal rotation)	These manoeuvres attempt to manipulate the fetus to rotate the anterior shoulder into an oblique plane and under the maternal symphysis.
R	Remove the posterior arm	Removing the posterior arm from the birth canal helps free the impaction by shortening the bisacromial diameter. Grasping and pulling directly on the fetal arm may fracture the humerus.
R	Roll the patient	Rolling the mother to the all-fours position often results in the dislodging of the shoulder during the act of turning. Gravity may also aid in the disimpaction of the fetal shoulders.

Manoeuvres to resolve shoulder dystocia

 The patient should be positioned with her buttocks flush with the edge of the bed to provide optimal access for executing manoeuvres that will bring about the delivery of the fetus.

The McRoberts' manoeuvre

- The McRoberts' manoeuvre is the initial step that most obstetricians utilise for the disimpaction of the shoulder.

- This is performed by sharply flexing the maternal thighs onto the abdomen with the help of an assistant or is done by the mother herself. This action straightens the sacrum, rotates the pubic symphysis anteriorly, and reduces the angle of inclination.
- About 40 per cent of cases of shoulder dystocia are resolved by the McRoberts' manoeuvre alone (Figure 30.1).

 Fundal pressure can further aggravate the impaction of the shoulder at the symphysis pubis and **should be avoided.**

The minimum necessary traction should be used to deliver the stuck shoulder. Excessive traction may lead to brachial plexus injury.

Suprapubic pressure

This is usually carried out along with the McRoberts' manoeuvre. Standing on one side of the mother, the assistant applies pressure with the heel of the hand or the fist moving in a downward and lateral motion on the posterior aspect of the anterior impacted shoulder (Figure 30.1). This helps adduct the shoulders, reduce the bisacromial diameter, and bring the shoulders to the oblique diameter of the pelvis.

Initially, the pressure can be continuous, but if delivery is not accomplished, a rocking motion is recommended to dislodge the shoulder from behind the pubic symphysis.

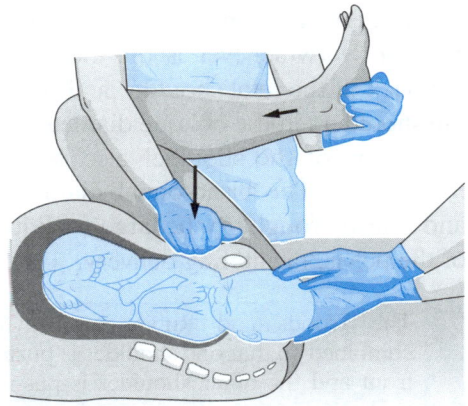

Figure 30.1 McRoberts' manoeuvre with suprapubic pressure.

Modified Woods screw method

- In the Woods screw manoeuvre, the fetus is rotated by exerting pressure on the anterior, clavicular surface of the posterior shoulder to turn the fetus until the anterior shoulder emerges from behind the maternal symphysis (Figure 30.2).
- In the modified Woods screw method, the same principle of rotating of the fetus is applied but the grasp is different.
  - The obstetrician grasps the fetal neck in a pincer-like hold between the index and middle fingers of each hand.
  - With gentle downward traction, the head, neck and the anterior shoulder are turned as a single unit towards the side of the fetal face. This rotational movement resembles the unscrewing of a bottle cap, with a diagonal torque being applied towards the floor.

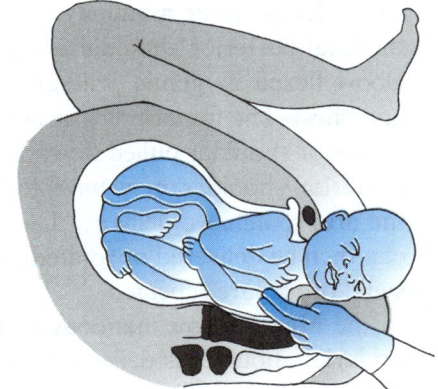

Figure 30.2 Woods corkscrew manoeuvre.

- The diagonal torque (or twist), combined with gentle downward traction, almost always disimpacts the anterior shoulder from behind the symphysis pubis.
- The head, neck, and shoulders may need to be rotated through 180° if necessary, until the posterior shoulder is under the symphysis and slips out.
- If the fetus is facing the mother's right thigh, the obstetrician's right hand is positioned on top, allowing the twist to be towards the right. If the fetus is facing the left, the grasp is reversed, with the left hand on top.

Rubin manoeuvre

The fingers of one hand are inserted anteriorly or posteriorly (whichever is the most accessible) to the back of the fetal shoulder and rotated to bring the shoulders in the oblique diameter of the pelvis. Adduction of the shoulder also occurs with this manoeuvre. The bisacromial diameter decreases and is also brought to the large (oblique) diameter of the pelvis, facilitating delivery.

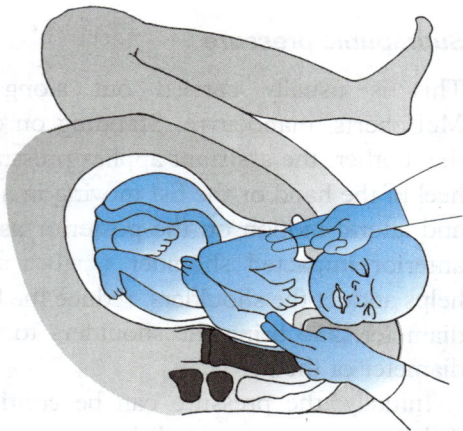

> The Woods and Rubin manoeuvres can be combined so that one shoulder is pushed from the front and the other shoulder is pushed from the back (Rubin manoeuvre) in the same clockwise or counterclockwise direction (Figure 30.3). This increases the rotational force on the shoulders.

Figure 30.3 Combined Rubin and Woods manoeuvre.

Delivery of the posterior arm

- Delivery of the posterior arm almost always relieves impaction of the anterior shoulder and resolves the dystocia. **However, this is technically more difficult and associated with greater neonatal morbidity**.
- In the **Jacquemier manoeuvre**, the operator's hand is passed into the sacral hollow and the fetal posterior shoulder is identified, the fingers moved along the humerus and the elbow flexed by gentle pressure on the cubital fossa. The arm slips over the fetal face and chest. The forearm is grasped and the arm and posterior shoulder pulled down into the pelvis. The posterior shoulder may have to be rotated using the arm to achieve delivery. The anterior shoulder can then be delivered or rotated posteriorly and the same procedure repeated.
- In the **Menticoglou manoeuvre** (Figure 30.4), the posterior shoulder is delivered before delivering the arm, especially if it is not possible to reach the elbow or forearm. An assistant gently flexes the fetal head toward the anterior shoulder, and the obstetrician

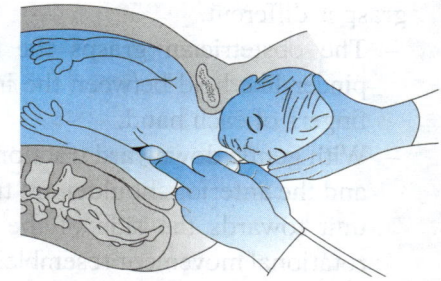

Figure 30.4 The Menticoglou manoeuvre.

uses the middle fingers of both hands to hook the fetus's posterior axilla. The two middle fingers in the axilla are then used to pull the posterior shoulder downwards, along the curve of the sacrum. Once the shoulder has been brought down sufficiently, the posterior arm can be grasped and delivered.

- A soft rubber catheter or tube may also be used as an alternative to hook the axilla and apply traction. This has the advantage of a better hold, and availability of more space since the hands are not inside the vagina/pelvis.

Gaskin all-fours manoeuvre

- Rolling the patient onto her hands and knees, known as the Gaskin all-fours manoeuvre, is a safe, rapid, and effective technique for the reduction of shoulder dystocia (Bruner et al., 1998).

- Once the patient is repositioned, the physician provides gentle downward traction to deliver the posterior shoulder with the aid of gravity (Figure 30.5).

- The all-fours position is compatible with all intravaginal manipulations for shoulder dystocia, which can then be reattempted in this new position.

The Zavanelli manoeuvre

This procedure involves the replacement of the fetal head in the pelvis followed by cesarean delivery. It is extremely difficult to carry out and is associated with both maternal and neonatal morbidity.

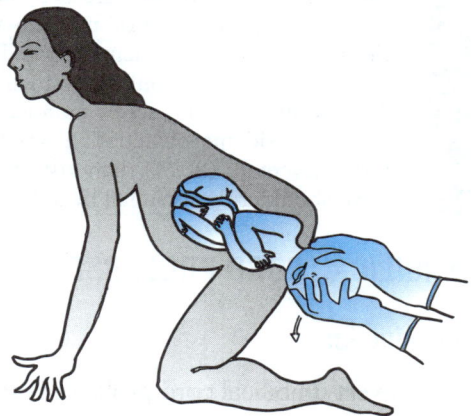

Figure 30.5   Gaskin all-fours manoeuvre.

The role of episiotomy in managing shoulder dystocia
- The primary problem in shoulder dystocia is bony impaction; an episiotomy by itself will not release the impaction.
- Episiotomy does provide additional room for the physician's hand when internal rotation manoeuvres are required.

Documentation of shoulder dystocia

- In the immediate postpartum period, it is important to record complete and accurate information regarding the difficulty in delivery, the manoeuvres used, and the condition of the neonate and the mother.
- Brachial plexus injury due to shoulder dystocia is one of the commonest causes of litigation. Proper documentation plays a major role in defending a legal case (Acker, 1991).
- The following facts need to be documented (Gherman et al., 2006):
  - Time of delivery of the head
  - Time of noticing shoulder dystocia
  - Who was called for help

- Which shoulder was anterior
- Manoeuvres performed and the order in which they were performed
- Time of delivery of the baby
- Condition of the baby
- Condition of the mother
- Communication about the difficult delivery to the parents

 Complete and accurate information regarding the difficulty in delivery, the manoeuvres used, and the condition of the neonate and the mother at the end of the delivery should be documented.

> **Shoulder dystocia drill**
> - All obstetric units should diligently practice a shoulder dystocia 'drill'.
> - The specific protocols for the management of shoulder dystocia should be written down and emphasised. The proper protocol should follow this order: McRoberts' position, suprapubic pressure, internal rotation manoeuvres, delivery of the posterior arm.
> - Several studies have demonstrated that simulated drills improve both management and documentation of shoulder dystocia (Deering et al., 2004; Goffman et al., 2008).
> - The modified Woods screw manoeuvre should be practised even during a normal delivery so that the residents/obstetricians are familiar with the manoeuvre.
> - Grobman et al. (2011) demonstrated that the frequency of brachial plexus injury associated with shoulder dystocia fell by at least two-thirds after training.

UMBILICAL CORD PROLAPSE

Introduction

- An **overt** umbilical cord prolapse is said to have occurred when the cord slips ahead of the presenting part of the fetus and protrudes into, or beyond, the cervical canal or vagina.
- An **occult** umbilical cord prolapse refers to a cord that is lying alongside the presenting part.
- It is an uncommon obstetric emergency, but can result in significant neonatal morbidity and mortality.

Risk factors

The risk factors that lead to cord prolapse are usually associated with the following conditions:
- The presenting part not filling the pelvis completely either due to maternal or fetal factors (see box below) leading to the cord slipping past it.

> **Fetal and maternal factors associated with umbilical cord prolapse**
> - Malpresentation (breech, transverse, oblique, or unstable lie)
> - Polyhydramnios
> - Low birth weight
> - Multiparity
> - Long umbilical cord
> - Prematurity
> - Second twin
> - Unengaged presenting part

- Obstetric interventions (see box below) that dislodge the presenting part may lead to cord prolapse. One study (Usta et al., 1999) found that obstetric interventions led to 50 per cent of the cases of cord prolapse.

> **Obstetric interventions that may lead to iatrogenic umbilical cord prolapse**
> - Artificial rupture of membranes in the presence of an unengaged presenting part
> - Artificial rupture of membranes in the presence of polyhydramnios
> - Cervical ripening with a balloon catheter
> - Upward displacement of the fetal head during manual rotation
> - Amnioinfusion
> - Internal podalic version
> - Application of forceps or vacuum

Prevention of umbilical cord prolapse

- A systematic review of the Cochrane Database that looked at amniotomy for shortening spontaneous labour (Smyth et al., 2013) found that routine amniotomy for labour augmentation in the general population is not associated with an increased risk of cord prolapse.
- In women in labour, a vaginal examination is recommended after spontaneous rupture of membranes to rule out cord prolapse. This is particularly important in women with the risk factors listed above.
- Amniotomy should be preferably performed only when the presenting part is well-applied to the cervix.
- An amniotomy should be done with great care in the presence of the following:
  - An unengaged fetal part
  - Polyhydramnios
  - Non-cephalic presentation
- In these situations, if an amniotomy is required, the following precautions should be taken:
  - A 'controlled' amniotomy may be done with a 22-gauge spinal needle to prevent a gush of fluid.
  - Care should be taken to leave the examining fingers in close contact with the break in the membranes. This will control the fluid and allow it to trickle instead of gushing out uncontrollably.

Diagnosis of umbilical cord prolapse

- The clinician may palpate the cord as it slips down past the cervical os immediately after an amniotomy.
- More commonly, the abrupt onset of severe, prolonged fetal bradycardia or moderate to severe variable decelerations in a patient with a previously normal tracing, alerts the clinician to a cord prolapse.

Consequences of cord prolapse

- Cord compression can lead to either profound acute asphyxia or subacute hypoxia with differing neonatal outcomes.
- However, short- and long-term neurological impairment are rare. Perinatal survival is currently 94 per cent due to the use of cesarean section as the recommended method of delivery (Gibbons et al., 2014).

Management of umbilical cord prolapse

- **Call for help:** The initial step would be to inform the concerned staff.
  - The nursing staff, anesthetist, and operating room should be alerted immediately for an emergency delivery.
  - Extra labour room staff are required for help with intrauterine resuscitation measures (see below).
- **Monitor fetal heart rate:** This is essential to direct further interventions.
- **Institute intrauterine resuscitative measures:**
  - Elevation of the presenting part manually is the first and most important intervention (Murphy and MacKenzie, 1995). An assistant or a nurse places gloved fingers in the vagina and gently elevates the fetal head until it is not compressing the cord. This is continued until the baby is delivered.
  - Manual replacement of the cord above the vertex may be attempted while elevating the presenting part. This should be followed with close monitoring of the fetal heart rate.
  - The patient is placed either in a steep Trendelenburg or the knee–chest position. This may assist in shifting the presenting part away from the cord and thereby, in relieving the compression.
  - Distending the bladder rapidly with 500 mL of saline using a Foley catheter may elevate the presenting part away from the cord (Lin, 2006).
- **Deliver by emergency cesarean:**
  - Unless vaginal delivery is imminent, the safest route of delivery in the presence of a cord prolapse would be a cesarean section.
  - If the mother already has an epidural catheter in place, it can be continued for the cesarean. In the absence of an epidural catheter, general anesthesia is speedier than regional anesthesia.

UTERINE RUPTURE

Introduction

- Uterine rupture is a rare but potentially life-threatening complication that can occur in labour or before the onset of labour. It is a major contributor to maternal morbidity and neonatal mortality, especially in a developing country like India.
- It is important to differentiate between rupture that occurs in a scarred uterus and that which occurs in an unscarred uterus.
- The four risk factors that contribute to 90 per cent of cases of uterine rupture in developing countries are as follows (Batra et al., 2016):
  - History of prior cesarean section
  - Obstructed labour
  - Fetal malpresentations
  - Higher parity

Incidence

- **Unscarred uterus**
  - In India, the incidence of uterine rupture in an unscarred uterus has been reported as ranging from 0.57 per 1000 births (Vernekar and Rajib, 2016) to 0.62 per 1000 births (Chhabra et al., 2002). These numbers are derived from small case studies and may vary depending on whether the woman delivers in a facility and whether the facility is well-equipped and staffed.
  - Higher parity, longer labours, a higher frequency of contracted pelvises and prolonged neglected obstructed labour in developing countries, along with the lack of access to emergency obstetrical services, contribute to the higher rate of uterine rupture in the unscarred uterus.

 Though uterine rupture is extremely rare in the primigravida, the increasing use of misoprostol has led to a rise in these cases. Since the symptoms and signs are very atypical and variable, it is important to have a high index of clinical suspicion (Walsh and Baxi, 2007).

- **Scarred uterus (prior cesarean section):**
  - Most studies describing uterine rupture following trial of labour after cesarean (TOLAC) do not differentiate between complete (**rupture**) and partial separation (**dehiscence**).
  - However, catastrophic rupture is most commonly associated with maternal morbidity and mortality (see **Chapter 25**, *Vaginal delivery after previous cesarean section*).
  - For practical purposes, it has been hypothesised that approximately 1 in 200 TOLACs will lead to uterine rupture. With elective repeat cesarean delivery (ERCD), the risk of uterine rupture is much lower. The risk has been calculated to be 26 per 100,000 cases (Metz, 2020).
  - In developing countries, unsupervised labour with a scarred uterus also contributes to the availability of the risk of uterine rupture.
  - In developed countries, though the incidence of uterine rupture was static due to the availability of better obstetric care, it is once again on the rise following the increase in the rate of cesarean sections and associated scar rupture.

Morbidity and mortality

Maternal mortality

- The incidence of maternal deaths in India due to uterine rupture has been reported to range from 3.33 per cent (Rashmi et al., 2001) to 5.88 per cent (Chhabra et al., 2002). However, the overall maternal mortality due to this cause is on the decline. Rajaram et al. (1995) found that uterine rupture accounted for 9.3 per cent of all maternal deaths in India.

 Maternal morbidity and mortality are higher in a **complete rupture** where the fetus is expelled into the peritoneal cavity. In **uterine dehiscence**, where the overlying peritoneum is still intact, the consequences are less severe.

- In developing countries, prolonged neglected obstructed labour continues to be the leading cause of uterine rupture in an unscarred uterus. The inability to access safe cesarean section is one of the leading causes of maternal mortality in resource-poor countries (Hofmeyr, 2004).
- Unfortunately, with the rising rates of cesarean section, the rate of rupture of the scarred uterus is also rising.

Perinatal mortality

The perinatal mortality rate is high—around 78 per cent (Rashmi et al., 2001; Chhabra et al., 2002).

Etiology of uterine rupture

Uterine rupture can occur in a scarred or unscarred uterus. In the unscarred uterus, the cause can be iatrogenic or spontaneous (Table 30.3).

Table 30.3   Causes of uterine rupture in a scarred and unscarred uterus

In a scarred uterus	In an unscarred uterus	
	Iatrogenic	**Spontaneous**
• Classical cesarean • Lower segment cesarean • Hysterotomy scar • Myomectomy scars • Metroplasty scar • Scars of previously repaired uterine rupture	• Induction and/or augmentation of labour (with oxytocin or misoprostol) • Internal podalic version and breech extraction • Difficult forceps delivery • Destructive surgeries on the fetus	• Following obstructed labour • Cephalopelvic disproportion • Malpresentations • Congenital abnormalities of the fetus, e.g., hydrocephalus • Blunt injury of the abdomen • Placenta accreta, increta, percreta • High parity • Disorders of collagen, e.g., Ehlers–Danlos syndrome • Uterine anomalies

Clinical manifestations of uterine rupture

- A high index of diagnostic suspicion should be present for the diagnosis of uterine rupture.
- Spontaneous uterine rupture is associated with highly variable and non-specific maternal complaints and fetal status.

> The main site of involvement in uterine rupture is the lower uterine segment in both the unscarred and scarred uterus, representing approximately 93 per cent of cases. However, cervical involvement is more common in the unscarred uterus as compared to a scarred uterus (Ofir et al., 2004).

Clinical manifestations include the following:

Fetal heart rate changes

- Sudden fetal heart abnormalities in labouring patients are a potential sign of danger (Ozdemir et al., 2005).
- *Bradycardia* is the most common fetal heart abnormality in uterine rupture.

Loss of station

When the uterus ruptures and the fetus is expelled into the peritoneal cavity, there might be a loss of station.

Abdominal pain

- Constant abdominal pain (unlike the periodic nature of labour pains) should be a warning sign.
- When constant pain is also accompanied by signs of intra-abdominal hemorrhage (e.g, hypotension, tachycardia, increasing abdominal girth), uterine rupture is highly likely.
- However, the degree, character, and location of pain may vary (Dow et al., 2009), and the clinician should be very alert to pick up subtle signs and symptoms of intra-abdominal bleeding.

Cessation of contractions

- As soon as uterine rupture occurs, the labour contractions will cease.
- This may be accompanied by a change in the shape of the uterine contour as the fetus is expelled into the peritoneal cavity.
- There might also be severe uterine tenderness on palpation.

Vaginal bleeding

In spite of significant intra-abdominal bleeding, vaginal bleeding may not be significant unless the cervix and upper vaginal wall are involved.

Hematuria

Hematuria is a strong indication that the rupture has involved the bladder.

Management of uterine rupture

Intervention in the presence of uterine rupture is almost always prompted by an abnormal fetal heart rate since it is the most common clinical manifestation of rupture. Management decisions are based on the following:
- Hemodynamic stability of mother
- Fetal condition as indicated by an abnormal pattern on fetal heart rate monitoring

Hemodynamically unstable mother and compromised fetus

- The mother is hemodynamically stabilised with appropriate fluids and blood transfusion as indicated, and prepared for laparotomy.
- The bladder is catheterised to monitor the urine output.
- Laparotomy is usually performed under general anesthesia.
- A vertical midline skin incision provides faster incision-to-delivery time and also better access to the uterine fundus and upper abdomen (Smith and Wax, 2020).
- A lower anterior uterine segment uterine rupture is usually apparent upon opening the abdomen. However, rupture at the fundus or posterior or lateral wall may not be immediately recognised.

- Hemoperitoneum may be significant.
- The fetal presenting part may be encountered floating freely in the peritoneal cavity. Extension of the abdominal wall incision and uterine incision may be necessary to facilitate delivery.

 Rupture at the fundus or posterior or lateral wall may not be immediately obvious at laparotomy. Hence a thorough inspection of the uterus is mandatory.

Hemodynamically stable mother and compromised fetus

- Decisions about neuraxial anesthesia vs. general anesthesia depend on the urgency of the situation and the fetal condition. If the mother is stable and fetal salvage is assured, spinal or epidural may be used.
- The choice of midline vs. transverse skin decision will depend on the obstetrician's assessment of how critical the incision-to-delivery time is to fetal health.
- A low transverse skin incision may be used if access to the upper abdomen is not believed to be necessary.

Surgical options

The surgical options available for the management of uterine rupture are as follows:
- Repair of rupture
- Hysterectomy

Repair of uterine rupture

- Repair of the uterine tear is undertaken in the following situations:
  - The patient is hemodynamically stable.
  - It is a clean and easily repairable rent.
  - A cesarean scar has given way.
  - The mother is a young woman desirous of further pregnancies.

 In women who do not desire a future pregnancy, it is advisable to perform tubal ligation since rent repair is associated with a higher rate of repeat rupture (Chibber et al., 2010; Usta et al., 2007).

- The uterine defect is repaired in two or three layers, as one would repair a hysterotomy. An absorbable suture is used.
- Consultation may be obtained from a urologist or surgeon depending on the nature of injury to the ureter, bladder, or bowel (Kapoor et al., 2003).

Hysterectomy

- A hysterectomy is usually resorted to in women who do not desire a future pregnancy.
- It may also be the only option in the presence of the following complications:
  - Rupture of an unscarred uterus
  - Ragged or spiral tears
  - Rupture involving the upper uterine segment
  - Colporrhexis
  - A hemodynamically unstable patient

Pregnancy after prior uterine rupture

- In a woman with a prior uterine rupture, there is an increased risk of recurrent rupture in a future pregnancy. If the rupture was surgically repaired, the couple should be counselled against another pregnancy.
- However, if the couple has lost the previous child and wants to attempt a pregnancy, the pregnancy should be followed in a fully-equipped tertiary care facility (Chibber et al., 2010).

> Though lower uterine scar thickness measurement by ultrasound imaging has been suggested as a means of predicting rupture in women attempting trial of labour following cesarean delivery, a systematic review (Kok et al., 2013) found that it was not useful in clinical practice. Routine assessment of the lower uterine segment thickness in women with a prior cesarean is not recommended (Landon and Frey, 2020).

- A study spanning 25 years (Usta et al., 2007) found that longitudinal ruptures (in an unscarred uterus) and short intervals (less than 2 years) between rupture and subsequent pregnancy predispose to recurrence of uterine rupture.
- In future pregnancies, cesarean delivery should be scheduled before labour. Delivery is recommended at 36^{+0} to 37^{+0} weeks (ACOG, 2019).

UTERINE INVERSION

Introduction

- Uterine inversion is the collapse of the uterine fundus into the endometrial cavity, either completely or partially. Though rare, it is a life-threatening situation, often following mismanagement of the third stage of labour. In one study (Hussain et al., 2004), mismanagement of the third stage of labour was found to be responsible for uterine inversion in 75 per cent of women.
- The incidence varies from 1 in 3700 to 20,000 at vaginal delivery and 1 in 1860 at cesarean delivery (Baskett, 2002; Witteveen et al., 2013).
- Puerperal uterine inversion can follow vaginal or cesarean delivery (Baskett, 2002) and is associated with significant blood loss and shock.

Precipitating factors

Risk factors associated with uterine inversion are as follows:
- Excessive umbilical cord traction
- Fundal pressure
- Fundal cord insertion
- Abnormal placentation

Diagnosis of uterine inversion

- Diagnosis is clinical and is based on the presence of a smooth, round mass protruding from the cervix or vagina (Figure 30.6), with the uterine fundus not being palpable abdominally.

- Excessive bleeding potentially resulting in shock, and lower abdominal pain are the other diagnostic features of uterine inversion.
- If there is a delay in identifying and diagnosing uterine inversion, the mother is at risk of hemorrhage and hypovolemic shock.

Management of uterine inversion

- Resuscitation of the patient and replacement of the inverted uterus to its normal position must be performed simultaneously and as soon as possible.
- The aims of management are:
    - Control of bleeding and treatment of shock
    - Repositioning of the fundus to its normal position
    - Prevention of recurrence

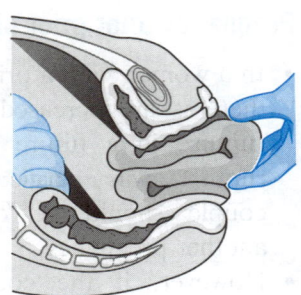

Figure 30.6   The presence of a smooth, round mass protruding from the cervix is diagnostic of uterine inversion.

Resuscitative measures

- **Help and extra assistance:** The first step is to call for help. It is important to have one team lead the resuscitative measures while the other team works at replacing the uterus.
- **Discontinuing oxytocin:** If oxytocin is being used, it should be discontinued since maximum uterine relaxation is required to replace the uterus.
- **Intravenous fluid infusion:** IV fluids should be started with lines in both arms, using large gauge needles (16–18 gauge). Fluid resuscitation with crystalloids must be aggressive, especially in the presence of shock.
- **Blood products:** At least four units of blood should be cross-matched. Blood transfusion should be started as soon as possible.
- **Covering the inverted uterus:** A moist sterile gauze or pad should be placed to cover the inverted uterus protruding outside the introitus.
- **Mechanical measures for correcting hypotension:** The foot end of the bed should be elevated.
- The mother should be rapidly shifted to the operating theatre where resuscitative measures can be continued.

Methods of repositioning of uterus

- Manual methods
- Hydrostatic methods
- Surgical correction

Tocolytics

- Tocolytics can be used for uterine relaxation while repositioning the inverted uterus (ACOG, 2017), but no clear evidence supports the use of one agent over the other.

- Agents commonly used are as follows:
  - Terbutaline 0.25 mg subcutaneously
  - Magnesium sulphate 4 to 6 g IV over 15–20 mins
  - Nitroglycerine 50 µg IV (can give up to four doses to achieve relaxation)
  - Halogenated general anesthetics, e.g., halothane, sevoflurane, and isoflurane have the advantage of being excellent uterine relaxants

Manual repositioning

- Manual replacement should be attempted as soon as the diagnosis is made and before the formation of the constriction ring.
- The palm of the hand or a closed fist is placed against the inverted fundus (Johnson's manoeuvre, Figure 30.7), as if holding a tennis ball, with the fingertips exerting upward pressure circumferentially at the utero-cervical junction (ACOG, 2017).
- The uterus is lifted out of the pelvis, well above the level of the umbilicus and held in this position for a few minutes. This stretches the uterine ligaments, and also widens the ring which aids in reduction.
- The part of the uterus that inverted last should be reduced first.
- Once reduced, the tocolytics are stopped and the placenta is removed, if still attached.
- Uterotonics such as ergometrine, oxytocin or $PGF_2\alpha$ are administered.
- The fisted hand is kept inside until the uterus contracts over it and then gently removed (Figure 30.8).
- Manual replacement with or without uterine relaxants is usually successful in the majority of cases.

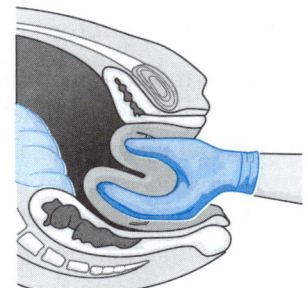

Figure 30.7 Palm of the hand placed against inverted fundus with fingertips exerting upward pressure.

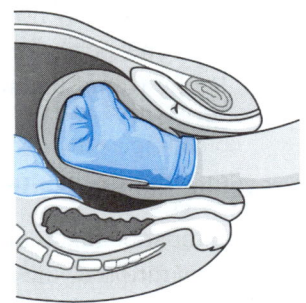

Figure 30.8 The fisted hand is kept inside until the uterus contracts over it and then gently removed.

Hydrostatic repositioning

- Hydrostatic reduction of acute uterine inversion is attempted if all other interventions have failed and before trying surgical intervention. This is performed using the O'Sullivan technique.
- A bag containing warm saline is placed 3 feet above the level of the woman. The nozzle at the end of the IV tubing is introduced into the posterior fornix of the vagina.
- The labia is closed over the tube to occlude the introitus and thus prevent fluid leak. A fist may also be used to occlude the vaginal introitus.
- A silastic ventouse cup (60 mm size) can also be used to occlude the vagina (Ogueh and Ayida, 1997; Tan and Luddin, 2005).
- The saline is run in so that it distends the vagina. Large amounts of fluid, up to 5L, may be required. Doing so increases the vaginal pressure, which aids in the repositioning of the uterine fundus.

- When the uterus flips back into position, a fisted hand is introduced into the uterus (Figure 30.8), oxytocin is administered, and the hand is withdrawn once the uterus contracts.

 If the placenta is still attached to the inverted uterus, it is not removed until the uterus is repositioned. This way, the bleeding can be reduced.

 Uterine rupture should be excluded before performing a hydrostatic repositioning of the uterus.

Surgical procedures

- When the aforementioned measures have failed, surgical repositioning may be required.
- General anesthesia helps with uterine relaxation.
- **Vaginal approach:** The constriction ring formed by the cervix is incised either anteriorly (*Spinelli procedure*) or posteriorly (*Cascarides procedure*). The incision is then repaired.
- **Abdominal approach:**
  - *Huntington's method:* At laparotomy, a Babcock or Allis clamp is inserted into the inverted cup formed by the fundal inversion. The round ligaments of the inverted corpus are held and progressively pulled up (ACOG, 2017). As the fundus starts moving upwards, the clamps are repeatedly released and applied to deeper levels until the fundus comes up.
  - *Haultain's procedure:* In the presence of a tough constriction ring, the previous technique may not work. The Haultain's procedure involves making a vertical incision over the posterior cervical ring to relieve the constriction. Traction is then applied to the round ligaments or an assistant may push the uterus up from below (ACOG, 2017).

Prevention of uterine inversion

- Care must be taken during the third stage to not apply undue traction on the cord before the separation of the placenta.
- The placenta should be delivered by controlled cord traction (*Brandt Andrew technique*).
- Excess fundal pressure should be avoided.

References

Shoulder dystocia

1. Acker DB. 1991. A shoulder dystocia intervention form. *Obstet Gynecol.* 78(1):150–1.
2. American College of Obstetricians and Gynecologists. 2017 (reaffirmed 2019). ACOG Practice Bulletin No. 178. Shoulder dystocia. *Obstet Gynecol.* 129:e123–33.
3. American College of Obstetricians and Gynecologists. 2020. ACOG Practice Bulletin No. 216. Macrosomia. *Obstet Gynecol.* 135:e18–35.
4. Baxley EG, Gobbo RW. 2004. Shoulder dystocia. *Am Fam Physician.* 69(7):1707-1714.

5. Bingham J, Chauhan SP, Hayes E, Gherman R, Lewis D. 2010. Recurrent shoulder dystocia: A review. *Obstet Gynecol Surv*. 65:183–8.

6. Boulvain M, Irion O, Dowswell T, Thornton JG. 2016. Induction of labour at or near term for suspected fetal macrosomia. *Cochrane Database Syst Rev*. Issue 5. Art. no.: CD000938.

7. Bruner JP, Drummond SB, Meenan AL, Gaskin IM. 1998. All-fours maneuver for reducing shoulder dystocia during labour. *J Reprod Med*. 43:439.

8. Chauhan SP, Rose CH, Gherman RB et al. 2005. Brachial plexus injury: A 23-year experience from a tertiary center. *Am J Obstet Gynecol*. 192:1795.

9. Deering S, Poggi S, Macedonia C et al. 2004. Improving resident competency in the management of shoulder dystocia with simulation training. *Obstet Gynecol*. 103:1224.

10. Gherman RB, Chauhan S, Ouzounian JG, Lerner H, Gonik B, Goodwin TM. 2006. Shoulder dystocia: The unpreventable obstetric emergency with empiric management guidelines. *Am J Obstet Gynecol*. 195;657–72.

11. Gherman RB, Ouzounian JG, Goodwin TM. 1998. Obstetric maneuvers for shoulder dystocia and associated fetal morbidity. *Am J Obstet Gynecol*. 178:1126–30.

12. Goffman D, Heo H, Pardanani S et al. 2008. Improving shoulder dystocia management among resident and attending physicians using simulations. *Am J Obstet Gynecol*. 199:294.e1.

13. Grobman WA, Miller D, Burke C et al. 2011. Outcomes associated with introduction of a shoulder dystocia protocol. *Am J Obstet Gynecol*. 205:513.

14. Gross SJ, Shime J, Farine D. 1987. Shoulder dystocia: Predictors and outcome. A five-year review. *Am J Obstet Gynecol*. 156(2):334–6.

15. Hoffman MK, Bailit JL, Branch DW et al. 2011. A comparison of obstetric maneuvers for the acute management of shoulder dystocia. *Obstet Gynecol*. 117:1272.

16. Langer O, Berkus MD, Huff RW, Samueloff A. 1991. Shoulder dystocia: Should the fetus weighing greater than or equal to 4000 grams be delivered by cesarean section? *Am J Obstet Gynecol*. 165:831–7.

17. Laughon SK, Berghella V, Reddy UM, Sundaram R, Lu Z, Hoffman MK. 2014. Neonatal and maternal outcomes with prolonged second stage of labor. *Obstet Gynecol*. 57–67.

18. Leung TY, Stuart O, Sahota DS et al. 2011. Head-to-body delivery interval and risk of fetal acidosis and hypoxic ischaemic encephalopathy in shoulder dystocia: A retrospective review. *BJOG*. 118:474.

19. Magro-Malosso ER, Saccone G, Chen M et al. 2017. Induction of labour for suspected macrosomia at term in non-diabetic women: A systematic review and meta-analysis of randomized controlled trials. *BJOG*. 124(3):414–421.

20. Nocon JJ, McKenzie DK, Thomas LJ, Hansell RS. 1993. Shoulder dystocia: An analysis of risks and obstetric maneuvers. *Am J Obstet Gynecol*. 168:1732–9.

21. Rouse DJ, Owen J, Goldenberg RL, Cliver SP. 1996. The effectiveness and costs of elective cesarean delivery for fetal macrosomia diagnosed by ultrasound. *JAMA*. 276(18):1480–6.

22. Rouse DJ, Owen J. 1999. Prophylactic cesarean delivery for fetal macrosomia diagnosed by means of ultrasonography—A Faustian bargain? *Am J Obstet Gynecol*. 181:332–8.

23. Torki M, Barton L, Miller DA, Ouzounian JG. 2012. Severe brachial plexus palsy in women without shoulder dystocia. *Obstet Gynecol*. 120:539–41.

24. Witkop CT, Neale D, Wilson LM et al. 2009. Active compared with expectant delivery management in women with gestational diabetes: A systematic review. *Obstet Gynecol*. 113:206

Umbilical cord prolapse

25. Gibbons C, O'Herlihy C, Murphy JF. 2014. Umbilical cord prolapse–changing patterns and improved outcomes: A retrospective cohort study. *BJOG.* 121:1705–1709.

26. Lin MG. 2006. Umbilical cord prolapse. *Obstet Gynecol Surv.* 61:269.

27. Murphy DJ, MacKenzie IZ. 1995. The mortality and morbidity associated with umbilical cord prolapse. *Br J Obstet Gynaecol.* 102:826.

28. Smyth RM, Markham C, Dowswell T. 2013. Amniotomy for shortening spontaneous labour. *Cochrane Database Syst Rev.* Issue 6, Art. no.: CD006167.

29. Usta IM, Mercer BM, Sibai BM. 1999. Current obstetrical practice and umbilical cord prolapse. *Am J Perinatol.* 16:479.

Uterine rupture

30. American College of Obstetricians and Gynecologists. 2019. ACOG Practice Bulletin No. 205. Vaginal birth after cesarean delivery. *Obstet Gynecol.*

31. Batra K, Gaikwad HS, Gutgutia I, Prateek S, Bajaj B. 2016. Determinants of rupture of the unscarred uterus and the related feto-maternal outcome: current scenario in a low-income country. *Tropical Doctor.* 46(2), 69–73.

32. Chhabra S, Bhagwat N, Chakravorty A. 2002. Reduction in the occurrence of uterine rupture in Central India. *J Obstet Gynaecol.* 22(1):39–42.

33. Chibber R, El-Saleh E, Al Fadhli R et al. 2010. Uterine rupture and subsequent pregnancy outcome–how safe is it? A 25-year study. *J Matern Fetal Neonatal Med.* 23:421.

34. Dow M, Wax JR, Pinette MG et al. 2009. Third-trimester uterine rupture without previous cesarean: A case series and review of the literature. *Am J Perinatol.* 26:739.

35. Hofmeyr GJ. 2004. Obstructed labor: Using better technologies to reduce mortality. *Int J Gynecol Obstet.* 85: S62–S72.

36. Kapoor DS, Sharma SD, Alfirevic Z. 2003. Management of unscarred ruptured uterus. *J Perinat Med.* 31:337.

37. Kok N, Wiersma IC, Opmeer BC et al. 2013. Sonographic measurement of lower uterine segment thickness to predict uterine rupture during a trial of labor in women with previous cesarean section: A meta-analysis. *Ultrasound Obstet Gynecol.* 42:132.

38. Landon MB, Frey H. 2020. Uterine rupture: After previous caesarean delivery. Berghella V (Ed). *UpToDate.* Waltham, MA.

39. Metz TD. 2020. Choosing the route of delivery after cesarean birth. Berghella V (Ed). *UpToDate.* Waltham, MA.

40. Ofir K, Sheiner E, Levy A et al. 2004. Uterine rupture: Differences between a scarred and an unscarred uterus. *Am J Obstet Gynecol.* 191:425.

41. Ozdemir I, Yucel N, Yucel O. 2005. Rupture of the pregnant uterus: a 9-year review. *Arch Gynecol Obstet.* 272:229.

42. Rashmi, Radhakrishnan G, Vaid NB, Agarwal N. 2001. Rupture uterus—changing Indian scenario. *J Indian Med Assoc.* 99(11):634-7.

43. Rajaram P, Agarwal A, Swain S. 1995. Determinants of maternal mortality: A hospital-based study from South India. *Indian J Matern Child Health.* 6(1):7–10.

44. Smith JF, Wax JR. 2020. Uterine rupture: Unscarred uterus. Lockwood CJ (Ed). *UpToDate.* Waltham, MA.

45. Usta IM, Hamdi MA, Musa AA, Nassar AH. 2007. Pregnancy outcome in patients with previous uterine rupture. *Acta Obstet Gynecol Scand.* 86:172.

46. Vernekar M, Rajib R. 2016. Unscarred uterine rupture: A retrospective analysis. *J Obstet Gynaecol India.* 66 (Suppl 1):51–54.

47. Walsh CA, Baxi LV. 2007. Rupture of the primigravid uterus: A review of the literature. *Obstet Gynecol Surv.* 62:327.

Uterine inversion

48. American College of Obstetricians and Gynecologists. 2017. ACOG Practice Bulletin No. 183. Postpartum hemorrhage. *Obstet Gynecol.* 130:e168–86.

49. Baskett TF. 2002. Acute uterine inversion: A review of 40 cases. *J Obstet Gynaecol Can.* 24:953.

50. Hussain M, Jabeen T, Liaquat N, Noorani K, Bhutta SZ. 2004. Acute puerperal uterine inversion. *J Coll Physicians Surg Pak.* 14(4):215-7.

51. Ogueh O, Ayida G. 1997. Acute uterine inversion: A new technique of hydrostatic replacement. *British Journal of Obstetrics and Gynaecology.* 104:951-2.

52. Tan KH, Luddin NS. 2005. Hydrostatic reduction of acute uterine inversion. *Int J Gynaecol Obstet.* 91:63.

53. Witteveen T, van Stralen G, Zwart J, van Roosmalen J. 2013. Puerperal uterine inversion in the Netherlands: A nationwide cohort study. *Acta Obstet Gynecol Scand.* 92:334–7.

Chapter 31

Antepartum Hemorrhage

INTRODUCTION

- Antepartum hemorrhage (APH) is defined as bleeding (ranging from spotting to obstetric hemorrhage) from or into the genital tract, occurring from 20 weeks of pregnancy to any time before delivery (Gyamfi-Bannerman, 2018). Some guidelines define it as bleeding occurring after 24 weeks (period of viability). It may also be referred to as *late pregnancy bleeding* or *bleeding in the second half of pregnancy*.
- Although antepartum hemorrhage (APH) accounts for fewer maternal deaths than postpartum hemorrhage, it is important to recognise this as a cause of feto-maternal morbidity.
- **Placenta previa** and **placental abruption** are the most important causes of APH.
- The prevalence of placenta previa is low—around 5 per 1000 pregnancies, with major placenta previa being 4.3 per 1000 pregnancies (Cresswell et al., 2013). Placental abruption complicates approximately 1 in 100–120 pregnancies (Ananth et al., 2015)
- APH can lead to very preterm delivery and accounts for up to 20 per cent of such deliveries. The strong association of cerebral palsy to APH can possibly be explained by the extreme prematurity of the neonates.

 Antepartum hemorrhage complicates 3–5 per cent of pregnancies and is a leading cause of perinatal and maternal mortality worldwide (Ananth et al., 2015). Arora et al. (2001) reported an incidence of 2.53 per cent in India.

CAUSES OF ANTEPARTUM HEMORRHAGE

- Placenta previa
- Placental abruption
- Unclassified
  - Marginal sinus rupture
  - Local lesions, e.g., cervical polyp, cervical carcinoma
  - Vasa previa
- Other underlying diseases may also contribute to antepartum bleeding; some diseases are as follows:
  - Bleeding disorders (e.g., von Willebrand disease)
  - Acquired hemostatic disorders due to liver failure (e.g., fulminant hepatitis, acute fatty liver of pregnancy)
  - Severe disseminated intravascular coagulation
  - Platelet dysfunction (e.g., severe preeclampsia, thrombotic thrombocytopenic purpura)

PLACENTA PREVIA

DEFINITION

- In placenta previa, the placental tissue is implanted partially or entirely in the lower uterine segment and extends upto or over the internal os, so that at the time of delivery, the placenta precedes the baby.
- The prevalence of placenta previa is low at around 5 per 1000 pregnancies, with major placenta previa being 4.3 per 1000 pregnancies in the second trimester (Cresswell et al., 2013). By term, the prevalence of placenta previa is 0.3–0.5 per cent (Oyelese, 2010).
- Placenta previa may be associated with the following:
  - Placenta accreta
  - Malpresentation due to the placenta occupying the lower pole and resulting in a non-cephalic presentation
  - Vasa previa and velamentous umbilical cord insertion

 The maternal mortality rate associated with placenta previa remains high in developing countries where pre-existing maternal anemia, lack of medical resources, and home births are common.

TYPES OF PLACENTA PREVIA

The classification of placenta previa is based on sonographic localisation, which is the gold standard for the diagnosis of placenta previa.

Earlier classification

Placenta previa was earlier classified into four types, as follows:
- **Total placenta previa:** The placenta covers the internal os completely (Figure 31.1a).
- **Partial placenta previa:** The placenta covers the internal os asymmetrically (Figure 31.1b).

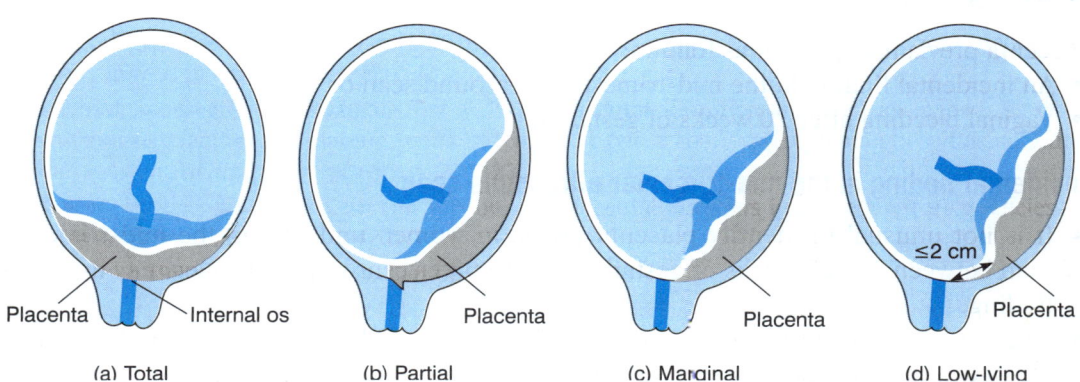

(a) Total   (b) Partial   (c) Marginal   (d) Low-lying

Figure 31.1   (a–d) The four types of placenta previa.

- **Marginal placenta previa:** The lower edge of the low-lying placenta reaches, but does not cover, the internal os (Figure 31.1c).
- **Low-lying placenta:** The placenta lies in the lower uterine segment, and the placental edge is ≤2 cm from the internal os (Figure 31.1d).

Current classification

The earlier classification has now been replaced by a simpler one.
- **True placenta previa:** The internal cervical os is covered by the placenta completely or partially (includes total and partial of earlier classification) (Figure 31.1a and b).
- **Low-lying placenta:** The placenta is in the lower segment; the edge of the placenta is within 2 cm of the os but does not cover it (Figure 31.1d).

RISK FACTORS FOR PLACENTA PREVIA

- **A previous cesarean section** is a major factor for the occurrence of placenta previa, increasing the risk of placenta previa by 50–60 per cent following a cesarean delivery (Ananth et al., 1997; Klar and Michels, 2014). A single cesarean delivery increases the incidence of placenta previa by 0.65 per cent, two increase the incidence by 1.5 per cent, three increase the incidence by 2.2 per cent, and four or more increase the incidence by 10 per cent (Naeye et al., 1980).
- **Previous placenta previa** has been associated with a recurrence risk of 4–8 per cent (Lavery, 1990).
- **Multiple pregnancy** also increases the risk of placenta previa. Twin pregnancies have a 40 per cent higher risk of placenta previa than singleton pregnancies. The risk is higher in dichorionic pregnancies than in monochorionic ones.

> In the presence of placenta previa in a woman who has had a previous cesarean delivery, other placental disorders like **placenta accreta** (including increta and percreta) should be anticipated.

CLINICAL PRESENTATION

Placenta previa may present as follows:
- An incidental finding in the mid-trimester ultrasound scan or
- Vaginal bleeding after 20 weeks of gestation

Incidental finding in the mid-trimester ultrasound scan

- It is not unusual to identify placenta previa in women undergoing the mid-trimester scan between 20–22 weeks of gestation. Up to 6 per cent of pregnancies may have this finding.
- Oyelese and Smulian (2006) found that 90 per cent of placenta previa identified before 20 weeks of gestation will resolve before delivery. This is due to the migration of the placenta towards the fundus (*trophotropism*).

- The risk of persistent placenta previa at delivery increases if:
  - The placenta extends over the internal os by 25 mm or more
  - The placenta previa is still present at 34–36 weeks
  - There is a history of a previous cesarean delivery

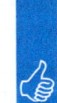 If a second-trimester ultrasound diagnosis of previa is made in the absence of bleeding, the mother may be reassured. There are no published studies to support or refute a recommendation of decreased activity or avoidance of intercourse.

Vaginal bleeding in the second half of gestation

- Women with persistent placenta previa may have their first episode of bleeding any time after 20 weeks. If the first episode occurs before 30 weeks, the bleeding can be more profuse and more likely to require a blood transfusion. These women are also at a greater risk of preterm delivery and perinatal mortality.
- 10 per cent of women with previa may reach term without any bleeding. The onset of labour may precipitate the first episode of bleeding.
- Jing et al. (2018) found that anterior placenta previas are more likely to be associated with the following complications:
  - Antepartum bleeding
  - Adverse pregnancy outcomes
  - Massive postpartum hemorrhage
- A complete placenta previa with the placenta located on the anterior wall also increases the risk of preterm delivery (Sekiguchi et al., 2013).

MATERNAL MORBIDITY AND MORTALITY IN PLACENTA PREVIA

- Placenta previa increases the risk of **antepartum** and **intrapartum hemorrhage**. In a systematic review, Fan et al. (2017) found that 52 per cent of women with placenta previa had antepartum hemorrhage.
- **Postpartum hemorrhage** (PPH) can occur due to inadequate occlusion of the sinuses in the lower segment after delivery. Approximately a quarter of women with placenta previa suffer from PPH.
- Placenta previa can be associated with a **morbidly adherent placenta** (accreta, increta, and percreta) in 1–5 per cent of pregnancies.
- The incidence of **cesarean section** increases in the presence of placenta previa.
- **Amniotic fluid embolism** is a rare complication, and has a strong association with placenta previa (Fong et al., 2015).
- Ascending infection of the raw placental bed can lead to **postpartum sepsis**.

NEONATAL MORBIDITY AND MORTALITY IN PLACENTA PREVIA

- **Preterm birth** is the principal cause of neonatal morbidity in placenta previa and triples the rate of neonatal mortality (Vahanian et al., 2015). Preterm labour is precipitated by the release of prostaglandin when the bleeding occurs.

- **Malpresentation** of the fetus is common in the presence of placenta previa. The presence of the placenta in the lower portion of the uterine cavity predisposes the fetus to assume a non-cephalic presentation (Sheiner et al., 2001).
- **Unexpected intrauterine death** (rupture of vasa previa, severe maternal hypovolemic shock) may occur, especially in the third trimester.

DIAGNOSIS

- Ultrasonography is the best diagnostic tool to rule out or confirm placenta previa in the presence of painless bleeding after 20 weeks (Figures 31.2–31.5).
- Transabdominal ultrasound is initially performed, and is followed by transvaginal or translabial (transperineal) examination if better definition of the leading edge of the placenta is required.

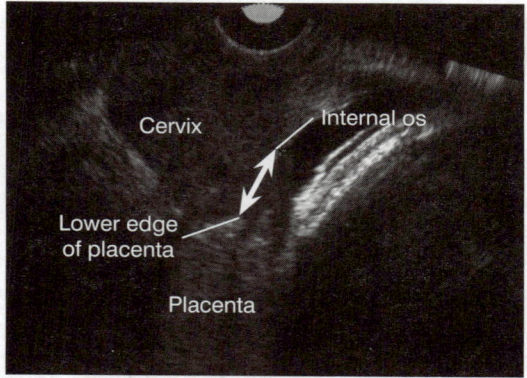

Figure 31.2 Transvaginal ultrasound image of low-lying placenta, with placental edge <2 cm from the internal os (arrow).

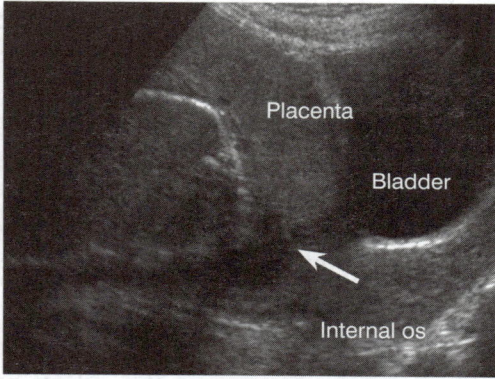

Figure 31.3 Transabdominal ultrasound image of marginal placenta previa, with placental edge extending just upto the internal os.

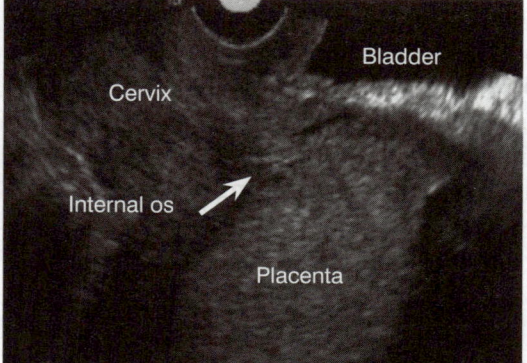

Figure 31.4 Transvaginal ultrasound image of partial placenta previa, with placental edge extending just beyond the internal os.

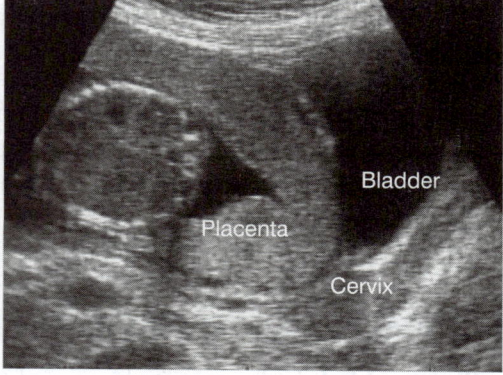

Figure 31.5 Transabdominal ultrasound image of complete placenta previa, with placental edge extending well beyond the internal os.

- The diagnosis is made with the imaging of echogenic homogeneous placental tissue extending upto or over the internal cervical os.
- Accuracy of diagnosis is better when imaging is done:
  - After the bladder has been emptied
  - After any lower uterine contraction has subsided
- Diagnosis may be more difficult with the following:
  - A low-lying fetal head
  - Posterior placenta
  - The presence of a hematoma, masking the edge of the placenta

> **Os-to-placental distance and mode of delivery**
> *When the placental edge-to-cervical os distance is >2.0 cm*
> - In this situation, vaginal delivery is successful in 82 per cent of cases. The incidence of emergency cesarean due to hemorrhage is 10 per cent (Jansen et al., 2019).
> - The decision to attempt vaginal delivery should be taken after discussion with the couple and must be based on the availability of blood products and immediate access to a theatre with a surgical team, including an anesthetist.
> - Even with a successful vaginal delivery, the incidence of postpartum hemorrhage remains high (Bhide and Thilaganatha, 2004).
>
> *When the placental edge-to-cervical os distance is ≤2.0 cm*
> - In this situation, the incidence of emergency sections for profuse bleeding is 45 per cent. Therefore, the mother should be offered an elective cesarean section.

PLACENTA PREVIA AND PLACENTA ACCRETA

- A diagnosis of placenta previa should always raise the possibility of an adherent placenta (**accreta, increta,** or **percreta**), especially in the presence of a previous cesarean scar.
- The normal interface between the placenta and bladder is characterised by a hypoechoic boundary that represents the myometrium and the normal retroplacental myometrial vasculature.
- When placenta accreta is present, this hypoechoic boundary is lost and the placenta appears contiguous with the bladder wall.

> **Ultrasound criteria for the diagnosis of placenta accreta**
> *Greyscale:*
> - Loss of the retroplacental sonolucent zone
> - Irregular retroplacental sonolucent zone
> - Thinning or disruption of the hyperechoic serosa–bladder interface
> - Presence of focal exophytic masses invading the urinary bladder
> - Abnormal placental lacunae (Figure 31.6)
>
> *Colour doppler:*
> - Diffuse or focal lacunar flow
> - Vascular lakes with turbulent flow
> - Hypervascularity of serosa–bladder interface
> - Markedly dilated vessels over peripheral subplacental zone

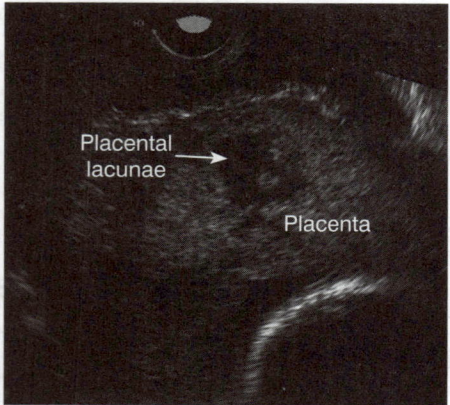

Figure 31.6 Adherent placenta showing abnormal placental lacunae.

MANAGEMENT OF PLACENTA PREVIA

Management of placenta previa differs for each of the following three presentations:
- Incidental diagnosis at routine 20–22 weeks scan
- Acute antepartum hemorrhage after 20 weeks
- Stable condition following episodes of bleeding after 20 weeks

Placenta previa diagnosed at routine 20–22 weeks' scan

- Asymptomatic women (no episodes of painless bleeding after 20 weeks of gestation) who have a low-lying placenta or placenta previa identified at the 20–22 weeks' ultrasound examination should undergo a follow-up scan between 34 and 36 weeks.
- An algorithm for interventions based on the findings at the 34–36 weeks' scan is presented in Figure 31.7 (Reddy et al., 2014; Lockwood and Russo-Stieglitz, 2020; ACOG, 2019).

Acute hemorrhage after 20 weeks

- An actively bleeding placenta previa is an obstetrical emergency and must be treated as such.
- Painless bleeding is the most common presentation of placenta previa. However, 10–20 per cent of women may present with contractions, pain, and bleeding that may mimic the presentation of placental abruption.
- If the mother has not had an earlier sonographic diagnosis of placenta previa, an ultrasound examination should be done to confirm or rule out placenta previa.
- The choice of management depends upon whether the bleeding is major or minor.

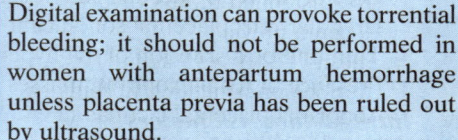

Digital examination can provoke torrential bleeding; it should not be performed in women with antepartum hemorrhage unless placenta previa has been ruled out by ultrasound.

- Women who have had a bleeding episode before 30 weeks of gestation tend to have more significant bleeding and are also at risk of preterm delivery, perinatal mortality, and the need for transfusion.

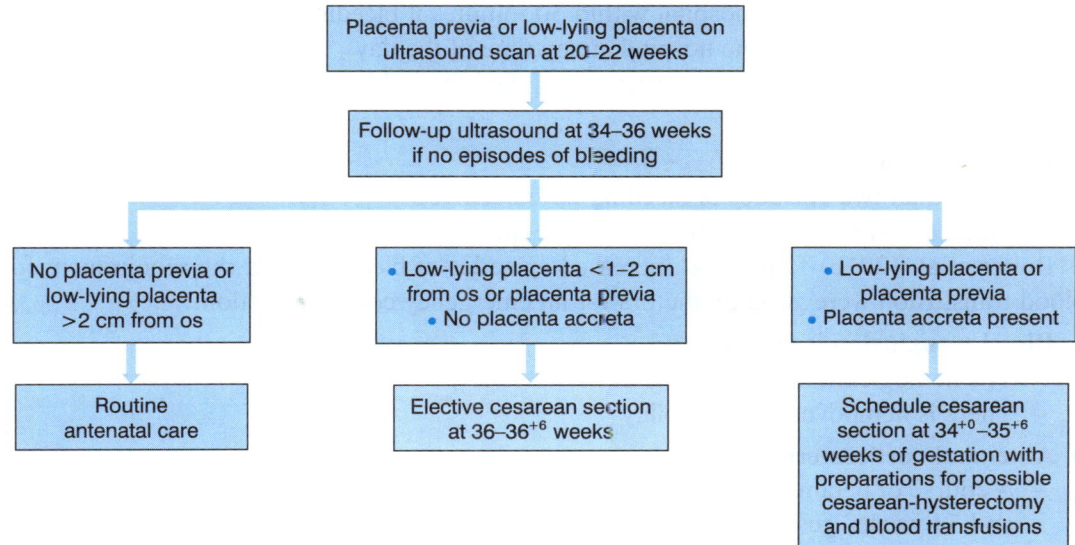

Figure 31.7   Follow-up of asymptomatic women with placenta previa or low-lying placenta diagnosed at routine 20– 22 weeks' ultrasound examination.

- Hospitalisation is recommended for close maternal and fetal monitoring and supportive care. With supportive care, 50 per cent of women with placenta previa who present with bleeding will not require an emergency cesarean section and will deliver at least four weeks after the bleeding episode.

 **Immediate delivery:** If the bleeding is heavy and compromising the feto-maternal condition, immediate delivery by emergency cesarean section is advised irrespective of the type of placenta previa, gestational age, and whether the fetus is dead or alive.

- An emergency cesarean section is indicated in the presence of the following:
  - Refractory, life-threatening maternal hemorrhage
  - Non-reassuring fetal status

Expectant management after an acute bleed

- Expectant management is offered to women:
  - Who are <34 weeks of gestation
  - Whose bleeding stopped sponta-neously
  - Who are hemodynamically stable
  - Who have no fetal heart rate abnormalities

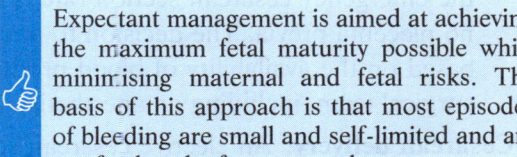 Expectant management is aimed at achieving the maximum fetal maturity possible while minimising maternal and fetal risks. The basis of this approach is that most episodes of bleeding are small and self-limited and are not fatal to the fetus or mother.

- **Outpatient management:** The mother may be sent home (Wing et al., 1996) if the following conditions are met:
  - She has had only one episode of bleeding that did not require a blood transfusion

- She can return to the hospital within 30 minutes if bleeding recurs and has someone who can bring her to the hospital at any time of the day
- She will be compliant with instructions (bed rest with limited activity, avoidance of sexual intercourse)

- **Hospitalisation** is advised if:
  - More than two episodes of bleeding have occurred
  - Blood transfusion was required with the episode of bleeding

Ruiter et al. (2016) found that increased episodes of bleeding, and the requirement for blood transfusion were good predictors for an emergency cesarean section.

- **Blood transfusion** is indicated if:
  - The hemoglobin level is <10 g/dL
  - There is hemodynamic instability

- **Antenatal corticosteroids**
  - A course of betamethasone is administered for accelerating lung maturity between 24 and 34 weeks' gestation.
  - A course of steroids is also recommended for women whose first bleed is at 34^{+0}–36^{+6} weeks of gestation and who have not received a prior course since these women have a significant risk of having a cesarean delivery before 37 weeks (Gyamfi-Bannerman, 2018).
  - However, in women with active hemorrhage in the late preterm period, delivery should not be delayed for the purpose of administering corticosteroids.

- **Tocolytics** are not routinely recommended (Lockwood and Russo-Stieglitz, 2020). If tocolysis is used to delay delivery for the administration of corticosteroids, they should be used with caution. Nifedipine can cause tachycardia and may confuse the clinical picture.

- **Anti-D immune globulin** should be given to Rh(D)-negative women to prevent possible alloimmunisation.

- **Vaginal delivery:**
  - Vaginal delivery may be safely attempted if the placental edge is lying ≥2 cms from the internal os.
  - A systematic review by Jansen et al. (2019) concluded that vaginal delivery is possible in 85 per cent of women if the placental edge is lying >2 cm from the os. However, the emergency cesarean section rate is still higher in such women than in those with no placenta previa. The decision to attempt vaginal delivery in this situation must be based on the availability of blood products and immediate access to a theatre with a surgical team, including an anesthetist.

- **Cesarean delivery:** An elective cesarean section should be offered if the placental edge is ≤2.0 cm from the internal os because, in these cases, the incidence of an emergency section for profuse bleeding is 45 per cent.

An algorithm for the immediate and expectant management of placenta previa is presented in Figure 31.8.

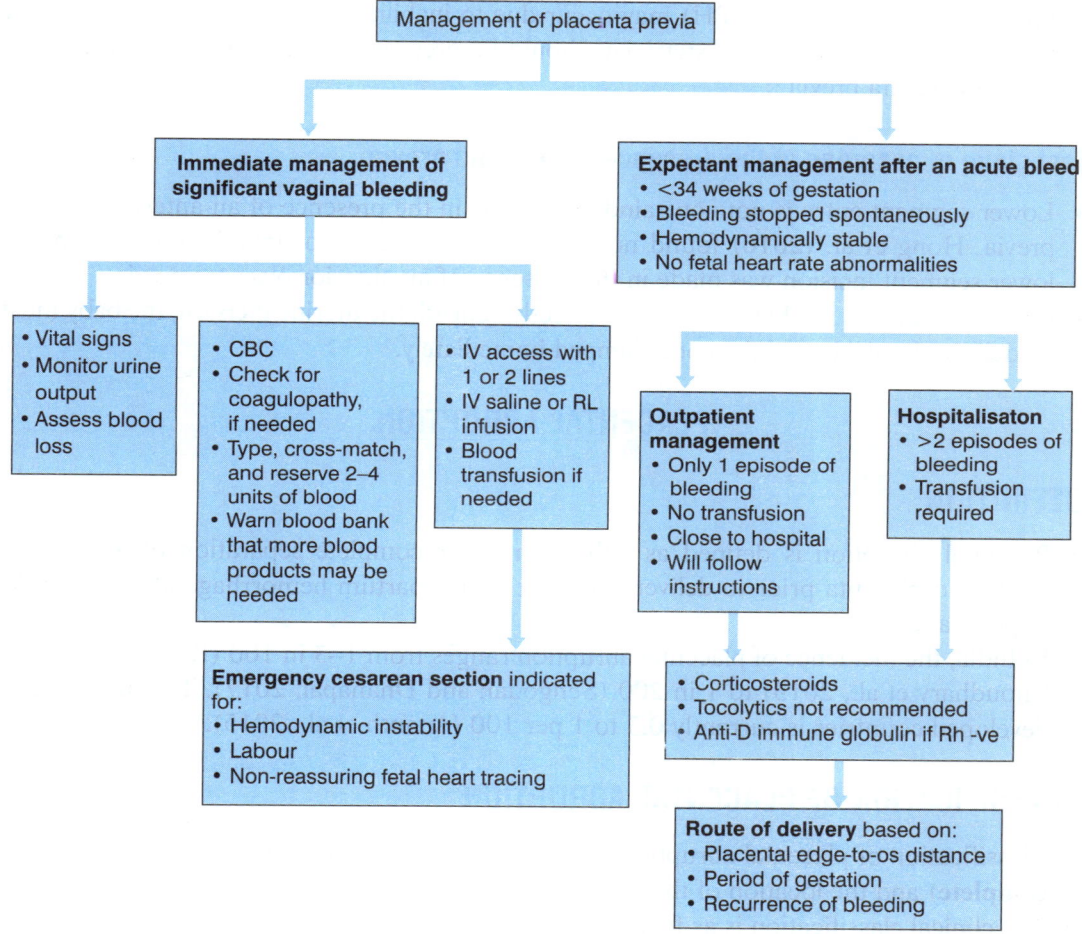

Figure 31.8   Management of placenta previa: Immediate management of significant vaginal bleeding and expectant management after an acute bleed. *CBC*, complete blood count; *IV*, intravenous; *Rh-ve*, Rh-negative blood type; *RL*, Ringer's lactated solution

Difficulties with cesarean section for placenta previa

Cesarean section for placenta previa may be complicated by the following factors:

- Fetal malpresentation
- Poorly developed lower uterine segment that may lead to the extension of the incision
- Difficulty in uterine entry with anterior placenta; there may be a need to cut through the placenta or separate it partially
- Excessive blood loss that further compromises the condition of the fetus and mother
- Placenta accreta (encountered in about 5 per cent of cases with no previous scar in the uterus and in up to 67 per cent of cases with multiple cesarean sections) may necessitate peripartum hysterectomy

- Postpartum hemorrhage (PPH) may occur due to inability of the lower uterine segment to contract efficiently; the obstetrician should be prepared to deal with PPH with every case of placenta previa

Technique of cesarean in the presence of placenta previa

- Lower segment entry is not contraindicated even in the presence of an anterior placenta previa. Hong et al. (2016) found no difference in maternal or fetal blood loss when a lower segment incision was made in the presence of an anterior placenta previa.
- Once the placenta has been transected directly beneath the uterine incision, the baby must be delivered quickly and the cord clamped immediately.

PLACENTAL ABRUPTION

DEFINITION

- Placental abruption is defined as either partial or complete separation of a normally implanted placenta prior to delivery, leading to antepartum hemorrhage after 20 weeks of pregnancy.
- In India, the incidence of placental abruption ranges from 1–3 in 100 (Khan et al., 2017; Choudhary et al., 2015) to 1 in 200 (Sengodan and Dhanapal, 2017). The incidence in developed countries is currently 0.3 to 1 per 100 (Ananth et al., 2015).

CLASSIFICATION OF PLACENTAL ABRUPTION

- Classification of placental abruption is based on the extent of separation (i.e., **partial** vs. **complete**) and the location of the separation (i.e., **marginal** vs. **central**).
- The clinical classification is as follows:
  - **Class 0 – Asymptomatic:** Diagnosis is made after delivery on finding an organised blood clot or a depressed area on a delivered placenta.
  - **Class 1 – Mild:** Occurs in 50 per cent of all cases. Characteristics include the following:
    - No vaginal bleeding or mild vaginal bleeding
    - Slightly tender uterus
    - Normal maternal BP and heart rate
    - No coagulopathy
    - No fetal distress
  - **Class 2 – Moderate:** Occurs in approximately 25 per cent of all cases. Characteristics include the following:
    - Ranging from no vaginal bleeding (concealed) to moderate vaginal bleeding
    - Moderate-to-severe uterine tenderness with possible tetanic contractions
    - Maternal tachycardia with orthostatic changes in BP and heart rate
    - Fetal distress
    - Hypofibrinogenemia (i.e., 50–250 mg/dL)

– **Class 3 – Severe:** Occurs in approximately 25 per cent of all cases. Characteristics include the following:
  - Ranging from no vaginal bleeding (concealed) to heavy vaginal bleeding
  - Very painful, tetanic uterus
  - Maternal shock
  - Hypofibrinogenemia (i.e., <150 mg/dL)
  - Coagulopathy
  - Fetal death

PATHOPHYSIOLOGY

The progression of placental abruption and its repercussions depend on the type of bleeding that occurs.

- **High-pressure arterial hemorrhage in the central portion** of the placenta results in acute signs and symptoms, which are as follows:
  – Extensive dissection of the placental–decidual plane by collection of blood
  – Severe bleeding
  – Thrombin production leading to:
    - Uterine hypertonus and contractions
    - Maternal disseminated intravascular coagulation
  – Fetal heart rate abnormalities or fetal death
- **Low-pressure venous hemorrhage at the periphery** of the placenta (marginal abruption) is usually self-limiting, and the separation tends to be over a small area. It may result in chronic morbidity, which may include the following:
  – Intermittent bleeding, usually in small quantities
  – Oligohydramnios
  – Fetal growth restriction

RISK FACTORS

Some of the maternal factors implicated in the etiology of placental abruption are as follows:
- Past history of abruption (the most significant risk factor)
- Pregnancy-induced hypertension (PIH), preeclampsia, and eclampsia
- Advanced maternal age
- Multiparity
- Premature rupture of membranes (PROM)
- Sudden uterine decompression resulting from:
  – Membrane rupture with polyhydramnios
  – The delivery of the first twin
- Uterine anomalies/fibroids
- Fetal growth restriction
- Intrauterine infections
- Abdominal trauma
- Smoking

First-trimester and second-trimester maternal serum biomarkers as predictors of placental abruption

Women with the following abnormal levels of analytes (estimated as part of Down screening) are at an increased risk of abruption (Ananth et al., 2017):
- Increased α-fetoprotein or human chorionic gonadotropin
- Decreased pregnancy-associated plasma protein A (PAPP-A) or unconjugated estriol
- Inhibin A ≤5th or ≥95th per centile

CLINICAL PRESENTATION OF PLACENTAL ABRUPTION

Most cases of placental abruption cannot be predicted or prevented. Placental abruption may present as follows:
- Acute abruption
- Chronic abruption

Acute abruption

- Acute abruption is an obstetric emergency, and unless managed aggressively, may result in fetal death, severe maternal morbidity, and possible maternal mortality.

When placental separation exceeds 50 per cent, acute disseminated intravascular coagulation and fetal death are common (Oyelese and Ananth, 2006).

- Acute abruption is of two types, which are as follows:
  - **Revealed abruption:** Blood trickles between the membranes and escapes through the vagina and cervix.
  - **Concealed abruption:** Blood collects behind the placenta with no evidence of vaginal bleeding. This occurs in 10–20 per cent of cases. In these women, vaginal bleeding may not be the presenting sign.

In concealed abruption, blood loss may be underestimated because bleeding may be retained behind the placenta and thus make it difficult to quantify.

- Acute abruption can present with the following signs and symptoms:
  - **Vaginal bleeding and pain:** Revealed abruption usually presents with a sudden onset of vaginal bleeding accompanied by the following:
    - Mild to moderate abdominal and/or back pain
    - A tense and rigid uterus that may be tender
    - Uterine contractions that may be very frequent and may lead to a rapid delivery

    Concealed abruption presents with the same symptoms but with no bleeding or only mild bleeding.
  - **Hemodynamic changes:** Maternal tachycardia and hypotension may be present. They may not correlate with the amount of vaginal bleeding present, especially in the presence of concealed abruption. The patient may be anxious, restless, and feel faint.

- **Fetal heart rate changes:**
  - ◆ The patient may report reduced fetal movements.
  - ◆ There may be significant fetal heart rate changes that signify fetal asphyxia.
  - ◆ Fetal heart tones may be absent in cases of fetal demise due to massive hemorrhage.

> **Couvelaire uterus**
> In severe abruption, blood may extravasate into the myometrium, turning the uterus deep purple. Because of the accumulation of blood between the muscle fibres, a Couvelaire uterus can lead to atonic postpartum hemorrhage. The atony may not respond to standard management, and a hysterectomy may be required to control the bleeding.

Chronic abruption

- Women with chronic abruption present with mild, intermittent bleeding.
- The low-pressure venous hemorrhage that leads to chronic abruption usually occurs at the periphery of the placenta (marginal abruption), is self-limiting, and results in a small area of separation.
- Over time, chronic abruption leads to placental ischemia and dysfunction that may result in the following:
  - Oligohydramnios (termed *chronic abruption-oligohydramnios sequence*)
  - Fetal growth restriction
  - Preeclampsia
- Women with chronic abruption are at risk of preterm prelabour rupture of membranes (PPROM).

MATERNAL CONSEQUENCES OF PLACENTAL ABRUPTION

- Maternal consequences are primarily related to the severity of the placental separation.
- Mild placental separation may result in no significant adverse effects.
- **Short-term consequences:** Increasing degrees of placental separation increase maternal risks. The consequences may be as follows:
  - Massive hemorrhage leading to:
    - ◆ Hypovolemic shock
    - ◆ Disseminated intravascular coagulation
    - ◆ Acute kidney injury due to tubular necrosis
    - ◆ Adult respiratory distress syndrome (ARDS)
    - ◆ Multiorgan failure
    - ◆ Peripartum hysterectomy
    - ◆ Death
  - Emergency cesarean section
- **Long-term consequences:** Riihimäki and colleagues (2017) concluded that overall, the mortality among women with a history of placental abruption is increased. These women were found more likely to die younger than the control population.

Placental abruption and disseminated intravascular coagulation (DIC)
- If a massive amount of the tissue factor (thromboplastin) is released, a massive amount of thrombin is generated, which rapidly enters the maternal circulation. Hemostatic control mechanisms are exhausted very quickly, leading to hypofibrinogenemia, elevated D-dimers and fibrin degradation products. The clinical consequence is DIC. As a result of widespread intravascular fibrin deposition, ischemic tissue injury and microangiopathic hemolytic anemia occur.
- DIC can lead to the following complications:
  - Couvelaire uterus which is unresponsive to oxytocin
  - Escalating hemorrhage
  - Acute kidney injury
  - Postpartum hemorrhage

FETAL CONSEQUENCES OF PLACENTAL ABRUPTION

Perinatal consequences related to hypoxemia, asphyxia, low birth weight, and/or preterm delivery are as follows:
- Fetal death
- Complications due to prematurity
- Growth restriction, which is reported in up to 80 per cent of infants (coexisting rather than as a sequel)

DIAGNOSIS OF PLACENTAL ABRUPTION

- **Clinical**: The diagnosis of placental abruption is essentially clinical. The abrupt onset of a combination of vaginal bleeding, abdominal pain and/or frequent labour pains, along with a hypertonic, tender uterus, is the classical presentation of abruption. It is important to differentiate placental abruption from placenta previa. Placenta previa is usually accompanied by *painless* bleeding.
- **Ultrasonography**:
  - Sonography has poor sensitivity (25–60 per cent) for the detection of placental abruption but is highly specific (Ananth and Kinzler, 2019).
  - A positive sonographic finding is the presence of a retroplacental hematoma that may be solid, complex, and hypo-, hyper-, or iso-echoic when compared with the placenta.
  - The identification of a retroplacental hematoma is associated with increased maternal morbidity and worse perinatal outcome because it represents an advanced stage of abruption (Shinde et al., 2016).
  - In the presence of a strong clinical suspicion of abruption with negative ultrasound findings, aggressive management results in better fetal and maternal outcomes.
  - Preterm patients with positive ultrasound and clinical findings of abruption have worse fetal outcome compared to term patients with abruption.

Ultrasound findings in placental abruption (Oyelese and Ananth, 2006)
- Preplacental collection under the chorionic plate (between the placenta and amniotic fluid)
- Jelly-like movement of the chorionic plate with fetal activity
- Retroplacental collection
- Marginal hematoma
- Subchorionic hematoma
- Increased heterogenous placental thickness (more than 5 cm in a perpendicular plane)
- Intra-amniotic hematoma

MANAGEMENT OF PLACENTAL ABRUPTION

As an obstetric emergency, abruption must be managed with immediate evaluation, supportive therapy, and interventions to deliver the fetus (Figure 34.9).

Immediate evaluation

- **Confirmation of fetal status**: If fetal heart tones are present, they must be monitored carefully because there is significant risk of fetal asphyxia.
- **Monitoring of maternal hemodynamic status** (heart rate, blood pressure, urine output, blood loss): Normal blood pressure in a known hypertensive may mask hypovolemia.
- **Evaluation and quantification of total blood loss**: This should be done to estimate the need for blood transfusion.
- **Hematological investigations:**
  - Complete blood count including platelet count
  - Blood type and crossmatch; four units of blood should be reserved
  - Coagulation studies (fibrinogen concentration, prothrombin time, activated partial thromboplastin time); a bedside **clot stability test** may be done while awaiting results

 In women with severe abruption and risk for DIC, the blood bank should be alerted to keep blood products available (red cells, fresh frozen plasma, cryoprecipitate, and platelets).

Supportive therapy

- Intravenous access should be secured with two 18-gauge intravenous lines. One line should have a blood transfusion set on it.
- A crystalloid solution like normal saline or Ringer's lactate should be administered at a rate that is adequate to maintain urine output at >30 mL/hour.
- Blood products should be replaced depending on the clinical situation. In the presence of DIC, fresh frozen plasma, cryoprecipitate, and platelets are required in addition to packed red blood cells.

Transfusion therapy aims to maintain:
- Hematocrit ≥25 to 30 per cent
- Platelet count ≥75,000/μL
- Fibrinogen ≥300 mg/dL
- Prothrombin and partial thromboplastin time <1.5 times control

Interventions to deliver the fetus

The mode of delivery depends on the following factors:
  - Hemodynamic stability of the mother
  - Gestational age
  - Fetal status
  - Stage of labour
- **Induction/augmentation:** When the maternal condition is stable and bleeding is not profuse, gestational age is >36 weeks, and fetal status is good, labour may be induced or augmented with the following:
  - Artificial rupture of membranes
  - Augmentation with oxytocin
  - Intensive fetal heart rate monitoring

- **Cesarean section:** This is indicated if the fetus is alive and there is:
  - Bleeding through an unfavourable cervix
  - Hemodynamic instability/significant coagulopathy/acute kidney injury
  - Non-reassuring fetal status as indicated by abnormal CTG
  - Malpresentation
  - Fetal growth restriction
  - Oligohydramnios
- **Fetal demise:** In the presence of fetal demise, the route of delivery depends on the maternal condition and whether the cervix is favourable. Since fetal demise is usually due to a massive abruption (placental separation > 50 per cent), a cesarean may be necessary to save the mother's life.
- **Conservative management:** Though some small studies have advocated tocolytics and steroids at <34 weeks' gestation (Towers et al., 1999; Bond et al., 1989) when the fetus and mother are both stable and there is no evidence of ongoing major blood loss or coagulopathy, the decision depends on the capacity to manage a recurrence of massive bleeding that may jeopardise the mother's life.

The management of placental abruption is summarised in Figure 31.9.

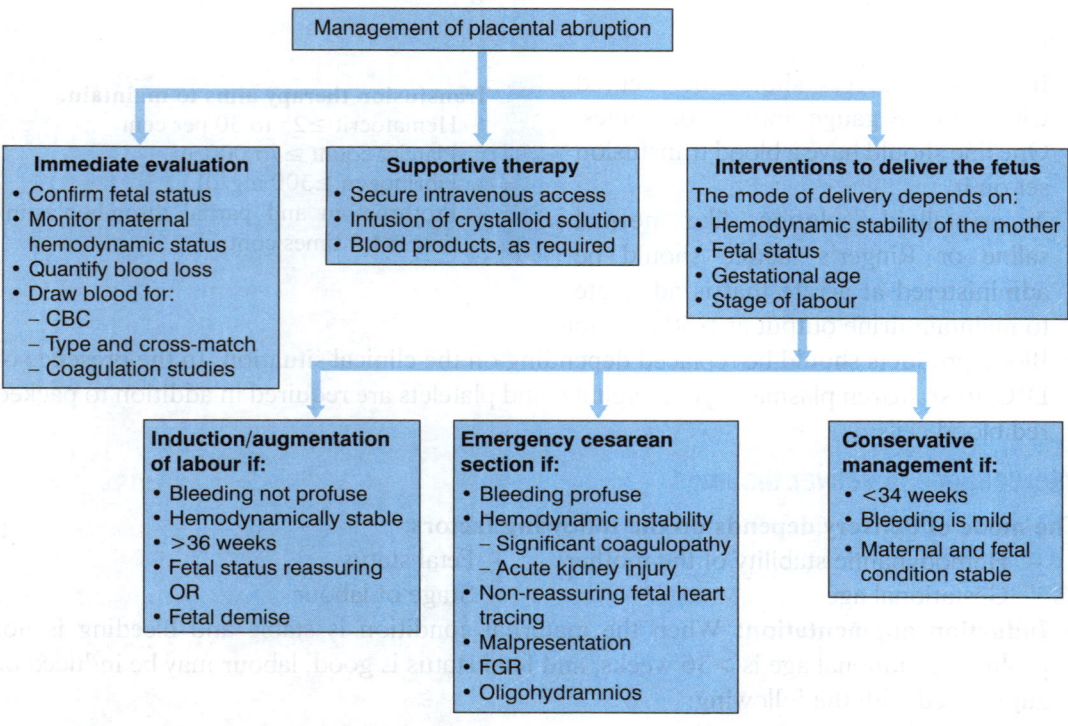

Figure 31.9 Management of placental abruption. As an obstetric emergency, abruption must be managed with immediate evaluation, supportive therapy and intervention to deliver the fetus. *FGR*, fetal growth restriction; *IV*, intravenous

References

1. American College of Obstetricians and Gynecologists. 2019. ACOG Committee Opinion No. 764. Medically indicated late-preterm and early-term deliveries. *Obstet Gynecol.* 133:e151–55.

2. Ananth CV, Keyes KM, Hamilton A et al. 2015. An international contrast of rates of placental abruption: An age-period-cohort analysis. *PLoS One.* 10:e0125246.

3. Ananth CV, Smulian JC, Vintzileos AM. 1997. The association of placenta previa with history of cesarean delivery and abortion: A metaanalysis. *Am J Obstet Gynecol.* 177:1071.

4. Ananth CV, Wapner RJ, Ananth S et al. 2017. First-trimester and second-trimester maternal serum biomarkers as predictors of placental abruption. *Obstet Gynecol.* 129:465.

5. Ananth CV, Kinzler WL. 2019. Placental abruption: Pathophysiology, clinical features, diagnosis, and consequences. Lockwood CJ (Ed). *UpToDate.* Waltham MA.

7. Arora R, Devi U, Majumdar R. 2001. Perinatal morbidity and mortality in antepartum haemorrhage. *J Obstet Gynecol India.* 51(30): 102-104.

8. Bhide A, Thilaganatha B. 2004. Recent advances in the management of placenta previa. *Curr Opin Obstet Gynecol.* 16:447–451.

9. Bond AL, Edersheim TG, Curry L et al. 1989. Expectant management of abruptio placentae before 35 weeks' gestation. *Am J Perinatol.* 6:121.

10. Choudhary V, Somani SR, Somani S. 2015. Evaluation of risk factors and obstetric and perinatal outcome in abruptio placenta. *IOSR Journal of Dental and Medical Sciences (IOSR-JDMS).* 14(5)(VII):36-39.

11. Cresswell JA, Ronsmans C, Calvert C, Filippi V. 2013. Prevalence of placenta praevia by world region: A systematic review and meta-analysis. *Trop Med Int Health.* 18:712.

12. Fan D, Wu S, Liu L et al. 2017. Prevalence of antepartum hemorrhage in women with placenta previa: A systematic review and meta-analysis. *Sci Rep.* 7:40320.

13. Fong A, Chau CT, Pan D, Ogunyemi DA. 2015. Amniotic fluid embolism: Antepartum, intrapartum and demographic factors. *J Matern Fetal Neonatal Med.* 28:793.

14. Gyamfi-Bannerman C. 2018. Society for Maternal-Fetal Medicine (SMFM) Consult Series #44: Management of bleeding in the late preterm period. *Am J Obstet Gynecol.* 218:B2.

15. Hong DH, Kim E, Kyeong KS, Hong SH, Jeong EH. 2016. Safety of cesarean delivery through placental incision in patients with anterior placenta previa. *Obstet Gynecol Sci.* 59(2):103–109.

16. Jansen C, de Mooij YM, Blomaard CM et al. 2019. Vaginal delivery in women with a low-lying placenta: A systematic review and meta-analysis. *BJOG.*126(9):1118.

17. Jing L, Wei G, Mengfan S, Yanyan H. 2018. Effect of site of placentation on pregnancy outcomes in patients with placenta previa. *PLoS One.* 13:e0200252.

18. Khan M, Saraswathi KS, Shyamala R et al. 2017. Placental abruption an obstetricians nightmare—a study of risk factors and maternofoetal outcomes at two tertiary care teaching hospitals in South India. *Asian Pacific J of Health Sci.* 4. 220–230.

19. Klar M, Michels KB. 2014. Cesarean section and placental disorders in subsequent pregnancies—a meta-analysis. *J Perinat Med.* 42:571.

20. Lavery JP. 1990. Placenta previa. *Clin Obstet Gynecol.* 33:414.

21. Lockwood CJ, Russo-Stieglitz K. 2020. Placenta previa: Management. Berghella V (Ed). *UpToDate.* Waltham, MA.

22. Naeye RL. 1980. Abruptio placenta and placenta previa: Frequency, perinatal mortality and cigarette smoking. *Obstet Gynecol.* 55:701-704.

23. Oyelese Y. 2010. Society for Maternal-Fetal Medicine. MFM consult: Evaluation and management of low-lying placenta or placenta previa on second-trimester ultrasound. *Contemp Ob/Gyn.* 30–33.

24. Oyelese Y, Smulian JC. 2006. Placenta previa, placenta accreta and vasa previa. Obstet Gynecol.107:927

25. Oyelese Y, Ananth CV. 2006. Placental abruption. *Obstet Gynecol.* 108:1005.

26. Reddy UM, Abuhamad AZ, Levine D et al. 2014. Fetal imaging: Executive summary of a joint Eunice Kennedy Shriver National Institute of Child Health and Human Development, Society for Maternal-Fetal Medicine, American Institute of Ultrasound in Medicine, American College of Obstetricians and Gynecologists, American College of Radiology, Society for Pediatric Radiology, and Society of Radiologists in Ultrasound Fetal Imaging workshop. *Obstet Gynecol.* 123:1070.

27. Riihimäki O, Paavonen J, Luukkaala T et al. 2017. Mortality and causes of death among women with a history of placental abruption. *Acta Obstet Gynecol Scand.* 96:1315.

28. Ruiter L, Eschbach SJ, Burgers M et al. 2016. Predictors for emergency cesarean delivery in women with placenta previa. *Am J Perinatol.* 33:1407.

29. Sekiguchi A, Nakai A, Kawabata I et al. 2013. Type and location of placenta previa affect preterm delivery risk related to antepartum hemorrhage. *Int J Med Sci.* 10:1683.

30. Sengodan SS, Dhanapal M. 2017. Abruptio placenta: A retrospective study on maternal and perinatal outcome. *Int J Reprod Contracept Obstet Gynecol.* 6:4389-92.

31. Sheiner E, Shoham-Vardi I, Hallak M et al. 2001. Placenta previa: Obstetric risk factors and pregnancy outcome. *J Matern Fetal Med.* 10:414.

32. Shinde GR, Vaswani BP, Patange RP et al. 2016. Diagnostic Performance of Ultrasonography for Detection of Abruption and its Clinical Correlation and Maternal and Foetal Outcome. *J Clin Diagn Res.*10:QC04.

33. Towers CV, Pircon RA, Heppard M. 1999. Is tocolysis safe in the management of third-trimester bleeding? *Am J Obstet Gynecol.* 180:1572.

34. Vahanian SA, Lavery JA, Ananth CV, Vintzileos A. 2015. Placental implantation abnormalities and risk of preterm delivery: A systematic review and meta-analysis. *Am J Obstet Gynecol.* 213:S78.

35. Wing DA, Paul RH, Millar LK. 1996. Management of the symptomatic placenta previa: A randomized, controlled trial of inpatient versus outpatient expectant management. *Am J Obstet Gynecol.* 175:806.

Chapter 32

Postpartum Hemorrhage

INTRODUCTION

- Obstetric hemorrhage is the world's leading cause of maternal mortality (Say et al., 2014). Approximately 127,000 women die of obstetric hemorrhage annually, accounting for 24 per cent of maternal deaths (WHO, 2007).
- Postpartum hemorrhage (PPH) is the most common type of obstetric hemorrhage and is the leading cause of maternal death in developing countries.
- The risk of maternal death from childbirth represents one of the greatest inequities in global health. While data are limited, studies have shown that PPH causes up to 60 per cent of all maternal deaths in developing countries.
- Even within developing countries, the risk of maternal death differs between women who have access to basic essential obstetrical care and those who do not.
- Women who survive severe postpartum hemorrhage experience significant morbidity, including problems caused by blood products, intensive care admission, further surgical interventions, infection, and prolonged hospitalisation (Zelop, 2011).

 Obstetric hemorrhage accounts for 25 per cent of the maternal mortality globally, and postpartum hemorrhage accounts for the majority of maternal deaths in developing countries.

DEFINITION

- **Postpartum hemorrhage is defined as bleeding that occurs within 24 hours after the birth process and that results in blood loss of ≥ 500 mL following a vaginal delivery and of ≥ 1000 mL following a cesarean section.**
- The World Health Organization (WHO) defines postpartum hemorrhage as blood loss of 500–1000 mL after vaginal delivery. When the blood loss is >1000 mL, it is defined as *severe PPH*.
- However, 30 per cent of women lose 500 mL or more of blood after a vaginal delivery with no consequences.
- Hence, the American College of Obstetricians and Gynecologists (2017) defined PPH as bleeding that occurs within 24 hours after the birth process and that results in the following:
  - A cumulative blood loss of greater than or equal to 1000 mL or
  - Signs or symptoms of hypovolemia
- Estimates of blood loss at delivery are quite often inaccurate, with significant underreporting being the rule. By the time the woman manifests tachycardia and hypotension, she may already have lost 25 per cent of her blood volume.

- Postpartum hemorrhage is further classified as follows:
  - **Primary PPH**, which occurs within 24 hours of delivery
  - **Secondary PPH**, which occurs between 24 hours and up to six weeks postpartum

Over the course of pregnancy, the plasma volume increases approximately 40 per cent and the red cell mass increases approximately 25 per cent (Chesley, 1972). This usually compensates for the blood loss that occurs at delivery. Unfortunately, in developing countries like India, pre-existing anemia and low basal blood volume may make the woman more susceptible to hemodynamic changes with even the usual amount of blood loss.

Primary PPH

Primary PPH is commonly due to abnormalities of one or more of the processes described in Table 32.1. The **4 Ts** mnemonic is used to summarise the principal causes.

Table 32.1   The '4 Ts' mnemonic (Anderson and Etches, 2007) for abnormalities leading to primary post-partum hemorrhage

4 Ts	Cause	Approximate incidence (%)
Tone	A non-contracting, atonic uterus	70
Tissue	• Retained products of conception • Adherent placenta	20
Trauma	• Genital tract lacerations and hematomas • Uterine rupture • Uterine inversion	10
Thrombin	Coagulation defects/abnormalities	1

Risk factors for primary PPH

- Investigators have tried to identify risk factors for the occurrence of primary PPH and found that it may occur unpredictably in women who have no apparent risk factor.
- Although the majority of postpartum hemorrhage is due to uterine atony, the rising incidence of cesarean delivery is leading to an increase in PPH due to retained placenta secondary to an abnormally adherent placenta (Silver et al., 2006).
- Obstetric risk factors for primary PPH include the following (Sheiner et al., 2005):
  - Induction of labour
  - Failure to progress during the second stage of labour
  - Instrumental delivery
  - Large-for-gestational age baby
  - Retained placenta/membranes
  - Morbidly adherent placenta
  - Lacerations
  - Hypertensive disorders (preeclampsia, eclampsia, HELLP syndrome [hemolysis, elevated liver enzymes, low platelets])

Secondary PPH

Secondary postpartum hemorrhage is commonly due to the following causes (Alexander et al., 2002):
- Abnormalities of placentation
  - Subinvolution of the placental site
  - Retained products of conception
  - Placenta accreta
- Infection
  - Endometritis, myometritis, parametritis
  - Infection/dehiscence of cesarean scar

PRIMARY POSTPARTUM HEMORRHAGE

ATONIC POSTPARTUM HEMORRHAGE

- Uterine atony or failure of the uterus to contract after delivery leads to atonic PPH. This accounts for 80 per cent of PPH (ACOG, 2017) and is the leading cause of maternal death.
- Myometrial contraction is responsible for placental separation and constriction of the blood vessels that supply the placental bed. In uterine atony, the myometrium fails to contract and retract effectively enough to occlude the spiral arterioles. This may result in uncontrolled, torrential bleeding. Clinically, the uterus feels flabby and relaxed.

Risk factors for atonic PPH

- Although there are known risk factors that may lead to atonic PPH (see box below), PPH is not always a predictable event.
- Women at high risk should be identified so that appropriate measures can be taken during labour. However, only 40 per cent of women with PPH following vaginal birth have an identifiable risk factor (Combs et al., 1991).
- Rouse and colleagues (2006) found that half the women who had atonic PPH after a primary cesarean section had no risk factors.

Risk factors for atonic PPH

Antepartum risk factors
- Overdistended uterus (hydramnios, twins, macrosomia)
- Placenta previa
- Obesity (BMI >35 kg/m²)
- Uterine abnormalities/fibroids

- Previous PPH
- Asian ethnicity
- Anemia (<9 g/dL)

Intrapartum risk factors
- Prolonged labour
- Prolonged use of oxytocin
- Precipitate labour
- Retained placental bits
- Halogenated anesthetics

Prevention of atonic PPH

Obstetric units should establish protocols for categorising women admitted to the labour room by the risk factors listed in the box below. This further helps identify the women for whom blood should be reserved.

Active management of the third stage of labour (AMTSL)

- The most effective method of preventing atonic PPH is the active management of the third stage of labour.
- A systematic review of the Cochrane Database (Begley et al., 2019) showed that active management reduced the risk of severe primary PPH (>1000 mL) at the time of birth, and also reduced the number of women with a postpartum hemoglobin of <9 gm/dL. These benefits were best demonstrated in women at high-risk for PPH. The benefit of these interventions in women at low risk for PPH is uncertain.
- AMTSL consists of the following set of interventions:
  - **Administration of uterotonics** (see box below)
    - This is the most important and useful part of AMTSL. Uterotonics should be administered at every birth.
    - Oxytocin is administered either as an intramuscular injection (10 units IM) or an IV infusion (10–20 units in 500 mL of saline). It is the uterotonic of choice (Mousa et al., 2014).

      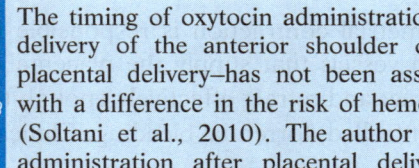 The timing of oxytocin administration–with delivery of the anterior shoulder or with placental delivery–has not been associated with a difference in the risk of hemorrhage (Soltani et al., 2010). The author prefers administration after placental delivery to reduce the risk of a retained placenta.

    - A network meta-analysis of the Cochrane Database (Gallos et al., 2018) concluded that a combination of ergometrine and oxytocin, or a combination of misoprostol and oxytocin may have some additional desirable effects over the current standard oxytocin.

Uterotonics
The following (in order of preference) are recommended as the most effective uterotonics for the prevention of PPH in all births (WHO, 2018; Gallos et al., 2018):
1. Oxytocin 10 units IM/IV
2. Oxytocin 10 units IM/IV + ergometrine (0.2 mg)/IV
3. Oxytocin 10 units IM/IV + misoprostol 400–600 mg orally, sublingually or 800–1000 mg rectally
- *Ergometrine is not effective by itself in preventing PPH. It should be avoided in women with hypertensive disorders.*
- *Misoprostol is the choice of drug when no injectable uterotonics are available and can be administered by a community health worker or even self-administered in a low-resource setting. It is associated with vomiting.*
- *Injectable prostaglandins are not effective as prophylaxis for preventing PPH. They are only effective for the treatment of atonic PPH.*

- In many developing countries including India, poor storage conditions and absence of cold chain facilities contribute to limited access to and utilisation of uterotonic drugs. The storage of oxytocin and ergometrine can be particularly challenging due to their instability in high temperatures and sensitivity to light.

- In low-resource settings, unskilled birth attendants may not be able to administer injectable uterotonics.

— **Controlled cord traction** for the delivery of the placenta has limited benefits for the prevention of PPH but does reduce the duration of the second stage (Hofmeyr et al., 2015).

— **Uterine massage** as a part of AMTSL has been recommended by some authors (Berghella, 2021) and is practiced by many obstetricians, but there are no randomised controlled studies that have proven its benefit in the prevention of PPH.

Management of atonic PPH

Well-established protocols should be in place in the labour room for the management of atonic PPH.

Assessing the severity of PPH

- Clinical assessment of the bleeding notoriously underestimates the amount of bleeding.
- Interpreting the signs and symptoms of PPH (Table 32.2) helps in identifying the magnitude of the problem.
- Excessive bleeding leading to hypovolemia (due to both inadequate hemoglobin level and circulatory volume) may lead to the following:
  - Tachypnea
  - Tachycardia
  - Hypotension
  - Low oxygen saturation
  - Air hunger
- In women who enter labour with pre-existing anemia and/or low blood volume, the signs and symptoms will manifest with a lesser volume of blood loss since they do not have the reserves to compensate for even the normal blood loss associated with delivery.

Table 32.2 Signs and symptoms associated with blood loss from postpartum hemorrhage

Blood loss in mL (% of normal blood volume)	Systolic blood pressure	Signs and symptoms
500–1000 (10–15%)	Normal	Palpitations, light-headedness, mild increase in heart rate
1000–1500 (15–25%)	Slightly low	Weakness, sweating, tachycardia (100–120 beats/minute)
1500–2000 (25–35%)	70–80 mmHg	Restlessness, confusion, pallor, oliguria, tachycardia (120–140 beats/minute)
2000–3000 (35–45%)	50–70 mmHg	Lethargy, air hunger, anuria, collapse, tachycardia (>140 beats/minute)

General measures

- **Calling for help:** Senior doctors, midwives, and nurses should be asked to come and assist in the resuscitation. The anesthetist, the theatre personnel, and the blood bank must be alerted.

- **Monitoring maternal vital signs:** Monitoring of the mother's pulse, blood pressure, and respiratory rate should be done concomitantly with investigation of the cause and measures to arrest the bleeding.

 The mother should be reassured at all times and the procedures being carried out should be explained to her in simple language.

- **Intravenous (IV) lines:** It is prudent to have two IV lines. If the mother already has an IV line in place, another should be started on the other arm, preferably with a blood set.
  - The IVs should be started with 16–18 gauge needles to facilitate large volume fluid infusions.

- **Laboratory investigations:** While starting the IV line, blood should be drawn for the following:
  - Complete blood count including platelet count
  - Blood group and type (if not on the medical record)
  - Cross-matching for at least four units of blood
  - Coagulation profile (including fibrinogen concentration, prothrombin time, activated partial thromboplastin time)

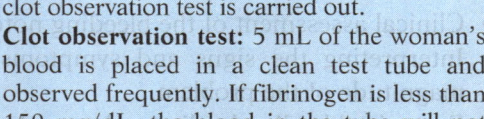 In low-resource areas, coagulation profile may not be available as a test. In such a situation, a clot observation test is carried out.
Clot observation test: 5 mL of the woman's blood is placed in a clean test tube and observed frequently. If fibrinogen is less than 150 mg/dL, the blood in the tube will not clot, or if it does, it will undergo partial or complete dissolution in 30–60 minutes.

- **Fluids for resuscitation:**
  - Isotonic crystalloids (normal saline or Ringer's lactate solution) should be infused to prevent hypotension (WHO, 2012). The goal should be to maintain the following parameters:
    - Systolic blood pressure at ≥90 mmHg
    - Urine output at >30 mL/hour

 Rapid infusion of large volumes of crystalloid (e.g., >3 to 4 L) may lead to dilutional coagulopathy and electrolyte imbalances, so careful monitoring is essential.

  - *Blood and blood product replacement* should be initiated as early as possible. It is essential to rapidly replace lost platelets and coagulation factors in order to avoid coagulopathy (see section below on *Resuscitation and the role of transfusion therapy in PPH*).

- **Urine output:** A Foley catheter should be inserted to monitor urine output.

 Women with preeclampsia are prone to have a contracted intravascular volume and therefore tissue hypoperfusion is difficult to overcome in hemorrhagic shock.

Pharmacological measures

- **Uterotonics** are the first line of management of atonic PPH (Table 32.3).
    - **Oxytocin** should always be offered as the first drug of choice.
        - An IV infusion of 500 mL of normal saline containing 20 units of oxytocin is started.
    - **Ergometrine** or an **oxytocin–ergometrine combination** should be offered as the second line of treatment.
    - **Injectable prostaglandin** ($PGF_{2\alpha}$) should be offered as the third line of treatment if bleeding continues despite oxytocin and ergometrine.
    - **Rectal misoprostol** (PGE_1) may be considered in the absence of injectable uterotonics because of its ease of administration and low cost. 800–1000 µg is administered rectally. Misoprostol may also be administered sublingually or orally at a dose of 400–800 µg.
- **Tranexamic acid** was found by the WOMAN trial (2017) to reduce death due to bleeding in women with postpartum hemorrhage, with no adverse effects. The WHO has adopted this recommendation. A recent study (Sentilhes et al., 2021) found that among women who underwent cesarean delivery and received prophylactic uterotonic agents, tranexamic acid treatment resulted in a significantly lower incidence of both calculated estimated blood loss > 1000 mL and blood transfusion.
    - Tranexamic acid reverses the fibrinolysis and depletion of fibrinogen that occur in the early stages of atonic and traumatic PPH.
    - The drug should be administered within 3 hours of a vaginal delivery to be effective. At a cesarean section in women at high risk of PPH, the recommendation is that tranexamic acid be administered just before the skin incision (Berghella, 2021).
    - *Dose and route:* Tranexamic acid 1 g is added to 100 mL of normal saline and infused IV over 10–20 minutes (at the rate of 1 mL/minute; faster infusions may result in

Table 32.3   Uterotonics used in the management of atonic postpartum hemorrhage

Drug	Dose/route	Frequency	Comment
Oxytocin	IV infusion: 10–20 units in 500 mL of normal saline or Ringer's lactate	Continuous	Avoid undiluted rapid IV infusion, which causes hypotension
Methylergometrine	IV: 0.2 mg	Every 2–4 hours	Avoid if the mother is hypertensive
$PGF_{2\alpha}$	IM: 0.25 mg	Every 15–90 minutes for a maximum of 8 doses	• Avoid in women with asthma, hepatic, renal, or cardiac disease • Diarrhea, fever, tachycardia may occur
Misoprostol (PGE_1)	400–800 µg sublingually or 800–1000 µg rectally	Single dose	• Used only if injectable uterotonics are not available • Rectal misoprostol takes up to 1 hour to act but its effect lasts longer

IM, intramuscularly; *IV*, intravenously; *PG*, prostaglandin

hypotension). If bleeding persists after 30 minutes, a second dose of 1 g may be infused.

Mechanical measures

The following mechanical measures are useful in the management of atonic PPH:
- Massaging the fundus
- Bimanual uterine compression
  The bladder should be emptied by catheterisation to facilitate uterine contraction.

Fundal massage

Gentle fundal massage stimulates the atonic uterus to contract. Massage should be continued while other interventions are being initiated and maintained until the uterus remains firm and bleeding has decreased or stopped.

Bimanual uterine compression

This is a simple, and usually effective, method of controlling bleeding from an atonic uterus. A hand on the abdomen massages the posterior aspect of the uterus while the fist of the other hand is in the vagina pushing against the anterior aspect of the uterus (Figure 32.1).

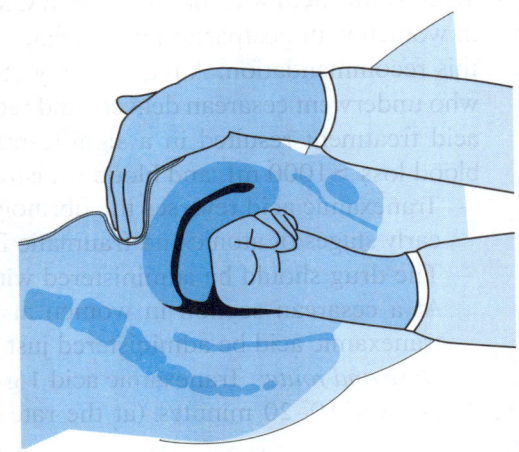

Tamponade techniques

Tamponade of the uterus can be attempted when uterotonics and massage fail to control bleeding. Both packing with gauze and balloon tamponade are recommended.

Figure 32.1   Bimanual uterine compression. The uterus is compressed between the operator's two hands.

Uterine packing

- Packing the uterus with gauze has made a limited comeback as an effective way of controlling PPH.
- Uterovaginal packing may be used to gain time to stabilise the mother while arranging for a surgical procedure or transporting her to a tertiary centre.

Uterine tamponade is particularly useful in controlling hemorrhage from uterine atony, and placental site bleeding caused by placenta previa or placenta accreta (Maier, 1993, Hsu et al., 2003).

- A long 4-inch gauze is layered tightly from side to side in the uterine cavity, beginning at the fundus and leaving no dead space. A Foley catheter is placed in the bladder, which helps avoid urinary retention while also monitoring urine output.
- Uterine balloon tamponade has replaced this procedure in most centres though it may still be useful in a low-resource facility.

Balloon tamponade

- Inserting an intrauterine balloon tamponade may help arrest the bleeding and provide time to transfer the mother to a tertiary centre.
- **Bakri balloon** is commercially available in India, though it is expensive. It consists of a silicone balloon connected to a 24 French silicone catheter. The collapsed balloon is inserted into the uterus and then filled with 500 mL of saline. When inflated with fluid, the balloon fills the uterine cavity and provides pressure against the vessels in the uterine wall.
- **Multiple Foley catheters** inserted into the uterine cavity have been used with the same effect.
- **Condom catheters** have been used in low-resource areas. A condom is placed over the end of a Foley catheter or a simple rubber catheter. A sterile suture is tightly tied around the base of the condom to prevent leakage. The tube with the condom is inserted into the uterine cavity and then the condom is filled with 500–600 mL of saline via the catheter. A vaginal pack is inserted to retain the tube in the vagina.
  - However, a recent study from low- and middle-income countries (Anger et al., 2019) concluded that *the introduction of condom-catheters in these settings did not improve maternal outcomes*. In fact, it was associated with an increase in the combined incidence of PPH-related surgery and maternal death because of a delay in management.

Surgical techniques for uterine atony

Surgical intervention is the next logical step when initial measures and uterine balloon tamponade fail. The woman is shifted to the operating theatre. Adequate blood and blood products must be kept available. The surgical options are as follows:
- Uterine compression sutures
  - B-Lynch suture
  - Other modifications
- Arterial ligation
  - Uterine artery ligation and stepwise devascularisation
  - Internal iliac artery ligation
- Hysterectomy

Uterine compression sutures

The B-Lynch technique and its modifications have been used successfully in atonic PPH. The suture compresses the anterior and posterior atonic walls of the uterus, achieving hemostasis.

B-Lynch compression suture

- The B-Lynch suture, also known as the 'brace suture', was described by B-Lynch and co-workers in 1997 as an The B-Lynch compression suture is simple, safe and life-saving and also preserves fertility.

alternative surgical method for controlling PPH due to uterine atony.

- The sutures compress the anterior and posterior atonic walls of the uterus, achieving hemostasis.
- **Materials:**
  - A large (70 mm), round-bodied, Mayo needle or a straight needle
  - #1 or # 2 chromic catgut (or any absorbable suture); using a thicker suture prevents breakage
- **Technique** (Figure 32.2):
  - The procedure is done under general anesthesia.
  - The woman is catheterised and placed in the dorsolithotomy position. This position allows an assistant to objectively evaluate bleeding from the vagina and assess whether it has been controlled at the end of the procedure.
  - The abdomen is opened by a low transverse incision if the mother has had a vaginal delivery. If the delivery was by a cesarean section, the same incision is reopened.
  - The uterovesical fold of the peritoneum is incised transversely and the bladder pushed down gently.
  - A lower segment incision is made, or sutures of a recent cesarean section are removed, and the uterine cavity is examined and swabbed out.
  - The uterus is exteriorised and rechecked to identify any bleeding points. A bimanual compression is first tried to assess the potential chance of success of the technique.
  - The needle with the suture is passed 3 cm from the right lower edge of the uterine incision and 3 cm from the right lateral border (point A in Figure 32.2). The catgut is re-threaded through the uterine cavity to emerge at the upper incision margin 3 cm above and 4 cm from the lateral border (point B) and is passed over to compress the uterine fundus approximately 3–4 cm from the right cornual border. The catgut is fed posteriorly and vertically to enter the posterior wall of the uterine cavity at the same level as the upper anterior entry point (point C). The suture is pulled under moderate tension along with bimanual compression exerted by the first assistant. The length of the catgut is passed back posteriorly through the same surface marking on the left side (point D). The suture is now passed over the left uterine cornu and passed through point E and point F of the anterior uterine wall.
  - The two lengths of suture are pulled taut, assisted by bimanual compression to minimise trauma and to aid compression, during which the vagina is checked for control of bleeding. The two ends are then knotted and tied.
  - The uterine incision is closed after ensuring control of vaginal bleeding.

Other compression sutures

- Various modifications of the B-Lynch suture have been introduced. However, no technique has been proven significantly more effective than another (Kayem et al., 2011).
- Transverse and vertical sutures are placed in the *Pereira technique* and multiple vertical sutures are used in the *Hayman technique*.

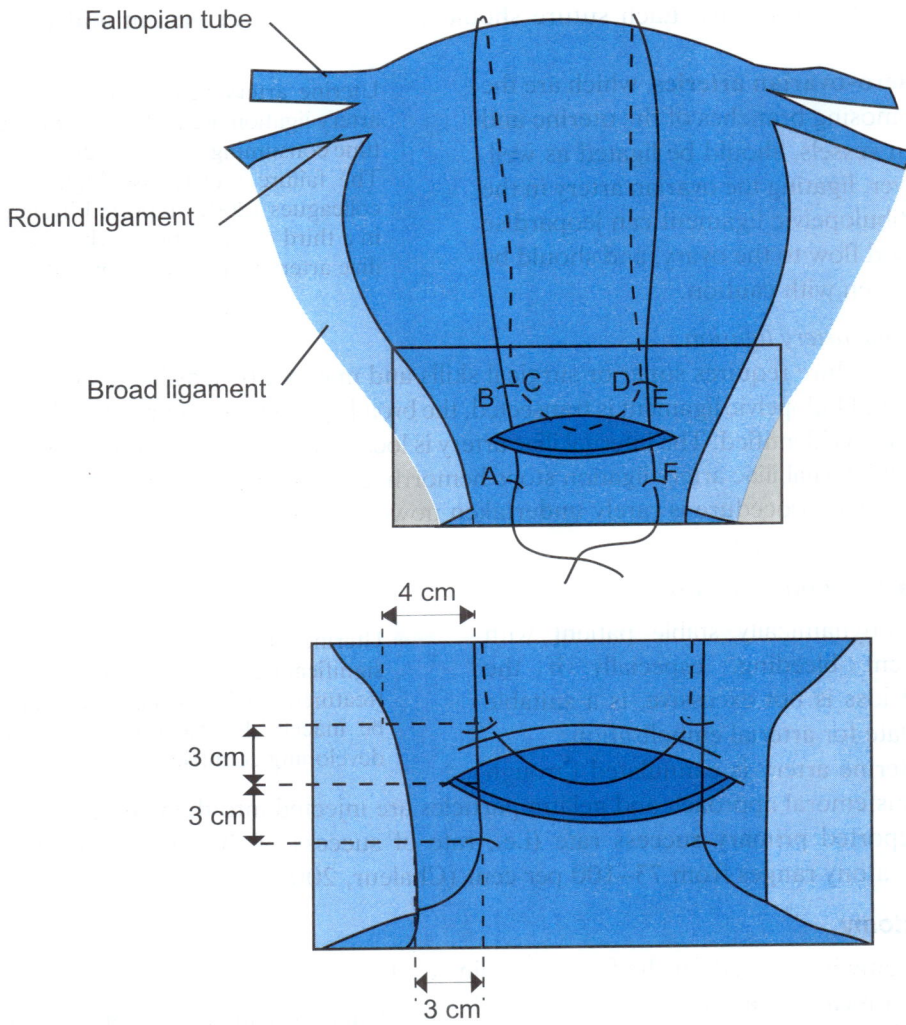

Figure 32.2 The B-Lynch uterine compression suture technique.

Arterial ligation

Arterial ligation may not completely control bleeding from an atonic uterus but will decrease bleeding and facilitate other interventions.

Uterine artery ligation and stepwise devascularisation

- Ligation of the **uterine arteries** decreases perfusion pressure in the myometrium. The *O'Leary technique* (O'Leary, 1995) involves ligating the uterine artery as it turns upward in the broad ligament, at the level of the uterovesical peritoneal reflection. Care should be taken to avoid the ureter.
- With continued bleeding, the **ascending uterine artery** is ligated bilaterally at intervals as it ascends in the broad ligament. This reduces the blood flow through the branches

that supply the uterus. Each suture should include the myometrium and the uterine vessel.

- The **utero-ovarian arteries**, which are the anastomosing branches of the uterine and ovarian vessels, should be ligated as well. However, ligating the ovarian artery in the infundibulopelvic ligament can jeopardise the blood flow to the ovary, and should be undertaken with caution.

 Uterine artery ligation and internal iliac artery ligation are technically difficult and time consuming in an already sick woman. The failure rate is also high. Joshi and colleagues (2007) reported hysterectomy in a third of the patients who had internal iliac artery ligation for atonic PPH.

Internal iliac artery ligation

- This procedure requires superior surgical skills and may not be feasible in an emergency.
- The infundibulopelvic ligament is transected, the broad ligament is opened, and the common iliac vessel is identified. The internal iliac artery is located and the anterior division is ligated. Bilateral internal iliac artery ligation stops hemorrhage in 80 per cent of cases.
- This surgical procedure is rarely undertaken now and has been replaced by the B-Lynch compression technique.

Uterine artery embolisation

- A hemodynamically stable patient with persistent bleeding, especially if the rate of loss is not excessive, is a suitable candidate for arterial embolisation.
- The uterine artery is cannulated through

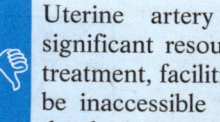 Uterine artery embolisation requires significant resources in terms of cost of treatment, facilities and training, and may be inaccessible to most obstetricians in developing countries.

the transfemoral approach and gelatin particles are injected into the vessel.
- The reported primary success rate (i.e., rate of success of the first embolisation) for uterine atony ranges from 73–100 per cent (Chaleur, 2008).

Hysterectomy

Hysterectomy is reserved for the following clinical situations:

- All other measures available have been tried and failed.
- Bleeding continues with a woman in severe hypovolemic shock.

 In most instances, a subtotal hysterectomy is adequate. It is quicker, simpler, safer and associated with less blood loss.

 Vaginal delivery and a delay between delivery and uterine suture placement of 2–6 hours have been found to be significantly associated with an increased risk of hysterectomy (Kayem et al., 2011).

TRAUMATIC POSTPARTUM HEMORRHAGE

- Bleeding from genital tract injuries is referred to as traumatic PPH. This is the second most common cause of PPH. Unlike atonic PPH where the bleeding could be profuse or torrential, traumatic PPH is usually associated with a continuous trickle of fresh blood. The uterus is well contracted.

- The common injuries that give rise to hemorrhage are as follows:
  - Lower genital tract
    - Perineal lacerations
    - Vaginal lacerations
    - Cervical tears
    - Vulvar hematoma
  - Upper genital tract
    - Uterine rupture
    - Broad ligament/retroperitoneal hematoma
- Lower genital tract injuries are often associated with the following risk factors:
  - Episiotomy
  - Instrumental delivery
  - Malpresentations, e.g., breech presentation
  - Fetal macrosomia
  - Shoulder dystocia
  - Prior surgery on the cervix, including cerclage and conisation

Identifying the source of bleeding

- Once atonic PPH is ruled out by the presence of a firm, well-contracted uterus, a meticulous examination must be carried out to identify the source of bleeding. Occasionally, more than one laceration may be present. It is essential to recognise all lacerations and tears.

 The mother must be positioned in stirrups for proper visualisation of the cervix and vagina. Good lighting and proper instruments must be utilised to carefully assess the lower genital tract.

- It is good clinical practice to shift the mother to the operation theatre where it is easier to place her in the dorsolithotomy position, the necessary lighting is available and, in extensive injury, anesthesia is readily administered.
- The suggested protocol for identifying the source of bleeding is as follows:
  - The perineum is inspected carefully for lacerations. Paraureteral tears may bleed out of proportion to the size of the tear since they occur in a very vascular area.
  - A speculum should then be inserted into the vagina for inspection of the vaginal walls and cervix. A second speculum placed in the anterior fornix is invaluable for proper visualisation.
  - Using a folded gauze in a sponge-holding forceps to push up the cervix, the vaginal walls should be carefully inspected all the way up to the fornices.
  - The cervix should then be carefully inspected for the presence of tears.
    - Two sponge-holding forceps are applied on the lips of the cervix, beginning anteriorly, at a distance of approximately 2 cm from each other.
    - The forceps are moved systematically around the circumference of the cervical lips. The part of the cervix between the two sponge-holding forceps should be inspected for tears.

- Vulvar hematoma may present as a fluctuant, discoloured swelling at the vulva that occurs after a vaginal delivery. It is associated with excruciating pain, urinary retention, and rectal pain. The mother may experience a persistent sensation of wanting to pass motion. A recto-vaginal examination will reveal a mass pushing into the vagina as well as the rectum. Hypovolemic shock may occur when the bleeding goes unnoticed.
- In the presence of shock without external hemorrhage, there should be a high suspicion for broad ligament or retroperitoneal hematoma.

Management of traumatic PPH

Perineal and vaginal lacerations/tears

- Perineal lacerations are sutured in layers in the same way as an episiotomy.
- Vaginal lacerations are commonly seen in the lower 2/3rds of the vagina, on the posterolateral walls. The upper 1/3rd of the vagina is less commonly involved. If the laceration is seen to extend upwards, the fornices must be meticulously inspected and the suturing should start above the apex of the tear. A vaginal tear extending into the fornix may be associated with a broad ligament or retroperitoneal hematoma.

Cervical lacerations/tears

- Cervical lacerations commonly occur at the 9 o'clock and 3 o'clock positions.
- Hemorrhage from cervical lacerations usually arises from the apex and edges.

The repair of perineal and cervical lacerations is discussed in detail in **Chapter 16**, *Prevention and repair of perineal trauma occurring in childbirth*.

Hematomas

- Small **vulvar hematomas** can be treated conservatively.
- **Expanding hematomas** with hemodynamic instability require surgical intervention. They should be opened, bleeding points should be secured and the dead space should be approximated with figure-of-eight sutures.
- **Broad ligament** or **retroperitoneal hematomas** are suspected when the hemodynamic instability is out of proportion to the external bleeding. A laparotomy is required to evacuate the hematoma and control the bleeding. A partial or complete rupture in the lower uterine segment should be looked for.

OTHER CAUSES OF POSTPARTUM HEMORRHAGE

Postpartum hemorrhage may also result from the following causes:
- Retained placenta
- Uterine inversion
- Uterine rupture

Uterine rupture and uterine inversion are discussed in detail in **Chapter 30**, *Obstetric emergencies*.

Retained placenta

- The placenta is said to be retained if it has not been expelled within 30 minutes of the delivery of the fetus.
- Retained placenta affects 0.6–3.3 per cent of normal deliveries.
- The risk of hemorrhage rises after 30 minutes have elapsed and the possibility of spontaneous delivery of the placenta after 60 minutes is non-existent.
- PPH may also result from a portion of the placenta or membranes being retained in the uterine cavity. After each delivery, the placenta should be placed on a flat surface and visually inspected for completeness. Even when the placenta appears intact, there may be additional remaining products of conception (e.g., succenturiate lobe) within the uterine cavity that may result in PPH.

Management of retained placenta

- If, despite controlled cord traction and the administration of uterotonics, the placenta is not delivered, manual extraction of the placenta should be offered as the definitive treatment.
- Injection of oxytocin, saline or $PGF_{2\alpha}$ into the umbilical vein has not been shown to be effective in reducing the need for manual removal of the placenta.
- The uterine cavity should be explored manually to rule out a retained portion of the placenta or membranes. The placenta accreta spectrum may also result in retained placenta. The management of postpartum hemorrhage is summarised in Figure 32.3.

RESUSCITATION AND THE ROLE OF TRANSFUSION THERAPY IN PPH

- In postpartum hemorrhage, maternal vital signs typically do not change severely until significant blood loss has occurred.
- If the obstetric team is not alert and fails to initiate adequate early resuscitation, the resulting hypoperfusion may lead to the following complications (Patil and Shetmahajan, 2014):
  - Lactic acidosis
  - Systemic inflammatory response syndrome (SIRS) with accompanying multiorgan dysfunction
  - Coagulopathy (disseminated intravascular coagulation)
  Left unattended, these complications lead to potentially preventable deaths.
- Hemoglobin levels will fall by approximately 1 g/dL for every 500 mL of blood loss. However, in PPH, the initial blood counts may not reflect this accurately.

Resuscitation measures

The RCOG Greentop-Guideline No. 52 (Mavrides et al., RCOG 2016) recommends the following:

In minor PPH (blood loss 500–1000 mL) without clinical shock

- Establish intravenous access with a large bore (16–18 gauge) cannula.
- Initiate infusion with crystalloid solution (0.9% normal saline or lactated Ringer's solution).
- Continue monitoring maternal vital signs every 15 minutes.

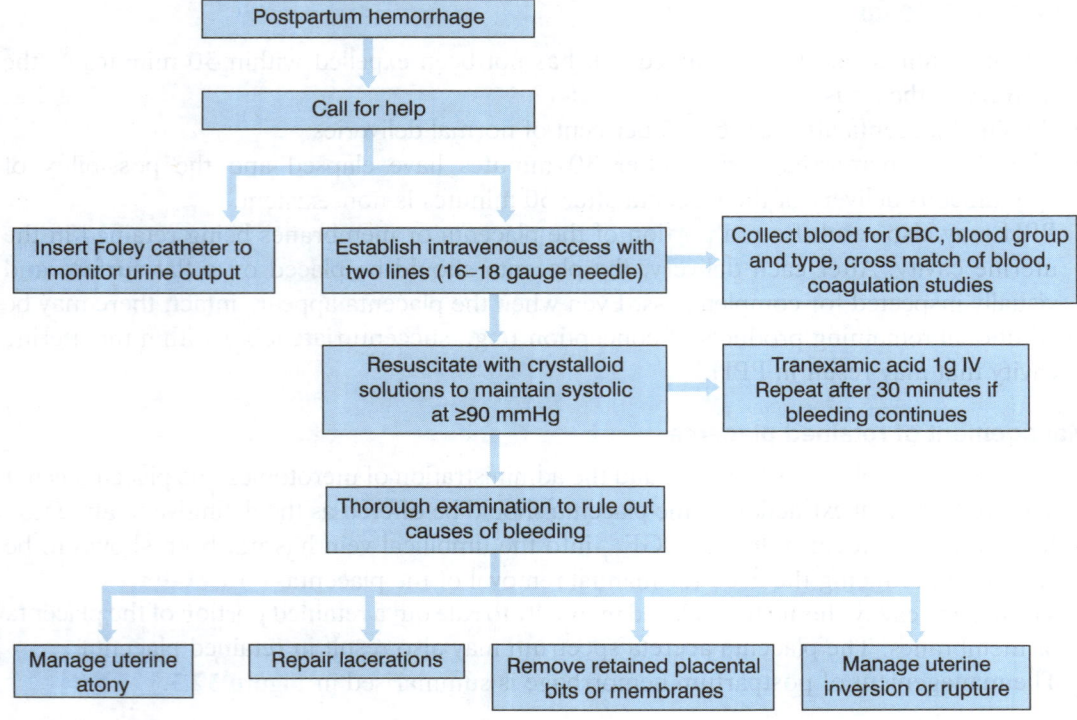

Figure 32.3 Algorithm for the management of postpartum hemorrhage.
CBC, complete blood count

In major PPH (blood loss greater than 1000 mL) and continued bleeding or clinical shock

- Compromise of airway and breathing must be assessed and corrected.
- Blood pressure and pulse rate must be monitored continuously.

 Restoration of both blood volume and oxygen-carrying capacity are vital in this situation.

- Oxygen should be administered by mask or nasal prongs at 10–15 litres/minute.
- The head end of the table should be flat. The head should not be propped up.
- The patient should be kept warm with blankets.
- Blood should be transfused as soon as possible.
- Until blood is available, up to 3.5 litres of fluids should be infused.
  - The initial 2 litres should be isotonic crystalloid.
  - Further fluid resuscitation can continue with additional isotonic crystalloid or colloid (succinylated gelatin). **Hydroxyethyl starch should not be used**.

Transfusion therapy

- All hospitals should have protocols in place for blood transfusion in PPH.

- When good blood bank facilities are available, massive blood transfusion is recommended as part of the management of severe PPH. It is defined as the transfusion of 4 units of packed red blood cells within 1 hour, when ongoing need for more blood is anticipated.
- Though there is not adequate evidence for the quantity of blood component therapy in obstetric hemorrhage, the consensus opinion is that the initial transfusion ratio for packed *red blood cells: fresh frozen plasma: platelets* be in the range of 1:1:1 (ACOG, 2017). This is designed to mimic replacement of whole blood.

SECONDARY POSTPARTUM HEMORRHAGE

- Secondary postpartum hemorrhage is defined as excessive bleeding that occurs more than 24 hours after delivery and up to 12 weeks postpartum.
- This may occur in approximately 2 per cent of pregnancies in developed countries. Data are not available from developing countries (Alexander et al., 2002).

CAUSES OF SECONDARY PPH

- Uterine atony (perhaps secondary to retained products of conception) may contribute to secondary PPH.
- Uterine infection (endometritis) may result in bleeding. The presence of uterine tenderness and a low-grade fever should raise a strong suspicion of this condition.

TREATMENT OF SECONDARY PPH

- Treatment depends on the etiology of the hemorrhage.
- Uterotonics, in combination with antibiotics, are usually indicated.
- Gentle uterine curettage with a broad curette may be indicated when retained products of conception are suspected.

Antibiotic regimens for the management of secondary PPH

- Postpartum endometritis is commonly a polymicrobial infection with the involvement of two to three aerobes and anaerobes.
- The current recommendation for the treatment of endometritis leading to PPH is as follows (Mackeen et al., 2015):
  - Clindamycin 900 mg every 8 hours plus gentamicin 5 mg/kg every 24 hours (preferred) or 1.5 mg/kg every 8 hours (without a loading dose)
  - The usual duration of treatment is 72 hours
  - Cephalosporins may also be used but are less effective

References

1. Alexander J, Thomas P, Sanghera J. 2002. Treatments for secondary haemorrhage. *Cochrane Database Syst Rev.* Issue 1. Art. no.: CD002867.

3. American College of Obstetricians and Gynecologists. 2017. Postpartum hemorrhage. *Obstet Gynecol.* 130:e168–86.

4. Anderson JM, Etches D. 2007. Prevention and management of postpartum hemorrhage. *Am Fam Physician.* 2007. 75:875–82.

5. Anger HA, Dabash R, Durocher J et al. 2019. The effectiveness and safety of introducing condom-catheter uterine balloon tamponade for postpartum haemorrhage at secondary level hospitals in Uganda, Egypt and Senegal: A stepped wedge, cluster-randomised trial. *BJOG.* 126:1612.

6. Begley CM, Gyte GM, Devane D et al. 2019. Active versus expectant management for women in the third stage of labour. *Cochrane Database Syst Rev.* Issue 2. Art. no.: CD007412.

7. Berghella V. 2021. Management of the third stage of labor: Prophylactic drug therapy to minimize hemorrhage. Lockwood CJ (Ed). *UpToDate.* Waltham, MA.

8. B-Lynch C, Coker A, Lawal AH, Abu J, Cowen MJ. 1997. The B-Lynch surgical technique for the control of massive postpartum haemorrhage: An alternative to hysterectomy? Five cases reported. *BJOG.* 104:372–5.

9. Chauleur C, Fanget C, Tourne G et al. Serious primary post-partum hemorrhage, arterial embolization and future fertility: A retrospective study of 46 cases. *Hum Reprod.* 2008; 23:1553.

10. Chesley LC. 1972. Plasma and red cell volumes during pregnancy. *Am J Obstet Gynecol.* 112:440–50

11. Combs CA, Murphy EL, Laros RK Jr. 1991. Factors associated with postpartum hemorrhage with vaginal birth. *Obstet Gynecol.* 77:69–76.

12. Gallos ID, Papadopoulou A, Man R et al. 2018. Uterotonic agents for preventing postpartum haemorrhage: A network meta-analysis. *Cochrane Database Syst Rev.* Issue 12. Art. no.: CD011689.

13. Hofmeyr GJ, Mshweshwe NT, Gülmezoglu AM. 2015. Controlled cord traction for the third stage of labour. *Cochrane Database Syst Rev.* Issue 1. Art. no.:CD008020.

14. Hsu S, Rodgers B, Lele A, Yeh J. 2003. Use of packing in obstetric hemorrhage of uterine origin. *J Reprod Med.* 48:69–71.

15. Kayem G, Kurinczuk JJ, Alfirevic Z et al. 2011. Uterine compression sutures for the management of severe postpartum hemorrhage. *Obstet Gynecol.* 117:14.

16. Mackeen AD, Packard RE, Ota E, Speer L. 2015. Antibiotic regimens for postpartum endometritis. *Cochrane Database Syst Rev.* Issue 2. Art. no.: CD001067.

17. Maier RC. 1993. Control of postpartum hemorrhage with uterine packing. *Am J Obstet Gynecol.* 169:317–321.

18. Mavrides E, Allard S, Chandraharan E et al., on behalf of the Royal College of Obstetricians and Gynaecologists. 2016. Prevention and management of postpartum haemorrhage. *BJOG.* 124: e106–e149.

19. Mousa HA, Blum J, Abou El Senoun G et al. 2014. Treatment for primary postpartum haemorrhage. *Cochrane Database Syst Rev.* Issue 2. Art. no.: CD003249.

20. O'Leary JA. 1995. Uterine artery ligation in the control of post-cesarean hemorrhage. *J Reprod Med.* 40(3):189–93.

21. Patil V, Shetmahajan M. 2014. Massive transfusion and massive transfusion protocol. *Indian J Anaesth.* 58:590–5.

22. Rouse DJ, MacPherson C, Landon M et al. 2006. Blood transfusion and cesarean delivery. *Obstet Gynecol.* 108:891.

23. Say L, Chou D, Gemmill A, Tuncalp O, Moller AB, Daniels J et al. 2014. Global causes of maternal death: A WHO systematic analysis. *Lancet Glob Health.* 2:e323–33.

24. Sentilhes L, Sénat MV, Le Lous M et al. 2021. Tranexamic acid for the prevention of blood loss after cesarean delivery. *N Engl J Med.* 384:1623.

25. Sheiner E, Sarid L, Levy A et al. 2005. Obstetric risk factors and outcome of pregnancies complicated with early postpartum hemorrhage: A population-based study. *J Matern Fetal Neonatal Med.* 18:149.

26. Silver RM, Landon MB, Rouse DT, Leveno KJ, Spong CY, Thom EA et al. 2006. Maternal morbidity associated with multiple repeat cesarean deliveries. *Obstet Gynecol.* 107:1226–32.

27. Soltani H, Hutchon DR, Poulose TA. 2010. Timing of prophylactic uterotonics for the third stage of labour after vaginal birth. *Cochrane Database Syst Rev.* Issue 8. Art. No.: CD006173.

28. WOMAN Trial Collaborators. 2017. Effect of early tranexamic acid administration on mortality, hysterectomy, and other morbidities in women with post-partum haemorrhage (WOMAN): An international, randomised, double-blind, placebo-controlled trial. Lancet.

29. World Health Organization. 2007. Reducing the global burden: postpartum haemorrhage. Making Pregnancy Safer. WHO, Geneva.

30. World Health Organization. 2012. WHO recommendations for the prevention and treatment of postpartum haemorrhage. WHO, Geneva.

31. World Health Organization. 2018. WHO recommendations: Uterotonics for the prevention of postpartum haemorrhage. WHO, Geneva.

32. Zelop CM. 2011. Postpartum hemorrhage: Becoming more evidence-based. *Obstet Gynecol.*

Chapter 33

Preterm Labour and Preterm Prelabour Rupture of Membranes

PRETERM LABOUR

INTRODUCTION

- Preterm labour is the onset of uterine contractions associated with cervical effacement and dilatation prior to 37 weeks' gestational age. **Preterm birth** (PTB) is defined as infants born alive before 37 completed weeks of gestation.
- Based on **gestational age**, preterm birth is categorised as follows:
  - Extremely preterm   : <28 weeks
  - Very preterm   : 28–31^{+6} weeks
  - Moderate to late preterm   : 32–36^{+6} weeks
- Preterm birth can also be categorised based on the **infant's birth weight**, as follows:
  - Low birth weight (LBW)   : <2500 g
  - Very low birth weight (VLBW)   : <1500 g
  - Extremely low birth weight (ELBW) : <1000 g
- Though more than 60 per cent of preterm births occur in Africa and South Asia, preterm birth is a global problem. In developing countries, approximately 12 per cent of babies are born preterm; the incidence is 9 per cent in developed countries. Within countries, families belonging to the lower socio-economic classes are at higher risk of preterm birth.
- India has the largest number of preterm births in the world with approximately 3.5 million preterm births in 2010 (Blencowe et al., 2012).
- The survival rate for preterm infants born in low-income countries differs dramatically from those born in high-income countries. In low-income settings, 50 per cent of infants born at or below 32 weeks die due to the lack of feasible, cost-effective care, including factors such as warmth, breastfeeding support, and basic care for infections and respiratory distress (WHO, 2012). In contrast, in high-income settings, more than 90 per cent of preterm infants survive.

RISK FACTORS FOR PRETERM LABOUR

Many preterm births occur in women with no risk factors, making it difficult to pinpoint the cause of preterm labour.

- **Prior spontaneous preterm labour** before 34 weeks is the strongest risk factor for subsequent preterm birth (Spong et al., 2007).
  - The risk of preterm birth increases two-fold with every subsequent preterm delivery (Mercer et al., 1996).

- – Recurrences also tend to occur at approximately the same gestational age.
- – If a preterm birth is followed by a term delivery, the risk of preterm birth in subsequent pregnancies decreases (McManemy, 2007).
- – A prior preterm twin birth is associated with an increased risk of preterm birth in a subsequent singleton pregnancy (Rafael et al., 2012).
- **Short cervical length** measured by transvaginal ultrasonography (<25 mm at 16–24 weeks of gestation) also has been associated with an increased risk of preterm birth (Mella and Berghella, 2009). Clinically, the shorter the cervix, the greater the risk of preterm birth. However, a short cervix on ultrasound examination is most predictive of preterm birth in women with a history of preterm birth.
- **Multiple pregnancy** or **polyhydramnios**, which cause uterine overdistension, may precipitate PTB.
- **Maternal medical disorders** leading to fetal growth restriction, fetal compromise, or worsening maternal condition leading to induction of labour or cesarean section may be the reason for PTB in women with gestational hypertension and preeclampsia, antiphospholipid syndrome or diabetes, especially pre-gestational. Asthma, seizure disorders, overweight and obesity, have also been implicated in the increased risk of PTB.
- **Urinary tract infection** (UTI), especially pyelonephritis, has been implicated in the causation of PTB.
  - – Asymptomatic bacteriuria in the first and early second trimester may lead to cystitis and pyelonephritis later in pregnancy. To avoid this, routine screening for asymptomatic bacteria at 12–16 weeks has been recommended in Western guidelines. However, this is not performed in many countries, including India.
  - – Systematic reviews of the Cochrane Database on the identification and treatment of asymptomatic bacteriuria (Smaill and Vasquez, 2007) and the treatment of established UTI in pregnancy (Vasquez and Abalos, 2011) failed to show a decrease in PTB following treatment.
- **Cervical surgical procedures** including conisation and loop electrosurgical excision procedure (LEEP) have been implicated in preterm birth because of associated cervical injury, but this relationship has not been established (ACOG, 2012).
- **Pregnancies following assisted reproductive techniques** are at a higher risk of preterm birth.
- **Factors in-low income countries** that increase the risk of preterm labour and are relevant in India include the following:
  - – Extremes of maternal age (<17 or >35 years)
  - – Low socio-economic status
  - – Low pre-pregnancy weight and poor weight gain in pregnancy
  - – Short inter-pregnancy interval
  - – Induced labour or planned cesarean section in women whose due date is not well-documented may result in iatrogenic preterm birth
  - – Malaria
  - – Periodontal disease

PREDICTION OF PRETERM LABOUR

- Though prediction of preterm birth is an important strategy in reducing neonatal morbidity and mortality, risk assessment for preterm delivery is difficult, particularly among women with no prior history of preterm birth.
- **A previous history of preterm labour** is one of the strongest risk factors for preterm labour. The rate of preterm birth is 12 per cent in the general population, but increases to 20–50 per cent in subsequent pregnancies in women who have had a previous preterm birth (Edlow et al., 2007).
- **Other factors** which have strong predictive values include the following:
  - Bleeding
  - Multiple pregnancy
  - History of cervical insufficiency

Assessment of cervical length

- The risk of spontaneous PTB increases as cervical length decreases. Shortening of the cervix precedes preterm labour by several weeks.
- The risk is highest when transvaginal ultrasound cervical length is ≤25 mm between 16 and 24 weeks of gestation. A short cervix in a woman admitted with suspected preterm labour also indicates a higher risk of progression to preterm birth.
- **Women with a history of preterm labour** are usually started on progesterone in the subsequent pregnancy. In women in whom the history of preterm labour is uncertain, the cervical length is assessed serially between 16 and 24 weeks to look for shortening of the cervix, which will indicate an increased risk of recurrence of preterm labour.
- **Women with no history of preterm labour**—routine measurement of cervical length is controversial in women with a singleton pregnancy and no history of PTB.
  - A 2019 meta-analysis of randomised trials (Berghella and Saccone) did not find sufficient evidence to recommend routine cervical length screening for all pregnant women.
  - However, the International Federation of Gynecology and Obstetrics (FIGO) recommends sonographic cervical length screening **in all women** at 19^{+0} to 23^{+6} weeks of gestation using transvaginal ultrasound.
- **Universal screening of cervical length is difficult to implement in low-resource countries like India**. Serial screening with cervical length is best restricted to the following:
  - Women with risk factors for preterm birth
  - Women with a short cervix identified during the routine second-trimester scan

PREVENTION OF PRETERM LABOUR

The two interventions available for the prevention of PTB are *progesterone* and *cervical cerclage*.

Progesterone

Progesterone supplementation may prevent preterm labour in women at risk for it. The following recommendations are made based on history of prior spontaneous preterm birth and cervical length in present pregnancy. Romero et al. (2018), in a meta-analysis, concluded that vaginal progesterone decreases the risk of preterm birth and improves perinatal outcomes in singleton gestations with a short cervix established by transvaginal ultrasound between 16 and 24 weeks of gestation.

- A recent meta-analysis (The EPPPIC group, 2021) established that progesterone supplementation reduces PTB <34 weeks by approximately 20 per cent *in singleton pregnancies with a short midtrimester cervical length or a previous history of PTB,* but **not** in *unselected multiple gestations.*

History-based recommendations

- Singleton pregnancy, **prior spontaneous preterm singleton birth** at 28 to 36 weeks' gestation:
  - Hydroxyprogesterone caproate 250 mg
    - Weekly by intramuscular injection
    - Starting at 16–20 weeks
- Singleton pregnancy, **prior spontaneous twin birth:**
  - If the prior twin preterm birth was ≥34 weeks, no progesterone
  - If the prior twin preterm birth was <34 weeks, hydroxyprogesterone as described above

Cervical measurement-based recommendations

- Singleton pregnancy, **no prior spontaneous preterm singleton birth** at 28 to 36 weeks' gestation, cervical length ≤20 mm at 20 weeks:
  - Daily vaginal micronised progesterone 100 mg until 36 weeks

Cervical cerclage

- Cervical cerclage is indicated in women with a history suggestive of preterm birth due to cervical insufficiency (multiple second-trimester pregnancy losses/PTBs associated with painless cervical dilatation).
- Women in whom the diagnosis of cervical insufficiency is uncertain should undergo cervical length measurement at 16 weeks in the current pregnancy. A cervical cerclage should be performed if the cervical length is ≤25 mm.
- Routine cervical cerclage is not indicated for the prevention of PTB in multiple pregnancy with a **normal cervical length**.

The recommendations based on history of prior spontaneous preterm birth, and/or cervical length in the current pregnancy are summarised in Table 33.1.

DIAGNOSIS OF PRETERM LABOUR

- Preterm labour is a difficult diagnosis to establish accurately. Suspected preterm labour is one of the common reasons for the hospitalisation of pregnant women. 50 per cent of

Table 33.1   Management of short cervix diagnosed by ultrasound imaging

History	Cervical length	Drug	Initiation	Dosage	Length of administration
Asymptomatic woman with no prior PTB	≤20 mm at 20 weeks	Vaginal micronised progesterone	At time of diagnosis	100 mg daily	Up to 36 weeks
Asymptomatic woman with prior PTB	Need not be measured	17-α-OHP	16–20 weeks	250 mg IM weekly	Up to 36 weeks
Asymptomatic woman with singleton pregnancy and prior twin delivery ≥34 weeks	Need not be measured	No progesterone	–	–	–
Asymptomatic woman with singleton pregnancy and prior twin delivery <34 weeks	Need not be measured	17-α-OHP	16–20 weeks	250 mg IM weekly	Up to 36 weeks
Asymptomatic woman with twin pregnancy	≤25 mm at 16–24 weeks	• Progesterone controversial • Vaginal micronised progesterone	At time of diagnosis	100 mg daily	Up to 36 weeks

17-α-OHP, 17 α-hydroxyprogesterone

women hospitalised with the suspicion of preterm labour will continue their pregnancy to term.

- The diagnosis is based on a careful history and clinical evidence of uterine contractions leading to cervical changes.

Prodromal signs and symptoms

Women may experience the following signs and symptoms that may precede true preterm labour:
- Period-like cramping
- Mild, irregular contractions
- Low backache
- Pressure sensation in the vagina or pelvis
- Increased mucoid vaginal discharge
- Spotting, light bleeding

Clinical diagnostic criteria

- Regular uterine activity, with contractions increasing in intensity and duration, is indicative of labour, be it preterm or at term.

- A threshold contraction frequency that effectively identifies women who will progress to true labour has not been defined (Lockwood, 2019). Uterine contractions are considered significant if there are **≥4 contractions every 20 minutes** or **≥8 in 60 minutes.**
- Preterm labour is confirmed if the contractions are associated with the following:
  - Cervical dilatation ≥3 cm
  - Cervical length <20 mm on transvaginal ultrasound
  - 'Show' or rupture of membranes

Transvaginal ultrasound examination

- A transvaginal ultrasound examination is only performed if the digital cervical examination is not definitive in confirming or ruling out preterm labour.
- A long cervix (≥30 mm) almost certainly rules out preterm labour.
- A short cervix before 34 weeks (<25 mm) may be indicative of an increased risk of preterm labour.
- When associated with uterine contractions, a cervical length <20 mm on transvaginal ultrasound may confirm preterm labour.

Measurement of fetal fibronectin (fFN)

- This test is not widely available in India. It is also expensive.
- fFN is an extracellular matrix glycoprotein present at the decidual-chorionic junction. When labour contractions disrupt this interface, fFN is released. The presence of fFN in cervicovaginal secretions is a marker for true preterm labour.
- In normal conditions, fFN is found at very low levels in cervicovaginal secretions. Levels ≥50 ng/mL at or after 22 weeks have been associated with an increased risk of spontaneous preterm birth.
- A systematic review of the Cochrane Database (Berghella and Saccone, 2019) showed that having fFN results available to clinicians had no effect on the following important outcomes:
  - Preterm birth less than 28 weeks
  - Gestational age at delivery (weeks)
  - Birthweight less than 2500 g
  - Perinatal death
  - Respiratory distress syndrome
  - Neonatal intensive care unit (NICU) admission and NICU days
- Knowledge of the fFN results was also found to have no impact on the following interventions:
  - Tocolysis
  - Steroids for fetal lung maturity
  - Time to evaluate

The measurement of fetal fibronectin is not widely available in India, and when available, is quite expensive. Even in countries where facilities are available to perform fFN, studies have shown that clinicians do not base their clinical management protocols on fFN results and that outcomes are not improved by knowing the fFN status.

INTERVENTIONS TO IMPROVE PRETERM BIRTH OUTCOMES

A woman with suspected or confirmed preterm labour should be hospitalised, and interventions that have been shown to improve perinatal outcomes should be initiated. These interventions include the following:
- Antenatal corticosteroids
- Tocolysis
- Magnesium sulphate for fetal neuroprotection

 If neonatal facilities are available to take care of the infant, and the mother has completed 34 weeks, interventions to inhibit labour at that gestation may not be worth the time and cost. The perinatal outcome is likely to be very good if neonatal care is available.

Antenatal corticosteroids

- The benefits of a single course of antenatal corticosteroids for women in preterm labour before 34 weeks have been validated by an updated systematic review of the Cochrane Database (Roberts et al., 2017).
- In preterm neonates, antenatal corticosteroids have been proven to decrease the risk of the following:
  - Respiratory distress syndrome
  - Intraventricular hemorrhage (IVH)
  - Necrotising enterocolitis
- The following are the recommended criteria for administering a single course of antenatal corticosteroids to women at risk of preterm labour between 24–34 weeks of gestation (WHO, 2015; ACOG, 2017):
  - Gestational age assessment is accurate
  - Preterm birth is considered imminent within seven days of starting treatment, and even as early as within the first 24 hours
  - It could be a singleton or multiple gestation
  - Membranes could be intact or ruptured
  - There is no clinical evidence of maternal infection (chorioamnionitis)
  - Antenatal corticosteroids are also recommended in the following clinical situations when preterm birth is imminent within seven days of starting treatment or even within the first 24 hours:
    - Women with hypertensive disorders
    - Women with pre-gestational and gestational diabetes (should be accompanied by strict maternal blood glucose control)
    - Women diagnosed with a fetus with growth restriction
  - Adequate childbirth care is available (including the capacity to recognise and safely manage preterm labour and birth)
  - The preterm newborn can receive adequate care if needed (including resuscitation, warmth to prevent hypothermia, nutritional support, infection treatment, and safe oxygen use)

Antenatal corticosteroids in the late preterm (34^{+0} weeks to 36^{+6} weeks)
The ACOG, in 2016, added a recommendation to administer one course of corticosteroids to women in the late preterm who are at imminent risk of preterm delivery. This recommendation was based on a multicentre study (Gyamfi-Bannerman et al., 2016) that indicated that betamethasone decreases newborn respiratory morbidity when given to women in the late preterm period between 34^{+0} and 36^{+6} weeks, who are at risk of preterm delivery within seven days and have not previously received corticosteroids. However, there is an increased risk of neonatal hypoglycemia in infants whose mothers received betamethasone.

Rescue (or repeat) course of corticosteroids

- Occasionally, after a course of steroids, the woman may not deliver in the next seven days. If the pregnancy progresses further, a single rescue (or repeat) course of antenatal corticosteroids should be considered (Garite et al., 2009; Crowther et al., 2015; ACOG, 2015) in a woman with intact membranes under the following conditions:
  - The woman is <34 weeks of gestation
  - She is still at risk of preterm delivery within the next 7 days
  - The prior course of antenatal corticosteroids was administered more than 14 days previously
- There is no evidence yet that there is any benefit to a repeat course of betamethasone in women in the late preterm (between 34^{+0} and 36^{+6} weeks) or with preterm premature rupture of membranes (ACOG, 2016).

Drugs and dosage

- Either betamethasone or dexamethasone may be used. Betamethasone is preferred because of the lesser number of doses required. Delivery is planned 24 hours after the last dose.
- The course of therapy is listed in Table 33.2.

Table 33.2 Dose and regimen for antenatal corticosteroids

Drug	Dose	Route	Interval	Number of doses	Total duration of course
Betamethasone	12 mg	Intramuscular	24 hours	2	24 hours
Dexamethasone	6 mg	Intramuscular	12 hours	4	48 hours

Both betamethasone and dexamethasone are effective for accelerating fetal lung maturity. Betamethasone is preferred for the following reasons:
- It is cheaper than dexamethasone.
- It requires fewer injections than dexamethasone.
- It has a shorter course (24 hours vs. 48 hours for dexamethasone).

Tocolysis

- In women in true preterm labour (in whom progressive cervical changes are documented), tocolytic therapy helps by inhibiting and stopping contractions

Maintenance (or long-term) tocolysis for more than 48 hours is not recommended since it does not improve neonatal outcomes.

temporarily. However, the underlying stimulus that initiated the process of labour is not affected.

- Tocolysis is administered for **48 hours** to arrest uterine contractions for **short-term prolongation of pregnancy**.

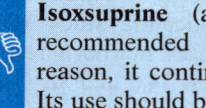 **Isoxsuprine** (a beta-mimetic) is **not** recommended for tocolysis. For some reason, it continues to be used in India. Its use should be actively discouraged.

- Arresting contractions allows for the following:
  - Administration of antenatal corticosteroids (for fetal lung protection)
  - Administration of magnesium sulphate (for fetal neuroprotection, see below)
  - Transport to a tertiary facility, if needed
- There is no available evidence to show that tocolytic therapy has a positive effect on neonatal outcomes.
- The recommended tocolytics and doses for tocolysis in women with preterm labour and intact membranes are as follows:
  - **Calcium channel blockers** (e.g., nifedipine) are the first-line of treatment at 32–34 weeks' gestation (ACOG, 2017; NICE, 2015; Simhan and Caritis, 2020).

 Bed rest has not been shown to reduce the risk of preterm birth and should not be prescribed routinely to women who are suspected of being in preterm labour.

    A systematic review of the Cochrane Database (Flenady et al., 2014) showed nifedipine to be superior to beta-mimetics and oxytocin receptor antagonists (e.g., atosiban).
  - **Beta-mimetics** (terbutaline) may be used, but have maternal side effects. NICE guidelines (2015) recommend against the use of beta-mimetics though the ACOG guidelines recommend injectable terbutaline as the second line of treatment.
  - **Cyclooxygenase inhibitors** (e.g., indomethacin) may be used for tocolysis at 24–32 weeks' gestation. Indomethacin is not recommended beyond 32 weeks' gestation and may lead to fetal kidney injury, oligohydramnios, and premature closure of the ductus arteriosus (PDA), if used for >48 hours.

Less effective tocolytic agents

- **Oxytocin receptor antagonists** (e.g., atosiban) were not shown to be superior to placebos, calcium channel blockers, or beta-mimetics in a systematic review of the Cochrane Database (Flenady et

 Nifedipine and atosiban should **not be administered** concomitantly with magnesium sulphate as they may produce maternal side effects.

al., 2014a). Atosiban is not easily available in India and is also expensive as compared to nifedipine.
- **Magnesium sulphate** is sometimes used as a tocolytic because of its ability to inhibit myometrial contractility. Its tocolytic efficacy is comparable to other tocolytics. It should not be used for >48 hours.

The mechanism of action, dosage, and maternal and fetal side effects of commonly used tocolytics are listed in Table 33.3.

Table 33.3   Commonly used tocolytics for women with preterm labour and intact membranes

Drug	Class of drug	Route and dose	Maternal side effects	Fetal/neonatal side effects
Nifedipine	Calcium channel blocker	• Loading dose 30 mg • Followed by 20 mg every 8 hours × 48 hours	Flushing, headache, dizziness, and palpitations	No known side effects
Terbutaline	Beta-mimetic	• 0.25 mg SC every 20 to 30 minutes up to 4 doses till tocolysis is achieved • Followed by 0.25 mg SC every 4 hours × 24–48 hours	Tachycardia, palpitations, and lower blood pressure	Neonatal tachycardia and hypoglycemia
Indomethacin (should not be given for >48 hours due to fetal side effects)	Cyclooxygen-ase inhibitor	• 50–100 mg loading dose (oral or per rectum) • Followed by 25 mg orally every 4–6 hours	Nausea, esophageal reflux, gastritis, and emesis; platelet dysfunction	Premature closure of ductus arteriosus, renal dysfunction, oligohydram-nios, necrotising enterocolitis in preterm newborns
Magnesium sulphate	Exact mechanism of action not known	• 6 g IV load over 20 minutes • Followed by a continuous infusion of 2 g/hour	Diaphoresis and flushing	Slight decrease in baseline fetal heart rate and fetal heart rate variability
Atosiban	Oxytocin receptor antagonist	• Initial IV bolus of 6.75 mg • Followed by 300 mg/minute infusion × 3 hours, then 100 mg/minute for up to 45 hours	Least side effects of all tocolytics	Good fetal safety profile

IV, intravenous; *SC*, subcutaneous

Magnesium sulphate for fetal neuroprotection

- When birth is anticipated **before 32 weeks of gestation**, magnesium sulphate reduces the severity and risk of cerebral palsy in surviving infants (Doyle et al., 2009).
- Magnesium sulphate is administered in the following clinical situations:
  - Singletons or twins at 24 through 31 weeks of gestation at high risk of spontaneous delivery because of:
    - Preterm rupture of the membranes occurring at 24 through 31 weeks of gestation
    - Advanced preterm labour with dilatation of 4–8 cm and intact membranes
    - Elective preterm delivery imminent within the next 2–24 hours for medical or obstetric indications
- **Dose**
  - 4 g intravenous loading dose of magnesium sulphate is administered over 20 minutes followed by a maintenance dose of 1 g/hour with an infusion pump.

– *The magnesium sulphate is stopped as soon as delivery occurs. It is administered for a maximum of 24 hours.*

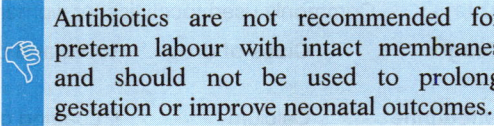 Antibiotics are not recommended for preterm labour with intact membranes and should not be used to prolong gestation or improve neonatal outcomes.

MANAGEMENT OF PRETERM LABOUR BASED ON GESTATIONAL AGE

The decisions regarding the management of preterm labour depend on the following factors:

- **Gestational age:** When the gestational age is ≥ 34 weeks, corticosteroids may be administered if time permits. If uterine contractions are not arrested, labour may be allowed to progress. At a gestational age >28 but <34 weeks, corticosteroids should be administered. For women <32 weeks pregnant, magnesium sulphate provides fetal neuroprotection.
- **Availability of resources:** The presence of neonatal intensive care facilities is useful in deciding the chances of neonatal salvage. In low-resource areas, neonatal salvage may be poor before 28 weeks. In such cases, the woman may be transferred to a tertiary centre with neonatal care facilities for a better outcome.

The management of preterm labour based on gestational age is depicted in Figures 33.1 and 33.2.

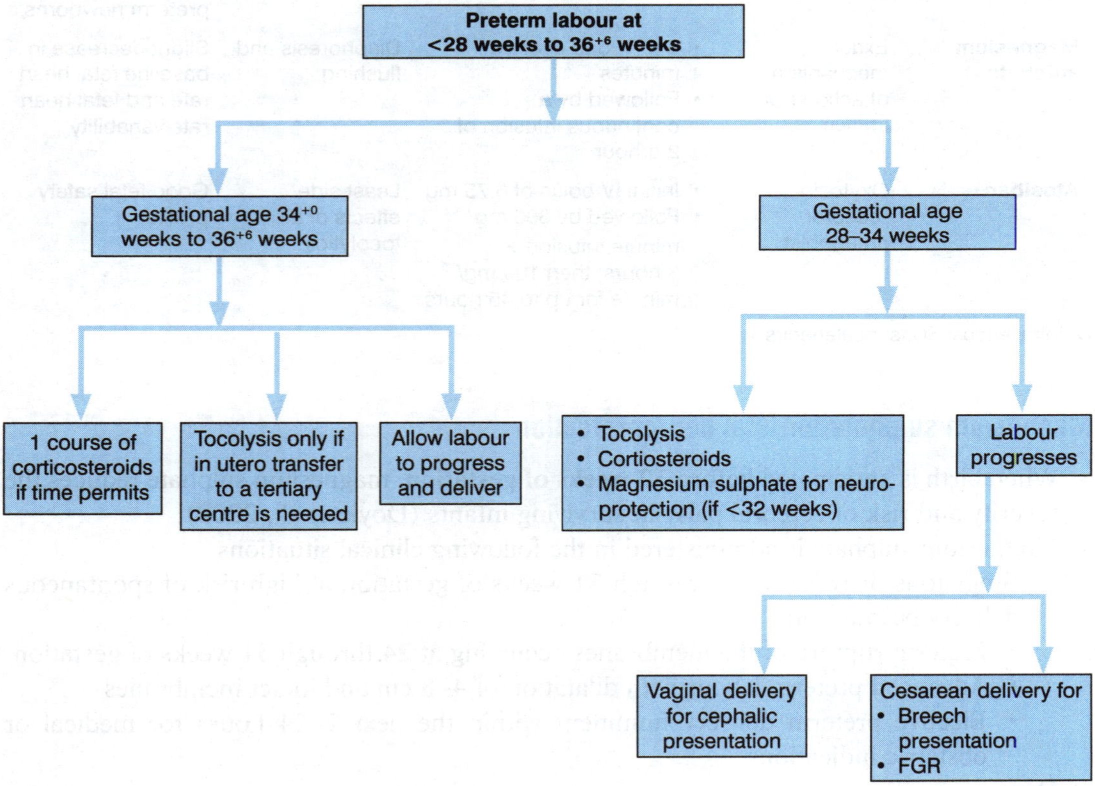

```
                    ┌─────────────────────────┐
                    │     Preterm labour at   │
                    │  <28 weeks to 36⁺⁶ weeks│
                    └─────────────────────────┘
            ┌──────────────────┴──────────────────┐
  ┌───────────────────────┐          ┌───────────────────────┐
  │  Gestational age 34⁺⁰  │          │   Gestational age     │
  │  weeks to 36⁺⁶ weeks   │          │     28–34 weeks       │
  └───────────────────────┘          └───────────────────────┘
```

| 1 course of corticosteroids if time permits | Tocolysis only if in utero transfer to a tertiary centre is needed | Allow labour to progress and deliver | • Tocolysis
• Cortiosteroids
• Magnesium sulphate for neuro-protection (if <32 weeks) | Labour progresses |

| Vaginal delivery for cephalic presentation | Cesarean delivery for
• Breech presentation
• FGR |

Figure 33.1   Management of preterm labour at gestational age of 28 weeks to 36⁺⁶ weeks. *FGR*, fetal growth restriction

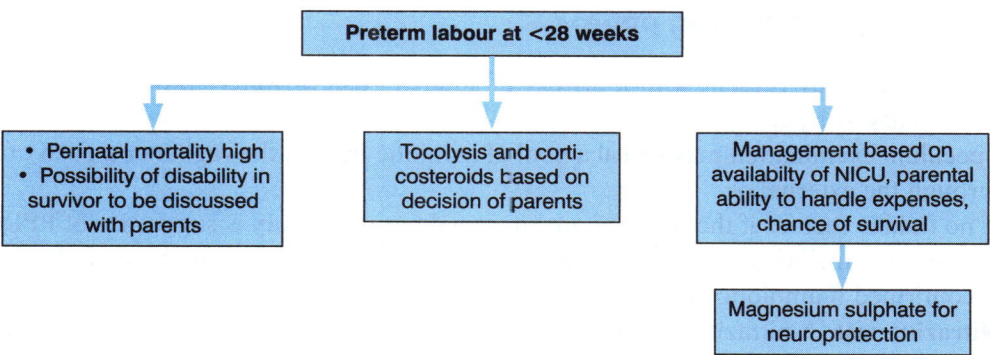

Figure 33.2 Management of preterm labour at <28 weeks of gestation. *NICU*, neonatal intensive care unit

TERM AND PRETERM PRELABOUR RUPTURE OF MEMBRANES

INTRODUCTION

- At term, **prelabour rupture of membranes** (PROM) complicates approximately 8 per cent of pregnancies (ACOG, 2018). Term PROM occurs at or after 37 weeks' gestation and is commonly followed by the spontaneous onset of labour and delivery.
- **Preterm prelabour rupture of membranes** (PPROM) occurs in 1–2 per cent of pregnancies and is defined as the spontaneous rupture of fetal membranes at ≥24 weeks but <37 completed weeks of gestation, and at least an hour prior to the onset of labour (Ugwumadu, 2009).
- PROM occurring between 16 and 24 weeks' gestation is termed **previable PROM**. This may occur in 0.3–0.7 per cent of pregnancies.

RISK FACTORS FOR PPROM

- A history of PPROM is a strong risk factor for recurrence. The Preterm Prediction Study (Mercer et al., 1999) found that women with a history of PPROM had a 13.5 per cent chance of PPROM in a subsequent pregnancy compared to 4.1 per cent in women with no such history.
- Genital tract infection has been implicated as a major etiological factor in the pathogenesis of PPROM (Gomez et al., 1997; Mercer, 2003). Infections of the urogenital tract with gonococcus, *Trichomonas*, *Chlamydia*, or colonisation with group B β-hemolytic *Streptococcus* (GBS) or *Gardnerella vaginalis*, have been implicated in PPROM.

> When PPROM is suspected, digital examination should be avoided because it may decrease the latency period (i.e., time from rupture of membranes to delivery) and increase the risk of intrauterine infection (Alexander et al., 2000).

- Antepartum bleeding in more than one trimester increases the risk of PPROM three- to seven-fold (Harger et al., 1990).
- Genetic susceptibility may be a risk factor for PPROM.

DIAGNOSIS OF PROM AND PPROM

- The woman may present with a history of sudden gush of watery fluid and continuing involuntary loss per vaginum.
- Speculum examination may reveal a pool of amniotic fluid in the vagina or a gush of fluid through the external os.
- If no fluid is seen or if the findings are equivocal but the history is suggestive of PPROM, the clinician may visualise the external cervical os and ask the patient to cough. Diagnosis is confirmed if amniotic fluid is observed trickling from the cervical os.
- **Nitrazine test**: A nitrazine paper strip is used to determine the vaginal pH as a means of confirming rupture of membranes (ROM). Normally, vaginal secretions have a pH between 3.8 and 4.2, whereas amniotic fluid is more alkaline (7.0–7.3). When the pH of the vaginal fluid as determined by nitrazine paper is found to be >6–6.5 (the colour turns blue), ROM can be confirmed. False-negative and false-positive results occur in up to 5 per cent of cases.
- **Ferning test:** Fluid from the posterior vaginal fornix is swabbed onto a glass slide and allowed to dry for at least 10 minutes and then examined under a microscope. Amniotic fluid produces a delicate ferning pattern.
- **Extended pad test**: If the diagnosis of ROM has still not been established, the extended pad test is offered. The mother is asked to wear a sanitary pad and walk around. On checking after a few hours, if the pad is wet, ROM may be confirmed. There are commercially available pads that will indicate with a colour change if amniotic fluid is leaking. These may be used, if available.
- **Commercial tests:** If, on speculum examination, no amniotic fluid is observed, clinicians should consider performing an **insulin-like growth factor-binding protein-1** (IGFBP-1) or **placental alpha microglobulin-1** (PAMG-1) test on the vaginal fluid to guide further management. *These test kits are not commonly available in India.*
- **Ultrasound:** Evidence of marked oligohydramnios or anhydramnios demonstrated by ultrasound may indicate a diagnosis of PPROM in the second and early third trimester. However, oligohydramnios can be confounded by other causes, including renal agenesis, renal dysplasia, and fetal growth restriction.

COMPLICATIONS OF PPROM

Maternal complications

- **Chorioamnionitis:** Ascending infection occurs in 15–25 per cent of women with PPROM, leading to chorioamnionitis. The risk of intrauterine infection increases with the duration of membrane rupture and with decreasing gestational age.
- **Endometritis:** 15–20 per cent of women develop postpartum infection following PPROM. The risk is more with cesarean than it is with vaginal delivery.
- **Placental abruption**: This occurs in 2–5 per cent of patients with PPROM (Ananth et al., 2004). The risk is 7- to 10-fold in women who have intrauterine infection and oligohydramnios.

- **Prolapse of the umbilical cord**: This is another complication of PPROM, especially in cases where there is a large gush of amniotic fluid.

Fetal and neonatal complications

- Infectious morbidity is high in the presence of chorioamnionitis. Fetal pneumonia or septicemia can lead to perinatal death.
- Fetal malpresentation is common because of the combination of prematurity and the frequent occurrence of oligohydramnios.
- Cord compression due to oligohydramnios can lead to fetal distress, increase in cesarean section rate, and fetal hypoxia.
- Respiratory distress syndrome is a consequence of preterm birth.
- Necrotising enterocolitis, intraventricular hemorrhage, and periventricular leukomalacia are seen in very-low-birth-weight neonates born with infection.
- Pulmonary hypoplasia may be a result of chronic loss of fluid if the PPROM occurs in the second trimester.
- Long-term sequelae such as cerebral palsy, intellectual and learning disabilities, periventricular leukomalacia, visual and hearing disabilities, and chronic lung disease may result from PPROM.

MANAGEMENT OF PPROM

Management depends on the following:
- Gestational age
- Associated sepsis
- Availability of neonatal intensive care
- Presence of uterine contractions
- Fetal presentation and condition

Once the diagnosis of PPROM is confirmed, the critical decision to be made is whether to **deliver immediately** or **manage expectantly**.

Initial evaluation

- *Confirmation of gestational age*
  Gestational age is confirmed by LMP and details of ultrasonography in the 1st and 2nd trimesters.
- *Identification of overt chorioamnionitis*
  Fever, uterine tenderness, and foul-smelling, purulent vaginal discharge indicate sepsis.
- *Evaluation of onset of labour*
  - Uterine contractions are watched for, cardiotocography is performed, and cervical effacement and dilatation are assessed on speculum examination.
  - Digital vaginal examination should be avoided unless the woman is in active labour.
- *Ascertaining fetal condition*
  - Ultrasonography is performed to check for the following:
    - Amniotic fluid volume
    - Fetal presentation
  - Fetal well-being should be monitored by cardiotocography and biophysical profile.

Subsequent management

- Depending on the combination of the factors mentioned above, management may be by one of the following two modalities:
  - **Immediate delivery** (by induction of labour or cesarean section)
  - **Expectant management**
- A systematic review of the Cochrane Database (Bond et al., 2017) concluded that in women with PPROM before 37 weeks' gestation with no contraindications to continuing the pregnancy, a policy of expectant management with careful monitoring was associated with better outcomes for the mother and baby. Further, the study did not find any clinically important difference in the incidence of neonatal sepsis between women who gave birth immediately and those who were managed expectantly.

Immediate delivery

- There does not seem to be much benefit in prolonging the pregnancy if PPROM has occurred between 34 and 37 weeks. The risk of neonatal sepsis after PPROM near term is low, and induction of labour does not reduce this risk (van der Ham et al., 2012).

 **Tocolysis is not recommended in PPROM** (ACOG, 2017). It is associated with an increased risk of chorioamnionitis without significant maternal or neonatal benefit.

- Prompt delivery of women with PPROM irrespective of gestational age is indicated in the presence of the following:
  - Active labour
  - Non-reassuring fetal status
  - Signs and symptoms of chorioamnionitis
  - Placental abruption
  - A high risk of cord prolapse

Expectant management of PPROM

- Expectant management is usually implemented to carry the pregnancy up to at least 34 weeks, and if possible, 37 weeks. A recent systematic review of the Cochrane Database (Bond et al., 2017) found that a policy of expectant management with careful monitoring was associated with better outcomes for the mother and baby. NICE Guideline no. 25 on preterm labour and birth (2019) also recommends expectant management until 37 weeks if there is no maternal or fetal indication for immediate delivery.
- Hospitalisation is recommended for at least 5–7 days for women who have a viable fetus. If necessary, this might be extended until the time of delivery. The majority of women enter labour within a week of PPROM (Duff, 2019).
- The mother is advised ambulation in the room since bed rest does not seem to change the course of management.

> The decision to manage the pregnancy expectantly beyond 34 weeks should be based on the facilities available to provide care for a preterm infant. If possible, the pregnancy should be prolonged till the gestational week when the chances of survival of the infant are most optimal.

Antenatal corticosteroids

- Women presenting with PPROM between 24 and 34 weeks' gestation should receive antenatal corticosteroids (Table 33.2). Either betamethasone or dexamethasone may be used.
- Antenatal corticosteroids reduce the risk of neonatal death, respiratory distress syndrome, intraventricular hemorrhage, necrotising enterocolitis, and the length of neonatal respiratory support without an increase in either maternal or neonatal infection (Roberts et al., 2017).
- Antenatal corticosteroids in PPROM do not increase the risks of maternal or neonatal infection regardless of gestational age (ACOG, 2018).

Prophylactic antibiotic therapy

- Administration of broad-spectrum antibiotics in PPROM is strongly recommended (Kenyon et al., ORACLE 1 study, 2001; ACOG, 2018) as it:
  - Prolongs pregnancy,
  - Reduces maternal and neonatal infections and
  - Reduces morbidity associated with prematurity.

> **Antibiotic regimens in PPROM**
> It is not clear which antibiotic regimen should be used. Any of the following may be used, with similar results:
> - Erythromycin 250 mg orally 4 times a day for 10 days (ORACLE 1 study, 2001; WHO, 2015) **OR**
> - Intravenous (IV) ampicillin (2 g every 6 hours) and IV erythromycin (250 mg every 6 hours) for 48 hours followed by oral amoxicillin (250 mg every 8 hours) and erythromycin base (333 mg every 8 hours) (ACOG, 2018; Mercer, 1997) **OR**
> - Azithromycin 1 g orally on admission PLUS IV ampicillin (2 g every 6 hours for 48 hours) followed by oral amoxicillin (500 mg 3 times daily) for another 5 days
> **Amoxicillin/clavulanic acid is contraindicated because of the increased risk of necrotising enterocolitis in neonates exposed to this antibiotic.**

Monitoring for maternal infection

- PPROM may be associated with ascending infection leading to chorioamnionitis and subsequent fetal and neonatal infection.
- Clinical assessment for infection includes monitoring of pulse, temperature, and blood pressure.
- Maternal blood tests (C-reactive protein and white cell count) may be used to confirm the presence of chorioamnionitis. These tests are not necessary in the presence of fever.
- Fetal tachycardia may be one of the earliest signs of chorioamnionitis.

> The white cell count rises 24 hours after the administration of corticosteroids and returns to baseline three days after administration. This must be kept in mind when monitoring for maternal infection (Danesh et al., 2012).

Fetal monitoring during expectant management

- There is no consensus on the tests and frequency of testing required during the expectant management of PPROM.
- The mother should be educated on fetal movement and should report decreased movements.
- Non-stress test may be performed daily but has poor sensitivity for predicting maternal or fetal infection.

References

1. Alexander JM, Mercer BM, Miodovnik M, Thurnau GR, Goldenberg RL, Das AF et al. 2000. The impact of digital cervical examination on expectantly managed preterm rupture of membranes. *Am J Obstet Gynecol.* 183:1003–7.

2. American College of Obstetricians and Gynecologists. 2012. ACOG Practice Bulletin No. 130. Prediction and prevention of preterm birth. *Obstet Gynecol.* 120:964–73.

3. American College of Obstetricians and Gynecologists. 2016 (reaffirmed 2018). ACOG Practice Bulletin No. 171. Management of preterm labor. *Obstet Gynecol.* 128:e155–64.

4. American College of Obstetricians and Gynecologists. 2017. ACOG Obstetric Care Consensus No. 6: Periviable birth. *Obstet Gynecol.* 130:e187–99.

5. American College of Obstetricians and Gynecologists. 2018. ACOG Practice Bulletin No. 188. Prelabor rupture of membranes. *Obstet Gynecol.* 131:e1–14.

6. Ananth CV, Oyelese Y, Srinivas N, Yeo L, Vintzileos AM. 2004. Preterm premature rupture of membranes, intrauterine infection, and oligohydramnios: Risk factors for placental abruption. *Obstet Gynecol.* 104:71–7.

7. Berghella V, Saccone G. 2019. Cervical assessment by ultrasound for preventing preterm delivery. *Cochrane Database Syst Rev.* Issue 9. Art. no.: CD007235.

8. Blencowe H, Cousens S, Oestergaard M et al. 2012. National, regional and worldwide estimates of preterm birth. *Lancet.* 9;379(9832):2162–72.

9. Bond DM, Middleton P, Levett KM et al. 2017. Planned early birth versus expectant management for women with preterm prelabour rupture of membranes prior to 37 weeks' gestation for improving pregnancy outcome. *Cochrane Database Syst Rev.* Issue 3. Art. no.:CD004735.

10. Crowther CA, McKinlay CJ, Middleton P, Harding JE. 2015. Repeat doses of prenatal corticosteroids for women at risk of preterm birth for improving neonatal health outcomes. *Cochrane Database Syst Rev.* Issue 7. Art. No.: CD003935.

11. Danesh A, Janghorbani M, Khalatbari S. 2012. Effects of antenatal corticosteroids on maternal serum indicators of infection in women at risk for preterm delivery: A randomized trial comparing betamethasone and dexamethasone. *J Res Med Sci.* 17:911.

12. Doyle LW, Crowther CA, Middleton P, Marret S, Rouse D. 2009. Magnesium sulphate for women at risk of preterm birth for neuroprotection of the fetus. *Cochrane Database Syst Rev.* Issue 1. Art. no.: CD004661.

13. Duff P. 2019. Preterm prelabor rupture of membranes: Clinical manifestations and diagnosis. Lockwood CJ (Ed). *UpToDate.* Waltham, MA.

14. Edlow AG, Srinivas SK, Elovitz MA. 2007. Second-trimester loss and subsequent pregnancy outcomes: What is the real risk? *Am J Obstet Gynecol.* 197:581.e1–581.e6.

15. FIGO Working Group on Best Practice in Maternal-Fetal Medicine, International Federation of Gynecology and Obstetrics. 2015. Best practice in maternal-fetal medicine. *Int J Gynaecol Obstet.* 128:80.

16. Flenady V, Reinebrant HE, Liley HG, Tambimuttu EG, Papatsonis DNM. 2014a. Oxytocin receptor antagonists for inhibiting preterm labour. *Cochrane Database Syst Rev.* Issue 6. Art. no.: CD004452.

17. Flenady V, Wojcieszek AM, Papatsonis DNM, Stock OM, Murray L, Jardine LA, Carbonne B. 2014. Calcium channel blockers for inhibiting preterm labour and birth. *Cochrane Database Syst Rev.* Issue 6. Art. no.: CD002255.

18. Garite TJ, Kurtzman J, Maurel K, Clark R. 2009. Impact of a 'rescue course' of antenatal corticosteroids: a multi-center randomized placebo-controlled trial. Obstetrics Collaborative Research Network. *Am J Obstet Gynecol.* 200:248.e1–9.

19. Gomez R, Romero R, Edwin SS et al. 1997. Pathogenesis of preterm labor and preterm premature rupture of membranes associated with intraamniotic infection. *Inf Dis Clin North Am.* 11:135.

20. Gyamfi-Bannerman C, Thom EA, Blackwell SC, Tita AT, Reddy UM, Saade GR et al. 2016. Antenatal betamethasone for women at risk for late preterm delivery. NICHD Maternal–Fetal Medicine Units Network. *N Engl J Med.* 374:1311–20.

21. Harger JH, Hsing AW, Tuomala RE et al. 1990. Risk factors for preterm premature rupture of fetal membranes: A multicenter case-control study. *Am J Obstet Gynecol.* 163(1 Pt 1):130.

22. Kenyon SL, Taylor DJ, Tarnow-Mordi W. 2001. Broad-spectrum antibiotics for preterm, prelabour rupture of fetal membranes: The ORACLE I randomised trial. ORACLE Collaborative Group [published erratum appears in *Lancet.* 2001; 358:156]. *Lancet.* 357:979–88.

23. Lockwood CJ. 2019. Preterm labor: Clinical findings, diagnostic evaluation, and initial treatment. Berghella V (Ed). *UpToDate.* Waltham, MA.

24. McManemy J, Cooke E, Amon E, Leet T. 2007. Recurrence risk for preterm delivery. *Am J Obstet Gynecol.* 196:576.e1–6.

25. Mella MT, Berghella V. 2009. Prediction of preterm birth: Cervical sonography. *Semin Perinatol.* 33:317–24.

26. Mercer BM, Goldenberg RI, Das A et al. 1996. The Preterm Prediction study: A clinical risk assessment system. *Am J Obstet Gynecol.* 174:1885–93.

27. Mercer BM, Goldenberg RL, Moawad AH et al. 1999. The preterm prediction study: Effect of gestational age and cause of preterm birth on subsequent obstetric outcome. National Institute of Child Health and Human Development Maternal–Fetal Medicine Units Network. *Am J Obstet Gynecol.* 181:1216.

28. Mercer BM, Miodovnik M, Thurnau GR, Goldenberg RL, Das AF, Ramsey RD et al. 1997. Antibiotic therapy for reduction of infant morbidity after preterm premature rupture of the membranes. A randomized controlled trial. National Institute of Child Health and Human Development Maternal–Fetal Medicine Units Network. *JAMA.* 278:989–95.

29. Mercer BM. 2003. Preterm premature rupture of the membranes. *Obstet Gynecol.* 101:178.

30. National Institute for Health and Care Excellence (NICE guideline 25). 2015. Preterm labour and birth.

31. NICE guideline [NG25]. 2015 (updated 2019). Preterm labour and birth.

32. Rafael TJ, Hoffman MK, Leiby BE. 2012. Gestational age of previous twin preterm birth as a predictor for subsequent singleton preterm birth. *Am J Obstet Gynecol.* Vol 206. Issue 2. pp156.e1-156.e6.

33. Roberts D, Brown J, Medley N, Dalziel SR. 2017. Antenatal corticosteroids for accelerating fetal lung maturation for women at risk of preterm birth. *Cochrane Database Syst Rev.* Issue 3. Art. no.: CD004454.

34. Romero R, Conde-Agudelo A, Da Fonseca E et al. 2018. Vaginal progesterone for preventing preterm birth and adverse perinatal outcomes in singleton gestations with a short cervix: A meta-analysis of individual patient data. *Am J Obstet Gynecol.* 218:161.

35. Simhan HN, Caritis S. 2020. Inhibition of acute preterm labor. Lockwood CJ (Ed). *UpToDate.* Waltham, MA.

36. Smaill F, Vazquez JC. 2007. Antibiotics for asymptomatic bacteriuria in pregnancy. *Cochrane Database Syst Rev.* Issue 2. Art. no.:CD000490.

37. Spong CY. 2007. Prediction and prevention of recurrent spontaneous preterm birth. *Obstet Gynecol.* 110:405–15.

38. The EPPPIC Group. 2021. Evaluating Progestogens for Preventing Preterm birth International Collaborative (EPPPIC): Meta-analysis of individual participant data from randomised controlled trials. *Lancet.* 397(10280), 1183-1194.

39. Ugwumadu A. 2009. Preterm prelabour rupture of membranes (pPROM). Best Practice in Labour and Delivery. Cambridge University Press. Chapter 19: 207–215.

40. van der Ham DP, van der Heyden JL, Opmeer BC, Mulder AL, Moonen RM, van Beek JH et al. 2012. Management of late-preterm premature rupture of membranes: The PPROMEXIL-2 trial. *Am J Obstet Gynecol.* 207:276.e1–276.10.

41. Vazquez JC, Abalos E. 2011. Treatments for symptomatic urinary tract infections during pregnancy. *Cochrane Database Syst Rev.* Issue 1. Art. No.: CD002256.

42. World Health Organization. 2012. Born Too Soon: The Global Action Report on Preterm Birth. The Partnership for Maternal, Newborn & Child Health. WHO Press, Geneva.

43. World Health Organization. 2015. WHO recommendations on interventions to improve preterm birth outcomes. WHO Press, Geneva.

Chapter 34

Management of Late-Term and Postterm Pregnancy

INTRODUCTION

- Singleton pregnancies usually have a gestation that lasts an average of 40 weeks (280 days) from the first day of the last menstrual period to the estimated date of delivery.
- Traditionally, the period from 37 weeks to 42 weeks of gestation was considered 'term' (WHO, 2004).
- Researchers have, in the past decade, realised that outcomes for neonates vary depending on when they are born within this five-week time frame.
- Tita et al. (2009), in a large multicentre study, found that the frequency of adverse neonatal outcomes is lowest among uncomplicated pregnancies delivered between 39^{+0} weeks of gestation and 40^{+6} weeks of gestation.
- In a study carried out in the United States that compared white, black, and Hispanic Americans, the lowest infant mortality rates across all race and ethnicities was reported at 40 weeks of gestation (Reddy et al., 2011).
- It has been shown that the rates of antepartum stillbirth begin to rise one week earlier in the South Asian population than in the Western population. **Therefore, it is prudent, in the Indian context, to begin monitoring the pregnancy at 40 weeks and plan delivery at 41 weeks.**

Length of gestation in Indian women
The median gestational age at delivery is <39 weeks in Indians.

- The WHO Multinational Longitudinal Study to establish growth charts for developing countries (Kiserud et al., 2017) found that the median gestational age at birth was 38 weeks +4 days in India.
- A large study (cohort of 122,000 women) done in a mixed population hospital in London (Patel et al., 2004), reported the following:
  - Normal gestational length is shorter in Indian, Pakistani, and Bangladeshi women
  - Meconium-stained amniotic fluid, which is a sign of fetal maturity, was significantly more frequent in preterm South Asian infants as compared to white European infants

---

DEFINITION

- Pregnancies at ≥42 weeks (294 days) are defined as **postterm, postdated,** or **prolonged.** Although 42 weeks is used as a cut-off for the definition of postterm pregnancy, it does not represent an absolute threshold.

- Term pregnancy (37–42 weeks) is classified into four subgroups (Table 34.1).
- Since Indian women have been found to have a median gestational age of 39 weeks with a shorter gestation than Caucasian women, studies are required to define late-term and postterm in Indian women. Until then, the current definitions may also be applied to Indian women.

Table 34.1   Classification of term and postterm pregnancy (ACOG, 2013)

Category	Gestation
Early-term	37^{+0} weeks through 38^{+6} weeks
Full-term	39^{+0} weeks through 40^{+6} weeks
Late-term	41^{+0} weeks through 41^{+6} weeks
Postterm	42^{+0} weeks and beyond

ETIOLOGY

- The etiology of prolonged pregnancy is largely unknown but certain factors are associated with an increased risk of prolonged pregnancy.
- A large number of postterm pregnancies seem to be genetically programmed, either due to maternal or fetal genetic influence (Oberg et al., 2013).
- Women at highest risk (relative risk ≥2) of postterm pregnancy are those with a previous postterm pregnancy.
- More modest risk factors (relative risk <2) include the following:
  - Nulliparity
  - Male fetus
  - Obesity
  - Older maternal age
  - Maternal race/ethnicity (Asian women have a lower risk of postterm birth)
- The absence of the fetal brain causing dysfunction of the HPA axis is considered responsible for prolonged pregnancy in *anencephalic pregnancies*.
- Placental sulphatase converts dehydroepiandrosterone sulphate (DHEAS) to estrogen, which is involved in triggering parturition. *Deficiency of placental sulphatase* has also been implicated in prolonged pregnancy.

 After one postterm pregnancy, the risk of a second postterm birth is increased two- to three-fold. After two prior postterm pregnancies, the risk of recurrence is quadrupled (Olesen et al., 2003).

COMPLICATIONS OF LATE-TERM AND POSTTERM PREGNANCY

Fetal and neonatal complications

- **Perinatal morbidity:** Late-term and postterm pregnancies are associated with an increased risk of perinatal morbidity (Clausson et al., 1999) which includes the following:
  - Neonatal convulsions
  - Meconium aspiration syndrome
  - 5-minute Apgar scores of less than 4

- **Perinatal mortality:** Neonates born at ≥ 41 weeks of gestation experience a 30 per cent greater risk of neonatal mortality than term neonates born at 38 to 40 weeks of gestation (Bruckner et al., 2008). The causes of perinatal deaths include the following:
  - Placental insufficiency due to placental aging
  - Cord compression leading to fetal hypoxia, asphyxia, and meconium aspiration
  - Intrauterine infection
- **Macrosomia:** Postterm fetuses have a higher incidence of macrosomia as a result of the longer duration of intrauterine growth. Macrosomia not only has an effect on labour and delivery (abnormal labour progression, increased risk of cesarean delivery, assisted vaginal delivery, shoulder dystocia, and maternal/postpartum hemorrhage) but also has an impact on the fetus and neonate (birth injury and neonatal metabolic problems).
- **Fetal dysmaturity (postmaturity) syndrome:** This is the opposite of macrosomia. Fetuses with dysmaturity are subject to chronic intrauterine malnutrition (Mannino, 1988) and after birth, face the morbidities associated with fetal growth restriction. Such neonates are small for gestational age and have:
  - A long, thin body; the absence of subcutaneous fat makes the skin loose, especially over the thighs and buttocks
  - Dry, meconium-stained, parchment-like, peeling skin with prominent creases
  - An increased risk of seizures and cerebral palsy

Maternal complications

- The mother too faces risks in a postterm pregnancy.
- Late-term and postterm pregnancies are associated with an increased risk of the following complications (Caughey and Musci, 2004):
  - Severe perineal laceration
  - Infection
  - Postpartum hemorrhage
  - Cesarean delivery

INTERVENTIONS TO PREVENT POSTTERM PREGNANCY

Accurate pregnancy dating

- The appropriate management of prolonged pregnancy begins with accurate assessment of gestational age.
- Error is associated with pregnancy dating by last menstrual period (LMP) alone. Dating gestational age based on LMP alone assumes both accurate recall of the LMP and that ovulation occurred on the 14th day of the menstrual cycle.
- In a systematic review of the Cochrane Database, Whitworth et al. (2015) found that women with their due date estimated by early routine ultrasound examination (before 24 weeks) had 40 per cent less incidence of labour induction for postterm pregnancy than women whose estimated delivery date was calculated based on their last menstrual period.

The most common reason for the diagnosis of postterm pregnancy is inaccurate dating of the pregnancy. The rates of postterm pregnancies decrease when ultrasonography is used to confirm LMP dating (Caughey et al., 2008).

Sweeping of fetal membranes

- A Cochrane Database review (Boulvain et al., 2005) assessed 22 trials involving the sweeping of membranes. The study found that the sweeping of membranes at term (38–41 weeks) reduced the frequency of

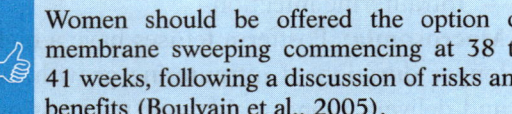 Women should be offered the option of membrane sweeping commencing at 38 to 41 weeks, following a discussion of risks and benefits (Boulvain et al., 2005).

pregnancies continuing after 41^{+0} and 42^{+0} weeks. The review estimated that eight women would need to undergo sweeping of membranes to prevent one induction of labour.
- Nulliparous women at 40 and 41 weeks and parous women at 41 weeks may be offered membrane sweeping (NICE Guidelines, 2008).
- The response to membrane sweeping is unpredictable and slow, and therefore, the method should be used only if the indication for induction is non-urgent.
- Sweeping of the membranes results in the release of endogenous prostaglandins, and consequently, of the softening the cervix, and augmentation of oxytocin-induced uterine contractions.
- Membrane sweeping has been associated with vaginal bleeding and maternal discomfort.
- Contraindications to membrane sweeping include placenta previa and other contraindications to labour and vaginal delivery.
- The method of membrane sweeping is explained in **Chapter 19**, *Induction of labour.*

ANTEPARTUM SURVEILLANCE IN THE POSTTERM PREGNANCY

- There is lack of data from randomised trials on the type and frequency of fetal surveillance recommended in postdated pregnancy.
- Fetal surveillance can be initiated at 40 weeks. Surveillance before 40 weeks is not required in an uncomplicated pregnancy.
- Though there are no randomised controlled trials for frequency of antenatal testing in postterm pregnancy, clinical consensus is that non-stress testing should be done twice weekly

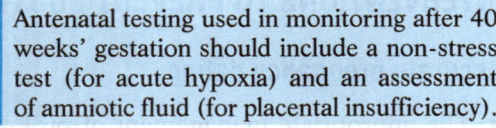 Antenatal testing used in monitoring after 40 weeks' gestation should include a non-stress test (for acute hypoxia) and an assessment of amniotic fluid (for placental insufficiency).

along with measurement of the amniotic fluid volume.
- It has been well-established that decreased amniotic fluid volume is associated with an increased risk of fetal demise (Chamberlain et al., 1984). Oligohydramnios in postterm pregnancies significantly increases the following:
  - Rates of meconium-stained amniotic fluid
  - Presence of growth restriction
  - Rates of fetal heart rate abnormalities and cesarean delivery

- If oligohydramnios (single deepest vertical pocket ≤ 2 cm) is detected at 41^{+0} weeks of gestation or beyond, delivery is usually indicated (ACOG, 2014).

MANAGEMENT OF THE POSTTERM PREGNANCY

- All women with a singleton fetus in vertex presentation and an uncomplicated pregnancy should be offered induction of labour if they have reached 41^{+0} weeks of gestation.
- A recent review of the Cochrane Database review on induction of labour for improving birth outcomes for women at or beyond term (Middleton et al., 2018) clearly concluded that when compared with a policy of expectant management, a policy of labour induction was associated with a 70 per cent reduction in perinatal mortality and stillbirth.
- The review found no clear differences between timing of induction (<41 versus ≥ 41 weeks' gestation) or the state of the cervix (ripe or unripe) on perinatal death, stillbirth, NICU admission, cesarean section, or perineal trauma.
- A systematic review and meta-analysis of cohort studies of 15 million pregnancies (Muglu et al., 2019) concluded that there is a significant additional risk of stillbirth with no corresponding reduction in neonatal mortality when term pregnancies continue to 41 weeks as compared to delivery at 40 weeks. The review included studies only from high-income countries, so this finding might be even more significant in low-income countries where the majority of stillbirths occur.

Management of the postterm pregnancy can be summarised as follows:
- Confirm gestational age early in all pregnancies
- Rule out associated medical/obstetric conditions that necessitate early delivery
- Perform sweeping of membranes at 39–40 weeks
- Fetal surveillance twice weekly from 40 weeks
    - Modified biophysical profile (NST + SDVP)*
 - Induction at 41 weeks
    - Pelvic examination for Bishop's score
    - Cervical ripening, if required
- Early artificial rupture membranes (AROM)
    - Rule out meconium staining
- Oxytocin infusion for augmentation
- Careful monitoring of fetal heart rate

*NST, non-stress testing; SDVP, single deepest vertical pocket

---

References

1. American College of Obstetricians and Gynecologists. 2013 (reaffirmed 2019). ACOG Committee Opinion No. 579. Definition of term pregnancy. *Obstet Gynecol.* 122:1139–40.

5. Boulvain M, Stan CM, Irion O. 2005. Membrane sweeping for induction of labour. *Cochrane Database Syst Rev.* Issue 1. Art. no.: CD000451.

2. Bruckner TA, Cheng YW, Caughey AB. 2008. Increased neonatal mortality among normal-weight births beyond 41 weeks of gestation in California. *Am J Obstet Gynecol.* 199:421.e1.

3. Clausson B, Cnattingius S, Axelsson O. 1999. Outcomes of post-term births: The role of fetal growth restriction and malformations. *Obstet Gynecol.* 94:758–62.

4. Caughey AB, Musci TJ. 2004. Complications of term pregnancies beyond 37 weeks of gestation. *Obstet Gynecol.* 103:57–62.

6. Caughey AB, Nicholson JM, Washington AE. 2008. First- vs second-trimester ultrasound: The effect on pregnancy dating and perinatal outcomes. *Am J Obstet Gynecol.*198:703. e1-703.e5.

7. Chamberlain PF, Manning FA, Morrison I, Harman CR, Lange IR. 1984. Ultrasound evaluation of amniotic fluid, Volume I. The relationship of marginal and decreased amniotic fluid volumes to perinatal outcome. *Am J Obstet Gynecol.* 150:245–9.

8. Doherty L, Norwitz ER. 2008. Prolonged pregnancy: When should we intervene? *Curr Opin Obstet Gyneco.* 20(6):519-27.

9. Kiserud T, Piaggio G, Carroli G et al. 2017. The World Health Organization fetal growth charts: A multinational longitudinal study of ultrasound biometric measurements and estimated fetal weight. *PLoS Med.* 14: e1002220.

10. Mannino F. 1988. Neonatal complications of postterm gestation. *J Reprod Med.* 33:271.

11. Middleton P, Shepherd E, Crowther CA. 2018. Induction of labour for improving birth outcomes for women at or beyond term. *Cochrane Database Syst Rev.* Issue 5. Art. no.: CD004945.

12. Muglu J, Rather H, Arroyo-Manzano D et al. 2019. Risks of stillbirth and neonatal death with advancing gestation at term: A systematic review and meta-analysis of cohort studies of 15 million pregnancies. *PLoS Med.*16:e1002838.

13. NICE clinical guideline 70. 2008. Induction of labour. National Institute for Health and Clinical Excellence.

14. Oberg AS, Frisell T, Svensson AC, Iliadou AN. 2013. Maternal and fetal genetic contributions to postterm birth: Familial clustering in a population-based sample of 475,429 Swedish births. *Am J Epidemiol.* 177:531.

15. Olesen AW, Westergaard JG, Olesen J. 2003. Perinatal and maternal complications related to postterm delivery: A national register-based study, 1978-1993. *Am J Obstet Gynecol.* 189:222–7.

16. Patel RR, Steer P, Doyle P et al. 2004. Does gestation vary by ethnic group? A London-based study of over 122,000 pregnancies with spontaneous onset of labour. *Int J of Epidemiology.* Vol 33, Issue 1. 107–113.

17. Reddy UM, Bettegowda VR, Dias T, Yamada-Kushnir T, Ko CW, Willinger M. 2011. Term pregnancy: A period of heterogeneous risk for infant mortality. *Obstet Gynecol.* 117:1279–87.

18. Tita AT, Landon MB, Spong CY, Lai Y, Leveno KJ, Varner MW et al. 2009. Timing of elective repeat cesarean delivery at term and neonatal outcomes. Eunice Kennedy Shriver NICHD Maternal-Fetal Medicine Units Network. *N Engl J Med.* 360:111–20.

19. World Health Organization. 2004. ICD-10: International statistical classification of diseases. and related health problems, 10th revision. Volume 2. 2nd ed. WHO, Geneva.

20. Whitworth M, Bricker L, Mullan C. 2015. Ultrasound for fetal assessment in early pregnancy. *Cochrane Database Syst Rev.* Issue 7. Art no.: CD007058.

Chapter 35

Multiple Pregnancy

INTRODUCTION

- Twin pregnancy is the most common form of multiple pregnancy, and is high-risk. Cheong and colleagues, in a systematic review and meta-analysis (2016), found that there was a five-fold increase in rates of stillbirth in dichorionic and a thirteen-fold increase in monochorionic twins as compared to singleton pregnancies.
- The risk of stillbirth in twin pregnancies can be decreased with intensive antenatal fetal surveillance (Burgess et al., 2014).
- Placental anastomoses, which are invariably present in the monochorionic placenta, contribute to the increased perinatal mortality and morbidity in monochorionic twin pregnancies as compared to dichorionic ones.
- Women with multifetal gestations are six times more likely to give birth preterm and 13 times more likely to give birth before 32 weeks of gestation than women with singleton gestations (Sebire et al., 1997).

INCIDENCE OF TWINNING

- India has one of the lowest rates of twinning in the world—9 per 1000 spontaneous conceptions (Smits and Monden, 2011). In comparison, the twinning rate in spontaneous conceptions is 19 per 1000 in the United States (ACOG, 2016).
- Dizygotic twins are more common (70 per cent) than monozygotic twins (30 per cent).
- The prevalence of monozygotic twins is stable at 3–5 per 1000 births globally. However, the incidence of dizygotic twin pregnancy is on the rise worldwide (Pison et al., 2015) due to the following factors:
  - Increasing use of fertility drugs
  - Assisted reproductive techniques (ART)
  - Increasing maternal age at childbearing

MANAGEMENT OF MULTIPLE PREGNANCY

The management of multiple pregnancy involves the following:
- General pregnancy advice
- Establishment of chorionicity and amnionicity
- Screening for aneuploidy
- Management in the first trimester
- Management in the second trimester
- Management in the third trimester
- Planning and management of labour and delivery

General pregnancy advice

Weight gain

- India does not have national guidelines for weight gain in pregnancy for either singleton or multiple gestation.
- Weight gain should be based on the mother's pre-pregnancy BMI. Table 35.1 lists the suggested weight gain in twin gestation in Indian women.
- Bodnar and colleagues (2019) studied weight gain in twin pregnancies and reported that both very low and very high weight gains were associated with adverse outcomes.

Table 35.1   Suggested weight gain in twin gestation based on pre-pregnancy BMI in Indian women

Pre-pregnancy BMI (kg/m²)	Suggested weight gain (kg)
Normal (18.5–23)	15–20
Overweight (23–27.5)	11–16
Class I obese (27.5–31)	10–14
Class II obese (31–35)	8–12
Class III obese (≥35)	8

BMI, body mass index

Nutritional recommendations

- Bricker et al. (2015) were unable to find any robust studies in the Cochrane Database to indicate whether specialised diets or nutritional advice for women with multiple pregnancies do more good than harm. There does not seem to be any advantage to artificially increasing calorie intake in these mothers.
- In women with multiple pregnancy, the Society for Maternal–Fetal Medicine (Goodnight and Newman, 2009) recommends a daily recommended caloric intake of 40–45 kcal/kg each day for normal-BMI women pregnant with twins. It also recommends a daily supplement of the following:
  - 60 mg elemental iron,
  - 1 mg folic acid, and
  - 2500 mg of calcium (1500 mg in the first trimester).

Activity and exercise

- Women with twin pregnancy are at a higher risk of preterm labour.
- In early pregnancy, their activity need not be curtailed and they may also exercise as much as women with a singleton pregnancy.
- However, from the late second trimester, a judicious restriction of activity is recommended.

Establishment of chorionicity and amnionicity

- Chorionicity and amnionicity are predictors of higher perinatal mortality in twins (Glinianaia et al., 2011). The shared fetoplacental circulation in monochorionic twins places them at a high risk of specific complications that can have serious repercussions on the pregnancy. It is therefore critical to determine chorionicity as early as possible. This evaluation is invaluable in determining the prognosis for the pregnancy and for planning obstetric management.

- Compared with dichorionic twins, monochorionic twins have a higher frequency of fetal and neonatal mortality as well as a higher risk of the following complications:
  - Congenital anomalies
  - Preterm birth
  - Fetal growth restriction
- A first-trimester transvaginal ultrasound (when the crown–rump length is between **45 mm** and **84 mm** and corresponding to 11^{+0} **weeks** to 13^{+6} **weeks**) can determine chorionicity in 95 per cent of cases (Lee et al., 2006). A study by Dias et al. (2011) in a tertiary centre showed that a scan at 11–14 weeks could achieve 100 per cent sensitivity for diagnosing monochorionic twin pregnancy.

- **Chorionicity** refers to the number of chorions surrounding the fetuses and denotes the number of placentas.
- **Zygosity** refers to the number of eggs from which the pregnancy develops.

Ultrasound features of dichorionic diamniotic (DCDA) twinning

- Two distinct placentas are the most dependable indicators of dichorionicity in early pregnancy.
- Discordant gender in the twins establishes dichorionicity reliably.

The pregnancy is definitely dichorionic if:
- Two placentas are seen
- The twins belong to different sexes

- **The presence of an intertwin membrane and its characteristic appearance is crucial in labelling the type of twinning.**
  - In DCDA twins, the intertwin membrane is thick (≥2 mm) because it consists of four layers (i.e., two layers each of both the amnion and chorion).
  - The **twin peak sign** or **lambda sign** (Figure 35.1) refers to a triangular projection of placental tissue between the dividing membranes. A systematic review and meta-analysis by Maruotti et al. (2016) clearly established that between 11 and 14 weeks, the presence of the twin peak sign indicates dichorionicity and that the absence of the twin peak sign indicates monochorionicity.
  - The twin peak sign may become less prominent or may even disappear after 20 weeks.

Ultrasound features of monochorionic diamniotic (MCDA) twinning

- An intertwin membrane with the **T sign** seen in MCDA twins refers to the appearance of the attachment of the thin dividing membrane to the placenta at a 90° angle (Figure 35.2).

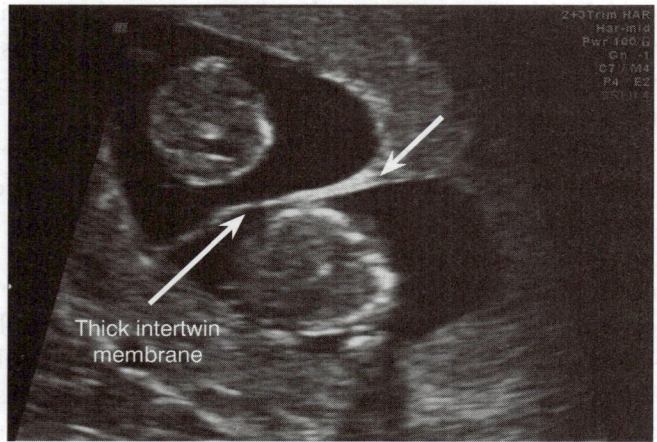

Figure 35.1   The twin 'peak' or 'lambda' sign in a dichorionic twin gestation. The long arrow points to the thick intertwin membrane. The short arrow points to the 'peak', which is the triangular projection of placental tissue between the dividing membranes (*Image courtesy:* Mediscan Systems, Chennai).

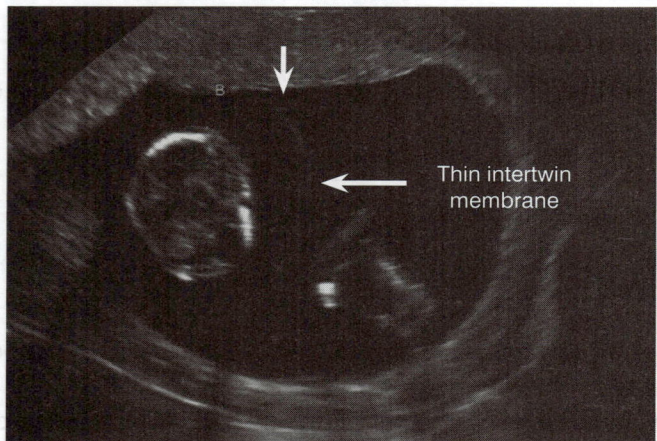

Figure 35.2   The 'T' sign in monochorionic twins (short arrow). The intertwin membrane is thin.

- The T sign has 100 per cent sensitivity and >98 per cent specificity for predicting MCDA twins (Dias et al., 2011).

Ultrasound features of monochorionic monoamniotic (MCMA) twinning

- The absence of an intertwin membrane is indicative of MCMA twinning.
- The intertwin membrane may be missed prior to 10 weeks' gestation and lead to an inaccurate diagnosis of monoamniotic twins. In such cases, counting the yolk sacs may help since monoamniotic twins usually have only a single yolk sac.
- The presence of intertwined umbilical cords is diagnostic of MCMA twins.

Screening for aneuploidy

- No method of aneuploidy screening is as accurate in twin gestations as it is in singleton pregnancies (ACOG, 2016).
- In the presence of fetal demise or an anomaly in one fetus of a multiple gestation, serum-based aneuploidy screening should not be offered for identifying aneuploidy.
- The following are the choices available for aneuploidy screening in multifetal pregnancy:

Chorionicity in assessing risk for aneuploidy
- Establishing chorionicity is an important first step for offering screening in twin gestation.
- In **monochorionic pregnancy**, either both the fetuses will be affected or both the fetuses will be unaffected. In **dichorionic pregnancy**, each fetus will have its own risk of Down syndrome.

- – *Nuchal translucency* measurement allows independent screening of each fetus in a twin or higher-order multifetal gestation. It has been recommended that greater reliance be placed on the nuchal translucency (NT) risk alone when counselling women about invasive testing (Spencer and Nicolaides, 2003).
- – *First-trimester combined screening* can be used for twin pregnancies. It gives the risk for the entire pregnancy and not for the individual fetus.
- – *Second-trimester serum screening* of twin gestations identifies approximately 50 per cent of pregnancies affected by Down syndrome at a 5 per cent false-positive rate.
- – *NIPT using cell-free DNA testing* is NOT recommended for aneuploidy screening in women with twin or higher-order multifetal gestations (ACOG, 2015).

Management in the first trimester

Establishment of diagnosis and gestational age

- The diagnosis of multiple pregnancy is best done in the first trimester, but may be diagnosed later in low-resource areas.
- Early ultrasound assessment provides an accurate estimation of gestational age (see **Chapter 9**, *Ultrasound in the first trimester*), and allows for the subsequent detection of growth discrepancy or growth restriction, timing of tests, and timing of delivery.
- The guidelines for accurate dating are as follows (FIGO, 2019):
  - – Twins conceived by in-vitro fertilisation should be dated using the date of fertilisation.
  - – In all other cases, the pregnancy should be dated according to the crown–rump length of the larger twin.
  - – Twin pregnancies presenting later than 14 weeks' gestation should be dated according to the head circumference of the larger twin.
- Discordance in crown–rump length may be observed as early as the first trimester and is predictive of later weight discordance.

 The $11-13^{+6}$ weeks' ultrasound should also be utilised for the detection of fetal anomalies.

Fetal complications in the first trimester

Vanishing twins

- In twin pregnancies diagnosed early in the first trimester, there is a high incidence of spontaneous fetal reduction. This has been termed 'vanishing twin'.
- Sampson and de Crespigny (1992) found that the vanishing twin syndrome occurs in 21–30 per cent of multifetal gestations and that the fetal loss rate was similar for IVF and non-IVF pregnancies.

> The risk of fetal death in one of the twins decreases after 7 weeks. If both twins are alive at 7–10 weeks, there is a 90 per cent chance of delivering two live babies (Sampson and de Crespigny, 1992).

Conjoined twins

- Prenatal diagnosis of conjoined twins in the first trimester has been well-established following the introduction of transvaginal and high-resolution ultrasound.
- Though rare (1 in 50,000 pregnancies), it is more common in monoamniotic twins (1 in 100).
- Ultrasonographic diagnosis depends on the presence of the following:
  - Monoamnionicity
  - Contiguous skin
  - Twins staying in the same orientation in relation to one another
  - Fetal scoliosis
  - Unusual limb position
  - More than three vessels in the umbilical cord

Maternal complications in the first trimester

- **Spontaneous miscarriage** occurs more commonly in monozygotic twins.
- **Hyperemesis gravidarum** is probably a result of the increased levels of circulating hCG.

Management in the second trimester

Ultrasound for anatomic survey

- All twin pregnancies should undergo an anatomic survey at 18–22 weeks.
- The incidence of congenital anomalies is higher in twins than it is in singleton pregnancies, with monochorionic twins having a greater incidence than dichorionic twins (Glinianaia et al., 2008). The incidence of congenital anomalies is as follows:
  - Monochorionic twins   634/10,000
  - Dichorionic twins   344/10,000
  - Singletons   238/10,000
- Monochorionic twins are at a higher risk of the following:
  - Twin-twin transfusion syndrome (TTTS)
  - Twin anemia-polycythemia sequence (TAPS)

- Twin reversed arterial perfusion sequence (TRAP)
- Selective fetal growth restriction (sFGR)
- Single fetal demise

Screening for complications in monochorionic twins

(See section on *Complications unique to monochorionic twins* below for a description of these disorders.)

- *Twin-twin transfusion syndrome (TTTS)*
  - The single deepest vertical pocket (SVDP) of amniotic fluid should be assessed at each scan to rule out oligohydramnios in one twin and polyhydramnios in the other.
- *Twin anemia-polycythemia sequence (TAPS)*
  - Middle cerebral artery peak systolic velocity should be considered from 28 weeks' gestation onwards to screen for TAPS.
- *Twin reversed arterial perfusion sequence (TRAP)*
  - Colour Doppler of the umbilical artery of the acardiac fetus will show blood flowing toward, rather than away from, the acardiac twin.
- *Selective fetal growth restriction (sFGR)*
  - Fetal biometry, amniotic fluid volume, and estimated fetal weight should be assessed for both twins at each scan.
  - An intertwin abdominal circumference difference ≥20 mm, irrespective of gestational age, has been reported to have 83 per cent positive predictive value of detecting a difference in birth weight ≥20 per cent (Sperling et al., 2001).
- *Single fetal demise*

The algorithm for the screening and monitoring of monochorionic twins presented in Figure 35.3 should be followed to ensure that no complication is missed.

Fetal complications in the second trimester

- The complications specific to monochorionic twins have been listed above.
- The complications common to both monochorionic and dichorionic twins are as follows:
  - Growth restriction/growth discordance
  - Congenital anomalies
  - Preterm delivery

Cervical length screening for preterm birth in twin pregnancy
- Routine cervical screening between 20–24 weeks for a short cervix is not recommended for women with twin pregnancy (Chasen and Chervenak, 2019; ISUOG Practice Guidelines 2016; ACOG, 2016).
- Asymptomatic women found to have a short cervix at the second-trimester ultrasound scan are known to be at an increased risk of spontaneous preterm birth. However, the sensitivity of this finding is low, and the cut-off of the cervical length used to define increased risk of preterm birth is controversial.
- There is no effective strategy to prevent preterm birth in these women. Bed rest, progesterone therapy, cervical pessary, cervical cerclage, or oral tocolytics do not reduce the risk of preterm delivery in twin gestation.

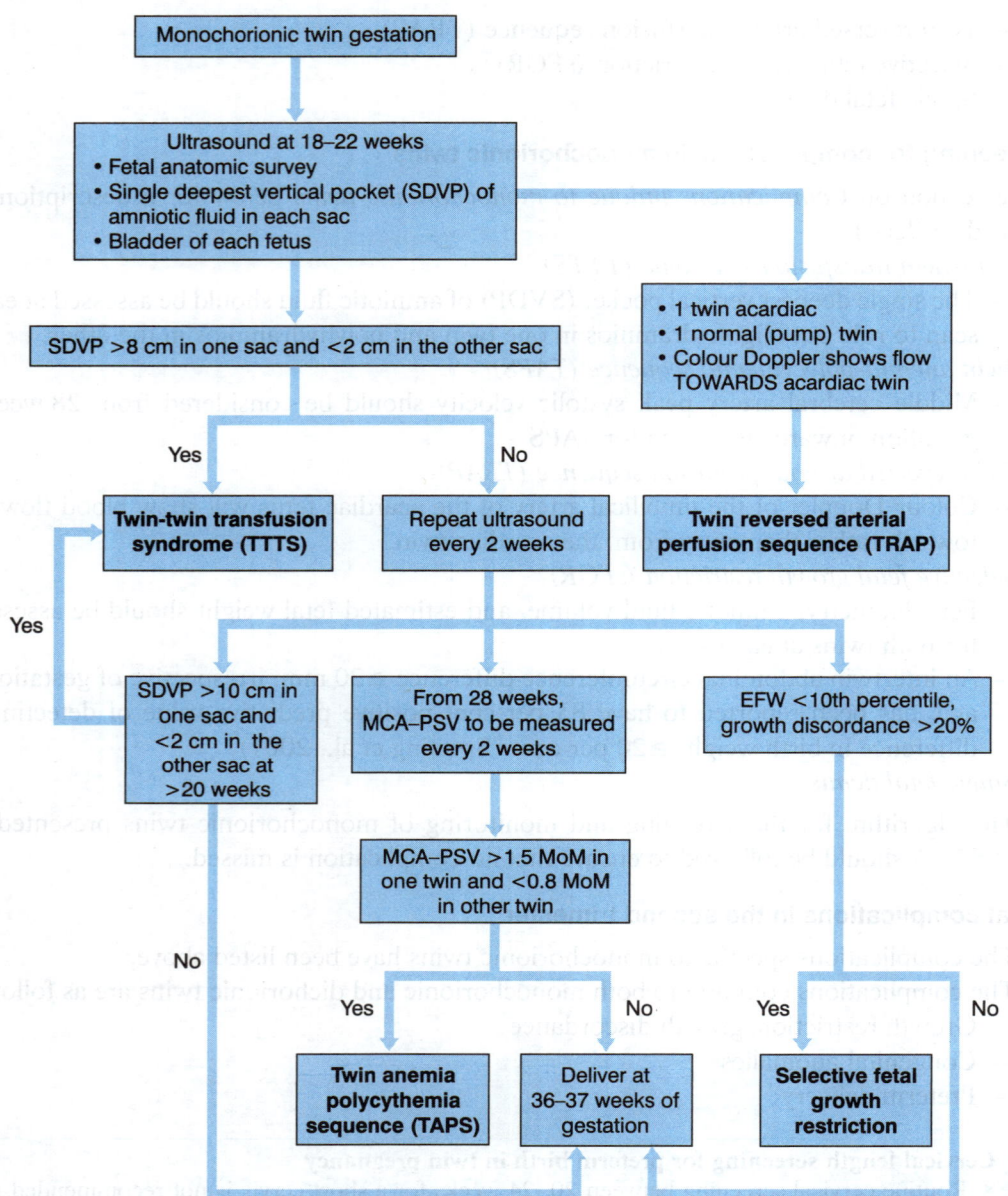

Figure 35.3   An algorithm for the screening of the complications associated with monochorionic twins, starting in the second trimester, based on the recommendations of the FIGO Committee report: Good clinical practice advice for the management of twin pregnancy (2019). *EFW*, estimated fetal weight; *MCA–PSV*, middle cerebral artery–peak systolic velocity; *MoM*, multiples of median; *SDVP*, single deepest vertical pocket

Maternal complications in the second trimester

- **Greater hemodynamic changes** occur in the late second trimester in a twin pregnancy. There is a 20 per cent higher cardiac output and 10–20 per cent greater increase in plasma volume in a twin pregnancy than in a singleton pregnancy.
- **Physiological anemia** is common, even though the red cell mass increases more in twin pregnancy than in singleton pregnancy.
- **Gestational hypertension** and **preeclampsia** are more common in women carrying twins (Francisco et al., 2017). Women with multiple pregnancy should be monitored more intensively for these complications.
- **Gestational diabetes:** There is no clear consensus on whether gestational diabetes is more common in twin pregnancy or not. Screening and diagnostic criteria are the same as they are for singleton pregnancy.
- **Other maternal disorders** observed in late second trimester in women with multiple gestations include the following:
  - Polymorphic eruption of pregnancy or PEP (earlier known as pruritic urticarial papules and plaques of pregnancy or PUPPP)
  - Intrahepatic cholestasis of pregnancy

Management in the third trimester

The evaluation and management in the third trimester includes the following:
- Prediction, prevention, and management of preterm birth
- Evaluation and management of fetal growth restriction/discordance
- Evaluation of the placental position
- Antenatal fetal surveillance

Prediction, prevention, and management of preterm birth

- Preterm birth is a major contributor to perinatal morbidity and mortality in twin pregnancy.
- Screening asymptomatic women with multifetal gestations has not proven effective for the prediction of preterm birth (see box on *Cervical length screening for preterm birth in twin pregnancy* above) (ACOG, 2016).
- Interventions (prophylactic cerclage, routine hospitalisation and bed rest, prophylactic tocolytics, and prophylactic pessary) have not proven to decrease neonatal morbidity

 Routine cervical cerclage is not beneficial in preventing preterm birth in multiple pregnancy.

  or mortality, and are **not recommended** in women with multifetal gestations (Chasen and Chervenak, 2019; ISUOG Practice Guidelines 2016; ACOG, 2016).
- Progesterone (including 17-α-hydroxyprogesterone) is not effective in preventing preterm labour in twin pregnancy (STOPPIT trial, Norman et al., 2009; Combs et al., 2011)
- Management of preterm labour may include tocolysis (though the risk of pulmonary edema is increased in multiple gestation). Corticosteroids may be administered as for a singleton pregnancy (see **Chapter 33**, *Preterm labour and preterm prelabour rupture of membranes*).

Evaluation and management of fetal growth restriction/discordance

- **Selective fetal growth restriction (sFGR):** In sFGR, the estimated fetal weight (EFW) of one twin is less than the 10th centile with EFW discordance of ≥20 per cent.
- **Growth discordance:** When there is a 20 per cent difference between the estimated fetal weights of the larger and the smaller twin, discordant fetal growth is said to be present (Breathnach et al., 2011). In almost two-thirds of discordant twin pairs, the smaller twin has a birth weight <10th percentile.
- **Growth abnormalities** in a twin pregnancy can present in the following ways (ISUOG Practice Guidelines, 2016):
  - One twin is small for gestational age (sFGR)
  - Both twins are small for gestational age
  - One twin is significantly smaller than the other twin (i.e., growth discordance), although neither is SGA

 Twin gestations with discordant but appropriate-for-gestational-age growth are not at increased risk of fetal or neonatal morbidity and mortality (Cohen et al., 2001; Kilic et al., 2006).

- Twin gestations with discordant growth and pregnancies with at least one growth-restricted fetus are associated with an approximately 8-fold increased risk of major neonatal morbidity.
- **Management:** There is very little published evidence on the best way to manage these pregnancies (RCOG, 2016; ISUOG Practice Guidelines, 2016).
  - **In dichorionic twin gestation with sFGR**, delivery of dichorionic twins should be delayed, if the condition of the sFGR fetus permits, in order to increase the gestational age of the normally growing fetus (Kaku et al., 2015).
  - **In monochorionic twin gestation with sFGR**, weekly follow-ups with ultrasound examinations are recommended.
    - Persistently absent/reversed umbilical artery Doppler flow pattern in the smaller twin indicates poorer outcomes.
    - Absent or reversed a-wave in the ductus venosus Doppler before 26 weeks of gestation indicates a substantial risk of fetal demise of the smaller twin. The option of selective termination should be considered in order to protect the normally grown fetus from serious harm, should the smaller twin die in utero.
    - In cases in which the ductus venosus Doppler is normal, early delivery at or beyond 32 weeks after a course of steroids is indicated.

Evaluation of the placental position

- Twin pregnancies should be monitored for the following placental abnormalities:
  - Placenta previa
  - Vasa previa
  - Velamentous attachment of the umbilical cord
- Identification and appropriate management of pregnancies with these complications can improve pregnancy outcome.

Antenatal fetal surveillance

- Giles et al. (2003) studied the value of adding umbilical artery Doppler ultrasound to standard ultrasound biometry measurements in the management of uncomplicated dichorionic multifetal gestations and found no difference in perinatal outcomes.
- Antenatal fetal surveillance is indicated in women with dichorionic twin gestations complicated by maternal or fetal disorders, e.g., fetal growth restriction (ACOG, 2016).

Planning and management of labour and delivery

- An experienced obstetrician should manage the labour and delivery of a twin gestation.
- The decision of the timing and route of delivery in women with twin gestations is based on the following factors:
  - Chorionicity and amnionicity of the twins
  - Gestational age
  - Fetal presentations (first twin cephalic or non-cephalic)
  - Presence of complications (maternal or fetal)

Timing of delivery

- Fifty per cent of women with twin pregnancies give birth at approximately **36 weeks of gestation** either spontaneously or for medical indications (Kogan et al., 2000).
- The recommended timing of elective delivery for twin pregnancies is as follows (ACOG, 2016):
  - Uncomplicated dichorionic diamniotic twin gestations: **38 weeks of gestation**
  - Uncomplicated monochorionic diamniotic twin gestations: **Between 34 weeks and 37^{+6} weeks of gestation**
  - Uncomplicated monochorionic monoamniotic twin gestations: **32–34 weeks of gestation**

 Cord entanglement is present at birth in practically 100 per cent of monoamniotic twins. It is an important diagnostic feature of monoaminionicity on sonography (Pasquini et al., 2006).

Route of delivery

The choice of route of delivery depends on the following:

- Amnionicity
- Fetal presentation at the onset of labour (80 per cent of first twins are cephalic)
- Gestational age
- The obstetrician's familiarity with internal podalic version, breech extraction, and external cephalic version

Vaginal delivery and trial of labour

- **Cephalic/cephalic diamniotic twins**: In the absence of any obstetric indication for cesarean, vaginal delivery is recommended.

- **Cephalic/non-cephalic diamniotic twins**: Trial of labour and breech extraction of the second twin (provided the obstetrician has experience in this) is recommended.
  - Non-cephalic second twins have comparable, if not higher, rates of vaginal delivery than second twins in cephalic presentation (Easter et al., 2016).

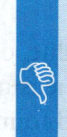 Elective cesarean delivery has no benefit over planned vaginal delivery in twin pregnancies between 32^{+0} weeks and 38^{+6} weeks of gestation if the first twin is in cephalic presentation (Barrett et al., 2013).

Delivery of the second twin
- After the delivery of the first twin, the heart rate and position of the second twin should be evaluated. As long as the fetal heart rate is reassuring, there are no specific recommendations on how soon to deliver the second twin.
- The membranes should not be ruptured until the presentation is confirmed and mode of delivery has been decided upon.
- Cord clamping should be done immediately after the delivery of the first twin but uterotonics should be avoided.
- If the contractions have reduced in frequency/intensity or ceased, augmentation with oxytocin may be initiated.

Second twin cephalic presentation, engaged: Augmentation and delivery
Second twin cephalic presentation, unengaged:
- Controlled amniotomy till head drops into pelvis, augmentation and delivery, **OR**
- Internal podalic version by grasping the feet of the second twin and performing breech extraction

Second twin breech or transverse presentation:
- Breech extraction
- External cephalic version followed by delivery

Cesarean delivery for the second twin: This may be required in approximately 10 per cent of twin deliveries and is associated with increased neonatal morbidity

Cesarean delivery

Cesarean delivery is recommended for:
- All monoamniotic twins
- Diamniotic twins with a non-cephalic presenting twin
- Pregnancies with standard obstetric indications for cesarean delivery (e.g., placenta previa)

 Women with monoamniotic twin gestations should undergo cesarean delivery to avoid an umbilical cord complication of the non-presenting twin at the time of the first twin's delivery.

Management of the third stage

- As soon as the second twin is delivered, ten units of oxytocin should be administered intramuscularly and ten units added to the infusion to prevent postpartum hemorrhage.
- Once the placentas are delivered, they should be examined. The layers in the inter-twin membrane should be counted. The presence of three (when two chorions have fused into a single layer) or four layers indicates DCDA twins; the presence of two layers indicates MCDA twins.

Management of pregnancy complications specific to twin pregnancy

Twin pregnancies may be complicated by issues unique to them, which are as follows:
- Anomalous twin
- Death of one twin
- Complications unique to monochorionic twins

Management of anomalous twin

Dichorionic twins

- The risk of a congenital anomaly is double (4 per cent) that in a singleton pregnancy (Glinianaia et al., 2008).
- Both fetuses are affected in only 10 per cent of cases. In 90 per cent, the twins are discordant for an anomaly, i.e., only one fetus is affected.
- **Management of discordant anomaly**:
  - If the anomaly is lethal, expectant management may be followed.
  - If the anomaly may result in a severe handicap or the anomaly is likely to jeopardise the normal twin during the pregnancy by causing the development of complications (e.g., polyhydramnios), selective termination should be offered.
  - **Selective termination** is carried out by intracardiac injection of potassium chloride.
    - *Termination at 11–14 weeks:* Risk of miscarriage is 7 per cent and risk of preterm birth at <32 weeks is 6 per cent.
    - *Termination at ≥16 weeks:* Risk of miscarriage is 14 per cent and risk of preterm birth at <32 weeks is 20 per cent.

Monochorionic twins

- The risk of a congenital anomaly in at least one fetus is 4 times as high (8 per cent) as that in a singleton pregnancy (Glinianaia et al., 2008).
- In 20 per cent of cases, both fetuses are affected, and in 80 per cent, only one fetus is affected (Chen et al., 1992).
- Management of discordant anomaly is more complex in monochorionic twins due to the shared circulation.
  - **Selective termination** in monochorionic twins can be carried out by occlusion of the umbilical cord vessels through endoscopic laser, ultrasound-guided bipolar forceps, or radiofrequency (Diehl and Hecher, 2007).
    - *Termination at ≥16 weeks* is associated with a 20 per cent risk of miscarriage and a 20 per cent risk of preterm birth at <32 weeks.

Management of death of one twin

- Single fetal death at ≥22 weeks occurs in 0.6 per cent of DCDA twin pregnancies and 1.7 per cent of MCDA twin pregnancies (Kristiansen et al., 2015).
- **Immediate intrauterine events** following the demise of one twin depend on the chorionicity of the gestation.

- **Dichorionic twins** have a much lower risk of morbidity and death in the surviving co-twin (Table 35.2).
- **Monochorionic twins** have placental vascular anastomoses. Therefore, there is instantaneous exsanguination into the low-pressure vascular system of the deceased twin; this results in the following:
  - ⬥ Acute hypotension, anemia, and ischemia in the co-twin lead to morbidity or occasional demise.
  - ⬥ In monochorionic pregnancies, 20 per cent of co-twin survivors have abnormal antenatal cranial imaging due to multicystic encephalomalacia.
  - ⬥ Approximately 30 per cent of surviving twins have neurodevelopmental impairment.
- Preterm birth is the most important consequence of fetal demise of one twin, and occurs in more than half the pregnancies.
- **Management:**
  - **Dichorionic twins**
    - ⬥ *Before 34 weeks:* With the mother's consent, and if there is no maternal complication requiring immediate delivery, it is better to delay delivery at least until 34 weeks so that the chances of survival are better. The surviving fetus should be monitored carefully.
    - ⬥ *After 34 weeks:* Timely delivery of the surviving twin helps prevent a second fetal loss. The pregnancy may be taken to term if there is no maternal indication for early delivery and if the monitoring of the surviving twin reveals no abnormality.
  - **Monochorionic twins**
    - ⬥ *Before 34 weeks:* Immediate delivery of the co-twin has not been demonstrated to be of benefit (Karageyim et al., 2005); management should be based on the condition of the mother and surviving fetus. If there is no maternal or fetal indication for immediate delivery, delivery can be delayed until 36–37 weeks.

       Though there are case reports about **maternal coagulopathy** in the presence of fetal demise of one twin, it is not necessary to test for it since it is rare (Chasen and Chervenak, 2019a).

    - ⬥ *After 34 weeks:* The parents should be informed about the possibility of severe neurological damage to the surviving twin. In an ongoing pregnancy, ultrasound

Table 35.2   Consequences of fetal demise of one twin based on a systematic review and meta-analysis by Mackie et al., 2019

Consequences of fetal demise of one twin	Dichorionic/diamniotic (DCDA) gestation	Monochorionic/diamniotic (MCDA) gestation
Preterm birth	54%	59%
Risk of demise in co-twin	22%	41%
Abnormal postnatal cranial imaging	12%	43%
Risk of neurological abnormality	10%	29%
Neonatal death of the co-twin	21%	28%

and MRI may be used to look for fetal intracranial changes that may predict poor prognosis. Delivery is decided upon after assessing fetal growth, and other indicators of fetal well-being. In the absence of maternal or fetal indications, pregnancy can be prolonged to 36–37 weeks.

COMPLICATIONS UNIQUE TO MONOCHORIONIC TWINS

Twin-to-twin transfusion syndrome (TTTS)

- Ten to 15 per cent of monochorionic twins may develop TTTS.
- Vascular communications exist between the two placentas in all monochorionic twins. These communications are usually artery-to-artery or vein-to-vein. If the pressure stays equal on both sides with no gradient, the blood supply to the fetuses is not compromised.
- *TTTS is thought to occur due to unidirectional flow through an arteriovenous anastomosis.* Blood from one fetus flows to the other, leading to hyperperfusion of the recipient twin and hypoperfusion of the donor twin. This occurs in 15 per cent of monochorionic twins.
- Since this condition usually manifests by mid-pregnancy, screening for TTTS starts in the second trimester (see Figure 35.3 in the section on *Management in the second trimester*). The risk of death in both fetuses is high in TTTS.
- The most serious form of TTTS is acute hydramnios in the recipient sac and anhydramnios in the donor sac. This typically presents by 18–26 weeks. With severe oligohydramnios, the dividing membrane appears closely applied to the fetal body, a condition called 'stuck twin'.
- **Ultrasonographic diagnosis** is based on the following:
  - Monochorionic twins of the same gender
  - Polyhydramnios with single deepest pocket of liquor (SDP) >8 cm in the recipient sac and oligohydramnios with SDP <2 cm in the donor sac
  - Discordant bladder appearance
  - Significant growth discordance
  - Hemodynamic and cardiac compromise in the recipient twin
- **Management**:
  - Amnioreduction may be performed when the condition is not severe.
  - Endoscopic laser ablation of communicating placental vessels is recommended for the management of advanced TTTS.

Twin anemia–polycythemia sequence (TAPS)

- Twin anemia–polycythemia sequence is defined by significant **intertwin hemoglobin discordance** without the amniotic fluid discordance that is characteristic of twin to-twin-transfusion syndrome (TTTS) in monochorionic twin pregnancies (Moaddab et al., 2016).
- TAPS may occur spontaneously in 5 per cent of monochorionic twins at >26 weeks' gestation. In 2–10 per cent of monochorionic twins, it may occur after laser ablation of placental vessels for TTTS.

- TAPS is thought to occur due to a slow transfusion of blood from the donor to the recipient twin through a few very small arteriovenous vascular (AV) anastomoses, leading to anemia in the donor and polycythemia in the recipient twin.
- **Ultrasound diagnosis** is based on the findings outlined in Table 35.3.

Table 35.3 Diagnostic criteria of twin anemia–polycythemia sequence based on ultrasound findings

Ultrasound findings	Anemic (donor) twin	Polycythemic (recipient) twin
Fetal size and amniotic fluid volume	Same	Same
Placenta	Thick and hyperechogenic	Thin and translucent
MCA–PSV*	Increased (>1.5 MoM*)	Decreased (<1 MoM)
Other signs	• Dilated heart • Tricuspid regurgitation • Ascites	• 'Starry sky pattern' of liver • Diminished echogenicity of liver parenchyma • Increased brightness of portal venule walls

*MCA–PSV, middle cerebral artery peak systolic velocity; MoM, multiples of median

- **Management** depends on the gestational age and severity of discrepancy between the twins (Papanna, 2019).
  - **<26 weeks:** Endoscopic laser ablation of communicating placental vessels is recommended. This should be followed by weekly scans to monitor fetal growth, brain anatomy, and MCA–PSV. If both babies are developing normally, vaginal delivery can be planned at 37 weeks.
  - **26–30 weeks:** Intrauterine blood transfusions to the anemic twin and exchange transfusion with Ringer's lactate solution/sterile saline for the polycythemic twin are recommended. Follow-up with Doppler assessment every 2–3 days will determine the necessity for further interventions. Delivery should be by cesarean section at 30–32 weeks.
  - **>30 weeks:** Delivery by cesarean section is recommended.
- **Prognosis**: Neurodevelopmental delay is seen in up to 20 per cent of cases (Slaghekke et al., 2014) and mainly depends on gestational age at birth. The risk is higher for the recipient twin.

Twin reversed arterial perfusion (TRAP) sequence

- Twin reversed arterial perfusion (TRAP) sequence is characterised by one fetus lacking a normally developed heart (acardiac) and head. It occurs in approximately 1 per cent of monochorionic twins (Sogaard et al., 1999).
- The *donor* (or *pump*) twin shunts blood into the *acardiac recipient*, which also lacks structures of the upper body. The deoxygenated blood from the pump twin enters the umbilical vessels of the acardiac twin and supplies mainly the lower half of the body.
- The pump twin has a mortality rate as high as 50 per cent due to a high cardiac output state and subsequent cardiac failure (van Gemert et al., 2005). Very preterm birth due to polyhydramnios also contributes to the high mortality.

- **Management** is by ablation of umbilical cord vessels by laser or diathermy, coagulation of placental anastomoses by laser, or ablation of intrafetal vessels by monopolar diathermy, laser, or radiofrequency. The survival rate of the pump twin is about 80 per cent when these methods are used (Lee et al., 2013).

Conjoined twins

- Conjoined twins are very rare (1/50,000 deliveries), and the mortality among such twins is very high. Conjoined twinning is the result of incomplete division of the embryo, occurring between 13 and 15 days after fertilisation. The twins may be connected at any level and may share a varying number of organs.
- When diagnosed early, termination of pregnancy is advised. If diagnosed in the third trimester, delivery by cesarean section is recommended. Surgical separation may be possible, but may be a very complex procedure depending on the number and the nature of organs shared.
- Once the diagnosis is made, one must evaluate the point of connection and the organs involved, along with the extent of the deformity. This helps in counselling the parents and in planning for the surgery required.

Monoamniotic twins

- Monochorionic monoamniotic placentation is found in approximately 1 per cent of all twin gestations and carries a high mortality rate of up to 50 per cent due to cord accidents, congenital anomalies, and prematurity.
- **Ultrasound diagnosis** is based on the following features:
  - In the early first trimester, the presence of two fetal poles with one yolk sac points to monoamnionicity (Bromley and Benacerraf, 1995).
  - In later pregnancy, monoamniocity is suggested by the absence of a dividing amniotic membrane, the presence of a single placenta, both fetuses of the same gender, adequate amniotic fluid surrounding each fetus, and both fetuses moving freely within the uterine cavity.
- **Management:** Though there is no evidence with regards to optimum management, it is prudent to administer antenatal steroids, undertake intensive fetal surveillance with frequent non-stress tests (NST), and perform elective cesarean section at 32 weeks (ACOG, 2016; Pasquini et al., 2006).

References

1. American College of Obstetricians and Gynecologists. 2016 (reaffirmed 2019). ACOG Practice Bulletin No. 169. Multifetal gestations: Twin, triplet, and higher-order multifetal pregnancies. *Obstet Gynecol.* 128:e131–46.
2. American College of Obstetricians and Gynecologists. 2016. ACOG Practice Bulletin 163. Screening for aneuploidy. *Obstet Gynecol.* 127(5):e123–37.

3. American college of obstetricians and gynecologists. 2015. ACOG Committee Opinion No. 640. Cell-Free DNA Screening For Fetal Aneuploidy. *Obstet Gynecol.* 126(3):e31–7.

4. Barrett JF, Hannah ME, Hutton EK et al. 2013. A randomized trial of planned cesarean or vaginal delivery for twin pregnancy. *N Engl J Med.* 369:1295.

5. Breathnach FM, McAuliffe FM, Geary M, Daly S, Higgins JR, Dornan J et al. 2011. Perinatal Ireland Research Consortium. Definition of intertwin birth weight discordance. *Obstet Gynecol.* 118(1):94–103.

6. Bodnar LM, Himes KP, Abrams B et al. 2019. Gestational weight gain and adverse birth outcomes in twin pregnancies. *Obstet Gynecol.* 134(5):1075–1086.

7. Bricker L, Reed K, Wood L, Neilson JP. 2015. Nutritional advice for improving outcomes in multiple pregnancies. *Cochrane Database Syst Rev.* Issue 11. Art. no.: CD008867.

8. Bromley B, Benacerraf B. 1995. Using the number of yolk sacs to determine amnionicity in early first trimester monochorionic twins. *Journal Am Inst Ultrasound in Med.* 14: 415–419.

9. Burgess JL, Unal ER, Nietert PJ, Newman RB. 2014. Risk of late-preterm stillbirth and neonatal morbidity for monochorionic and dichorionic twins. *Am J Obstet Gynecol.* 210(578):e1–e9.

10. Chasen ST, Chervenak FA. 2019. Twin pregnancy: Prenatal issues. Levine D, Simpson LL (Eds). *UpToDate.* Waltham, MA.

11. Chasen ST, Chervenak FA. 2019a. Twin pregnancy: Labor and delivery. Simpson LL (Ed). *UpToDate.* Waltham, MA.

12. Chen CJ, Wang CJ, Yu MW, Lee TK. 1992. Perinatal mortality and prevalence of major congenital malformations of twins in Taipei city. *Acta Genet Med Gemellol* (Roma). 41:197.

13. Cohen SB, Elizur SE, Goldenberg M, Beiner M, Novikov I, Mashiach S et al. 2001. Outcome of twin pregnancies with extreme weight discordancy. *Am J Perinatol.* 18:427–32.

14. Combs CA, Garite T, Maurel K, Das A, Porto M. 2011. 17-hydroxyprogesterone caproate for twin pregnancy: A double-blind, randomized clinical trial. Obstetric Collaborative Research Network. *Am J Obstet Gynecol.*

15. Cheong-See F, Schuit E, Arroyo-Manzano D et al. 2016. Global Obstetrics Network (GONet) Collaboration. Prospective risk of stillbirth and neonatal complications in twin pregnancies: Systematic review and meta-analysis. *BMJ.* 354:i4353.

16. Dias T, Arcangeli T, Bhide A et al. 2011. First-trimester ultrasound determination of chorionicity in twin pregnancy. *Ultrasound Obstet Gynecol.* 38:530.

17. Diehl W, Hecher K. 2007. Selective cord coagulation in acardiac twins. *Semin Fetal Neonatal Med.* 12:458.

18. Easter SR, Lieberman E, Carusi D. 2016. Fetal presentation and successful twin vaginal delivery. *Am J Obstet Gynecol.* 214:116.e1.

19. FIGO Committee report. 2019. Good clinical practice advice: Management of twin pregnancy. *Int J Gynecol Obstet.* 144: 330-337.

20. Francisco C, Wright D, Benkö Z et al. 2017. Hidden high rate of pre-eclampsia in twin compared with singleton pregnancy. *Ultrasound Obstet Gynecol.* 50:88.

21. Giles W, Bisits A, O'Callaghan S, Gill A. 2003. The Doppler assessment in multiple pregnancy randomised controlled trial of ultrasound biometry versus umbilical artery Doppler ultrasound and biometry in twin pregnancy. DAMP Study Group. *BJOG.* 110:593–7.

22. Goodnight W, Newman R. 2009. Society of Maternal-Fetal Medicine Recommendations. Optimal nutrition for improved twin pregnancy outcome. *Obstet Gynecol.* 114:1121.

23. Glinianaia SV, Obeysekera MA, Sturgiss S, Bell R. 2011. Stillbirth and neonatal mortality in monochorionic and dichorionic twins: A population-based study. *Hum Reprod.* 26:2549–57.

24. Glinianaia SV, Rankin J, Wright C. 2008. Congenital anomalies in twins: A register-based study. *Hum Reprod.* 23:1306.

25. Khalil A, Rodgers M, Baschat A et al. 2016. Ultrasound ISUOG Practice Guidelines: Role of ultrasound in twin pregnancy. *Obstet Gynecol.* 47:247

26. Karageyim Karsidag AY, Kars B, Dansuk R, Api O, Unal O, Turan MC et al. 2005. Brain damage to the survivor within 30 min of co-twin demise in monochorionic twins. *Fetal Diagn Ther.* 20:91–5.

27. Kristiansen MK, Joensen BS, Ekelund CK et al. 2015. Perinatal outcome after first-trimester risk assessment in monochorionic and dichorionic twin pregnancies: A population-based register study. *BJOG.* 122:1362.

28. Kaku S, Kimura F, Murakami T. 2015. Management of fetal growth arrest in one of dichorionic twins: Three cases and a literature review. *Obstet Gynecology Int.* Article ID 289875.

29. Kilic M, Aygun C, Kaynar-Tuncel E, Kucukoduk S. 2006. Does birth weight discordance in preterm twins affect neonatal outcome? *J Perinatol.* 26:268–72.

30. Kogan MD, Alexander GR, Kotelchuck M et al. 2000. Trends in twin birth outcomes and prenatal care utilization in the United States, 1981-1997. *JAMA.* 284:335.

31. Lee YM, Cleary-Goldman J, Thaker HM, Simpson LL. 2006. Antenatal sonographic prediction of twin chorionicity. *Am J Obstet Gynecol.* 195:863–7.

32. Lee H, Bebbington M, Crombleholme TM. 2013. North American Fetal Therapy Network. The North American Fetal Therapy Network Registry data on outcomes of radiofrequency ablation for twin-reversed arterial perfusion sequence. *Fetal Diagn Ther.* 33:224.

33. Mackie FL, Rigby A, Morris RK, Kilby MD. 2019. Prognosis of the co-twin following spontaneous single intrauterine fetal death in twin pregnancies: A systematic review and meta-analysis. *BJOG.* 126:569.

34. Moaddab A, Nassr AA, Espinoza J et al. 2016. Twin anemia polycythemia sequence: a single center experience and literature review. *Eur J Obstet Gynecol Reprod Biol.* 205:158.

35. Maruotti GM, Saccone G, Morlando M, Martinelli P. 2016. First-trimester ultrasound determination of chorionicity in twin gestations using the lambda sign: A systematic review and meta-analysis. *Eur J Obstet Gynecol Reprod Biol.* 202:66.

36. Norman JE, Mackenzie F, Owen P, Mactier H, Hanretty K, Cooper S et al. 2009. Progesterone for the prevention of preterm birth in twin pregnancy (STOPPIT): A randomised, double-blind, placebo-controlled study and meta-analysis. *Lancet.* 373:2034–40.

37. Papanna R. 2019. Twin-twin transfusion syndrome: Management and outcome. Levine D, Simpson LL (Eds). *UpToDate.* Waltham, MA.

38. Pasquini L, Wimalasundera RC, Fichera A, Barigye O, Chappell L, Fisk NM. 2006. High perinatal survival in monoamniotic twins managed by prophylactic sulindac, intensive ultrasound surveillance, and Cesarean delivery at 32 weeks' gestation. *Ultrasound Obstet Gynecol.* 28: 681–687.

39. Pison G, Monden C, Smits J. 2015. Twinning rates in developed countries: Trends and explanations. Population and Development Review, Wiley-Blackwell. 41(4). pp. 629–649.

40. Royal College of Obstetricians and Gynaecologists (RCOG). 2016. Green-top Guideline No. 51. Management of monochorionic twin pregnancy.

41. Sampson A, de Crespigny LC. 1992. Vanishing twins: The frequency of spontaneous fetal reduction of a twin pregnancy. *Ultrasound Obstet Gynecol.* 2(2):107–9.

42. Sebire NJ, Snijders RJ, Hughes K, Sepulveda W, Nicolaides KH. 1997. The hidden mortality of monochorionic twin pregnancies. *Br J Obstet Gynaecol.* 104:1203–1207.

43. Slaghekke F, van Klink JM, Koopman HM et al. 2014. Neurodevelopmental outcome in twin anemia-polycythemia sequence after laser surgery for twin-twin transfusion syndrome. *Ultrasound Obstet Gynecol.* 44:316.

44. Sogaard K, Skibsted L, Brocks V. 1999. Acardiac twins: Pathophysiology, diagnosis, outcome and treatment. Six cases and review of the literature. *Fetal Diagn Ther.* 14:53–9.

45. Smits J, Monden C. 2011. Twinning across the Developing World. *PLoS ONE.* 6(9): e25239.

46. Spencer K. Nicolaides KH. 2003. Screening for Trisomy 21 in twins using first trimester ultrasound and maternal serum biochemistry in a one-stop clinic: A review of three years' experience. *BJOG.* 110:276–80.

47. Sperling L, Tabor A. 2001. Twin pregnancy: The role of ultrasound in management. *Acta Obstet Gynecol Scand.* 80:287.

48. van Gemert MJ, Umur A, van den Wijngaard JP, VanBavel E, Vandenbussche FP, Nikkels PG. 2005. Increasing cardiac output and decreasing oxygenation sequence in pump twins of acardiac twin pregnancies. *Phys Med Biol.* 50:N33–42.

Chapter 36

Fetal Growth Disorders: Growth Restriction and Macrosomia

INTRODUCTION

- Fetal growth restriction (FGR; also referred to as intrauterine growth restriction or IUGR) and macrosomia are the two ends of the spectrum of fetal growth disorders. In fetal growth restriction, the fetus fails to reach its full growth potential. In macrosomia, the fetus exhibits excessive growth with disproportionate fat deposition.

- FGR is the single largest contributing factor to perinatal mortality in fetuses that have no congenital anomalies. Better understanding of antenatal fetal surveillance and the availability of advanced neonatal critical care have resulted in a reduction in neonatal deaths. However, stillbirth rates have remained unchanged.

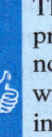 There is a high risk of perinatal death in pregnancies where fetal growth restriction has not been recognised antenatally. Pregnancies with unrecognised FGR carry over an 8-fold increased risk of stillbirth when compared to pregnancies without FGR (Gardosi et al., 2013).

- In India, the incidence of low-birth-weight (LBW) babies has been reported to be 26 per cent; half of these are due to fetal growth restriction (Pinheiro et al., 2001; Antonisamy et al., 1996).

- Fetal growth restriction is linked to an increased risk of perinatal morbidity and mortality. Growth-restricted fetuses are more prone to the following:
  - Intrauterine hypoxia/asphyxia
  - Stillbirth and hypoxic–ischemic encephalopathy (HIE)

- Barker (2006) emphasised the adult consequences of FGR. Low birth weight in relation to the length of gestation is now known to be associated with the following long-term complications:
  - Increased rates of coronary heart disease
  - Hypertension and stroke
  - Type 2 diabetes

- Macrosomia, on the other hand, is associated with both maternal and fetal morbidity.
  - *Immediate risks* associated with macrosomia are as follows:
    - **Fetal risks:** Perinatal asphyxia, death, and shoulder dystocia
    - **Maternal risks:** Cesarean section, prolonged labour, postpartum hemorrhage, and perineal trauma
  - *Long-term consequences* associated with macrosomia are as follows (Johnsson et al., 2015):
    - Early obesity
    - Increased cardiovascular and metabolic risk

WHAT DETERMINES FETAL GROWTH AND BIRTH WEIGHT?

- The natural growth potential of the fetus is impacted on one hand by the fetal genome and on the other, by the intrauterine environment (Figure 36.1).
- The intrauterine environment is under the influence of both maternal and placental factors.
- **Maternal factors** that have been shown to have an impact on fetal growth are as follows:
  - Parity (the second baby will weigh more than the first)
  - Body mass index (BMI) at the beginning of pregnancy (Abu–Saad and Fraser, 2010; HAPO study, 2010)
  - Weight gain in pregnancy—suboptimal weight gain is associated with low-birth-weight infants and high weight gain with macrosomic infants
  - Maternal fasting glucose levels have an effect on birth weight; hyperglycemia is associated with macrosomia (HAPO study, 2008)
- **Placental factors** that play a major role in fetal growth are as follows:
  - Placental perfusion, which allows the placenta to transfer substrates across to the fetus
  - Placental size and weight (Roland et al., 2012)
- **Fetal hormones** also play a role in promoting normal growth as follows:
  - In the third trimester, insulin-like growth factors (IGFs) coordinate a precise and orderly increase in growth.
  - Insulin and thyroxine (T4) are required through late gestation to regulate appropriate growth in both normal and abnormal nutritional circumstances.

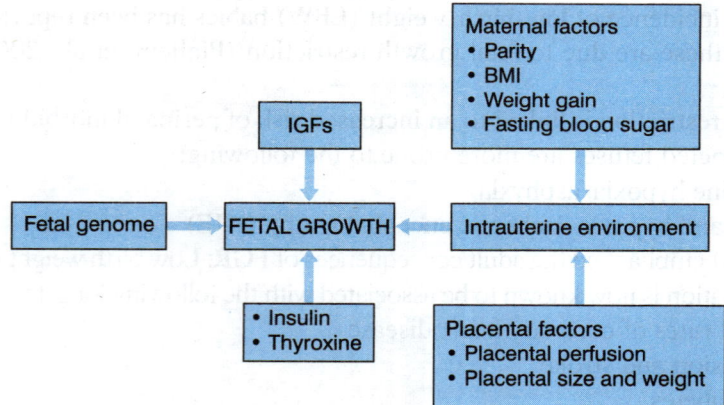

Figure 36.1   Factors that influence fetal growth.
BMI, body mass index; *IGF*, insulin-like growth factors

Fetal growth velocity over the trimesters
The total substrate needs of the fetus are relatively small in the first half of pregnancy. The rate of fetal growth is much more in the late third trimester as compared to early pregnancy. Fetal weight increases from 5 g/day at 14–15 weeks of gestation to 10 g/day at 20 weeks, and to 30–35 g/day at 32–34 weeks. Between 32 and 34 weeks, the fetus gains approximately 230–285 g per week. The rate of weight gain decreases after that. After 41 weeks, there may even be a slight loss of weight.

FETAL GROWTH RESTRICTION

DEFINITION

- A fetus is said to be growth-restricted if it does not achieve its intrinsic growth potential due to a pathologic process that could be fetal, placental, or maternal in origin.
- The term small-for-gestational age (SGA) is sometimes used for a fetus exhibiting less than expected growth (<10th percentile). However, 50–70 per cent of SGA fetuses are *constitutionally small but healthy fetuses*. Only 20 per cent of SGA fetuses are actually growth-restricted. **To avoid confusion, the term fetal growth restriction (FGR) should be applied to the fetus, while small-for-gestational age (SGA) should be used while referring to the newborn infant** (ACOG, 2019).
- Fetal growth restriction is usually defined by the statistical deviation of fetal size from a population-based standard. ACOG (2021) and the RCOG (2013) define a fetus as having FGR if its estimated fetal weight (EFW) is below the 10th percentile for a given gestational age. The RCOG and ACOG also consider a fetus to be growth-restricted if the abdominal circumference (AC) is below the 10th percentile.

> Estimated fetal weight and abdominal circumference perform similarly in predicting smallness for gestational age. However, sensitivity is higher for abdominal circumference (Caradeux et al., 2019).

- Clinically, hypoxia and acidemia are more common when the AC is **below the 5th percentile** for gestational age. Fetuses with the AC **below the 3rd percentile** are at the highest risk of an adverse outcome.
- More recent definitions have included Doppler abnormalities that also help differentiate **early-onset** (at <32 weeks' gestational age) from **late-onset** (at >32 weeks' gestational age) FGR. These findings are as follows (Table 36.1):
  - EFW < 5th percentile and umbilical artery pulsatility index (PI) >95th percentile (Unterscheider et al., PORTO study, 2013)
  - Fetal abdominal circumference (AC) <10th percentile and umbilical artery PI >95th percentile (Lees et al., TRUFFLE study, 2013)

Table 36.1   Definitions for early and late fetal growth restriction (FGR) in the absence of congenital anomalies (Based on 'Consensus definition of fetal growth restriction: A Delphi procedure', Gordijn et al., 2016)

Early-onset FGR at <32 weeks' gestational age	Late-onset FGR at >32 weeks' gestational age
AC or EFW <3rd percentile or UA-absent/reversed end-diastolic flow **Or**	AC/EFW <3rd percentile **Or**
AC/EFW <10th percentile **combined with** UtA-PI >95th percentile **and/or** UA-PI >95th percentile	**At least two out of the following three:** AC/EFW <10th percentile AC/EFW crossing centiles >2 quartiles on growth percentiles CPR <5th percentile or UtA-PI >95th percentile

AC, fetal abdominal circumference; *CPR*, cerebroplacental ratio; *EFW*, estimated fetal weight; *PI*, pulsatility index; *UtA*, uterine artery; *UA*, umbilical artery.

– AC or EFW <3rd centile or absent/reversed end-diastolic flow in the umbilical artery or both of the following: i. EFW or AC < 10th centile and ii. uterine artery PI >95th centile and/or umbilical artery PI >95th centile (Gordijn et al., 2016)

INCIDENCE

- FGR is a major health concern in developing countries like India. The incidence of FGR is 23 per cent, or approximately 30 million term newborns per year in developing countries. Nearly 75 per cent of all affected newborns are born in Asia, mainly in South–Central Asia.
- On the other hand, the prevalence of FGR is about 10 per cent of the general population in developed countries.

ETIOLOGY OF FETAL GROWTH RESTRICTION

A single risk factor or a combination of risk factors can result in fetal growth restriction. Maternal, placental, and fetal causes, singly or in combination, have been implicated in the pathophysiology of FGR.

Maternal factors

Maternal factors usually result in **asymmetric FGR**. Poor fetal growth can result from one or more of the following mechanisms:
- Decreased uteroplacental perfusion
- Chronic maternal hypoxemia
- Reduced availability of nutritional substrates

Decreased uteroplacental perfusion

- This can occur in maternal medical conditions associated with vascular disease. Placental underperfusion is the most common cause of FGR in a fetus with no congenital anomalies.
- Placental microthrombi and occlusion of vessels and infarcts may decrease placental perfusion.
- The common disorders resulting in reduced uteroplacental perfusion include the following (ACOG, 2021):
    – Pregnancy-related hypertensive diseases of pregnancy (e.g., chronic hypertension, gestational hypertension, or preeclampsia)
    – Pre-gestational diabetes mellitus
    – Renal insufficiency
    – Autoimmune disease (e.g., systemic lupus erythematosus)
    – Antiphospholipid antibody syndrome

Chronic maternal hypoxemia

- Chronic maternal hypoxemia can lead to fetal hypoxemia and FGR.

- Common disorders resulting in maternal hypoxemia include the following:
  - Cyanotic cardiac disease
  - Pulmonary disease (including severe, uncontrolled asthma)
  - Severe anemia
  - Living at a high altitude
  - Smoking

Reduced availability of nutritional substrates

- If the mother herself is undernourished, there is decreased nutrition for the fetus.
- However, unless there is severe malnourishment with a caloric intake as low as 600–900 calories, there is no high-quality evidence to indicate that additional nutrient intake increases fetal weight or improves the outcome in cases of suspected FGR (Say et al., 2003).
- Common indicators of the risk for FGR include the following:
  - Low pre-pregnancy weight
  - Poor weight gain in pregnancy
  - Pregnancy at the extremes of reproductive age
  - Short interpregnancy interval

Fetal factors

- Fetal factors usually result in **early and symmetric IUGR**. The growth restriction may be identified in the first and second trimesters.
- Since fetal factors cause a global decrease in fetal growth, all fetal measurements are below expected, resulting in symmetric growth restriction.

Genetic factors

- Chromosomal abnormalities contribute to 20 per cent of all FGR. This usually affects fetal growth early in gestation rather than late.
- Fetal weight is influenced greatly by the fetal genome. Though the maternal genes contribute more to the final fetal weight, paternal genes also have an effect.
- The common chromosomal abnormalities associated with FGR are as follows:
  - Aneuploidy (e.g., trisomy 18 or 13, Turner 45 X, triploidy). At least 50 per cent of fetuses with trisomy 13 or trisomy 18 have fetal growth restriction
  - Partial deletions, duplications, and mutations
  - Ring chromosomes
  - Confined placental mosaicism

Congenital anomalies

- In the presence of major or multiple structural congenital anomalies, the fetus is unable to maintain normal growth velocity.
- Several congenital anomalies associated with FGR result from chromosomal abnormalities.

Multiple pregnancy

In multiple pregnancy, FGR is usually seen in the third trimester, when fetal nutritional requirements are not met. Fetal growth in multiple pregnancy depends on the following:
- Number of fetuses present
- Type of placentation (monochorionic versus dichorionic)
- Presence of complications like the following:
  - Twin-to-twin transfusion syndrome
  - Congenital anomalies

Congenital infection

- Transplacental transmission of maternal infection early in pregnancy may result in FGR.
- Approximately 5–15 per cent of FGR are associated with infection with *T. gondii*, rubella, cytomegalovirus (CMV), herpes simplex virus (HSV), varicella-zoster virus (VZV), and *Treponema* (Longo et al., 2014).

Placental factors (including umbilical cord abnormalities)

Abnormal placentation

Abnormal placentation resulting in poor placental perfusion and placental insufficiency is the most common pathophysiology associated with asymmetric FGR (Salafia et al., 1995).

Structural abnormalities of the placenta

- Placental abnormalities like abruption, infarction, circumvallate placenta, hemangioma, and chorioangioma have also been associated with FGR.
- However, placenta accreta and placenta previa do not result in FGR.

Umbilical cord abnormalities

Cord abnormalities like velamentous or marginal cord insertion and single umbilical artery have been associated with FGR.

The etiological factors for fetal growth restriction are listed in Table 36.2.

CLASSIFICATION OF FETAL GROWTH RESTRICTION

- **Morphological classification**
  Fetal growth restriction is classified according to morphology as follows:
  - Symmetric growth restriction
  - Asymmetric growth restriction
- **Functional or phenotypical classification:**
  Depending on the time of onset, FGR is classified as follows:
  - Early-onset growth restriction
  - Late-onset growth restriction

Table 36.2 Etiological factors associated with fetal growth restriction

Maternal factors	Fetal factors	Placental factors
Decreased placental perfusion Hypertensive disorders Diabetes APA syndrome Systemic lupus erythematosus Renal disorders	**Genetic disorders** Aneuploidy Deletions, duplications Ring chromosomes Mosaicism	Abnormal placentation Structural abnormalities Abnormalities of the cord
Maternal hypoxemia Cyanotic heart disease Anemia Pulmonary disease High altitude	**Congenital malformations** **Multifetal pregnancy** **Infections** *Toxoplasma* *Rubella* Cytomegalovirus Syphilis Herpes simplex Varicella-zoster	
Decreased nutrition Low pre-pregnancy weight Poor weight gain Short interpregnancy interval		

Symmetric FGR

- Symmetric FGR occurs in 20–30 per cent of growth-restricted fetuses.
- This growth pattern results from a universal impairment of early fetal cellular hyperplasia caused by infection, teratogens, or chromosomal abnormality. The insult usually happens early in fetal development and therefore affects the fetus uniformly.
- In symmetric FGR, there is a proportionate decrease in the growth of all fetal organs. The head size and abdominal size are proportionately small.

Asymmetric FGR

- 70–80 per cent of growth-restricted fetuses have asymmetric FGR.
- When the insult (usually placental insufficiency) to the fetus happens in the late second trimester or in the early third trimester, it results in asymmetric FGR. The fetal head size stays normal but the abdominal circumference decreases.
- The decrease in abdominal size is due to the decrease in liver volume (caused by reduced glycogen storage in the liver) and subcutaneous fat.
- Faced by a hostile environment, the fetus compensates by redistributing blood flow to vital organs like the brain, heart, and placenta (Bahado-Singh, 1999) and decreasing flow to non-vital fetal organs like the abdominal viscera, lungs, skin, and kidneys.

Constitutionally small fetus
- These are fetuses whose EFW is <10th percentile for the gestational age but who are otherwise healthy. They are small due to constitutional factors like ethnicity, body mass index, or female gender.
- Other ultrasound findings like amniotic fluid volume and Doppler studies are normal in these fetuses.
- These fetuses are associated with normal perinatal outcome. It is generally considered that active management or elective delivery before full term offers no benefit to such fetuses (Figueras et al., 2014).

Early-onset fetal growth restriction

- Early-onset FGR, by definition, is diagnosed **at or below 32 weeks** (Gordijn et al., 2016; Figueras et al., 2018) and differs from late-onset FGR in the following aspects:
  - Clinical manifestations
  - Association with hypertension
  - Patterns of deterioration
  - Severity of placental dysfunction
- Early-onset FGR represents 20–30 per cent of all FGR and is associated with gestational hypertension and/or preeclampsia in up to 70 per cent of cases.
- It is associated with high impedance uteroplacental perfusion, which in turn leads to elevated umbilical artery blood flow resistance once villous damage exceeds 30 per cent.
- A systematic review of the Cochrane Database (Alfirevic et al., 2017) confirmed that evaluation of the placental function by umbilical artery (UA) Doppler studies is the clinical standard for identifying early-onset FGR and that its use in these pregnancies improves a number of obstetric care outcomes and reduces perinatal deaths.

Late-onset fetal growth restriction

- Late-onset fetal growth restriction is diagnosed **at >32 weeks** (Gordijn et al., 2016; Figueras et al., 2018).
- As compared to early-onset FGR, only 10 per cent of late-onset FGR is associated with hypertensive disorders of pregnancy (Unterscheider et al., PORTO study, 2013).
- Universal screening with an ultrasound in the late third trimester triples the detection rate of late-onset FGR (Sovio et al., 2015). As opposed to early third-trimester ultra sound, scanning late in pregnancy (around 36 weeks) increases the detection rate for birth weight <3rd centile. However, there has been no improvement in outcomes with universal late third-trimester screening for FGR (Divon, 2019; ACOG, 2021).
- Adding another screening ultrasound scan in late pregnancy is an extra intervention that may not be economically feasible in a low-resource country like India. For every small fetus identified, there are two false-positive diagnoses (Sovio et al., 2015).
- This condition is mildly associated with a higher risk of perinatal hypoxic events and suboptimal neurodevelopment. Consequences of late FGR include the following:
  - Late, unexpected stillbirth
  - Cesarean delivery for fetal distress
  - Neonatal acidosis
  - Admission to the neonatal unit

> Early- and late-onset FGR represent two distinct clinical phenotypes of placental dysfunction and differ significantly in clinical progression. The definitions are applicable only to fetuses without congenital abnormalities.
>
> This classification helps identify a fetus that requires fetal surveillance and is most likely to be compromised. It also helps direct the utilisation of the most appropriate surveillance modalities and decide on the timing of delivery based on the findings of antenatal surveillance.

The differentiation between early- and late-onset FGR is described in Table 36.3.

Table 36.3 Clinical differences between presentation and course of disease in early- and late-onset fetal growth restriction

Early-onset FGR	Late-onset FGR
Less common (30 per cent) but more severe	More common (70 per cent) but less severe
More difficult to manage	More difficult to diagnose
Associated with hypertensive disorders and placental dysfunction	Usually not associated with hypertensive disorders or placental dysfunction
Confirmed with umbilical artery abnormalities that precede decreased middle cerebral artery (MCA) impedance	Confirmed with decreased middle cerebral artery (MCA) impedance rather than umbilical artery Doppler flow, which may be normal
Associated with earlier deterioration of the fetal condition	Associated with late unexpected stillbirth

CONSEQUENCES OF FETAL GROWTH RESTRICTION

- A growth-restricted fetus faces an **increased risk of perinatal mortality and morbidity**. The greater the severity of the FGR, the greater the risk of complications.

> **Severity of fetal growth restriction and perinatal outcome**
> - Clinically, the perinatal outcome of FGR fetuses is largely dependent on the severity of the growth restriction.
> - Hypoxia and acidemia are more common when the EFW or AC is below the 5th percentile for gestational age.
> - Those below the 3rd percentile by biometry alone and without any Doppler abnormalities are still at high risk of adverse outcome (Unterscheider et al., PORTO study, 2013; Figueras et al., 2008).
> - The risk is highest when there are associated abnormal umbilical artery Doppler measurements (Unterscheider et al., PORTO study, 2014).

- **Prematurity** is a major issue because preterm delivery is more common in the presence of FGR. In many cases, the intrauterine environment is more hostile to the fetus than the extrauterine environment. In this situation, the infant is delivered early because staying in-utero is riskier than prematurity.
- **Stillbirth** is a major complication of FGR. Gardosi et al. (2013) found that stillbirth rates were five-fold greater if FGR was not detected antenatally than when it was.
- **Intrapartum consequences** associated with FGR include the following:
  - Non-reassuring fetal status
  - Operative vaginal delivery
  - Cesarean section
- **The infant born with FGR** can have the following complications:
  - Hypoxic–ischemic encephalopathy (HIE)
  - Meconium aspiration
  - Neonatal hypothermia
  - Hypoglycemia
  - Necrotising enterocolitis
  - Bronchopulmonary dysplasia

- **Long-term consequences** have been emphasised by Barker (2006), who extensively researched the adult consequences of fetal growth restriction, which may present in adulthood. Low birth weight in relation to the length of gestation is now known to be associated with the following:
  - Increased rates of coronary heart disease
  - Hypertension and stroke
  - Type 2 diabetes

 Slow growth during infancy and rapid weight gain after the age of two years exacerbate the adult consequences of fetal growth restriction.

SCREENING FOR FETAL GROWTH RESTRICTION

- All pregnancies should be screened for the presence of fetal growth restriction by evaluating the fundal height at each visit. Clinical assessment of fundal height is adequate screening for growth restriction in low-risk pregnancies.
- Pregnancies with risk factors for FGR (Table 36.2) should be especially screened for fetal growth discrepancies.
- **Palpation:** Uterine size can be determined by abdominal palpation and comparing fundal height to anatomical landmarks such as the pubic symphysis, umbilicus, and xiphisternum.
- **Symphysio-fundal height (SFH):** A systematic review of the Cochrane Database (Robert et al., 2015) found insufficient evidence to indicate that measuring the symphysio-fundal height (SFH) with a tape measure is effective in detecting fetal growth restriction. However, in low-resource areas where access to ultrasound (the most accurate method of detecting fetal growth restriction) is limited, the WHO (2016) recommends SFH measurement as a low-cost method of detecting growth abnormalities.

 For fetuses growing normally, from 24 weeks of gestation, the SFH measurement in centimetres should correspond to the number of weeks of gestation. A difference of ±2 cm is considered normal. A suspicion of FGR is raised when the fundal height is at least 3 cm below the gestational age in weeks.

- **Uterine artery Doppler:** Notching or increased pulsatility index (PI) in uterine artery Doppler in the first or second trimester has been studied as a screening test. A positive test is associated with a three-fold increase in the risk of FGR. However, the sensitivity of the test is higher for predicting FGR with preeclampsia. *The test is not recommended for routine screening.*

DIAGNOSIS OF FETAL GROWTH RESTRICTION

- Ultrasound is the most effective modality for the diagnosis of FGR (see **Chapter 12**, *Ultrasound in the third trimester*). Fetal growth is usually assessed with serial ultrasound examinations every 3–4 weeks. Interval growth assessment in the severely growth-restricted fetus may sometimes be indicated as frequently as every two weeks.

- **Abdominal circumference** is the single most sensitive parameter for the diagnosis of FGR.
  - Since there is depletion of abdominal adipose tissue and decreased hepatic size as a result of reduced glycogen storage in the liver of the growth-restricted fetus, the abdominal circumference will decrease in the third trimester.
  - AC is more sensitive when the interval between measurements is more than two weeks (Mongelli et al., 1998).
- **Estimated fetal weight (EFW)** is one of the most common and reliable methods of identifying the growth-restricted fetus.
  - Fetal weight is estimated by using equations that incorporate two or more biometric parameters. Equations that incorporate AC, BPD, and FL seem to provide the most accurate estimates of fetal weight, especially in the growth-restricted fetus (Guidetti et al., 1990).
  - EFW varies with ethnicity and race. It is therefore important to calculate estimated fetal weight using charts specific to the racial background of the mother. The World Health Organization has published the WHO Fetal Growth Charts, which include the common ultrasound biometric measurements based on longitudinal data derived from ten countries, including India (Kiserud et al., 2017). The **Intergrowth-21 growth chart** is also becoming a global standard because it incorporates the WHO recommendations. The standards and tools of the Intergrowth-21 project are available for clinicians on the Intergrowth-21 website.

> Birth weight differs from one country to the next, e.g., India has significantly smaller neonates than other countries, even after adjusting for gestational age. It is therefore important to use country-specific charts (Kiserud et al., 2017).

  - EFW is most sensitive for predicting FGR and adverse outcome associated with FGR in infants with severe growth restriction, i.e., birth weight <3rd percentile, which is consistently associated with adverse outcome (Divon, 2019).
- **Fetal growth charts** are invaluable in the diagnosis of FGR. Fetal biometric parameters are plotted on a growth chart that helps in identifying FGR.
  - A constitutionally small but otherwise healthy fetus will have all its biometric parameters at <10th percentile but will maintain normal growth velocity.
  - The growth chart in a pregnancy with asymmetric FGR will show slowing of the growth of the AC. The growth restriction starts in the third trimester and affects the AC, which is unable to maintain growth velocity and will start dropping.

See **Chapter 12,** *Ultrasound in the third trimester* for the explanations of growth charts and growth velocity in the diagnosis of FGR.

IDENTIFYING THE AT-RISK GROWTH-RESTRICTED FETUS

- Clinically, the perinatal outcome of FGR fetuses is largely dependent on the severity of growth restriction. A fetus whose EFW is <10th percentile but has normal Doppler indices and normal amniotic fluid is at low risk for a poor outcome.

- Hypoxia and acidemia are more common when the AC is below the 5th percentile for gestational age. Those below the 3rd percentile by biometry are at high risk for adverse outcome (Unterscheider et al., PORTO study, 2013; Figueras et al., 2008).

> In the PORTO study (Unterscheider et al., 2014), nearly 17 per cent of fetuses with EFW <3rd percentile and abnormal umbilical artery Doppler developed the following complications:
> - Intraventricular hemorrhage
> - Periventricular leukomalacia
> - Hypoxic–ischemic encephalopathy
> - Necrotising enterocolitis
> - Bronchopulmonary dysplasia
> - Sepsis
> - Death

- The risk from FGR is highest when there are associated abnormal umbilical artery Doppler measurements (Unterscheider et al., PORTO study, 2014).
- To identify placental dysfunction across the phenotypes of early- and late-onset FGR, besides umbilical artery Doppler, the inclusion of the MCA Doppler is mandatory.
- The tests performed to evaluate the health of a growth-restricted fetus and to identify the fetus at risk are as follows:
  - Doppler velocimetry
  - Amniotic fluid assessment
  - Non-stress test (NST) and biophysical profile (BPP)

Doppler indices for surveillance in FGR

Umbilical artery (UA) Doppler

- This is useful both for diagnosis (see Table 36.1) and prognostication in FGR. The use of UA indices reduces perinatal deaths in FGR (Alfirevic et al., 2017).
- UA pulsatility index (PI) is used for surveillance and decision-making in the growth-restricted fetus. When it is **>95th percentile**, it denotes placental dysfunction.
- **Absent** or **reversed end-diastolic velocities**, the end of the spectrum of the abnormalities of the UA Doppler, have been reported to be present on average one week before acute decompensation (Ferrazzi et al., 2002). 40 per cent of acidotic fetuses exhibit these findings.
- The interpretation of umbilical artery Doppler findings in decision-making in a pregnancy with FGR is detailed in Table 36.4.

Middle cerebral artery (MCA) Doppler

- MCA Doppler is a surrogate for fetal hypoxia (Figueras et al., 2014). It reflects the '**brain sparing' effect** of FGR where the fetus redistributes its cardiac output to maximise oxygen and nutrient supply to the brain.
- Cerebral vasodilation and thus lowered cerebral vascular resistance lead to increased end-diastolic flow velocity in the cerebral arteries. The middle cerebral artery (MCA) is used as the gold standard, and a MCA–PI <5th percentile is generally classified as abnormal.

Table 36.4 Interpretation of umbilical artery Doppler findings for decision-making in a pregnancy with fetal growth restriction

Findings	Clinical Intervention
Normal indices	• Continue to observe with weekly Doppler studies, NST, and SDP/AFI
Reduced end-diastolic flow	• Early sign of fetal compromise • Increase frequency of fetal surveillance • Can manage pregnancy expectantly
Absent end-diastolic flow	• Ominous finding with increased risk of perinatal mortality • Immediate delivery should be considered if beyond 34 weeks' gestation
Reversed end-diastolic flow	• Preterminal event associated with poor perinatal outcome • Immediate delivery is warranted

AFI, amniotic fluid index; *NST*, non-stress test; *SDP*, single deepest pocket

- There is an association between abnormal MCA–PI and adverse perinatal and neurological outcome.
- In late-onset FGR, MCA–PI is extremely important for the identification and prediction of adverse outcome because the UA–PI may very well be normal in these cases.

- Fetuses with abnormal MCA–PI have a six-fold risk of emergency cesarean section for fetal distress (Cruz-Martinez et al., 2011).
- Late FGRs with abnormal MCA–PI have poorer neurobehavioral competence at birth and at two years of age.

Cerebroplacental ratio (CPR)

- The cerebroplacental ratio is calculated as the simple ratio between the middle cerebral artery pulsatility index (MCA–PI) and the umbilical artery pulsatility index (UA–PI). The CPR is an extremely important diagnostic index. It becomes abnormal even when its individual components are still within the normal ranges.
- **Low CPR** (a fetal hypoxemic response) is related to the following:
  - Impaired placental perfusion
  - Placental dysfunction
  - Poor fetal growth
- At term, CPR is more diagnostic of placental insufficiency and fetal compromise than birth weight.
- **Fetal CPR <5th percentile in the third trimester is an independent predictor of stillbirth and perinatal mortality** (Khalil et al., 2016), **especially in late-onset FGR**.

Ductus venosus (DV) Doppler

- DV flow waveforms become abnormal only in advanced stages of fetal compromise.
- **In early-onset FGR, DV is the strongest single Doppler parameter to predict the short-term risk of fetal death** (Figueras et al., 2014).
- A DV >95th percentile is associated with higher risk of perinatal mortality.
- Absent or reversed 'a' wave is associated with a perinatal mortality risk ranging from 40–100 per cent in early-onset FGR.

Aortic isthmus (AoI) Doppler

- The aortic isthmus (AoI) Doppler is associated with increased fetal mortality and neurological morbidity in early-onset FGR (Fouron et al., 1999).
- This vessel reflects the balance between the impedance of the brain and systemic vascular systems.
- Reversed AoI flow is a sign of advanced deterioration and follows changes in the UA and MCA Dopplers.

Uterine artery (UtA) Doppler

- Recent studies have shown that in late-onset SGA, UtA–PI >95th percentile is associated with a higher frequency of placental underperfusion (Parra-Saavedra et al., 2014).
- In late FGR, abnormal UtA Doppler may predict the development of abnormal MCA and CPR.
- However, the value of serial uterine artery Doppler assessment as a surveillance tool for late-onset FGR is doubtful (Oros et al., 2011).

Amniotic fluid volume

- Ultrasound examination helps in assessing amniotic fluid volume.
- Oligohydramnios is a sign of fetal compromise.

Non-stress test and biophysical profile

- Decelerations during an NST or a low score on the BPP indicates fetal compromise. Fetal surveillance with these tests improves perinatal outcome.
- Frequency of testing varies with the severity of FGR. For fetuses with mild growth restriction (>5th to <10th percentile) and normal Doppler indices, testing may be done once in two weeks. More severe growth restriction warrants weekly or bi-weekly testing. See **Chapter 6**, *Antepartum fetal surveillance* for a detailed explanation of the different tests.

Antenatal interventions in FGR
- There are very few antenatal interventions that have been shown to improve the perinatal outcome in the presence of FGR. Treatment of infections such as malaria in endemic areas and discontinuation of smoking may be effective in preventing fetal growth restriction.
- **Interventions with no benefits**: Bed rest, protein supplementation, IV fluids, fructodex, L-arginine, zinc supplementation, calcium supplementation, plasma volume expansion, sildenafil, maternal oxygen therapy, heparin, and low-dose aspirin (in the absence of the risk of preeclampsia) are not beneficial and may be potentially harmful in the prevention and treatment of FGR.

TIMING OF DELIVERY OF THE GROWTH-RESTRICTED FETUS

- Delivery is recognised to be the only treatment for FGR at present. Landmark studies (GRIT Study Group, 2003; Lees et al., TRUFFLE study, 2013) have focused on how to monitor and when to deliver FGR fetuses in order to optimise perinatal outcomes.
- Early-onset FGR is more likely to present with marked placental blood flow abnormalities (as reflected in umbilical artery indices) and significant cardiovascular findings (DV Doppler abnormalities) as deterioration progresses.

- Late-onset FGR may have minimal or no elevation in placental flow resistance and subtle signs of deterioration (abnormal CPR and MCA indices).

 The primary goal of management is delaying delivery in the preterm growth-restricted fetus with the intention of gaining gestational age (Baschat, 2018). The anticipated increase in neonatal survival for each day gained in utero is 2 per cent.

Early-onset FGR

- Early-onset FGR is usually associated with maternal hypertensive disease. **In fetuses with severe FGR and fetal compromise on evaluation, the aim is to delay delivery till 34 completed weeks, when the chances of fetal survival are better**.
- In early-onset FGR, placental disease affects >30 per cent of the placenta; this is reflected in changes in the UA Doppler in the majority of cases.
- A fetus with an EFW/AC <3rd percentile is at a high risk for poor outcomes. When this is associated with worsening UA Doppler indices, the perinatal mortality is highest (Unterscheider et al., PORTO study, 2014).
- Weekly surveillance should be instituted when UA–PI is the >95th percentile. The goal is for the fetus to reach a gestational age of 34 weeks.
- Fetal deterioration in FGR can manifest itself in Doppler, amniotic fluid, fetal heart rate, and biophysical parameters. Delivery by cesarean is recommended in the presence of one or more of the following findings:
  – The UA end-diastolic flow is absent/reversed
  – Single deepest pocket of amniotic fluid is 2 cm or less
  – The NST is non-reactive or shows late decelerations
  – The BPP score is low
- A course of **antenatal steroids** should be administered when there is deterioration in the Doppler indices indicating delivery at <34 weeks.
- **Magnesium sulphate** should be given for fetal neuroprotection if delivery is expected at <32 weeks.

Timing of delivery

- If the UA end-diastolic flow (UA-EDF) is **decreased** but not absent or reversed, delivery may be delayed beyond 34 weeks.
- If the UA end-diastolic flow (UA-EDF) is **absent** or **reversed**, delivery should not be delayed beyond one week.
  – **If ≤28 weeks,** the neonatal prognosis is poor. The parents must be given a clear idea about the poor prognosis for the fetus.
  – **At 28–32 weeks**, ductus venosus Doppler helps identify a fetus that is having cardiovascular deterioration.
    • Immediate delivery is indicated in the presence of absent or reversed 'a' wave on ductus venosus Doppler even if the fetus is <32 weeks.
    • If the ductus venosus Doppler is normal, the fetus can be delivered within a week, after a course of steroids.
  – **At ≥34 weeks,** delivery is indicated. A course of steroids may be administered to the mother.

- The three **absolute indications for delivery**, regardless of gestational age, are as follows:
  - **Worsening of maternal condition**, for example, preeclampsia with severe features
  - **Obstetric emergencies** (e.g., abruption) requiring delivery
  - **Evidence of fetal compromise** as indicated by fetal surveillance testing (NST is nonreactive or shows late decelerations, or single deepest pocket of amniotic fluid is ≤2 cm).

Route of delivery

- Cesarean delivery is the optimal route of delivery for early-onset FGR.
- A suggested algorithm for the management and delivery of early-onset FGR is presented in Figure 36.2.

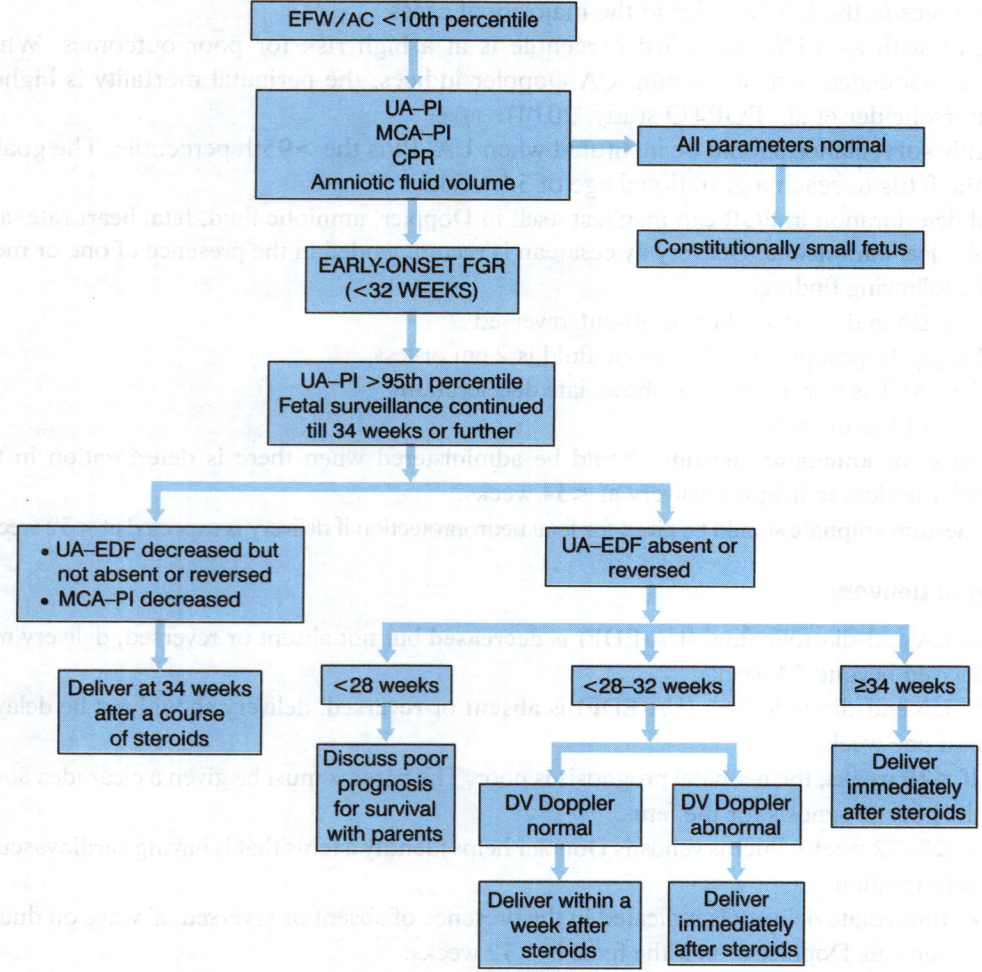

Figure 36.2 Management algorithm for early-onset FGR. *CPR*, cerebroplacental ratio; *DV*, ductus venosus; *MCA–PI*, middle cerebral artery pulsatility index; *UA–EDF*, umbilical artery end-diastolic flow; *UA–PI*, umbilical artery pulsatility index

Late-onset FGR

- The fetus should be delivered when continuation of pregnancy increases the risk of fetal compromise.
- In late-onset FGR, MCA Doppler abnormalities predict deterioration and stillbirth, in contrast to early-onset FGR, where UA Doppler abnormalities arise first. MCA Doppler findings determine the frequency of fetal surveillance (Baschat, 2018; Figueras et al., 2018)
- Even in the absence of UA Doppler abnormalities, 'brain sparing' as denoted by MCA Doppler indices should alert the clinician to the risk of sudden late stillbirth after 37 weeks.
- MCA–PI <5th percentile is indicative of hypoxia. Since placental reserve is already minimal, sudden severe deterioration may occur. The term-mature fetus is much more susceptible to hypoxia than the preterm fetus. There is a high risk of intrauterine fetal death after 37 weeks in these cases.

Timing of delivery

- Delivery may be induced at 37–38 weeks though robust evidence on optimal delivery timing is lacking.

 The term-mature fetus is much more susceptible to hypoxia than the preterm fetus. This explains the high risk of intrauterine fetal death after 37 weeks in late-onset FGR (Figueras et al., 2018).

Route of delivery

- Vaginal delivery is safe in late-onset FGR.
- Immediate cesarean delivery is indicated when there is significant oligohydramnios, spontaneous late decelerations on the non-stress test, or other obstetric causes.
  A suggested algorithm for the management and delivery of late-onset FGR is presented in Figure 36.3.

POSTNATAL CONCERNS FOR INFANTS BORN WITH FGR

The problems for a growth-restricted fetus do not end with delivery. Infants with fetal growth restriction (FGR) are at risk of several complications in the perinatal period.

- **Perinatal asphyxia:** Poor placental function leads to perinatal hypoxia and acidemia. The infant may be at risk of hypoxic–ischemic encephalopathy, meconium aspiration, and persistent pulmonary hypertension.
- **Hypothermia:** Due to poor deposition of subcutaneous fat and very low reserves of thermogenic nutrients, these infants struggle to maintain body temperature. They require careful attention to the maintenance of their body temperature post-delivery.
- **Hypoglycemia:** Serum glucose levels must be monitored carefully and intravenous fluids containing glucose must be administered. Hypoglycemia usually manifests within the first 12 hours of life.

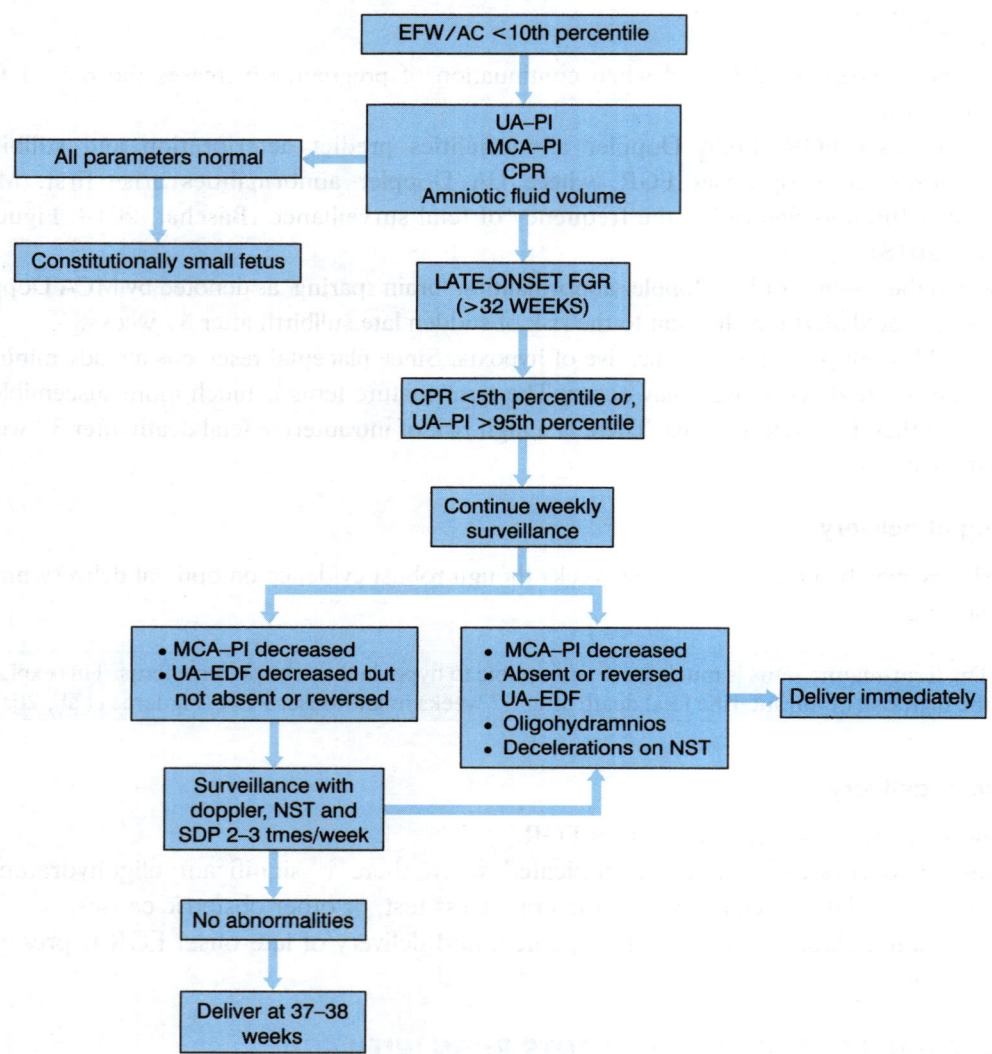

Figure 36.3 Management algorithm for late-onset FGR.
CPR, cerebroplacental ratio; *MCA–PI*, middle cerebral artery pulsatility index; *NST*, non-stress test;
UA–EDF, umbilical artery end-diastolic flow; *UA–PI*, umbilical artery pulsatility index

- **Hypocalcemia:** An infant with FGR and prematurity is at risk for hypocalcemia in the first 2–3 days following delivery. Calcium levels must be carefully monitored and calcium replacement should be started if found to be low.
- **Necrotising enterocolitis (NEC):** Infants with FGR are at a high risk for developing NEC. The combination of prematurity and low birth weight makes them susceptible to developing this complication. Absent or reversed UA–EDF is a good predictor of NEC. Oral feeds should be delayed in infants who are considered to be at a high risk for this complication.

MACROSOMIA

DEFINITION

- The term macrosomia describes a very large fetus or neonate. A macrosomic or large-for-gestational-age (LGA) infant is one whose **birth weight is equal to or greater than the 90th percentile for a given gestational age**. This definition is based on the average birth weight at each gestational age, and is country-specific.
- The World Health Organization (Kiserud et al., 2017), and the International Fetal and Newborn Growth Consortium for the 21st Century (Intergrowth-21 project) have published weight tables that should be applicable worldwide (Stirnemann et al., 2017).
- Though Western countries define macrosomia as an infant born at term and weighing ≥4000–4500 g (ACOG, 2016), this is not applicable to Indian babies. The data from the WHO's Global Survey on Maternal and Perinatal Health showed that only 0.5 per cent of babies in India are born weighing >4000 g as compared to 5–20 per cent in developed countries (Koyanagi et al., 2013).

 Given that macrosomia is defined by birth weight greater than the 90th percentile, in India, a fetus weighing ≥3250 g at term is said to have macrosomia. Even if the cut-off were the 95th percentile, a fetus weighing ≥3250 g would be considered macrosomic (Koyanagi et al., 2013).

- Even within a country, the definition of macrosomia may differ between the urban and the rural population, and between different socio-economic classes.
- In Western countries, the incidence of LGA babies has shown a continuous upward trend. However, a study from South India demonstrated that the incidence of macrosomia remained nearly the same over one and a half decades (Jeyaseelan et al., 2016).

FACTORS ASSOCIATED WITH MACROSOMIA

- The commonest factors associated with macrosomia are as follows:
  - **Maternal overweight and obesity:** Pre-pregnancy overweight and obesity account for a high proportion of LGA, even in the absence of GDM (Black et al., 2013).
  - **Gestational diabetes (GDM):** Pre-gestational and gestational diabetes are associated with fetal macrosomia. Unrecognised and untreated/poorly-controlled GDM has the highest risk of fetal macrosomia (ACOG, 2016; HAPO study, 2008).
  - **Excessive weight gain in pregnancy:** This is a modifiable risk factor for macrosomia.
  - Previous macrosomic baby
  - Parental height
  - Higher maternal age
  - Postterm pregnancy
  - Male fetus
- To prevent macrosomia, interventions should focus on managing maternal pre-pregnancy overweight/obesity and excessive gestational weight gain, regardless of GDM status. This will have a greater impact on a larger segment of women at risk for macrosomia.

CONSEQUENCES OF MACROSOMIA

- **Maternal consequences** of macrosomia include the following:
  - Increased risk of cesarean delivery
  - Protracted or arrested labour
  - Operative vaginal delivery
  - Two- to three-fold increase in risk of third-degree and fourth-degree lacerations
  - Postpartum hemorrhage
  - Uterine rupture
- **Fetal consequences:** The most important problems associated with macrosomia are those that are a result of shoulder dystocia, which are as follows:
  - Brachial plexus injury (Erb–Duchenne paralysis)
  - Clavicular fracture
  - Asphyxia
- **Neonatal problems** that may present themselves are as follows:
  - Increased risk of depressed 5-minute Apgar scores leading to admission and stay in a neonatal intensive care unit
  - Hypoglycemia
  - Respiratory problems
  - Polycythemia
- **Long-term consequences** which manifest in adulthood include the following:
  - Obesity
  - Impaired glucose tolerance
  - Metabolic syndrome
  - Cardiac remodelling

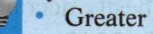

> **Diabetes, macrosomia, and shoulder dystocia**
> Macrosomia in fetuses caused by glucose intolerance is different from macrosomia that results from other causes. Babies born to diabetic mothers tend to have an increased risk of shoulder dystocia because of the following factors:
> - Greater total body fat
> - Greater shoulder and upper extremity circumferences
> - Chest circumference much larger than the head
> - Altered fetal body shape—barrel-chested infant with a short neck and broad shoulders

DIAGNOSIS OF MACROSOMIA

- The antenatal diagnosis of macrosomia, either clinically or by ultrasound, is an imprecise science.
- **Clinical assessment:** When there is clinical suspicion of a large fetus near term, fundal height measurement has poor diagnostic performance. Palpation through the abdominal wall is made difficult by the following factors:
  - Quantity of amniotic fluid
  - Uterine size
  - Maternal body fat (in overweight and obese women)

- **Ultrasound assessment:** Though ultrasonography has better diagnostic accuracy than clinical examination, Kayem et al. (2009) found the diagnostic performance of both methods to be quite low.
  - Ultrasound examination involves the measurement of the biparietal diameter (BPD), abdominal circumference (AC), and femur length (FL) and incorporating these into a formula for calculating estimated fetal weight (EFW). The larger the fetus, the less accurate is the ultrasound estimation of fetal weight.
  - Ultrasonography is also poor in predicting fetal weight in multiple gestation and diabetic pregnancies.
  - Attempts have been made to use subcutaneous fat measurements of the abdominal or thigh soft tissue to predict fetal weight but these have not proved useful.

 Abdominal circumference (AC) is the most important parameter for the assessment of the risk for macrosomia.

MANAGEMENT OF MACROSOMIA

- The suspicion of macrosomia alerts the clinician to the possibility of complications, the most important being shoulder dystocia (see the section on *Shoulder dystocia* in **Chapter 30**, *Obstetric emergencies*).
- Complications associated with macrosomia, however, also depend on other factors including maternal and fetal anatomy.
- **Vaginal delivery:** The majority of macrosomic infants do well with vaginal delivery, even if there is shoulder dystocia. A trial of vaginal delivery can be offered to women with suspected macrosomia.
- **Cesarean section:** Cesarean delivery reduces but does not eliminate the risk of birth trauma and brachial plexus injury associated with fetal macrosomia. A cesarean delivery should be offered to women with suspected macrosomia in the presence of the following:
  - A previous macrosomic baby with poor obstetric outcome
  - Prolonged second stage of labour
  - Midpelvic arrest
  - Suspected fetopelvic disproportion
- **Special situations:**
  - *A previous cesarean delivery* is a relative contraindication for attempting vaginal delivery (VBAC). Macrosomia, especially in the presence of diabetes, may be an indication for elective repeat cesarean delivery.
  - *Diabetes mellitus:* When macrosomia is suspected in a mother with gestational diabetes, a cesarean section may be offered electively if the EFW is >3500 g. The risk of shoulder dystocia is higher in infants of diabetic mothers because of the abnormal fat distribution. The labour should be monitored carefully for signs of fetopelvic disproportion.
  - *Previous shoulder dystocia:* Since the recurrence of shoulder dystocia in the subsequent pregnancy is low, a woman with a previous history of shoulder dystocia may be allowed to deliver vaginally, as long as there is no significant fetal macrosomia.

References

Fetal growth restriction

1. Abu-Saad K, Fraser D. 2010. Review: Maternal nutrition and birth outcomes. *Epidemiol Rev.* 32:5-25.

2. American College of Obstetricians and Gynecologists. 2019. ACOG Practice Bulletin No. 204. Fetal growth restriction. *Obstet Gynecol.* 133:e97–109.

3. American College of Obstetricians and Gynecologists. 2021. ACOG Practice Bulletin No. 227. Fetal growth restriction. *Obstet Gynecol.*

4. Alfirevic Z, Stampalija T, Dowswell T. 2017. Fetal and umbilical Doppler ultrasound in high-risk pregnancies. *Cochrane Database Syst Rev.* Issue 6. Art. No.: CD007529.

5. Antonisamy B, Sivaram M, Richard J, Rao PSS. 1996. Trends in intra-uterine growth of single live births in Southern India. *J Trop Pediatr.* pp. 339–341.

6. Barker D. 2006. Adult consequences of fetal growth restriction. *Clinical Obstetrics and Gynecology.* Vol 49. Issue 2. pp. 270–283.

7. Bahado-Singh RO, Kovanci E, Jeffres A et al. 1999. The Doppler cerebroplacental ratio and perinatal outcome in intrauterine growth restriction. *Am J Obstet Gynecol.* 180:750.

8. Baschat AA. 2018. Planning management and delivery of the growth-restricted fetus. *Best Practice & Research Clinical Obstetrics and Gynaecology.* 49; 53–65.

9. Caradeux J, Martinez-Portilla RJ, Peguero A et al. 2019. Diagnostic performance of third-trimester ultrasound for the prediction of late-onset fetal growth restriction: A systematic review and meta-analysis. *Am J Obstet Gynecol.* 220:449.

10. Cruz-Martinez R, Figueras F, Hernandez-Andrade E et al. 2011. Fetal brain Doppler to predict cesarean delivery for non-reassuring fetal status in term small-for-gestational-age fetuses. *Obstet Gynecol.* 117:618-626.

11. Divon MY. 2019. Fetal growth restriction: Screening and diagnosis. Levine D (Ed). *UpToDate.* Waltham, MA.

12. Ferrazzi E, Bozzo M, Rigano S, Bellotti M, Morabito A, Pardi G, Battaglia FC, Galan HL. 2002. Temporal sequence of abnormal Doppler changes in the peripheral and central circulatory systems of the severely growth-restricted fetus. *Ultrasound Obstet Gynecol.* 19: 140–146.

13. Fouron JC, Skoll A, Sonesson SE et al. 1999. Relationship between flow through the fetal aortic isthmus and cerebral oxygenation during acute placental circulatory insufficiency in ovine fetuses. *Am J Obstet Gynecol.* 181:1102–1107.

14. Figueras F, Eixarch E, Meler E, Iraola A, Figueras J, Puerto B, Gratacos E. 2008. Small-for-gestational-age fetuses with normal umbilical artery Doppler have suboptimal perinatal and neurodevelopmental outcome. *Eur J Obstet Gynecol Reprod Biol.* 136: 34–38.

15. Figueras F, Caradeux J, Crispi F et al. 2018. Diagnosis and surveillance of late-onset fetal growth restriction. *Am J Obstet & Gynec.* Volume 218. Issue 2. S790–802. e1.

16. Figueras F, Gratacos E. 2014. Update on the diagnosis and classification of fetal growth restriction and proposal of a stage-based management protocol. *Fetal Diagn Ther.* 36:86–98.

17. Gardosi J, Madurasinghe V, Williams M, Malik A, Francis A. 2013. Maternal and fetal risk factors for stillbirth: Population-based study. *BMJ.* 346: f108-10.

18. Gordijn SJ, Beune IM, Thilaganathan B et al. 2016. Consensus definition for placental fetal growth restriction: A Delphi procedure. *Ultrasound Obstet Gynecol.* 48: 333–339.

19. GRIT Study Group. 2003. A randomized trial of timed delivery for the compromised preterm fetus: Short-term outcomes and Bayesian interpretation. *BJOG.* 110: 27–32.

20. Guidetti DA, Divon MY, Braverman JJ et al. 1990. Sonographic estimates of fetal weight in the intrauterine growth retardation population. *Am J Perinatol*. 7:5.

21. HAPO Study Cooperative Research Group. 2010. Hyperglycaemia and Adverse Pregnancy Outcome (HAPO) Study: Associations with maternal body mass index. *BJOG*.117(5):575-84.

22. HAPO Study Cooperative Research Group. 2008. Hyperglycaemia and Adverse Pregnancy Outcome (HAPO) Study. *N Engl J Med*. 358(19):1991–2002.

23. Johnsson IW, Haglund B, Ahlsson F, Gustafsson J. 2015. A high birth weight is associated with increased risk of type 2 diabetes and obesity. *Pediatr Obes*. 10: 77–83.

24. Khalil A, Morales-Roselló J, Townsend R, Morlando M, Papageorghiou A, Bhide A, Thilaganathan B. 2016. Value of third-trimester cerebroplacental ratio and uterine artery Doppler indices as predictors of stillbirth and perinatal loss. *Ultrasound Obstet Gynecol*. 47: 74–80.

25. Kiserud T, Piaggio G, Carroli G et al. 2017. The World Health Organization Fetal Growth Charts: A Multinational Longitudinal Study of Ultrasound Biometric Measurements and Estimated Fetal Weight. *PLoS Med*. 14(1): e1002220.

26. Lees C, Marlow N, Arabin B, Bilardo CM, Brezinka C, Derks JB et al. 2013. Perinatal morbidity and mortality in early-onset fetal growth restriction: Cohort outcomes of the trial of randomized umbilical and fetal flow in Europe (TRUFFLE). *Ultrasound Obstet Gynecol*. 42:400–8.

27. Longo S, Borghesi A, Tzialla C, Stronati M. 2014. IUGR and infections. *Early Hum Dev*. 90 Suppl 1. S42–4.

28. Mongelli M, Ek S, Tambyraja R. 1998. Screening for fetal growth restriction: A mathematical model of the effect of time interval and ultrasound error. *Obstet Gynecol*. 92:908.

29. Oros D, Figueras F, Cruz-Martinez R, Meler E, Munmany M, Gratacos E. 2011. Longitudinal changes in uterine, umbilical and fetal cerebral Doppler indices in late-onset small-for-gestational age fetuses. *Ultrasound Obstet Gynecol*. 37: 191–195.

30. Parra-Saavedra M, Crovetto F, Triunfo S et al. 2014. Association of Doppler parameters with placental signs of under-perfusion in late-onset small-for-gestational-age pregnancies. *Ultrasound Obstet Gynecol*. 44: 330–337.

31. Pinheiro A, David A, Joseph B. 2001. Pregnancy weight gain and its correlation to birth weight. *Indian J Med Sci*. 55(5):266–70.

32. Robert PJ, Ho J, Valliappan RJ, Sivasankari S. 2015. Symphysial fundal height (SFH) measurement in pregnancy for detecting abnormal fetal growth. *Cochrane Database Syst Rev*. Issue 9. Art. no.: CD008136.

33. Roland MC, Friis CM, Voldner N et al. 2012. Fetal growth versus birthweight: The role of placenta versus other determinants. *PLoS One*. 7(6):e39324.

34. Royal College of Obstetricians and Gynaecologists (RCOG). 2013. The investigation and management of the small for gestational age fetus. Green-top Guideline No. 31.

35. Salafia CM, Minior VK, Pezzullo JC, Popek EJ, Rosenkrantz TS, Vintzileos AM. 1995. Intrauterine growth restriction in infants of less than thirty-two weeks' gestation: Associated placental pathologic features. *Am J Obstet Gynecol*. 173:1049–57.

36. Say L, Gulmezoglu AM, Hofmeyr GJ. 2003. Maternal nutrient supplementation for suspected impaired fetal growth. *Cochrane Database Syst Rev*. Issue 1. Art. no.: CD000148.

37. Sovio U, White IR, Dacey A, Pasupathy D, Smith GCS. 2015. Screening for fetal growth restriction with universal third trimester ultrasonography in nulliparous women in the Pregnancy Outcome Prediction (POP) study: A prospective cohort study. *Lancet*.

38. Unterscheider J, Daly S, Geary MP, McAuliffe FM, Kennelly MM et al. 2013. Optimizing the definition of intrauterine growth restriction–results of the multicenter prospective PORTO study. *AJOG*. 208 (4): 290.

39. Unterscheider J, O'Donoghue K, Daly S, Geary MP, Kennelly MM, McAuliffe FM, Hunter A, Morrison JJ, Burke G, Dicker P, Tully EC, Malone FD. 2014. Fetal growth restriction and the risk of perinatal mortality – case studies from the multicentre PORTO study. *BMC Pregnancy Childbirth*. 14: 63.

Macrosomia

40. American College of Obstetricians and Gynecologists. 2016 (reaffirmed 2018). ACOG Practice Bulletin No. 173. Fetal macrosomia. *Obstet Gynecol*. 128:e195–209.

41. Black MH, Sacks DA, Xiang AH, Lawrence JM. 2013. The relative contribution of prepregnancy overweight and obesity, gestational weight gain, and IADPSG-defined gestational diabetes mellitus to fetal overgrowth. *Diabetes Care*. 36:56.

42. Jeyaseelan L, Yadav B, Silambarasan V et al. 2016. Large for gestational age births among south Indian women: Temporal trend and risk factors from 1996 to 2010. *J Obstet Gynaecol India*. 66 (Suppl 1):42–50.

43. Kayem G, Grange G, Breart G, Goffinet F. 2009. Comparison of fundal height measurement and sonographically measured fetal abdominal circumference in the prediction of high and low birth weight at term. *Ultrasound Obstet Gynecol*. 34:566–71.

44. Koyanagi A, Jun Zhang, Amarjargal Dagvadorj et al. 2013. Macrosomia in 23 developing countries: An analysis of a multicountry, facility-based, cross-sectional survey. *Lancet*. 381:476.

45. Stirnemann J, Villar J, Salomon LJ et al. 2017. International estimated fetal weight standards of the INTERGROWTH-21st Project. *Ultrasound Obstet Gynecol*.

46. The Hyperglycemia and Adverse Pregnancy Outcome (HAPO) Study. 2002. *Int J of Gynec & Obstet*. 78: 69-77.

47. World Health Organization. 2016. WHO recommendations on antenatal care for a positive pregnancy experience. WHO, Geneva.

Chapter 37

Late Intrauterine Fetal Death and Stillbirth

INTRODUCTION

- Late fetal death or stillbirth is devastating, not only for the couple and their family but also for the obstetrician taking care of them. The couple needs emotional support, empathetic counselling, and the obstetrician's help in finding the cause of stillbirth. Help should also be sought from a neonatologist and a geneticist as part of counselling. The cause of death must be identified and explained to the couple, and further management must be discussed.
- In 2015, there were 2.6 million stillbirths recorded globally. Ninety-eight per cent of these deaths occurred in low- and middle-income countries. Of these, approximately half occured during labour and delivery (intrapartum). Approximately 50 per cent of stillbirths in South Asia (including India) are **intrapartum**, as compared to 10 per cent in developed countries.

DEFINITION

- **Intrauterine fetal death** refers to a fetus with no signs of life in utero.
- **Stillbirth** refers to a baby born/delivered with no signs of life, known to have died in utero after the period of viability.
  - The definition of stillbirth varies across countries.
  - The World Health Organization recommends defining stillbirth as a baby born with no signs of life at or after 28 weeks' gestation or fetal weight of ≥ 1000 g. This definition is used in India.
  - In the United States of America, stillbirth is defined as the loss of pregnancy after 20 weeks; in the United Kingdom, it is defined as the loss of pregnancy after 24 completed weeks' gestation.
- **Fetal deaths have been defined as early** and **late, antepartum** or **intrapartum.**
  - **Early fetal death** refers to the death of a fetus between 20 and 27 weeks' gestation (fetal weight >500 g).
  - **Late fetal death** (discussed in this chapter) refers to fetal death after 28 weeks, birth weight of 1000 g or more, or crown–heel length of ≥ 35 cm.
  - **Antepartum fetal death** is usually defined as fetal death occurring before the onset of labour.
  - **Intrapartum fetal death** is defined as fetal death after the onset of labour.

Intrapartum stillbirths in low-income countries occur predominantly due to the lack of skilled birth attendants and restricted access to cesarean delivery.

In this chapter, **intrauterine fetal death will refer to late fetal demise after the period of viability**. The terms intrauterine fetal death, fetal demise, stillbirth, and stillborn are used interchangeably.

ETIOLOGY

Stillbirth results from maternal, fetal, and placental disorders that may be present singly or in combination. However, a large number of fetal deaths may not have an identifiable etiology (*unexplained IUFD*). This could be attributed to the lack of essential information or the non-availability of diagnostic tests to reach a conclusion.

- An **unexplained late fetal death** (intrauterine fetal demise or IUFD) occurring near term is one that cannot be attributed to any specific fetal, placental, maternal, or obstetric cause. This can account for anywhere from 25–60 per cent of stillbirths (Stillbirth Collaborative Research Network Writing Group, 2011). Huang and colleagues (2000) found that two-thirds of the unexplained fetal deaths in their series occurred after 35 weeks' gestation.
- **Fetal growth restriction (FGR)** is the second most common cause of IUFD. Unrecognised growth restriction is considered the single largest risk factor for stillbirth (Gardosi et al., 2013). Growth-restricted fetuses have a five- to seven-fold risk of stillbirth as compared to normally grown fetuses (Bukowski et al., 2014).

In developing countries, hypertensive disorders contribute to a large number of stillbirths because of the associated growth restriction, placental dysfunction, and abruption.

- **Placental dysfunction** resulting from various etiologies like hypertensive disorders or the antiphospholipid antibody syndrome can lead to fetal demise.
- **Placental abruption** is uncommon but results in 10–20 per cent of all stillbirths. The larger the area of placental separation, the greater is the risk of fetal demise. Hypertension and preeclampsia are significant contributors to abruption and stillbirth.
- **Diabetes** is associated with an increased risk of stillbirth. The risk for stillbirth results from two mechanisms (Fretts, 2019):
  - Fetal hyperglycemia and hyperinsulinemia increase fetal oxygen consumption, leading to fetal hypoxemia and acidosis.
  - Maternal vasculopathy and hyperglycemia can lead to reduced placental function resulting in FGR.
- **Postterm pregnancy** is known to contribute to stillbirth. A systematic review and meta-analysis of cohort studies of 15 million pregnancies (Muglu et al., 2019) concluded that there is a significant additional risk of stillbirth if a woman does not deliver by 40 weeks and her pregnancy continues to 41 weeks. If spontaneous labour does not occur, the woman should be monitored after 40 weeks and labour should be induced by 41 weeks to avoid the risk of stillbirth (see **Chapter 34**, *Management of the postterm pregnancy*).

- **Infections** play an important role in the etiology of IUFD, especially in developing countries. Maternal malaria, hepatitis, herpes simplex, toxoplasmosis, and cytomegalovirus infection are established causes of intrauterine fetal demise. Infection with Zika virus has been associated with stillbirth (Sarno et al., 2016). The stillbirth rate has increased during the SARS-CoV-2 pandemic (see **Chapter 49**, *COVID-19 in Pregnancy*). However, this does not seem to be as a direct result of infection. Studies in developed and developing countries have surmised that stillbirth may result from women not being able to access healthcare, either due to the fear of disease transmission or due to the lack of public transport during lockdown (Khalil et al., 2020; Ashish et al., 2020).
- **Congenital anomalies** are commonly seen in stillborn fetuses. This rate is lower in areas where a routine second-trimester ultrasound is done, and pregnancy is terminated in cases where there are lethal anomalies.
- **Chromosomal abnormalities** are usually lethal, and end in an early pregnancy loss. The commonest association of late fetal death and chromosomal abnormality is with trisomies 13, 18, 21, and sex chromosome aneuploidies. If a congenital abnormality is noted in a stillborn fetus, the risk of a chromosomal anomaly is higher (Korteweg et al., 2008).
- **Immune or non-immune hydrops** may lead to IUFD.
- **Cord entanglement** is often blamed for an unexplained fetal death. Nuchal cord occurs in 1 out of 3 pregnancies, but very rarely causes fetal death. Postnatal examination of the umbilical cord around the neck allows for the assessment of how tight it was and whether it could have been the cause of death. **True knots** are sometimes seen. Nuchal cord or knots in the cord must be considered the cause of fetal death only after thorough assessment for other etiologies.

DIAGNOSIS OF FETAL DEATH

- The mother may present with an absence of previously perceived fetal movements; this usually raises the first suspicion of an IUFD.
- Often, IUFD may be suspected when fetal heart sounds are not audible on auscultation at a routine antenatal check-up.
- The mother may also present with vaginal bleeding with or without uterine contractions.
- Auscultation of the fetal heart by stethoscope or Doppler is insufficient to confirm an IUFD.

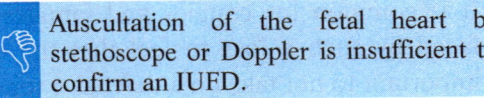

Auscultation of the fetal heart by stethoscope or Doppler is insufficient to confirm an IUFD.

- Real-time USG enables direct visualisation of the fetal heart movement. The absence of cardiac activity confirms fetal death.
- Other ultrasound features that may help confirm the diagnosis of IUFD are seen when fetal death has occurred earlier than the diagnosis. These features are as follows:
  - Collapse of the fetal skull (Spalding sign) with overlapping bones (Zeit, 1976) (Figure 37.1)
  - Hydrops
  - Maceration resulting in an unrecognisable fetal mass

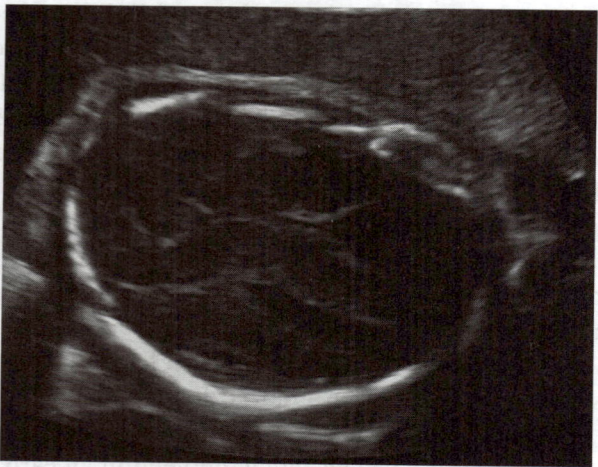

Figure 37.1 Intrauterine fetal death with collapse and overlapping of the skull bones (arrows) on ultrasound imaging.

- Intrafetal gas (within the heart, great vessels, joints) called Robert's sign
- Hyperflexion of the spine
- Crowding of the rib shadow

INFORMING THE COUPLE

- Intrauterine fetal death is an emotionally wrenching event for the woman and her family. It must be handled with great sensitivity.
- The woman and her husband/partner should be informed about the problem in privacy and with great empathy.
- Other family members whom the couple want to include in the discussion may be called in after the initial breaking of the news.

> Breaking bad news is a skill that may not come naturally. It is a clinical competence that can be taught and should be a part of training. Senior doctors must teach their junior colleagues empathy and the right words to be used in such a tragic situation.
>
> An intrapartum fetal death may also have medicolegal implications and must be dealt with great sensitivity.

- It is common for couples and families faced by such a loss to feel that the obstetrician has been negligent. However, it is important to not take on a defensive tone. There should be no attempt to place the blame on the woman, even by implication.
- All the proceedings should aim to support the couple's choices. The following points must be discussed:
    - Need to establish cause of death by evaluation
    - Expectant management and its implications
    - Mode of delivery
    - Timing of delivery
    - Need for postmortem examination and other tests on the fetus after it is delivered

– Management of death rituals (cremation/burial)
– Timing and management of subsequent pregnancy

FURTHER EVALUATION

- Though no cause may be found in 30–50 per cent of antepartum deaths even after complete evaluation (Stillbirth Collaborative Research Network Writing Group, 2011), every attempt must be made to ascertain the cause of death.
- Sometimes, clinical findings strongly suggest a cause of the fetal demise. In such a case, further testing may not be required, or may be limited to a fewer number of tests. For example, an obvious cause could include cord prolapse, a true knot, or anencephaly.
- Identification of the cause of fetal death requires both maternal and fetal evaluation.

Maternal evaluation

- A thorough **history** is the first step in investigating the cause of the IUFD.
- **Physical examination** should rule out the presence of hypertensive disorders.
- **Ultrasonography** may help establish *fetal growth restriction* or the presence *of fetal structural abnormalities*.
- **Blood tests** are important to rule out certain causes that may have resulted in the IUFD. The following tests are recommended:
  - Screening for diabetes
  - Screening for antiphospholipid antibody syndrome (especially in the presence of fetal growth restriction or early onset preeclampsia)

 Certain basic investigations should be performed in all women with IUFD. Special tests are ordered only when indicated.

  - Kleihauer–Betke test to rule out massive fetal–maternal hemorrhage, though it is a rare cause of stillbirth
  - Indirect Coombs test to rule out Rh alloimmunisation (see **Chapter 43**, *Management of Rh alloimmunisation in pregnancy*)
  - Coagulation tests if the fetal demise is suspected to have occurred 2–3 weeks earlier. However, coagulopathies associated with prolonged fetal retention are uncommon for at least four weeks after the event. Coagulation workup is, therefore, not required immediately after a recent stillbirth.
  - Inherited thrombophilias have not been associated with stillbirths and do not need to be tested for (ACOG, 2020).

 DIC occurs in 10 per cent of IUFDs and usually occurs after four weeks. The risk may be increased in the presence of maternal sepsis, preeclampsia, or abruption.

- **Amniocentesis** may be advised to rule out a chromosomal or infective cause of IUFD.
  - Saal and colleagues (1987) showed that performing an amniocentesis immediately after fetal death allows successful cytogenetic studies, whereas the culture of fetal tissues after delivery is not as successful.
  - Other studies have also shown an 80–100 per cent success rate of cell culture from

amniotic fluid obtained before delivery versus a rate of 10–30 per cent from skin or umbilical cord blood after delivery (Khare et al., 2005; Korteweg et al., 2008).

– Chromosomal abnormalities may be identified with these studies. *Microarray analysis* improves the detection of genetic anomalies as compared to conventional karyotyping (ACOG, 2020).

– Polymerase chain reaction (PCR) for viral infection and amniotic fluid culture may also be carried out if infection with cytomegalovirus, Toxoplasma or Parvovirus B$_{19}$ is suspected.

Fetal and stillborn evaluation

• **Examination of the placenta, cord, and membranes** is essential since some placental abnormalities are associated with clinical causes of stillbirth (Heazell and Martindale, 2009). A detailed examination may reveal one of the following possible causes of IUFD:

– Placenta

♦ Retroplacental clots suggestive of abruption

♦ Placental infarction which may be associated with FGR

 Placental and cord samples must not be placed in formalin. They should be sent to the lab in a sterile tissue medium of lactated Ringer's solution (ACOG, 2020).

♦ Leukocyte infiltration due to chorioamnionitis

♦ Velamentous attachment of the cord

♦ Vasa previa

– Cord

♦ True knot with signs of umbilical cord thrombosis

• **Examination** of the fetus includes a general examination and a postmortem examination.

– *General examination* of the fetus should document the following:

♦ A detailed external examination of the fetus

♦ Fetal weight and length, head and abdominal circumference

♦ Measurement of the limbs

♦ Anatomical abnormalities, dysmorphic features, and relevant negative findings

♦ Detailed photographs of the entire fetus and a facial photograph, which would be useful for future reference

– *Postmortem examination* of the fetus is a very important part of the investigation for the etiology of stillbirth and has the highest diagnostic yield (RCOG, 2010; ACOG, 2020).

• The need for a postmortem should be discussed with the parents with great sensitivity and compassion.
• Their cultural values must be treated with respect.
• An informed consent should be obtained.
• Families may hesitate to proceed with a postmortem examination if they feel that the fetus will not be handled with respect. Most parents will agree to the examination when they are told that the information obtained may help prevent a fetal death in the next pregnancy.
• Following the autopsy, some parents may want to follow rituals specific to their culture or religion.

- The postmortem should ideally be performed by a specialised perinatal pathologist (RCOG, 2010; ACOG, 2020). If the required facilities are not available, the fetus or organs can be sent to a centre where these facilities are available.
  - Histological examination of the placenta may yield findings of clinical relevance (Kidron et al., 2009).
- If the parents do not agree to a postmortem, the following may be performed; however, they are not substitutes for a complete autopsy:
  - Photographs of the fetus
  - Whole body radiography
  - Ultrasonography
  - Needle biopsies
  - Magnetic resonance imaging (MRI)

> **Time of fetal demise**
> Most parents will want to know when the fetus died. Estimating the time of fetal death is difficult. Genest et al. (1992) have suggested the following guidelines for the estimation of the time of fetal death:
> - Brown or red discolouration of the umbilical cord or desquamation ≥1 cm suggests that the fetus has been dead at least six hours.
> - Desquamation of the face, back, and abdomen suggests that the fetus has been dead at least 12 hours.
> - Desquamation ≥5 per cent of the body or ≥2 body zones suggests that the fetus has been dead at least 18 hours (body zones – scalp, face, neck, chest, back, arms, hands, legs, feet, and scrotum).
> - Brown or tan colouration of skin suggests that the fetus has been dead at least 24 hours.
> - Mummification (i.e., reduced soft tissue volume, leathery skin, deeply brown-stained tissues) suggests that the fetus has been dead for at least two weeks.

MANAGEMENT OF LABOUR AND DELIVERY

- Fetal demise is an extremely difficult diagnosis to accept. Parents usually struggle to come to terms with the diagnosis.
- If there is no immediate medical complication putting the mother's health at risk, the couple should be allowed to make an informed decision about the timing of the delivery.
- It is important to reassure the couple and their families that the fetal demise will not negatively impact the mother's health.
- The method and timing of delivery depends on the following:
  - Gestational age at which the IUFD occurred
  - History of previous hysterotomy
  - Maternal preference
- The following must be borne in mind in such a situation:
  - Delaying delivery may aggravate maternal anxiety.
  - 85–90 per cent of women deliver spontaneously within three weeks of IUFD (RCOG, 2010).
  - Vaginal delivery should be attempted unless there are definite indications for cesarean section.

- Surgical induction should be avoided since it is associated with an increased risk of sepsis.
- Coagulopathies associated with prolonged fetal retention are uncommon. 10–30 per cent of women develop disseminated intravascular coagulation (DIC) if undelivered for four weeks after IUFD (Parasnis et al., 1992; Fontenot Ferriss et al., 2016). However, in current obstetrics, the risk of hemorrhage due to DIC following IUFD is very low—reportedly 2 per cent (Kerns et al., 2019).

Immediate delivery

Immediate delivery is indicated in women with the following complications:
- Severe preeclampsia
- Antepartum hemorrhage
- Infection
- Rupture of membranes

Indications for cesarean section

Cesarean section should be considered in the following clinical situations:
- Major degree of placenta previa
- Transverse lie
- Two or more scars on the uterus
- Significant macrosomia

Delivery by induction within 24–48 hours

- Induction of labour should be offered soon after the diagnosis of fetal death is made since this is less distressing for the woman and her family. The prospect of carrying a dead baby may cause severe anxiety and emotional anguish.

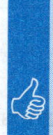 Most women with IUFD opt for delivery within 24–48 hours. A systematic review has shown that 90 per cent of women with IUFD in the second and third trimesters deliver within 24 hours of induction and 100 per cent deliver within 48 hours (Gómez Ponce de León and Wing, 2009).

- **Misoprostol** is recommended in the presence of IUFD after 28 weeks of gestation and an unfavourable cervix. An initial dose of 50 µg misoprostol should be placed vaginally, and if effective contractions with cervical changes occur, then the dose should be repeated every four hours for a maximum of six doses. In a systematic review, Gómez Ponce de León and Wing (2009) concluded that this regimen was successful in effecting delivery within 48 hours.

- **Oxytocin** can be initiated four hours after the administration of the last misoprostol dose, if required for the

 Antibiotic prophylaxis is **not** indicated during induction for IUFD.

augmentation of labour. It is most effective once the cervix has dilated to 3–4 cm.
- Induction of labour has the following advantages:
  - 90 per cent of women deliver within 24 hours of induction (Wagaarachchi, 2002) and 100 per cent deliver within 48 hours (Gómez Ponce de León and Wing, 2009).

- There is less maternal anxiety.
- Postmortem examination will be more informative since there is less chance of autolysis or maceration of the baby.
- The risk of DIC is low.

See **Chapter 19**, *Induction of labour* for methods of induction in the second trimester following fetal demise.

> **Viewing or holding the baby after delivery**
> Two studies (Hughes et al., 2002; Turton et al., 2009) found that viewing and holding the stillborn baby after delivery resulted in more depression, anxiety, and posttraumatic stress disorder (PTSD) in mothers as compared to those who had not. This is in strong contrast to some guidelines that say that viewing and holding the baby helps in the grieving process. Unless the mother absolutely insists, it may be better not to show the baby to the mother.

Prolonged expectant management

- Though the majority of women will choose not to postpone delivery, a policy of wait-and-watch is acceptable if the mother, after being counselled regarding risks and benefits, opts for this.
- Plasma fibrinogen levels should be monitored twice a week. Spontaneous labour usually begins within three weeks.
- If undelivered after 3–4 weeks, labour should be induced after ruling out coagulation defects.

Women with previous cesarean section

- Women who have had a previous cesarean delivery are at higher risk of uterine rupture when labour is induced. Though the absolute risk of uterine rupture in labour following a previous cesarean is low, a trial of labour after prior cesarean delivery is associated with a greater risk of uterine rupture as compared to elective repeat cesarean delivery without labour (Landon et al., 2004).
- Mechanical methods of cervical ripening like transcervical Foley catheter are preferred over misoprostol for cervical ripening as the risk of uterine rupture is lower, and no more than with spontaneous labour (Bujold et al., 2004; Grunebaum and Chervenak, 2019).
- Women with a scarred uterus should be closely monitored for scar rupture.

POSTNATAL MANAGEMENT

- Lactation should be suppressed with cabergoline.
- Rh-negative mothers should be administered Rh immunoglobulin. If

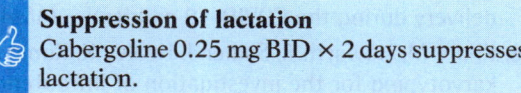

> **Suppression of lactation**
> Cabergoline 0.25 mg BID × 2 days suppresses lactation.

possible, an attempt should be made to ascertain the baby's blood group.
- Psychological support should be provided to the parents and family. The mother usually carries a huge burden of guilt, and every effort should be made to reassure her and provide her comfort.

- The couple should be counselled during follow-up visits regarding the risks of recurrence, contraception, plans for future pregnancy, and preventive measures, if any.

References

1. American College of Obstetricians and Gynecologists. 2020. ACOG Obstetric Care Consensus No. 10. Management of stillbirth. *Obstet Gynecol.* 135:e110–32.

2. Bujold E, Blackwell SC, Gauthier RJ. 2004. Cervical ripening with transcervical Foley catheter and the risk of uterinerupture. *Obstet Gynecol.* 103:18–23.

3. Bukowski R, Hansen NI, Willinger M et al. 2014. Fetal growth and risk of stillbirth: A population-based case-control study. *PLoS Med.* 11:e1001633.

4. Fontenot Ferriss AN, Weisenthal L, Sheeder J et al. 2016. Risk of hemorrhage during surgical evacuation for second-trimester intrauterine fetal demise. *Contraception.* 94:496.

5. Fretts RC. 2019. Prenatal care: Late fetal death and stillbirth: Incidence, etiology, and prevention. Lockwood CJ (Ed). *UptoDate.* Waltham, MA.

6. Gardosi J, Madurasinghe V, Williams M et al. 2013. Maternal and fetal risk factors for stillbirth: A population-based study. *BMJ.* 346:f108.

7. Genest DR, Singer DB. 1992. Estimating the time of death in stillborn fetuses: III. External fetal examination: A study of 86 stillborns. *Obstet Gynecol.* 80:593.

8. Gómez Ponce de León R, Wing DA. 2009. Misoprostol for termination of pregnancy with intrauterine fetal demise in the second and third trimester of pregnancy - a systematic review. *Contraception.* 79:259.

9. Grunebaum A, Chervenak FA. 2019. Late fetal death and stillbirth: Maternal care. Lockwood CJ (Ed). *UptoDate.* Waltham, MA.

10. Heazell AE, Martindale EA. 2009. Can post-mortem examination of the placenta help determine the cause of stillbirth? *J Obstet Gynaecol.* 29:225–8.

11. Huang DY, Usher RH, Kramer MS et al. 2000. Determinants of unexplained antepartum fetal deaths. *Obstet Gynecol.* 95:215.

12. Hughes P, Turton P, Hopper E et al. 2002. Assessment of guidelines for good practice in psychosocial care of mothers after stillbirth: A cohort study. *Lancet.* 360: 114-118.

13. KC Ashish, Gurung R, Kinney MV et al. 2020. Effect of the COVID-19 pandemic response on intrapartum care, stillbirth, and neonatal mortality outcomes in Nepal: A prospective observational study. *Lancet Glob Health.* 8: e1273-e1281.

14. Kerns JL, Ti A, Aksel S et al. 2019. Disseminated Intravascular Coagulation and hemorrhage after dilation and evacuation abortion for fetal death. *Obstet Gynecol.* 134:708.

15. Khalil A, von Dadelszen P, Draycott T et al. 2020. Change in the incidence of stillbirth and preterm delivery during the COVID-19 pandemic. *JAMA.* 324: 705.

16. Khare M, Howarth E, Sadler J, Healey K, Konje JC. 2005. A comparison of prenatal versus postnatal karyotyping for the investigation of intrauterine fetal death after the first trimester of pregnancy. *Prenat Diagn.* 25:1192–5.

17. Kidron D, Bernheim J, Aviram R. 2009. Placental findings contributing to fetal death, a study of 120 stillbirths between 23 and 40 weeks gestation. *Placenta.* 30(8):700–4.

18. Korteweg FJ, Bouman K, Erwich JJ et al. 2008. Cytogenetic analysis after evaluation of 750 fetal deaths: Proposal for diagnostic workup. *Obstet Gynecol.* 111:865.

19. Landon MB, Hauth JC, Leveno KJ, Spong CY, Leindecker S, Varner MW et al. 2004. Maternal and perinatal outcomes associated with a trial of labor after prior cesarean delivery. *N Engl J Med.* 351:2581–9.

20. Muglu J, Rather H, Arroyo-Manzano D et al. 2019. Risks of stillbirth and neonatal death with advancing gestation at term: A systematic review and meta-analysis of cohort studies of 15 million pregnancies. *PLoS Med.* 16(7):e1002838.

21. Parasnis H, Raje B, Hinduja IN. 1992. Relevance of plasma fibrinogen estimation in obstetric complications. *J Postgrad Med.* 38:183–5.

22. Royal College of Obstetricians and Gynaecologists. 2010. RCOG Green-top Guideline No. 55. Late intrauterine fetal death and still birth.

23. Saal HM, Rodis J, Weinbaum PJ, DiMaggio R, Landrey TM. 1987. Cytogenetic evaluation of fetal death: The role of amniocentesis. *Obstet Gynecol.* 70:601–3.

24. Sarno M, Sacramento GA, Khouri R et al. 2016. Zika virus infection and stillbirths: A case of hydrops fetalis, hydranencephaly and fetal demise. *PLoS Negl Trop Dis.* 10:e0004517.

25. Stillbirth Collaborative Research Network Writing Group. 2011. Causes of death among stillbirths. *JAMA.* 306:2459.

26. Turton P, Evans C, Hughes P. 2009. Long-term psychosocial sequalae of stillbirth: Phase II of a nested case-control cohort study. *Arch Womens Ment Health.* 12:35-41.

27. Wagaarachchi PT, Ashok PW, Narvekar NN, Smith NC, Templeton A. 2002. Medical management of late intrauterine death using a combination of m fepristone and misoprostol. *BJOG.* 109: 443–7.

28. World Health Organization (WHO).http://www.who.int/maternal_child_adolescent/epidemiology/stillbirth/en/

29. Zeit RM. 1976. Sonographic demonstration of feta death in the absence of radiographic abnormality. *Obstet Gynecol.* 48 1 Suppl:49S–52S.

Chapter 38

Pregnancy in Women with Fibroids

INTRODUCTION

- Myomas (fibroids) are the most common benign smooth muscle tumours of the uterus. They have been found to be associated with menstrual disorders and pelvic pain and can negatively affect fertility and pregnancy outcome.
- Fibroids affect approximately 35–77 per cent of reproductive-age women (Cramer and Patel, 1990).

 The majority of women with uterine fibroids have normal pregnancy outcomes (Segars et al., 2014; Parker, 2007).

- The reported incidence of fibroids in pregnancy ranges from 1.6–10.7 per cent of all pregnancies (Ouyang and Norwitz, 2021). Fibroids during pregnancy are more likely to be encountered with advanced maternal age (≥35 years). Nulliparas are more likely to present with a fibroid since increasing parity and prolonged duration of breastfeeding reduce the prevalence of fibroids (Terry et al., 2010; Qidwai et al., 2006).
- Segars and colleagues, in a comprehensive review (2014), found that the majority of women with uterine fibroids have normal pregnancy outcomes. A review by Parker (2007) also concluded that myomas only very rarely affect pregnancy outcomes.
- Obstetricians must be aware of the behaviour of fibroids in pregnancies, the associated complications, and their management in pregnancy.
- Ultrasound plays a major role in the detection of fibroids in pregnancy.

BEHAVIOUR OF FIBROIDS IN PREGNANCY

- One of the most common misconceptions is that fibroids increase in size during pregnancy. However, several studies, using ultrasonographic monitoring of fibroids during pregnancy (Neiger et al., 2006; Rosati et al., 1992) have shown that this is not true. Data from these studies suggest that fibroid size remains stable (<10 per cent change) through the pregnancy in 50–60 per cent of cases, increases in 22–32 per cent, and decreases in 8–27 per cent (Table 38.1). Very few fibroids will increase more than 25 per cent in volume.
- Larger fibroids (>5 cm in diameter) have a greater chance of growing as compared to smaller ones (Strobelt et al., 1994).
- **Postpartum regression:** The majority (90 per cent) of fibroids detected in the first trimester will undergo regression within 3–6 months following delivery. 10 per cent may show an increase in size. Postpartum regression may be less in women who use progestin-only contraception.

Table 38.1 Change in size of fibroids during pregnancy as noted with ultrasound follow-up (based on data from studies conducted by Neiger et al., 2006; Rosati et al., 1992)

Change in fibroid size during pregnancy	Percentage of fibroids
Stable with <10 per cent change	50–60%
Increase	22–32%
Decrease	8–27%

 Fibroids that do grow tend to grow most in the first trimester with very little further growth in the second and third trimesters (Ciavattini et al., 2016).

COMPLICATIONS IN PREGNANCIES WITH FIBROIDS

Most women do not have any problems in pregnancy from the fibroid itself. Of those who do, pain is the most common problem. However, there may be a slightly increased risk of obstetrical complications such as miscarriage, premature labour and delivery, abnormal fetal position, and placental abruption.

Spontaneous miscarriage

- The presence of fibroids was not associated with an increased risk of spontaneous miscarriage in an analysis of more than 20,000 pregnant women (Sundermann et al., 2017). This is an important finding and is reassuring both for pregnant women with fibroids and their obstetricians.
- Evidence suggests that multiple fibroids may increase the miscarriage rate as compared to the presence of a single fibroid (Benson et al., 2001).
- Subserosal and pedunculated fibroids clearly have no effect on the risk of miscarriage.
- The effect of intramural fibroids is debated, but Lee et al. (2010) stated that early miscarriage may be more common in women with large fibroids located in the uterine corpus than in those who had fibroids in the lower uterine segment.
- Submucosal fibroids may interfere with placentation and the development of normal uteroplacental circulation (Ouyang and Norwitz, 2021). Large submucosal fibroids that distort the cavity may cause infertility, but if implantation does occur, the risk of early miscarriage is increased.

 Early miscarriage is more common in women with large submucosal fibroids that distort the cavity.

Bleeding in early pregnancy

- The location of the fibroid determines the risk of bleeding.
- Winer–Muram et al. (1984) found that bleeding in early pregnancy is significantly more common if the placenta implants close to the fibroid as compared to pregnancies in which there is no contact between the placenta and fibroid (60 per cent vs. 9 per cent, respectively).

Pain

Pain from fibroids in pregnancy can be due to increase in size, red degeneration, or rarely, torsion of a pedunculated fibroid.

Increase in size

- The most commonly reported complaint associated with uterine fibroids during pregnancy is pain. This is seen most often in women with large fibroids (>7–10 cm).
- Women are usually admitted with pain in the **late first** or **early second trimester**, which corresponds to the time when fibroids are most likely to grow rapidly.

Red degeneration

Acute pain during pregnancy can arise as a result of red degeneration. This type of degeneration is found usually, but not exclusively, during pregnancy and is associated with pain, fever, and leukocytosis (Parker, 2007).

- Three main theories have been proposed to explain the severe pain associated with red degeneration.
  - Rapid fibroid growth results in the tissue outgrowing its blood supply, leading to tissue anoxia, necrosis, and infarction.
  - Even in the absence of fibroid growth, the growth of the uterus results in a change in the architecture (kinking) of the blood supply to the fibroid, leading to ischemia and necrosis.
  - The pain results from the release of prostaglandins from cellular damage within the fibroid. This is supported by the observation that ibuprofen and other prostaglandin synthetase inhibitors effectively and rapidly control fibroid pain.
- Degenerating fibroids may have a complex appearance on ultrasound with areas of cystic change (Wilde and Scott-Barrett, 2009).

Torsion

Rarely, pain arises because of the torsion of a subserous pedunculated fibroid.

Pain management

- Pain due to fibroids during pregnancy is usually managed conservatively with bed rest, hydration, and simple analgesics like paracetamol.
- If there is no improvement, ibuprofen (400 mg 6–8 hourly) usually provides good relief.
- When NSAIDs are used for more than 48 hours, it may be prudent to monitor for oligohydramnios by ultrasound.
- Severe pain may necessitate inpatient admission, additional pain medication (narcotic analgesia), or in rare instances, epidural analgesia.
- In cases of intractable pain from the torsion of a subserous pedunculated fibroid, a myomectomy may be performed.

Placental abruption

- Though there are conflicting reports, the risk of placental abruption is increased three-fold in women with fibroids (Klatsky et al., 2008).
- The highest risk of abruption is with retroplacental fibroids, submucosal fibroids, and fibroids measuring >7–8 cm in diameter (Ouyang and Norwitz, 2021).

 Retroplacental fibroids, submucosal fibroids, and fibroids >7–8 cm diameter are independent risk factors for placental abruption.

Placenta previa

Most studies have not shown any association between fibroids and placenta previa.

Malpresentation

- Breech presentation is slightly increased in pregnancies with fibroids.
- The risk of malpresentation increases with a large submucosal fibroid, multiple fibroids, a fibroid located behind the placenta or in the lower uterine segment, or a large fibroid (e.g., >10 cm in diameter).

Preterm labour

- Fibroids may increase the risk of preterm labour (Pritts et al., 2009) if:
  - They are large.
  - There are multiple fibroids.
  - Placentation occurs next to or overlying a fibroid.
- In contrast, fibroids do not appear to be a risk factor for preterm premature rupture of membranes (PPROM).

Fetal growth restriction

Fibroids have not been shown to have any effect on fetal growth (Klatsky et al., 2008).

MODE OF DELIVERY IN PREGNANCIES WITH FIBROIDS

- Most women with fibroids will have a successful vaginal delivery. A trial of labour should be offered unless there is a clear obstetric indication for a cesarean delivery, e.g., failure to progress, or breech or transverse presentation.

 Even though there is a higher cesarean section rate in women with fibroids (Zhao et al., 2017), the presence of even large fibroids (>5 cm) should not be regarded as a contraindication to a trial of labour (Coronado et al., 2000).

- When women with large fibroids go into labour with a cephalic presentation, their likelihood of having a successful vaginal delivery remains high (Vergani et al., 2007). It is good clinical practice to offer these women a trial of labour (Ouyang and Norwitz, 2021).

- Elective cesarean delivery may be considered in women with large fibroids (cervical or in the lower uterine segment) that may potentially obstruct the descent of the fetal head.

TECHNICAL ISSUES AT CESAREAN SECTION

- It is extremely important to obtain a good quality ultrasound to map the location of the fibroids before proceeding with an elective cesarean section. This is particularly important in the case of large fibroids.
- A vertical skin incision may sometimes be required if a large fibroid is occupying the lower uterine segment. In this situation, the hysterotomy scar may have to be placed either in the upper segment, or in rare cases, on the posterior uterine surface.

Myomectomy at cesarean section

- A systematic review and meta-analysis (Pergialiotis et al., 2017) found that women undergoing myomectomy during a cesarean section had greater falls in hemoglobin and higher risks of requiring blood transfusion than women who did not.
- Myomectomy at the time of cesarean delivery should only be performed in the following conditions:
  - If the fibroid is along the site of, or makes access difficult for the uterine incision
  - To facilitate safe delivery of the fetus
  - To facilitate the closure of the hysterotomy
- Hasan et al. (1991), in a large series of 60 cases of fibroids in pregnancy, found that pedunculated subserosal fibroids could be safely removed at the time of cesarean delivery. However, removal of non-pedunculated fibroids resulted in severe hemorrhage, leading to the risk of hysterectomy.

POSTPARTUM COMPLICATIONS

- Pregnant women with uterine fibroids are at an increased risk for postpartum hemorrhage (PPH).
- This is most likely caused by decreased uterine contractility in women with fibroids. In their series, Zhao et al. (2017) found that the rates of PPH were significantly higher with increasing size of the uterine fibroid and its location, with large intramural fibroids having the highest risk of PPH.

PREGNANCY AFTER MYOMECTOMY

- One of the major concerns about prior myomectomy is the risk of uterine rupture during pregnancy or labour.
- While uterine rupture can occur following myomectomy performed either by laparoscopy or laparotomy, the rate of rupture following abdominal myomectomy is extremely low (Miller, 2000).

- There are concerns that laparoscopic myomectomy has an increased risk of uterine rupture during labour due to the technical difficulties of achieving good apposition of the edges with laparoscopic suturing (Nezhat, 1996).
- The ACOG (2019) recommends elective cesarean at 37^{+0} to 38^{+6} weeks of gestation for women who have had a previous myomectomy. This can be as early as 36^{+0} weeks in cases where the myomectomy resulted in a uterine scar that extended deep into the myometrium.

References

1. American College of Obstetricians and Gynecologists. 2019. ACOG Committee Opinion No. 764. Medically indicated late-preterm and early-term deliveries. *Obstet Gynecol.* 133:e151–55.

2. Benson CB, Chow JS, Chang-Lee W et al. 2001. Outcome of pregnancies in women with uterine leiomyomas identified by sonography in the first trimester. *J Clin Ultrasound.* 29:261–264.

3. Cramer S, Patel A. 1990. The frequency of uterine leiomyomas. *Am J Clin Pathol.* 94:435–8.

4. Ciavattini A, Delli Carpini G, Clemente N et al. 2016. Growth trend of small uterine fibroids and human chorionic gonadotropin serum levels in early pregnancy: An observational study. *Fertil Steril.* 105:1255.

5. Coronado G, Marshall L, Schwartz S. 2000. Complications in pregnancy, labor, and delivery with uterine leiomyomas: A population-based study. *Obstet Gynecol.* 95:764–9.

6. Hasan F, Arumugam K, Sivanesaratnam V. 1991. Uterine leiomyomata in pregnancy. *Int J Gynaecol Obstet.* 34:45–48.

7. Klatsky PC, Tran ND, Caughey AB, Fujimoto VY. 2008. Fibroids and reproductive outcomes: A systematic literature review from conception to delivery. *Am J Obstet Gynecol.* 198:357–366.

8. Lee HJ, Norwitz ER, Shaw J. 2010. Contemporary management of fibroids in pregnancy. *Rev Obstet Gynecol.* 3(1):20–27.

9. Miller CE. Myomectomy. 2000. Comparison of open and laparoscopic techniques. *Obstet Gynecol Clin North Am.* 27:407–420.

10. Nezhat C. 1996. The "cons" of laparoscopic myomectomy in women who may reproduce in the future. *Int J Fertil Menopausal Stud.* 41:280.

11. Neiger R, Sonek JD, Croom CS, Ventolini G. 2006. Pregnancy-related changes in the size of uterine leiomyomas. *J Reprod Med.* 51:671.

12. Ouyang DW, Norwitz ER. 2021. Uterine fibroids (leiomyomas): Issues in pregnancy. Lockwood CJ (Ed). *UpToDate.* Waltham, MA.

13. Parker WH. 2007. Etiology, symptomatology, and diagnosis of uterine myomas. *Fertil Steril.* 87:725.

14. Pergialiotis V, Sinanidis I, Louloudis IE et al. 2017. Perioperative complications of cesarean delivery myomectomy: A meta-analysis. *Obstet Gynecol.* 130:1295.

15. Pritts EA, Parker WH, Olive DL. 2009. Fibroids and infertility: An updated systematic review of the evidence. *Fertil Steril.* 91:1215–23.

16. Qidwai G, Caughey A, Jacoby A. 2006. Obstetric outcomes in women with sonographically identified uterine leiomyomata. *Obstet Gynecol.* 107:376–82.

17. Rosati P, Exacoustòs C, Mancuso S. 1992. Longitudinal evaluation of uterine myoma growth during pregnancy: A sonographic study. *J Ultrasound Med*. 11:511.

18. Strobelt N, Ghidini A, Cavallone M et al. 1994. Natural history of uterine leiomyomas in pregnancy. *J Ultrasound Med*. 13:399.

19. Segars JH, Parrott EC, Nagel JD et al. 2014. Proceedings from the Third National Institutes of Health International Congress on Advances in Uterine Leiomyoma Research: A comprehensive review, conference summary and future recommendations. *Hum Reprod Update*. 20:309.

20. Sundermann AC, Velez Edwards DR, Bray MJ et al. 2017. Leiomyomas in Pregnancy and spontaneous abortion: A systematic review and meta-analysis. *Obstet Gynecol*. 130:1065.

21. Terry KL, De Vivo I, Hankinson SE, Missmer SA. 2010. Reproductive characteristics and risk of uterine leiomyomata. *Fertil Steril*. 94:2703.

22. Vergani P, Locatelli A, Ghidini A, AndreaniM, Sala F, Pezullo JC. 2007. Large uterine leiomyomata and risk of cesarean delivery. *Obstet Gynecol*. 109:410–4.

23. Winer-Muram HT, Muram D, Gillieson MS. 1984. Uterine myomas in pregnancy. *J Can Assoc Radiol*. 35:168–170.

24. Wilde S, Scott-Barrett S. 2009. Radiological appearances of uterine fibroids. *Indian J Radiol Imaging*. 19(3):222–231.

25. Zhao R, Wang X, Zou L et al. 2017. Adverse obstetric outcomes in pregnant women with uterine fibroids in China: A multicenter survey involving 112,403 deliveries. *PLoS One*. 12:e0187821.

Chapter 39

Hypertensive Disorders in Pregnancy

INTRODUCTION

- Hypertensive disorders in pregnancy are a major cause of maternal deaths worldwide. In Africa and Asia, nearly one-tenth of all maternal deaths are associated with hypertensive disorders of pregnancy (WHO, 2011).

 Hypertension and preeclampsia complicate 5–10 per cent of pregnancies globally (ACOG, 2020) and 7–8 per cent of pregnancies in India (Mehta et al., 2015; Magee et al., 2019).

- Every year, 70,000 women die due to hypertensive disorders of pregnancy; half a million stillbirths or neonatal deaths are related to these disorders (FIGO, 2016). The vast majority of these deaths are in the developing world.
- The Third Report of Confidential Review of Maternal Deaths, Kerala, India (Paily et al., 2021), found that hypertensive disorders in pregnancy were the second commonest cause of maternal deaths in the state of Kerala, India, between 2010 and 2020. Between 2010 and 2020, 9.8 per cent of maternal deaths were caused by hypertensive disorders.
- A diagnosis of hypertension in pregnancy increases a woman's risk of developing chronic hypertension and an increase in lifetime risk of cerebrovascular and cardiovascular events, leading to premature death. This risk is highest in women with early-onset preeclampsia (Steegers et al., 2010).

DEFINITIONS

The hypertensive disorders that occur in pregnant women are classified as follows (ACOG, 2020):

- **Gestational hypertension**: This is defined as a systolic blood pressure (BP) ≥140 mmHg or diastolic BP ≥90 mmHg, or both, on two occasions at least 4 hours apart after 20 weeks of gestation, in a woman with a previously normal blood pressure.

 The term pregnancy-induced hypertension (PIH) is no longer used since it confusingly denotes both hypertension with or without proteinuria (FIGO, 2016).

- **Severe gestational hypertension:** This is characterised by a sustained systolic BP ≥160 mmHg or diastolic BP ≥110 mmHg.
- **Preeclampsia**: This is a disorder of pregnancy associated with new-onset hypertension, which occurs most often after 20 weeks of gestation and frequently near term. Although often accompanied by new-onset proteinuria, hypertension, and other signs or symptoms, preeclampsia may present in some women in the absence of proteinuria.

- **HELLP syndrome:** The clinical presentation of hemolysis, elevated liver enzymes, and low platelet count (HELLP) syndrome is a severe form of preeclampsia and is associated with increased rates of maternal morbidity and mortality.
- **Eclampsia:** Eclampsia is hypertension accompanied by convulsions in pregnancy. It is defined by new-onset tonic-clonic, focal, or multifocal seizures in the absence of other causative conditions such as epilepsy, cerebral arterial ischemia and infarction, intracranial hemorrhage, or drug use.
- **Chronic (pre-existing) hypertension:** Chronic hypertension is defined as systolic pressure ≥140 mmHg and/or diastolic pressure ≥90 mmHg that antedates pregnancy, is present before the 20th week of pregnancy, or persists longer than 12 weeks postpartum.

 Reassessment of blood pressure up to 12 weeks postpartum is necessary to establish a final definitive diagnosis of chronic hypertension.

- **Preeclampsia–eclampsia superimposed upon chronic hypertension:** Preeclampsia–eclampsia superimposed upon chronic hypertension is diagnosed when a woman with chronic hypertension develops worsening hypertension with new-onset proteinuria or other features of preeclampsia (e.g., elevated liver enzymes, low platelet count).

 White coat hypertension is defined as blood pressure that is consistently elevated when taken by a doctor or nurse but does not meet diagnostic criteria for hypertension based upon out-of-hospital readings. It is important to take repeat readings after helping the patient relax.

Technique for measuring blood pressure
1. **Position:** The woman should be still and seated with her legs uncrossed, her feet flat on the floor, and her back resting against the back of the chair. Her arm should be resting at the level of her heart. Supine positioning should be avoided.
2. **Relaxation:** The woman should rest for five minutes before her blood pressure is taken. She should not talk, read, look at her phone/computer, or watch television.
3. **The BP cuff:** The blood pressure cuff must be the right size. It must be long enough (i.e., length should be 1.5 times the circumference of the arm) and wide enough. The cuff should cover two-thirds of the distance between the shoulder and elbow; the bottom edge of the cuff should end up approximately 1–2 cm above the elbow. The blood pressure cuff should be placed on the woman's bare upper arm, and not over clothing.
4. **Designation of diastolic BP:** Korotkoff phase V (disappearance of Korotkoff sounds) should be used for designation of the diastolic BP. Korotkoff phase IV (muffling of sounds) should be used only if Korotkoff sounds are audible as the diastolic BP level approaches 0 mmHg (as may happen in pregnancy).
5. **Equipment:** Since mercury sphygmomanometers have been banned, well-calibrated aneroid devices or good quality automated BP devices may be used.

GESTATIONAL HYPERTENSION

- Clinicians must remember that gestational hypertension is not necessarily a 'milder' disease than preeclampsia and requires the same degree of maternal and fetal surveillance.

- Though the maternal and perinatal outcomes with gestational hypertension are usually good, up to 50 per cent of women with gestational hypertension eventually develop proteinuria or other end-organ dysfunction and progress to preeclampsia. When the hypertension presents before 34 weeks of gestation (early-onset), it indicates pregnant women at substantial perinatal and maternal risk (Sibai and Stella, 2009; Magee et al., 2003).
- In terms of long-term cardiovascular disease, including chronic hypertension, both gestational hypertension and preeclampsia carry the same risk (Williams, 2011).

The absence of proteinuria does not exclude preeclampsia (see below). Non-proteinuric hypertension may also progress to eclampsia (Homer et al., 2008). Thornton et al. (2010) found that the perinatal mortality rate was higher in women with non-proteinuric preeclampsia when compared to proteinuric women.

SEVERE GESTATIONAL HYPERTENSION

- A sustained systolic BP ≥160 mmHg or diastolic BP ≥110 mmHg is an indication of the severity of the condition. There is no necessity to wait for four hours to confirm the readings.
- In 2018, the American College of Obstetricians and Gynecologists classified this as **'preeclampsia with severe features'** (ACOG, 2020).
- This change of definition from severe gestational hypertension to preeclampsia with severe features emphasises the fact that severely elevated pregnancy-related hypertension carries the risk for serious adverse events even in the absence of proteinuria (Homer et al., 2008).

PREECLAMPSIA

Preeclampsia is defined as the new onset of systolic blood pressure ≥140 mmHg or diastolic blood pressure ≥90 mmHg on at least two occasions at least four hours apart after 20 weeks of gestation in a previously normotensive patient AND the new onset of one or more of the following:

- **Proteinuria**
  - ≥300 mg in a 24-hour urine specimen or
  - Protein/creatinine ratio ≥0.3 in a random urine specimen or
  - Dipstick ≥2+ if a quantitative measurement is unavailable

Even though hypertension and proteinuria are considered the classical criteria for the diagnosis of preeclampsia, 10 per cent of women with preeclampsia may not have proteinuria. In these cases, the diagnosis is based on the presence of any of the following severe features:

- **Platelet count** <100,000/μL
- **Serum creatinine**
  - >1.1 mg/dL or
  - Doubling of the creatinine concentration in the absence of other renal disease

- **Impaired liver function**
  - Severe, persistent right upper quadrant or epigastric pain unresponsive to medication and not accounted for by an alternative diagnosis and/or
  - Liver transaminases twice the normal concentration
- **Pulmonary edema**
- **Cerebral or visual symptoms**
  - New-onset and persistent headaches not accounted for by alternative diagnoses and not responding to usual doses of analgesics
  - Blurred vision, flashing lights or sparks, scotomata

> **Early- and late-onset preeclampsia**
> When preeclampsia presents before 34 weeks of gestation, it is termed early-onset. This presentation is often associated with fetal growth restriction. It poses a high risk to both the mother and fetus (Paruk and Moodley, 2000). It usually results from developmental abnormalities of the uteroplacental circulation.
> Preeclampsia occurring after 34 weeks is called late-onset and may present with less severe clinical symptoms.

Preeclampsia with severe features

This is diagnosed when a blood pressure of $\geq 160/110$ mmHg is associated with symptoms, signs, and laboratory features that indicate multiorgan involvement. The criteria for preeclampsia with severe features and the organ involvement are listed in Table 39.1.

Table 39.1 Criteria for preeclampsia with severe features and the organ involvement that results in the symptoms, signs or laboratory findings

Blood pressure ≥160/110 mmHg with any of the following criteria	
Criteria	**Causative organ involvement**
Severe headache despite analgesic therapy	Cerebral edema
Photophobia, cortical blindness, scotomata, retinal vasospasm	Changes in the optic fundus
Severe and persistent right upper quadrant or epigastric pain	Stretching of liver capsule
Thrombocytopenia (<100,000/μL)	Platelet aggregation and activation
Elevated liver enzymes >twice the upper limit of normal range	Liver ischemia
Serum creatinine >1.1 mg/dL or doubling of the serum creatinine	Impaired renal function
Pulmonary edema	Left ventricular failure due to hypertension and extravasation of fluid into the interstitial space

Prediction of preeclampsia

- Screening tests for predicting preeclampsia, especially early-onset preeclampsia, have been investigated.

- To date, **no single test has reliably predicted preeclampsia**. Further prospective studies are required to demonstrate its application in clinical practice (ACOG, 2019).
- Poon and colleagues (2009) reported that a combination of low maternal serum concentrations of placental growth factor (PlGF), high uterine artery pulsatility index, and other maternal parameters could be used to identify 93 per cent of patients who would develop preeclampsia requiring delivery before 34 weeks of gestation. However, it was found that these indices had a poor positive predictive value and that 80 per cent of screen-positive women would not develop preeclampsia.
- Uterine artery Doppler velocimetry, both in the first and second trimester, is more useful for the prediction of fetal growth restriction than for the prediction of preeclampsia, and is **not recommended for routine screening for preeclampsia**.

 First-trimester uterine artery Doppler studies have a low predictive value for the development of early-onset preeclampsia. (ACOG, 2019; Cnossen et al., 2008).

Prevention of preeclampsia

- Currently, no intervention exists that has been proved unequivocally effective at eliminating the risk of preeclampsia (ACOG, 2019).
- Based on a systematic review of the Cochrane Database (Hofmeyr et al., 2014), the WHO recommends **calcium supplementation** (in women with low dietary calcium intake) for the prevention of preeclampsia in women at a high risk of developing preeclampsia. A dose of 1.5–2.0 g elemental calcium/day is recommended.
- **Low-dose aspirin** has proved effective in the prevention of preeclampsia, especially early-onset preeclampsia. One of the causes implicated in the pathogenesis of preeclampsia is an imbalance in prostacyclin and thromboxane A2 metabolism. Low-dose aspirin

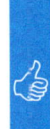 In a systematic review of the Cochrane Database, Duley et al. (2019) found that low-dose aspirin started at <16 weeks' gestation in high-risk women leads to reductions in preeclampsia, preterm birth, fetal growth reduction, and fetal or neonatal death.

preferentially inhibits thromboxane A2 and so has been used as prophylaxis against preeclampsia.
  - The recommended dose is 75–150 mg per day (the effect seems to be better with the higher dose).
  - It is best started as soon as pregnancy is confirmed, and definitely before 16 weeks for it to be effective (Roberge et al., 2017; Duley et al., 2019).
  - The ASPRE trial (Rolnik et al., 2017) demonstrated that in women with singleton pregnancy who were identified by means of first-trimester combined screening as being at a high risk for early-onset preeclampsia, the administration of aspirin at a dose of 150 mg per day from 11–14 weeks until 36 weeks' gestation reduces the incidence of early-onset preeclampsia by >60 per cent.
  - The risk factors for preeclampsia and the recommendations regarding the administration of aspirin are presented in Table 39.2.

Table 39.2   Clinical risk factors associated with preeclampsia and the recommendations regarding low-dose aspirin prophylaxis (ACOG, 2019)

Clinical level of risk (based on history)	Risk factors	Recommendation
High-risk (factors that are consistently associated with the greatest risk of preeclampsia)	• Previous history of preeclampsia (especially if it had an adverse outcome) • Twin gestation • Chronic hypertension • Type 1 or 2 diabetes • Renal disease • Antiphospholipid antibody syndrome, systemic lupus erythematosus	Low-dose aspirin recommended in the presence of **1 or more of these factors**
Moderate-risk	• Nulliparity • Mother or sister with history of preeclampsia • Age ≥35 years • Pregnancy interval >10 years • Personal history factors (low birth weight, previous adverse pregnancy outcome)	Low-dose aspirin recommended in the presence of **>1 of these factors**
Low-risk	Previous uncomplicated term delivery	Low-dose aspirin **not recommended**

- The following are **not recommended** for the prevention of preeclampsia:
  - Vitamins C, E, and D
  - Fish oil
  - Garlic supplementation
  - Folic acid
  - Sodium restriction
  - Bed rest
  - Metformin, sildenafil, and statins

HELLP SYNDROME

- The clinical presentation of hemolysis, elevated liver enzymes, and low platelet count (HELLP) syndrome is considered a very severe form of preeclampsia.
- HELLP develops in 0.1–1.0 per cent of pregnant women overall.
- Microangiopathy and activation of intravascular coagulation can account for all of the laboratory findings in HELLP syndrome.

 Women with HELLP syndrome are at an increased risk of pulmonary edema, acute respiratory distress syndrome, and acute kidney injury (AKI).

- The onset of symptoms is usually rapid after which, they progressively worsen.
- **Colicky abdominal pain** is the most common symptom and is present in most patients. It may be present in the epigastrium, right upper quadrant, or below the sternum.
- Though it is associated with hypertension and proteinuria in 85 per cent of cases, severe HELLP syndrome may present without either of these signs (Sibai, 2004).

- Women with HELLP syndrome require intensive monitoring until delivery and in the postpartum period. Laboratory testing should be repeated at least at 12-hour intervals.
- The disease may worsen during the first two days after delivery, with a possible downward trend in hematocrit.

> **Mortality risk is increased if:**
> - Aspartate aminotransferase levels are >2000 IU/L and
> - LDH is >3000 IU/L

- With supportive care alone, 90 per cent of women with HELLP syndrome recover **within seven days of delivery** (ACOG, 2019). The thrombocytopenia reverses by this time, and a platelet count of >100,000/μL is reached. The liver enzymes values also start trending downward.

ECLAMPSIA

- The occurrence of new-onset, generalised, tonic-clonic seizures, or coma in a woman with preeclampsia is referred to as eclampsia. It is the most severe form of the preeclampsia spectrum.
- Eclampsia occurs in 2–3 per cent of women with preeclampsia with severe features who are not receiving magnesium sulphate for seizure prophylaxis. However, it may rarely occur in women who do not have proteinuria or other signs of preeclampsia with severe features.
- Seizures in the second half of pregnancy and up to 48 hours postpartum, not attributable to any other cause, are always considered to be eclampsia.
- The treatment of eclampsia with magnesium sulphate is described below in the section on *Seizure prophylaxis and treatment*.

> **Symptoms of imminent eclampsia**
> - Headache
> - Visual disturbances
> - Vomiting
> - Epigastric pain

MANAGEMENT OF HYPERTENSIVE DISORDERS IN PREGNANCY

The goals of the management of hypertensive disorders in pregnancy include the following:
- Early identification of worsening of the disease
- Treatment of hypertension
- Seizure prophylaxis and treatment
- Timing and route of delivery

Early identification of worsening of disease

Maternal evaluation

When a pregnant woman is first diagnosed with hypertension, she must be evaluated for increasing hypertension and to rule out preeclampsia, with or without severe features.

- The blood pressure should be recorded at least every four hours and more frequently in case of severe disease.
- The urine must be tested for proteinuria. A dipstick test should be performed first, and if it is 2+ or more, then protein in a 24-hour urine specimen should be assessed, along with a protein/creatinine ratio.
- A history should be elicited for new onset of cerebral or visual disturbances, or epigastric or right upper quadrant pain.
- Laboratory evaluation should include:
  - Platelet count
  - Renal function tests
  - Liver function tests

Fetal evaluation

Fetal evaluation should include:

- Non-stress test with amniotic fluid estimation (see **Chapter 6**, *Antepartum fetal surveillance*)
- Estimation of fetal weight by ultrasound biometry
- Doppler velocimetry is reserved for fetuses with growth restriction (see **Chapter 36**, *Fetal growth disorders: Fetal growth restriction and macrosomia*)

Treatment of hypertension

- Women who have gestational hypertension can be managed on an outpatient basis. They should be educated regarding signs and symptoms of severe hypertension/preeclampsia.
- Salt restriction is not recommended.
- Bed rest is not recommended for non-severe hypertension as it does not prevent progression to severe preeclampsia. However, women may be advised restriction of activity, and rest for varying periods of time in the day in non-severe preeclampsia.
- Since antihypertensives reduce the risk of the development of severe hypertension by 40–50 per cent, oral antihypertensives are now recommended when the hypertension is ≥150/100 mmHg or persists between 140–150/90–100 mmHg.

Treatment of mild–moderate hypertension

- Mild (140–150 mmHg/90–100 mmHg) to moderate hypertension (150–159 mmHg/100–109 mmHg) should be treated with oral medication.

 Tight control of mild–moderate hypertension reduces the risk of severe hypertension and consequently, adverse maternal and perinatal outcomes (Magee et al., 2016).

- The Control of Hypertension in Pregnancy Study (CHIPS) trial (Magee et al., 2015) showed that lower blood pressure was associated with a reduced occurrence of severe maternal hypertension during pregnancy but did not result in less preeclampsia.
- A follow-up study on the CHIPS data (Magee et al., 2016) and a 2018 systematic review of the Cochrane Database (Abalos et al.) showed that tight control with medications resulted

in reduced risk of severe hypertension and consequently, reduced adverse maternal and perinatal outcomes.

Treatment of severe hypertension

- Severe hypertension ($\geq$160 mmHg/$\geq$110 mmHg) persisting for $\geq$15 minutes is an obstetric emergency requiring immediate treatment.
- Treatment reduces the risk of congestive heart failure, myocardial ischemia, renal injury or failure, and ischemic or hemorrhagic stroke.
- Though acute severe hypertension should ideally be treated with intravenous labetalol, it is not always available in low-resource facilities. A 2019 multicentre trial from India (Easterling et al.) showed that oral medications are equally effective in under-resourced facilities where intravenous drugs may not be available. Their findings confirmed the following:
  - All three oral drugs (**nifedipine retard, labetalol**, and **methyldopa**) are viable initial options for treating severe hypertension in low-resource settings.
  - Each drug reduced blood pressure to the desired range within six hours in most women, with no adverse outcomes.
  - Nifedipine retard was most successful in reducing blood pressure.

Choice of drug

- The most effective antihypertensive drugs that are used in pregnancy and recommended by the WHO are the following:
  - Nifedipine
  - Methyldopa
  - Labetalol
- All these drugs have an acceptable safety profile in pregnancy.

Drugs to be avoided in pregnancy:
- Angiotensin-converting enzyme (ACE) inhibitors
- Angiotensin II receptor blockers (ARBs)

The sublingual route of nifedipine is best avoided since it may cause a sudden drop in blood pressure.

The dosages and side-effects of anti-hypertensive drugs used for the management of moderate and acute severe hypertension are listed in Table 39.3.

Seizure prophylaxis and treatment

- Eclampsia is best prevented by immediate delivery.
- Magnesium sulphate has proved to be an excellent prophylaxis against the occurrence of seizures during labour and delivery and in the postpartum period.
- The MAGPIE trial (Altman et al., 2002) and a subsequent systematic review of the Cochrane Database (Duley et al., 2010) have clearly demonstrated that magnesium sulphate reduces the risk of

Magnesium sulphate should be used for the prevention and treatment of seizures in women with gestational hypertension and preeclampsia with severe features or eclampsia.

Table 39.3   Antihypertensives used for hypertension in pregnancy—drugs and dosage

Drug	Dose and route	Side effects	Onset of action
Nifedipine or nifedipine retard	**Moderate hypertension** 10–20 mg **orally** every 6–8 hours **Acute severe hypertension** • 10 mg **orally** initially • If BP exceeds 155/105 mmHg after 1 hour, an additional 10 mg dose can be provided each hour for 2 additional doses (to a total of 30 mg)	• The retard preparation is preferred, though immediate-release nifedipine may also be used • Headache and tachycardia may occur	5–10 minutes
Labetalol	**Moderate hypertension** 200 mg orally twice daily **Acute severe hypertension** • 200 mg orally initially. If target BP is not reached in 1 hour, an additional 200 mg dose may be provided each hour for 2 additional doses (to a total of 600 mg) **OR** • 10–20 mg **IV**, then 20–80 mg every 10–30 minutes to a maximum of 300 mg	Tachycardia less common	1–2 minutes
Methyldopa	**Moderate hypertension** 250–500 mg orally every 6–8 hours **Acute severe hypertension** Single dose of 1000 mg **orally**	Drowsiness	3–6 hours

seizures by 50 per cent. Magnesium sulphate also reduces the risk of placental abruption and maternal mortality.

- Magnesium sulphate can be administered intravenously or intramuscularly (if there is difficulty in establishing IV access or if an infusion pump is not available). The dosage of magnesium sulphate for the prevention and treatment of eclampsia is described in Table 39.4.

- For women requiring cesarean delivery (before the onset of labour), the infusion should ideally begin before surgery and continue during surgery, as well as for 24 hours

Table 39.4   Dosage of magnesium sulphate for the prevention and treatment of eclampsia

Route	Dosage	Timing
Intramuscular	**Loading dose** 10 g of 50% solution (5 g IM in each buttock) **Followed by** 5 g of 50% solution every 4 hours, alternate buttocks (May be mixed with 1 mL of 2% xylocaine to reduce pain)	**Cesarean delivery** (before onset of labour): Initiate before surgery, continue during surgery, maintain for 24 hours afterwards **Vaginal delivery:** Continue for 24 hours after delivery
Intravenous (with infusion pump)	**Loading dose** 4 g diluted in 100 mL of IV fluid over 20–30 minutes **Followed by** a maintenance dose of 1 g/hour	**If convulsions recur:** Additional 2 g of 20% solution IV over 3–5 minutes

IM, intramuscular; *IV*, intravenous

afterwards. For women who deliver vaginally, the infusion should continue for 24 hours after delivery.

- Before administering the next dose, the mother should be monitored for the presence of magnesium toxicity (Table 39.5).

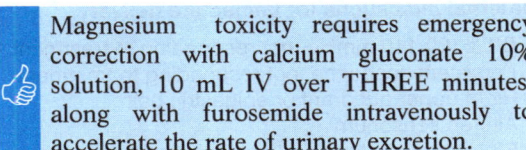 Magnesium toxicity requires emergency correction with calcium gluconate 10% solution, 10 mL IV over THREE minutes, along with furosemide intravenously to accelerate the rate of urinary excretion.

- Magnesium sulphate is a smooth muscle relaxant and can cause respiratory depression and cardiac arrest. Deep tendon reflexes are lost at a serum magnesium level of 9 mg/dL, respiratory depression occurs at 12 mg/dL, and cardiac arrest at 30 mg/dL. The presence of deep tendon reflexes rules out the risk of more serious toxicity. Because magnesium sulphate is excreted almost exclusively in the urine, measuring urine output should be part of the clinical monitoring.

Table 39.5 Monitoring for magnesium sulphate toxicity

To be monitored before each dose	Clinical significance
Patellar reflex should be present	Lost at serum magnesium level of 9 mg/dL
Respiratory rate should be >20/minute	Depressed at serum magnesium level of 12 mg/dL
Urine output should be >100 mL in 4 hours	Magnesium is excreted in the urine and good renal function is required to avoid toxicity

Timing of delivery

- The only known cure for preeclampsia is the delivery of the baby.
- However, when the pregnancy is remote from term, the clinician has to decide whether delaying delivery by expectant management may help salvage the baby.
- The baby's health has to be weighed against the very real dangers of serious maternal complications such as eclampsia and acute kidney injury.

Immediate delivery

- In women with gestational hypertension or preeclampsia without severe features at or beyond 37^{+0} weeks of gestation, delivery rather than expectant management is recommended upon diagnosis.

 Hospitalisation is appropriate for women with severe features and for women in whom frequent maternal and fetal monitoring is required.

- Immediate delivery is indicated when gestational hypertension or preeclampsia **with severe features** is diagnosed at or beyond 34^{+0} of gestation (Table 39.6), after maternal stabilisation or, with labour or prelabour rupture of membranes.
- If the mother is <34 completed weeks, but the disease is rapidly deteriorating or if facilities are not available for intensive maternal monitoring, immediate delivery is indicated because that is the only way to control the progression.

Table 39.6   Maternal and fetal indications for immediate delivery at or beyond 34 completed weeks of pregnancy

Maternal indications for immediate delivery	Fetal indications for immediate delivery
• BP ≥160/110 mmHg, not responding to treatment • Persistent headache, not responding to treatment • Right upper quadrant or epigastric pain • Altered sensorium • Blurred vision, flashing lights or sparks, scotomata • HELLP syndrome • Renal dysfunction • Pulmonary edema • Eclampsia • Placental abruption or vaginal bleeding	• Abnormalities on NST/amniotic fluid volume • Fetal demise • Extreme prematurity • Lethal anomaly • Fetal growth restriction with persistent reversed end-diastolic flow in the umbilical artery

Expectant management

- Expectant management up to 37^{+0} weeks of gestation is recommended in women with gestational hypertension or preeclampsia **without severe features**. Frequent fetal and maternal evaluation is recommended with expectant management.

 Expectant management should only be attempted when there are intensive care facilities to monitor the mother. Neonatal survival also depends on the availability of a neonatal intensive care unit. This may not be possible in a low-resource setting.

- When the pregnancy is between 28 and 34 weeks, expectant management may be considered in an attempt to take the pregnancy to 34 weeks and beyond. **Expectant management is not advised when neonatal survival is doubtful**.

- A systematic review of the Cochrane Database (Churchill et al., 2018) concluded that an expectant approach to the management of women with severe early-onset preeclampsia may be associated with decreased morbidity for the baby.

- However, Vigil-De Gracia et al. (2013) did not demonstrate neonatal benefit with expectant management of severe preeclampsia from 28–34 weeks. Additionally, they found that a conservative approach may increase the risk of abruption and small-for-gestational age babies. **This may be true in all low-resource settings**.

  – In addition to intense maternal and fetal surveillance, laboratory testing (complete blood count including platelets, liver enzymes, and serum creatinine) should be performed serially (Balogun et al., 2017).

  – Immediate delivery, irrespective of fetal age, is indicated with the appearance of any of the factors listed in Table 39.6.

 Corticosteroid therapy
If delivery is indicated at <34 weeks of gestation, administration of corticosteroids for fetal lung maturation is recommended (see **Chapter 33**, *Preterm labour and preterm prelabour rupture of membranes*).

Mode of delivery

- The Hypertension and Preeclampsia Intervention Trial At Term (HYPITAT) trial (Koopmans et al., 2009) showed that women with gestational hypertension or mild preeclampsia had better maternal outcomes and equivalent neonatal outcomes with induction at ≥37 weeks when compared to those who underwent expectant management.

Induction of labour is associated with improved maternal outcome and should be advised for women with mild hypertensive disease beyond 37 weeks' gestation.

- In early-onset preeclampsia with severe features, induction of labour may not be effective in very preterm pregnancies; in such cases, cesarean may be opted for.
- In women with chronic hypertension and superimposed preeclampsia or other pregnancy complications (e.g., fetal growth restriction, previous stillbirth), the timing and mode of delivery should be individualised.
- Indications for cesarean section are as follows:
  - Prematurity <32 weeks
  - Unfavourable cervix, not responding to ripening
  - Severe fetal growth restriction/oligohydramnios
  - Abnormal fetal surveillance tests
  - Maternal complications that jeopardise her health
  - Obstetric indications (malpresentations, cephalopelvic disproportion, intrapartum non-reassuring fetal status)

Anesthesia

- Regional anesthesia is the preferred technique for labour and delivery in women with preeclampsia with severe features or with eclampsia.
- Both spinal and epidural anesthesia are safe, even in women with preeclampsia

Platelet count and neuraxial anesthesia
Epidural or spinal anesthesia is considered acceptable, and the risk of epidural hematoma is exceptionally low in patients with platelet counts of ≥70,000/μL (ACOG, 2019).

with severe features (Aya et al., 2005; Hogg et al., 1999).
- General anesthesia carries the risk of aspiration and failed intubation because of pharyngolaryngeal edema, and stroke secondary to increased systemic and intracranial pressures during intubation and extubation (Huang et al., 2010).

POSTPARTUM MANAGEMENT

- Women with preeclampsia must be monitored carefully for at least 48 hours after delivery as they may develop severe features of preeclampsia or eclampsia.
- Even women without the preceding symptoms might develop postpartum eclampsia or stroke.

Breastfeeding

Antihypertensive medication used antenatally can be continued since methyldopa, nifedipine, and labetalol are all safe during breastfeeding.

Screening of women with early-onset preeclampsia

Primiparas who develop early-onset severe preeclampsia (before 34 weeks) should be screened in the postpartum period for pre-existing hypertension, underlying renal disease, and antiphospholipid syndrome.

Risk of recurrence

- The risk of recurrence of gestational hypertension ranges from 13–52 per cent.
- Preeclampsia can recur in a subsequent pregnancy in 16 per cent of pregnancies. When a pregnancy has been complicated by severe preeclampsia, HELLP, or eclampsia needing delivery before 34 weeks, the risk of developing preeclampsia in a future pregnancy is 25 per cent. This rises to 55 per cent if the delivery took place before 28 weeks' gestation (NICE, 2010).

Lifetime risk of cardiovascular disease and preventive measures

- Preeclampsia (especially early-onset preeclampsia) is associated with an increased risk of cardiovascular disease in subsequent years (Stuart et al., 2018; Brown et al., 2013).
- The odds of developing hypertension, myocardial infarction, congestive heart failure, cerebrovascular events (stroke), peripheral arterial disease, and cardiovascular mortality are doubled.
- These women should be counselled about lifestyle modifications to better manage risk factors for cardiovascular disease. They must focus on achieving and maintaining an optimal weight by adopting regular exercise and a healthy diet. Smoking should be strictly avoided.

References

1. Abalos E, Duley L, Steyn DW, Gialdini C. 2018. Antihypertensive drug therapy for mild to moderate hypertension during pregnancy. *Cochrane Database Syst Rev.* Issue 10. Art no.: CD002252.

2. Altman D, Carroli G, Duley L, Farrell B, Moodley J, Neilson J et al. 2002. Do women with preeclampsia and their babies benefit from magnesium sulphate? The Magpie Trial: A randomised placebo-controlled trial. Magpie Trial Collaboration Group. *Lancet.* 359:1877–90.

3. American College of Obstetricians and Gynecologists. 2020. ACOG PracticeBulletin No. 222. Gestational hypertension and preeclampsia. *Obstet Gynecol.* 135:e237–60

4. Aya AG, Vialles N, Tanoubi I, Mangin R, Ferrer JM, Robert C et al. 2005. Spinal anesthesia-induced hypotension: A risk comparison between patients with severe preeclampsia and healthy women undergoing preterm cesarean delivery. *Anesth Analg.* 101:869–75.

5. Balogun OA, Sibai BM. 2017. Counseling, management and outcomes in women with severe preeclampsia at 23 to 28 weeks' gestation. *Clin Obstet Gynecol.* 60:183–9.

6. Brown MC, Best KE, Pearce MS, Waugh J, Robson SC, Bell R. 2013. Cardiovascular disease risk in women with preeclampsia: Systematic review and meta-analysis. *Eur J Epidemiol.* 28:1–19.

7. Churchill D, Duley L, Thornton JG, Moussa M, Ali HS, Walker KF. 2018. Interventionist versus expectant care for severe preeclampsia between 24 and 34 weeks' gestation. *Cochrane Database Syst Rev.* Issue 10. Art. no.: CD003106.

8. Cnossen JS, Morris RK, Ter Riet G, Mol BW, van der Post J A, Coomarasamy A et al. 2008. Use of uterine artery Doppler ultrasonography to predict preeclampsia and intrauterine growth restriction: A systematic review and bivariable meta-analysis. *CMAJ.* 178:701–11.

9. Duley L, Gülmezoglu AM, Henderson-Smart DJ, Chou D. 2010. Magnesium sulphate and other anticonvulsants for women with preeclampsia. *Cochrane Database Syst Rev.* Issue 11. Art. no.: CD000025.

10. Duley L, Meher S, Hunter KE, Seidler AL, Askie LM. 2019. Antiplatelet agents for preventing preeclampsia and its complications. *Cochrane Database Syst Rev.* Issue. 10. Art. no.: CD004659.

11. Easterling T, Mundle S, Bracken H, Parvekar S, Mool S, Magee LA, von Dadelszen P, Shochet T, Winikoff B. 2019. Oral antihypertensive regimens (nifedipine retard, labetalol, and methyldopa) for management of severe hypertension in pregnancy: An open-label, randomised controlled trial. *Lancet.* 394(10203):1011.

12. Hofmeyr GJ, Lawrie TA, Atallah ÁN, Duley L, Torloni MR. 2014. Calcium supplementation during pregnancy for preventing hypertensive disorders and related problems. *Cochrane Database Syst Rev.* Issue 6. Art. no.: CD001059.

13. Hogg B, Hauth JC, Caritis SN, Sibai BM, Lindheimer M, Van Dorsten JP, et al. 1999. Safety of labor epidural anesthesia for women with severe hypertensive disease. National Institute of Child Health and Human Development Maternal–Fetal Medicine Units Network. *Am J Obstet Gynecol.* 181:1096–101.

14. Homer CS, Brown MA, Mangos G, Davis GK. 2008. Non-proteinuric preeclampsia: A novel risk indicator in women with gestational hypertension. *J Hypertens.* 26:295–302.

15. Huang CJ, Fan YC, Tsai PS. 2010. Differential impacts of modes of anaesthesia on the risk of stroke among pre-eclamptic women who undergo Caesarean delivery: A population-based study. *Br J Anaesth.* 105:818–26.

16 Koopmans CM, Bijlenga D, Groen H et al. 2009. Induction of labour versus expectant monitoring for gestational hypertension or mild preeclampsia after 36 weeks' gestation (HYPITAT): A multicentre, open-label randomised controlled trial. *Lancet.* 374:979.

17. Magee LA, Sharma S, Nathan HL et al. 2019. The incidence of pregnancy hypertension in India, Pakistan, Mozambique, and Nigeria: A prospective population-level analysis. *PLoS Med.* 16(4):e1002783.

18. Magee LA, von Dadelszen P, Bohun CM, Rey E, El-Zibdeh M, Stalker S et al. 2003. Serious perinatal complications of non-proteinuric hypertension: An international, multicentre, retrospective cohort study. *J Obstet Gynaecol Can.* 25:372–82.

19. Magee LA, von Dadelszen P, Rey E et al. 2015. Less-tight versus tight control of hypertension in pregnancy. *N Engl J Med.* 372:407–417.

20. Magee LA, von Dadelszen P, Singer J et al. 2016. The CHIPS Randomized Controlled Trial (Control of Hypertension in Pregnancy Study): Is Severe Hypertension Just an Elevated Blood Pressure? *Hypertension.* 68(5):1153–1159.

21. Mehta B, Kumar V, Chawla S, Sachdeva S, Mahopatra D. 2015. Hypertension in Pregnancy: A Community-Based Study. *Indian J Community Med.* 40(4):273–278.

22. NICE Guidelines no. 107. 2010. Hypertension in pregnancy. National Institute for Health and Clinical Excellence. London.

23. Paily VP, Ambujam K, Thomas B et al. 2021. Why mothers die, Kerala, 2010-2020. Observations, recommendations. Third report of confidential review of maternal deaths, Kerala.

24. Paruk F, Moodley J. 2000. Maternal and neonatal outcome in early- and late-onset preeclampsia. *Seminars in Neonatology,* Vol. 5, no. 3, pp. 197–207.

25. Poon LC, Kametas NA, Maiz N, Akolekar R, Nicolaides KH. 2009. First-trimester prediction of hypertensive disorders in pregnancy. *Hypertension.* 53:812–8.
26. Roberge S, Nicolaides K, Demers S, Hyett J, Chaillet N, Bujold E. 2017. The role of aspirin dose on the prevention of preeclampsia and fetal growth restriction: systematic review and meta-analysis. *Am J Obstet Gynecol.* 216:110–20.e6.
27. Rolnik DL, Wright D, Poon LCY et al. 2017. ASPRE trial: Performance of screening for preterm preeclampsia. *Ultrasound Obstet Gynecol.* 50: 492-495.
28. Sibai BM, Stella CL. 2009. Diagnosis and management of atypical preeclampsia-eclampsia. *Am J Obstet Gynecol.* 200:481.e1–7.
29. Sibai BM. 2004. Diagnosis, controversies, and management of the syndrome of hemolysis, elevated liver enzymes, and low platelet count. *Obstet Gynecol.* 103:981.
30. Steegers EA, von Dadelszen P, Duvekot JJ, Pijnenborg R. 2010. Preeclampsia. *Lancet.* 376:631–44.
31. Stuart JJ, Tanz LJ, Missmer SA, Rimm EB, Spiegelman D, James-Todd TM et al. 2018. Hypertensive disorders of pregnancy and maternal cardiovascular disease risk factor development: An observational cohort study. *Ann Intern Med.* 169:224–32.
32. The FIGO textbook of pregnancy hypertension – an evidence-based guide to monitoring, prevention and management. International Federation of Gynecology and Obstetrics (FIGO). 2016.
33. Thornton CE, Makris A, Ogle RF, Tooher JM, Hennessy A. 2010. Role of proteinuria in defining preeclampsia: Clinical outcomes for women and babies. *Clin Exp Pharmacol Physiol.* 37:466–70.
34. Vigil-De Gracia P, Reyes Tejada O, Calle Minaca A, Tellez G, Chon VY, Herrarte E et al. 2013. Expectant management of severe preeclampsia remote from term: The MEXPRE Latin Study, a randomized, multicenter clinical trial. *Am J Obstet Gynecol.* 209:425.e1–8.
35. Williams D. 2011. Long-term complications of preeclampsia. *Semin Nephrol.* 31:111–22.
36. World Health Organization. 2011. WHO recommendations for prevention and treatment of preeclampsia and eclampsia. WHO, Geneva.

Chapter 40

Gestational and Pre-gestational Diabetes

INTRODUCTION

- As the prevalence of diabetes increases in the general population in India, there is a concomitant rise in gestational diabetes (diabetes diagnosed during pregnancy).
- The prevalence of gestational diabetes mellitus (GDM) varies in different cities/regions in India and has been reported to range from 6.2 per cent in Mysore, 9.5 per cent in Western India to 17.9 per cent in Tamil Nadu. Recent studies have shown alarmingly high prevalence in Punjab (35 per cent) and Lucknow (41 per cent) (Mithal et al., 2015).
- The prevalence of GDM also varies between urban and rural areas. In a community-based survey, Seshiah and colleagues (2008) ascertained the prevalence of GDM in a South Indian population. The prevalence of GDM in urban, semi-urban, and rural areas was found to be 17.8 per cent, 13.8 per cent, and 9.9 per cent, respectively.
- Gestational diabetes is associated with a greatly increased future risk of type 2 diabetes (Noctor and Dunne, 2015).
- Planned pregnancies, pre-pregnancy counselling, and tight glycemic control have made it possible for women with pre-gestational and gestational diabetes to expect outcomes similar to women who do not have diabetes.
- Maternal consequences of diabetes in pregnancy include preeclampsia, gestational hypertension, hydramnios, birth trauma, and operative delivery (cesarean or instrumental).
- Fetal and neonatal consequences include macrosomia and large-for-gestational age infant, birth trauma, perinatal mortality, neonatal respiratory problems, and metabolic complications after birth (hypoglycemia, hyperbilirubinemia, hypocalcemia, polycythemia).

Screening, detection, counselling and follow-up of diabetes in pregnancy can decrease the burden of future diabetes in women with GDM; good glycemic control can decrease, prevent, or delay the onset of diabetes in the offspring.

- An obstetrician taking care of women with gestational diabetes needs to have a good understanding of the maternal and fetal concerns arising from GDM, the management of hyperglycemia, monitoring of the fetus, and the timing of delivery.

More than 90 per cent of cases of hyperglycemia in pregnancy are estimated to occur in low- and middle-income countries (Guariguata et al., 2014).
The epidemic of obesity and diabetes, a trend towards pregnancies at an older age, the decrease in physical activity, and the adoption of modern lifestyles in developing countries may all be factors that contribute to this increase in the prevalence of GDM.

TYPES OF DIABETES COMPLICATING PREGNANCY

Diabetes complicating pregnancy is of two distinct types:

- **Gestational diabetes mellitus (GDM):** Women who develop glucose intolerance during their pregnancy have GDM. Gestational diabetes is further classified as follows (ACOG, 2018):
  - *Diet-controlled GDM* or *class A1GDM:* Gestational diabetes that is adequately controlled without medication
  - *Medication-controlled* or *class A2GDM:* Gestational diabetes mellitus that requires medication to achieve euglycemia
- **Pre-gestational diabetes:** Women who have type 1 or type 2 diabetes before conception are classified as having pre-gestational diabetes.

DEFINITION OF GESTATIONAL DIABETES MELLITUS (GDM)

Differing definitions of GDM have been postulated. It is important to choose any ONE of the definitions, and follow it for **all** women being cared for. This will ensure uniform management.

- **ACOG (2018)** — The term gestational diabetes mellitus (GDM) is used with the presence of any degree of glucose intolerance/hyperglycemia with onset in or first recognition in pregnancy. This may include previously unrecognised diabetes, which may have antedated pregnancy.
- **WHO (2018)** — Hyperglycemia first detected at any time during pregnancy should be classified as either gestational diabetes mellitus (GDM) or diabetes mellitus in pregnancy according to the WHO diagnostic criteria (see below).

  Diabetes mellitus in pregnancy differs from GDM in that the hyperglycemia is more severe in the former and does not resolve after pregnancy as it does with GDM.
- **American Diabetes Association (ADA, 2019)** — Since many women may have unrecognised or undiagnosed glucose intolerance prior to pregnancy, the American Diabetes Association (2019) defines GDM as diabetes diagnosed in the second or third trimester of pregnancy that was not clearly either pre-existing type 1 or type 2 diabetes.
- **The International Association of Diabetes and Pregnancy Study Groups (IADPSG, 2010)** — Diabetes in pregnancy is classified into two categories – overt and gestational (Metzger et al., 2010). Overt diabetes refers to pre-existing diabetes that is diagnosed at the initial visit, and gestational diabetes is diagnosed either by the initial fasting blood sugar level or at 24–28 weeks' gestation.

DIAGNOSTIC CRITERIA FOR DIABETES IN PREGNANCY

The following diagnostic criteria are recommended by the IADPSG (2010) and endorsed by the WHO (2018) and ADA (2019).

- **Overt diabetes/diabetes in pregnancy**—A diagnosis of overt diabetes can be made in women who meet any of the following criteria at their initial prenatal visit:

- Fasting plasma glucose ≥126 mg/dL (7.0 mmol/L)
- A1C ≥6.5 per cent using a standardised assay
- Random plasma glucose ≥200 mg/dL (11.1 mmol/) that is subsequently confirmed by elevated fasting plasma glucose or A1C, as described above
- **Gestational diabetes**—A diagnosis of gestational diabetes can be made in women who meet either of the following criteria (IADPSG, 2010; ADA, 2019):
  - **Any gestational age:** Fasting plasma glucose ≥92 mg/dL (5.1 mmol/L) but <126 mg/dL (7.0 mmol/L)
  - **At 24 to 28 weeks of gestation:** 75 g 2-hour oral glucose tolerance test (OGTT) with at least one abnormal value

SCREENING FOR GESTATIONAL DIABETES

Many professional bodies had differing opinions on what was the best screening and indeed, diagnostic test. The Hyperglycemia and Adverse Pregnancy Outcome (HAPO) study clearly established that there is a linear association between rising blood glucose levels and adverse pregnancy outcome, even with minor degrees of glucose intolerance not amounting to diabetes mellitus. Currently, it is standard of care to screen all pregnant women for glucose intolerance.

Who should be screened?

Though certain factors place women at high-risk for gestational diabetes (see box below), **universal screening for all pregnant women**, irrespective of risk factors is recommended currently by the Gestational Diabetes Mellitus guidelines, Government of India (2018), and the IADPSG (2010).

 In India, given the high incidence of type 2 diabetes and an incidence of 12–15 per cent of GDM, universal screening is recommended.

Risk factors for developing gestational diabetes mellitus (GDM)
- Maternal age >25 years
- Ethnicity (high rate of type 2 diabetes)
  - Indian subcontinent – 11-fold
  - Southeast Asia – 8-fold
- Pre-pregnancy weight >80 kg or BMI >28 kg/m², significant weight gain in early adulthood and between pregnancies or excessive gestational weight gain
- Family history of diabetes in first-degree relative
- Previous macrosomia/polyhydramnios
- Previous unexplained perinatal loss or birth of a malformed infant
- Polycystic ovarian syndrome
- Metabolic syndrome

Which screening test?

Outside the United States, most professional bodies agree on a single-step screening and diagnostic process.

The single-step approach

- The single-step approach proposed by the IADPSG (2010) and endorsed by the ADA (2019) is most commonly used. A 75 g 2-hour oral glucose tolerance test (OGTT) is performed as follows:
  - At 24–28 weeks of gestation in women not previously diagnosed with diabetes
  - In the morning after an overnight fast of at least 8 hours
  - Plasma glucose measurement is done in the fasting state and at 1 and 2 hours after glucose
- Gestational diabetes is diagnosed if any one value is abnormal (Table 40.1).

Table 40.1   Diagnostic values for GDM after 75 g oral GTT according to the recommendations of the IADPSG and ADA. Any one abnormal value is diagnostic of gestational diabetes.

Fasting plasma glucose	≥92 mg/dL (5.1 mmol/L), but <126 mg/dL (7.0 mmol/L)
One hour value	≥180 mg/dL (10.0 mmol/L)
Two hour value	≥153 mg/dL (8.5 mmol/L)

- Adoption of these screening criteria significantly increased the reported incidence of GDM from 5–6 per cent to 15–20 per cent (Sacks et al., 2012), primarily because only one abnormal value, not two, became sufficient to make the diagnosis.
- Duran and colleagues (2014), in a large study, found that the application of the IADPSG criteria was associated with significant improvements in pregnancy outcomes, and was cost-effective. They recommended adoption of these criteria universally.
- A recent follow-up study of women who were diagnosed with GDM by the one-step approach OGTT, found that 11 years after their pregnancies, these women were at a 3.4-fold higher risk of developing pre-diabetes and type 2 diabetes, and had children with a higher risk of obesity and increased body fat (Lowe et al., 2018).

 Women diagnosed as GDM by the one-step, single abnormal value screening are at a high risk of developing glucose intolerance and should have long-term follow-up (Lowe et al., 2018).

DIPSI Guidelines and National Guidelines, Ministry of Health and Family Welfare, Government of India (MoHFW), India (2018)

- The Diabetes in Pregnancy Study Group India (DIPSI) guidelines (Seshiah et al., 2006), recommend a simplified screening diagnostic test.
- The Guidelines for the Diagnosis and Management of Gestational Diabetes, Ministry of Health, Government of India (2018), endorse the one-step testing using the DIPSI method and recommend the following:
  - Performed when a pregnant woman presents at the antenatal clinic in the fasting or non-fasting state, irrespective of timing of her last meal
  - 75 g oral glucose load in 150–200 mL of water or lime juice
  - Plasma glucose level at 2 hr of ≥140 mg/dL confirms GDM
  - A glucometer may be used in facilities where women may not be able to return the next day for the report

- If vomiting occurs within 30 minutes of oral glucose intake, the test has to be repeated the next day. If vomiting occurs after 30 minutes, the test can be continued
- The criteria for the diagnosis of GDM, based on plasma glucose at 2 hours, are as follows:
  - ≥140 mg/dL: Gestational diabetes
  - ≥120 mg/dL: Decreased gestational glucose tolerance
  - ≥200 mg/dL: Pre-gestational diabetes mellitus

The two-step approach

The ACOG recommends **a two-step approach** as proposed by the National Institutes of Health (Vandorsten et al., 2013) and Carpenter and Coustan (1982).

Step 1: Perform a 50 g glucose load test (GLT):
- At 24–28 weeks of gestation in women not previously diagnosed with diabetes
- In the non-fasting state
- Plasma glucose measurement at 1 hour

If the plasma glucose level measured 1 hour after the load is ≥130 mg/dL or 140 mg/dL (7.2 mmol/L or 7.8 mmol/L, respectively), a 100 g OGTT should be performed. The ACOG recommends that either cut-off can be used, since no data exists to support one over the other. Obstetricians should select one of these as a single consistent cut-off for their practice.

Step 2: The 100 g 3-hour OGTT should be performed when the patient is fasting. The diagnosis of GDM is made if **at least two of the four plasma glucose levels** listed in Table 40.2 **are met or exceeded** (ADA, 2019).

Table 40.2 Diagnostic values for GDM screening with the 100 g 3-hour OGTT; GDM is diagnosed when any two of the four values is exceeded

Blood sugar	Carpenter and Coustan criteria		NDDG criteria
Fasting	95 mg/dL (5.3 mmol/L)		105 mg/dL (5.8 mmol/L)
1 hour	180 mg/dL (10.0 mmol/L)	**OR**	190 mg/dL (10.6 mmol/L)
2 hour	155 mg/dL (8.6 mmol/L		165 mg/dL (9.2 mmol/L)
3 hour	140 mg/dL (7.8 mmol/L)		145 mg/dL (8.0 mmol/L)

NDDG, National Diabetes Data Group

CONSEQUENCES OF DIABETES IN PREGNANCY

Gestational diabetes

- **Gestational hypertension and preeclampsia:** Women with GDM are at an increased risk for gestational hypertension and preeclampsia (Yogev et al., HAPO study, 2010; Hauth et al., 2011). This association is related to the increased insulin resistance in women with GDM.
- **Macrosomia:** Macrosomia is the most common adverse neonatal outcome associated with GDM.

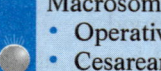

Macrosomia increases the risk of the following complications:
- Operative vaginal delivery
- Cesarean section
- Shoulder dystocia
- Maternal and fetal injury

- In a recent study, Sovio et al. (2016) found that in women who have GDM, excessive growth of the fetal abdominal circumference (AC) between 20 and 28 weeks' gestational age occurs even before the diagnosis of GDM.
- Macrosomic fetuses in pregnancies with glucose intolerance are different from macrosomic fetuses from other causes. They tend to have an increased risk of shoulder dystocia because of the following features:
  - Greater total body fat
  - Greater shoulder and upper-extremity circumferences
  - Chest circumference much larger than the head
  - Altered fetal body shape—barrel-chested infant with a short neck and broad shoulders (see **Chapter 36**, *Fetal growth disorders: growth restriction and macrosomia*)
- **Polyhydramnios** is also seen in women with GDM but does not in itself impact outcomes. Though fetal polyuria may be implicated, the etiology of polyhydramnios in GDM is unclear.
- **Neonatal morbidity** in pregnancies complicated by GDM includes hypoglycemia, hyperbilirubinemia, hypocalcemia, polycythemia, and respiratory distress syndrome (Metzger et al., 2008).
- **Stillbirth** risk is also increased in women with GDM (Rosenstein et al., 2012). However, the relationship of stillbirth to glycemic control is not clear.
- **The risk of cesarean delivery** increases in women with GDM. 25 per cent of women with GDM who require insulin and 17 per cent of women with GDM controlled by lifestyle modification underwent cesarean delivery as compared to 9.5 per cent of the controls (Ehrenberg et al., 2004).
- **The risk of type 2 diabetes later in life** increases in women with GDM.
  - Bellamy et al. (2009), in a meta-analysis, showed that women with gestational diabetes have a greatly increased risk of developing type 2 diabetes. More disturbingly, in a recent study from North India, Jindal et al. (2015) found that a large proportion of women who had GDM and who were tested with an OGTT at 6 weeks postpartum had some persistent glucose abnormality after birth, with nearly 7 per cent having overt type 2 diabetes.
  - The following additional factors influence the risk of diabetes later in life in women with GDM (Noctor and Dunne, 2015):
    - *Breastfeeding* improves glycemic indices in the postpartum period but its long-term influence on the occurrence of type 2 diabetes is unclear.
    - *BMI and waist* circumference have shown an association with future risk of diabetes. Women should be counselled about excess weight gain after the pregnancy. Excessive weight gain in each pregnancy further increases the risk.

- *Progesterone-only* oral contraceptives are thought to confer a higher risk of developing type 2 diabetes later in life.
- **The risk of type 2 diabetes in children born to mothers with uncontrolled diabetes** is increased. Children born to mothers with GDM are four to eight times more likely to develop diabetes in later life as compared to other children (siblings) born to the same parents in a non-GDM pregnancy (Damm, 2009). The development of **obesity** and **metabolic syndrome** is also increased in the offspring of women who have GDM.

Pre-gestational diabetes

- **Miscarriage and congenital anomalies:** In addition to the above-mentioned risks of gestational diabetes, women with pre-existing diabetes have an increased risk of miscarriage and congenital anomalies.
  - The risk of early miscarriage is higher and is associated with the level of hyperglycemia. Hyperglycemia may possibly be associated with an increased risk of fetal abnormalities (Jovanovic et al., 2005).
  - The main congenital defects associated with pre-gestational diabetes are in the cardiovascular, central nervous, and musculoskeletal systems, and are linearly related to maternal glycemic control in the periconceptional period (Gabbay-Benziv, 2015). The risk of anomalies is linked to the degree of hyperglycemia in the early weeks of pregnancy. Even with good glycemic control, the risk remains marginally higher than in non-diabetic women (Correa et al., 2008).
- **Preterm birth:** Pre-gestational diabetes mellitus predisposes to both induced and spontaneous preterm birth (Sibai et al., 2000). Inductions in the preterm period are dictated by factors such as preeclampsia, macrosomia, and poor glycemic control. Delivery is hastened in these cases to avoid the risk of late fetal death.

MANAGEMENT OF DIABETES IN PREGNANCY

The diagnosis and treatment of GDM has conclusively been proven to reduce maternal and fetal morbidity, especially fetal macrosomia. Management consists of the following:
- Pre-pregnancy counselling
- Antenatal glycemic control
- Obstetric management

Pre-pregnancy counselling for diabetic women planning pregnancy

- Diabetic women planning a pregnancy require specific counselling to ensure a safe and successful pregnancy outcome.
- All women of childbearing age with diabetes should be counselled about the importance of tight glycemic control prior to conception. Elevations in A1C during the first 10 weeks of pregnancy are directly related to the risk of diabetic embryopathy, especially anencephaly, microcephaly, congenital heart disease, and caudal regression (Guerin et al., 2007).

- **Periconceptional glycemic control:** The following preconception glucose targets are recommended by the ADA (2019).
  - A1C <6–6.5 per cent (if it can be achieved without significant hypoglycemia)
  - Fasting capillary blood glucose concentration 80–110 mg/dL

  > Preconceptional high-dose folic acid (5 mg/day) is recommended up to 12 weeks' gestation in women with diabetes to reduce the risk of birth defects, especially neural tube defects (NICE, 2016).

  - Two-hour postprandial glucose concentration <155 mg/dL
- Medication should be reviewed at the preconception visit, and the possible need to increase or change medication should also be discussed.
- Diabetic women also need to be assessed for established complications of diabetes, especially of the eyes and kidneys. Women with pre-existing type 1 or type 2 diabetes who are planning pregnancy or who have become pregnant should be counselled on the risk of development and/or progression of diabetic retinopathy.

> Unfortunately, >50 per cent of pregnancies are unplanned. Women with diabetes who have not had preconception planning or those who have had an unexpected pregnancy, should have their glycemic control assessed as soon as practical, and advice on risk should be offered on the basis of this result.

Antenatal glycemic control

Benefits of treating gestational diabetes

- There are proven benefits to managing hyperglycemia in pregnancy.
- The Australian Carbohydrate Intolerance Study in Pregnant Women Trial Group (Crowther et al., 2005) demonstrated that diagnosing and treating GDM improves both maternal and fetal outcomes. There was a significant decrease in perinatal death, shoulder dystocia, and birth trauma, including fracture or nerve palsy. Treatment also reduced preeclampsia and macrosomia. A randomised, multicentre trial by Landon et al. (2009) also confirmed this.
- Though a meta-analysis (Hartling et al., 2013) did show benefits of treating mild GDM, it did not show a treatment effect on clinical neonatal hypoglycemia or future poor metabolic outcomes of the offspring.

The treatment of gestational diabetes includes the following:
- Lifestyle modification therapy
- Pharmacological therapy

Lifestyle modification therapy

- 85–90 per cent of women diagnosed with GDM can control hyperglycemia with lifestyle modification alone.
- A systematic review of the Cochrane Database (Brown et al., 2017) concluded that lifestyle interventions including nutritional therapy, exercise, and self-monitoring of blood glucose concentrations are useful as the primary therapeutic strategy in GDM.

Nutritional therapy

- Nutritional therapy is the mainstay in the management of GDM. The aims of nutritional therapy are as follows (Durnwald, 2019):
  - To achieve normoglycemia
  - To prevent ketosis
  - To provide adequate gestational weight gain based on maternal body mass index (BMI)
  - To ensure adequate fetal growth and development

> All women with GDM should have nutritional counselling and a diet plan that is based on their BMI. The aim should be to achieve adequate weight gain along with good glycemic control.

- Yamamoto and colleagues (2018), in a systematic review and meta-analysis, showed that dietary interventions favourably influenced outcomes related to maternal glycemia and birth weight.
- It is important for the mother to receive nutritional counselling from a trained dietitian. Commonly, three meals and two to three snacks are recommended to distribute carbohydrate intake and to reduce postprandial glucose fluctuations.
- The total caloric requirement is calculated based on the mother's BMI. This may vary from 30 kcal/kg/day for those with ideal body weight, to 12–14 kcal/kg/day for morbidly obese women.
- The meal plan is made based on the normal eating pattern of the woman and is adjusted based on the results of self-glucose monitoring, appetite, and weight gain patterns to maintain target glucose levels.
- Once the total calories are calculated, the carbohydrate intake distributed across meals is limited to <40 per cent of the total calorie requirement. The carbohydrate restriction helps blunt the postprandial glucose rise. The remaining calories come from protein (<20 per cent) and fat (40 per cent), with saturated fat intake kept at <7 per cent.
- While it is important to achieve good control, one must be careful to avoid hypoglycemia. There is evidence that overly tight control can result in an increase in the incidence of small-for-gestational age offspring (Langer et al., 1989).

Exercise and activity

- Exercise helps in maintaining normoglycemia largely by reducing insulin resistance.
- A moderate exercise programme is beneficial as part of the treatment plan for women with GDM. The goal should be to include 30 minutes of brisk walking at least five days a week or a minimum of 150 minutes per week.
- Simple exercise such as walking for 10–15 minutes after each meal can lead to improved glycemic control and is commonly recommended since it reduces both fasting and postprandial blood glucose concentration. Anjana et al. (2016) found that in their cohort of Indian women, those with GDM were more sedentary than those without. Recreational walking was associated with a 70 per cent decreased risk of adverse neonatal outcomes.

Monitoring of plasma glucose levels

- Women with GDM should be taught to self-monitor their glucose levels with a glucometer where possible, and ideally Urine glucose monitoring is not useful in GDM. check levels four times in a day to see if there is hyperglycemia that can increase fetal risk.
- In low-resource areas, a fasting blood sugar and 1-hour or 2-hour postprandial level may be measured every 2–3 days (Government of India Guidelines, 2018).
- A combination of fasting, pre-meal, and post-meal glucose levels should be checked, staggered over different meals in a day. This, of course, is more important for women who are on medication.
- Once good glycemic control is achieved, especially for women who are only on nutritional therapy, the frequency of monitoring can be reduced to once in two weeks.
- When comparing 1-hour postprandial with preprandial glucose levels, 1-hour postprandial monitoring was associated with the following benefits (de Veciana et al., 1995):
  - Better glycemic control
  - A lower incidence of large-for-gestational age infants
  - A lower rate of cesarean delivery for cephalopelvic disproportion

> **Goals of therapy (ADA, 2019; ACOG, 2018)**
> Fasting or or preprandial blood glucose values   <95 mg/dL
> Postprandial blood glucose values   <140 mg/dL at 1 hour or
>   <120 mg/dL at 2 hours
>
> A fasting plasma glucose level >105 mg/dL is associated with a risk of macrosomia that was five-fold greater than that with a fasting glucose level <75 mg/dL (Metzger et al., HAPO study, 2010).

Pharmacological therapy

- Insulin is the preferred medication for treating hyperglycemia in gestational diabetes mellitus as it does not cross the placenta to a measurable extent.

> The ADA (2019) recommends that metformin, when used to treat polycystic ovary syndrome and induce ovulation, should be discontinued once pregnancy has been confirmed. The clinician should make an individualised decision based on the feasibility of insulin therapy.

- The ADA (2019) does not recommend metformin and glyburide as first-line agents as both cross the placenta to the fetus. All oral agents lack long-term safety data.
- The ACOG (2018), NICE (2015), and Government of India Guidelines (2018) consider metformin a reasonable alternative choice in the following women:
  - Those who decline insulin therapy
  - Those who will be unable to safely administer insulin
  - Those who cannot afford insulin

Insulin

- When insulin is initiated, an endocrinologist should be involved in the management of the disease.

- Administration of insulin is recommended if:
  - Nutritional intervention and exercise alone are not successful in achieving optimal blood glucose levels.
  - The fetal abdominal circumference (AC) on ultrasound examination at 28–32 weeks is >75th percentile, since this is a sign of fetal

 It is good clinical practice to hospitalise the patient for at least 48 hours when insulin is initiated. This allows for calculating the optimal dose and immediate correction of the dose if hypoglycemia is encountered. This also provides the mother/her partner the opportunity to learn how to administer insulin.

  hyperinsulinemia, and there is evidence that insulin may reduce the risk of macrosomia (Bonomo et al., 2004).
- Using the same rationale, in women who have mild hyperglycemia and whose fetuses have a small AC (<75th percentile) at 28–32 weeks, a more relaxed insulin dose or even the avoidance of insulin may minimise the risk of iatrogenic growth restriction (Kjos, 2001).

Type and timing of insulin

- The dose and type of insulin is decided based on the degree of hyperglycemia and obesity. The dose is then divided through the day depending on the specific abnormality of glucose levels on monitoring and modified based on the self-glucose monitoring results.
- A combination of intermediate- and rapid-acting insulin is initiated for women with postprandial glucose elevations. A premixed human insulin 30:70 is commonly used.
- Insulin analogues (insulin lispro and insulin aspart) are short-acting insulins, and do not cross the placenta. Insulin

 Insulin analogues are very expensive and may not be feasible in low-resource areas.

  lispro and insulin aspart are preferred over regular insulin for the following reasons:
  - The rapid onset of action
  - Insulin can be administered at the time of a meal rather than 10–15 minutes before an anticipated meal

 Even when insulin is required in pregnancy to normalise glucose levels, only a minority of these women will need any insulin during labour (Barrett et al., 2009).

  - Better glycemic control
  - Fewer hypoglycemic episodes

Oral hypoglycemic agents (OHA)

- Traditionally, insulin was the only drug used for the medical management of diabetes in pregnancy. However, there has been increasing use and evidence on the safety of oral hypoglycemic agents in the management of GDM. Metformin is the most commonly used OHA in pregnancy.
- The safety of glyburide has not been established. Balsells et al. (2015) found that glyburide was associated with a higher rate of neonatal hypoglycemia and macrosomia than either insulin or metformin.
- In two systematic reviews, metformin was associated with a lower risk of neonatal hypoglycemia and less maternal weight gain than insulin (Balsells et al., 2015; Jiang et al., 2015).

 Glyburide and metformin fail to provide adequate glycemic control in up to 30 per cent of women with GDM.

- Though current data demonstrate no adverse short-term effects of metformin therapy during pregnancy on maternal or neonatal health, demonstrated long-term outcomes on the body composition of offspring include higher BMI and increased obesity in offspring exposed to metformin (Rowan et al., 2018).

> The **ADA (2019)** does not endorse the use of oral anti-hyperglycemic agents in pregnancy. The **ACOG (2018)** recommends its use with caution and advises it only if insulin therapy is not available or if it is refused. **NICE guidelines (2015)** endorse the safety of use and efficacy of metformin and glyburide in pregnancy but add that informed consent needs to be obtained and documented before initiating or continuing these drugs in pregnancy. **The Government of India Guidelines (2018)** recommend metformin for GDM after 20 weeks of gestation as an alternative to insulin.

Obstetric management

Obstetric management consists of the following:
- Antepartum management
- Intrapartum management

Antepartum management

- There is no robust data on when to initiate and how often to perform fetal surveillance in diabetic pregnancies. Antepartum surveillance reduces the risk of stillbirth in complicated diabetic pregnancies.
- Fetal surveillance is not routinely required in the following since the risk of stillbirth is very low:
  - Women who are euglycemic on diet and exercise alone
  - Women with no obstetric complications (e.g., macrosomia, preeclampsia, growth restriction, polyhydramnios, or oligohydramnios)
- Tests for fetal surveillance should be done weekly or twice weekly starting at 32 weeks (ACOG, 2018) for the following:
  - Women on insulin/OHA
  - Women with poor glycemic control
  - Women with obstetric complications
- Fetal surveillance consists of the following:
  - Serial ultrasound examinations for fetal growth
  - Tests to identify fetal compromise
    - Non-stress test
    - Biophysical profile score
    - Assessment of amniotic fluid volume in the third trimester

Serial ultrasound for assessing fetal growth

20–22 weeks' scan with a detailed cardiac evaluation
A mid-trimester scan is routinely done to:
- Rule out structural abnormalities

- Obtain a baseline AC for monitoring fetal growth later in pregnancy

Monitoring fetal growth

- It is well known that fetal hyperglycemia causes reactive hyperinsulinemia and that the resulting increase in insulin-like growth factor (IGF) is the chief cause of accelerated fetal growth.

- A fetal echo must be offered to all diabetics in pregnancy given the increased incidence of cardiac anomalies in fetuses of diabetic mothers.
- Since some women with GDM/DM are obese, the scan and fetal echo may be done at 20–22 weeks for better visualisation of the fetal organs.

- An ultrasound early in the third trimester is useful to identify fetal growth acceleration, as this appears to be a sign of non-optimal glycemic control. Abdominal circumference is the parameter best correlated with the nutritional state of the fetus. Insulin may be initiated at this point to prevent macrosomia (Bonomo et al., 2004).
- Amniotic fluid assessment helps identify polyhydramnios, which is commonly associated with macrosomia.
- Routine estimation of fetal weight at 36 weeks has been recommended by some (Caughey, 2019), but no method of fetal growth assessment performs well. Current methods are neither sensitive nor specific in identifying the macrosomic fetus.

The decision to deliver a baby by cesarean section based solely on an ultrasound diagnosis of macrosomia may result in unnecessary cesarean sections.

Tests to identify fetal compromise

- Three pathological processes have been implicated as causes of fetal compromise in complicated diabetic pregnancies.
  - Fetal hypoxia
  - Fetal acidemia
  - Alterations in maternal–fetal metabolism

In diabetic pregnancies without growth restriction or hypertension, surveillance with Doppler does not add value. Doppler studies are not useful in LGA babies.

- The reactive fetal hyperinsulinemia causes increased fetal oxygen consumption and decreased arterial oxygen levels, thus contributing to hypoxia.
- The tests to identify fetal compromise (NST, biophysical profile, and amniotic fluid assessment) are described in detail in **Chapter 6,** *Antepartum fetal surveillance*.

Intrapartum management

Timing of delivery

- The timing of delivery has to be balanced between prematurity and complications arising from delay. Early delivery is associated with an increase in the risk of respiratory distress syndrome, whereas prolonging the pregnancy in the presence of maternal or fetal compromise increases perinatal mortality and morbidity.
- The risks of late fetal death and macrosomia are higher in pre-gestational diabetics. With good metabolic control, the risk of fetal death near term is significantly decreased.

- A study that compared induction of labour between 38 and 39 weeks of gestation with expectant management, irrespective of whether they were insulin-dependent or not, demonstrated a reduction in cesarean delivery among women with GDM who were induced (Melamed et al., 2016).

Women with good glycemic control and no obstetric complication

- These women may be allowed to wait for spontaneous onset of labour but should not be allowed to go past 40 completed weeks.
- Labour may be induced at 40 weeks if there is no spontaneous onset of labour.
- However, Niu et al. (2014) showed that delivery of women with GDM (euglycemic on diet alone) at 38 or 39 weeks of gestation would reduce overall perinatal mortality without increasing cesarean delivery rates.

Women on insulin for glycemic control

- For women with GDM that is well-controlled by insulin, delivery is recommended at 38 weeks of gestation.
- For women with poorly-controlled GDM, the timing of delivery should take into consideration the risk–benefit ratio between prematurity and sudden stillbirth. In such a setting, delivery between 37^{+0} weeks and 38^{+6} weeks of gestation may be justified (ACOG, 2018).

Mode of delivery

Vaginal delivery

- Vaginal delivery is safe in uncomplicated diabetic pregnancies.
- Vaginal delivery may be attempted in a woman who is believed to have a fetus at an appropriate weight for gestational age.
- Macrosomia and shoulder dystocia are more common in pregnancies complicated by diabetes than they are in those not complicated by diabetes. It is good clinical practice to assess fetal growth by ultrasonography or by clinical examination late in the third trimester in an attempt to identify macrosomia among women with GDM.

Elective cesarean section

- An elective cesarean section may be indicated when there is strong suspicion of macrosomia (which may lead to shoulder dystocia) or an associated obstetric complication like severe preeclampsia.
- The evidence is insufficient to determine whether cesarean delivery should be performed to reduce the risk of birth trauma in cases of suspected macrosomia.
- It is not clear at what fetal weight the risk of shoulder dystocia increases to offset the risks of a failed induction in diabetic women. The ACOG recommends cesarean section if fetal weight is >4500 g in diabetics.
- In the Indian context, when average birth weights are lower in non-diabetic women, there is no clear cut-off for fetal weight at which an elective cesarean section or induction of

labour may be offered to minimise risk of shoulder dystocia. Taking the average weight of Indian babies, ≥3500 g can be considered to be macrosomia.

 Diabetes by itself is not an indication for elective cesarean delivery.

Glycemic control during labour and delivery

- In general, the need for insulin decreases in labour due to reduced intake and increased expenditure of calories from the physical exertion.
- It is important to maintain euglycemia during labour and delivery, although intrapartum maternal hyperglycemia leading to an adverse neonatal outcome is infrequent in GDM.
- A recent study (Hamel et al., 2019) in women with GDM undergoing vaginal delivery concluded that glucose levels may be checked every four hours, and blood sugar levels maintained between 60 mg/dL and 120 mg/dL.

Postpartum management

- Screening at 6–12 weeks postpartum (with a 75 g 2-hour OGTT) is recommended for all women with GDM. This helps to identify women with diabetes, impaired fasting glucose levels, or impaired glucose tolerance (IGT).
- Women with impaired fasting glucose, IGT, or diabetes should be referred for preventive or medical therapy.
- The ADA and ACOG recommend repeat testing every 1–3 years for women who had a pregnancy affected by GDM and normal postpartum screening test results.
- Because of the increased risk of developing diabetes, lifestyle modifications and diet are emphasised in the postpartum period and at discharge.
- In the postpartum period, the insulin requirements drop, and so the dosage of medications will need to be changed. Most women with GDM can be taken off medications and managed on diet alone. It is important to continue to maintain good glycemic control in the postpartum period.
- Breastfeeding is the preferred option for all women with GDM and pre-gestational diabetes. Along with nutritional and immunological advantages, breastfeeding has been associated with a reduction in the rates of childhood obesity in the general population.

CONTRACEPTION

- An intrauterine device is the ideal contraceptive for women who had diabetes in pregnancy.
- Low-dose combined oral contraceptive pills may be safely prescribed in women with a history of GDM (Damm et al., 2007). Formulations that contain the lowest dose of ethinyl estradiol and the lowest dose/potency progestin should be prescribed.
- In the presence of coexisting hypertension or other cardiovascular risk factors, non-estrogen-containing methods should be prescribed.

References

1. Anjana RM, Sudha V, Lakshmipriya N, Anitha C, Unnikrishnan R, Bhavadharini B et al. 2016. Physical activity patterns and gestational diabetes outcomes—the wings project. *Diabetes Res Clin Pract.* 116:253–62.

2. American Diabetes Association. 2019. Classification and Diagnosis of Diabetes: Standards of medical care in diabetes. *Diabetes Care.* 42:S13.

3. American College of Obstetricians and Gynecologists. 2018. ACOG Practice Bulletin No. 190. Gestational diabetes mellitus. *Obstet Gynecol.* 131:e49–64.

4. Bellamy L, Casas JP, Hingorani AD, Williams D. 2009. Type 2 diabetes mellitus after gestational diabetes: A systematic review and meta-analysis. *Lancet.* 373:1773–9.

5. Barrett HL, Morris J, McElduff A. 2009. Watchful waiting: A management protocol for maternal glycaemia in the peripartum period. *Aust N Z J Obstet Gynaecol.* 49:162.

6. Balsells M, García-Patterson A, Solà I et al. 2015. Glibenclamide, metformin, and insulin for the treatment of gestational diabetes: a systematic review and meta-analysis. *BMJ.* 350:h102.

7. Bonomo M, Cetin I, Pisoni MP et al. 2004. Flexible treatment of gestational diabetes modulated on ultrasound evaluation of intrauterine growth: A controlled randomized clinical trial. *Diabetes Metab.* 30:237.

8. Brown J, Alwan NA, West J, Brown S, McKinlay CJ, Farrar D et al. 2017. Lifestyle interventions for the treatment of women with gestational diabetes. *Cochrane Database Syst Rev.* Issue 5. Art. no.: CD011970.

9. Carpenter MW, Coustan DR. 1982. Criteria for screening tests for gestational diabetes. *Am J Obstet Gynecol.* 144:768.

10. Caughey AB. 2019. Gestational diabetes mellitus: Obstetric issues and management. Werner EF (Ed). *UpToDate.* Waltham, MA.

11. Crowther CA, Hiller JE, Moss JR, McPhee AJ, Jeffries WS, Robinson JS. 2005. Effect of treatment of gestational diabetes mellitus on pregnancy outcomes. Australian Carbohydrate Intolerance Study in Pregnant Women (ACHOIS) Trial Group. *N Engl J Med.* 352:2477–86.

12. Correa A, Gilboa SM, Besser LM et al. 2008. Diabetes mellitus and birth defects. *Am J Obstet Gynecol.* 199:237.e1.

13. Damm P. 2009. Future risk of diabetes in mother and child after gestational diabetes mellitus. *Int J Gynaecol Obstet.*104:S25–6.

14. Damm P, Mathiesen ER, Petersen KR, Kjos S. 2007. Contraception after gestational diabetes. *Diabetes care.* 30 (Supplement 2). S236–S241.

15. de Veciana M, Major CA, Morgan MA et al. 1995. Postprandial versus preprandial blood glucose monitoring in women with gestational diabetes mellitus requiring insulin therapy. *N Engl J Med.* 333:1237.

16. Diagnosis and management of gestational diabetes mellitus. Technical and operational guidelines. Maternal health division, MoHFW, Government of India. 2018.

17. Durnwald C. 2019. Gestational diabetes mellitus: Glycemic control and maternal prognosis. Nathan DM, Werner EF (Eds). *UpToDate.* Waltham, MA.

18. Duran A, Sáenz S, Torrejón MJ et al. 2014. Introduction of IADPSG criteria for the screening and diagnosis of gestational diabetes mellitus results in improved pregnancy outcomes at a lower cost in a large cohort of pregnant women: The St. Carlos Gestational Diabetes Study. *Diabetes Care.* 37:2442–2450.

19. Ehrenberg HM, Durnwald CP, Catalano P, Mercer BM. 2004. The influence of obesity and diabetes on the risk of cesarean delivery. *Am J Obstet Gynecol.* 191:969–74.

20. Gabbay-Benziv R, Reece EA, Wang F, Yang P. 20˙5. Birth defects in pregestational diabetes: Defect range, glycemic threshold and pathogenesis. *World J Diabetes.* 6(3):481–488.

21. Guariguata L, Linnenkamp U, Beagley J et al. 2014. Global estimates of the prevalence of hyperglycaemia in pregnancy. *Diabetes Res Clin Pract.* 103:176.

22. Government of India. 2018. Maternal and Health Division, Diagnosis and Management of Gestational Diabetes Mellitus: Technical and Operational Guidelines. Ministry of Health & Family Welfare, New Concept Information Systems. New Delhi, India.

23. Guerin A, Nisenbaum R, Ray JG. 2007. Use of maternal GHb concentration to estimate the risk of congenital anomalies in the offspring of women with pre-pregnancy diabetes. *Diabetes Care.* 30:1920–1925.

24. Hamel MS, Kanno LM, Has P et al. 2019. Intrapartum glucose management in women with gestational diabetes mellitus: A randomized controlled trial. *Obstet Gynecol.* 133:1171.

25. Hartling L, Dryden DM, Guthrie A, Muise M, Vandermeer B, Donovan L. 2013. Benefits and harms of treating gestational diabetes mellitus: A systematic review and meta-analysis for the U.S. Preventive Services Task Force and the National Institutes of Health Office of Medical Applications of Research. *Ann Intern Med.* 159:123–9.

26. Hauth JC, Clifton RG, Roberts JM et al. 2011. Maternal insulin resistance and preeclampsia. *Am J Obstet Gynecol.* 204:327.e1.

27. Jindal R, Siddiqui MA, Gupta N, Wangnoo SK. 2015. Prevalence of glucose intolerance at 6 weeks postpartum in Indian women with gestational diabetes mellitus. *Diabetes Metab Syndr.* 9:143–6.

28. Jiang YF, Chen XY, Ding T et al. 2015. Comparative efficacy and safety of OADs in management of GDM: network meta-analysis of randomized controlled trials. *J Clin Endocrinol Metab.* 100:2071–2080.

29. Jovanovic L, Knopp RH, Kim H et al. 2005. Elevated pregnancy losses at high and low extremes of maternal glucose in early normal and diabetic pregnancy: Evidence for a protective adaptation in diabetes. *Diabetes Care.* 28:1113.

30. Kjos SL, Schaefer-Graf U, Sardesi S et al. 2001. A randomized controlled trial using glycemic plus fetal ultrasound parameters versus glycemic parameters to determine insulin therapy in gestational diabetes with fasting hyperglycemia. *Diabetes Care.* 24:1904.

31. Landon MB, Spong CY, Thom E, Carpenter MW, Ramin SM, Casey B et al. 2009. A multicenter, randomized trial of treatment for mild gestational diabetes. Eunice Kennedy Shriver National Institute of Child Health and Human Development Maternal-Fetal Medicine Units Network. *N Engl J Med.* 361:1339–48.

32. Langer O, Levy J, Brustman L et al. 1989. Glycemic control in gestational diabetes mellitus–how tight is tight enough: small for gestational age versus large for gestational age? *Am J Obstet Gynecol.* 161:646.

33. Lowe WL Jr, Scholtens DM, Lowe LP et al. 2018. HAPO Follow-up Study Cooperative Research Group. Association of gestational diabetes with maternal disorders of glucose metabolism and childhood adiposity. *JAMA.* 320:1005–1016.

34. Metzger BE, Gabbe SG et al. 2010. International Association of Diabetes and Pregnancy Study Groups Consensus Panel. International association of diabetes and pregnancy study groups recommendations on the diagnosis and classification of hyperglycemia in pregnancy. *Diabetes Care.* 33:676.

35. Mithal A, Bansal B, Kalra S. 2015. Gestational diabetes in India: Science and society. *Indian J Endocr Metab.* 19:701–4.

36. Metzger BE, Lowe LP, Dyer AR, Trimble ER, Chaovarindr U, Coustan DR et al. 2008. Hyperglycemia and adverse pregnancy outcomes. HAPO Study Cooperative Research Group. *N Engl J Med*. 358:1991–2002.

37. Melamed N, Ray JG, Geary M, Bedard D, Yang C, Sprague A et al. 2016. Induction of labor before 40 weeks is associated with lower rate of cesarean delivery in women with gestational diabetes mellitus. *Am J Obstet Gynecol*. 214:364.e1–8.

38. National Institute for Health and Care Excellence. 2015. NICE Guideline NG3. Diabetes in pregnancy: Management from preconception to the postnatal period.

39. National Institute for Health and Care Excellence. 2016. NICE Quality Standard No. 109. Diabetes in pregnancy.

40. Niu B, Lee VR, Cheng YW, Frias AE, Nicholson JM, Caughey AB. 2014. What is the optimal gestational age for women with gestational diabetes type A1 to deliver? *Am J Obstet Gynecol*. 211: 418.e1–6.

41. Noctor E, Dunne FP. 2015. Type 2 diabetes after gestational diabetes: The influence of changing diagnostic criteria. *World J Diabetes*. 6(2):234–244.

42. Rosenstein MG, Cheng YW, Snowden JM, Nicholson JM, Doss AE, Caughey AB. 2012. The risk of stillbirth and infant death stratified by gestational age in women with gestational diabetes. *Am J Obstet Gynecol*. 206:309.e1–7.

43. Rowan JA, Rush EC, Plank LD et al. 2018. Metformin in Gestational Diabetes: The Offspring Follow-Up (MiG TOFU): body composition and metabolic outcomes at 7-9 years of age. *BMJ open diabetes res care*. 6:e000456

44. Sovio U, Murphy HR, Smith GC. 2016. Accelerated Fetal Growth Prior to Diagnosis of Gestational Diabetes Mellitus: A Prospective Cohort Study of Nulliparous Women. *Diabetes Care*. 39:982.

45. Sacks DA, Hadden DR, Maresh M et al. 2012. HAPO Study Cooperative Research Group. Frequency of gestational diabetes mellitus at collaborating centers based on IADPSG consensus panel-recommended criteria: The hyperglycemia and adverse pregnancy outcome (HAPO) study. *Diabetes care*. 35:526–528.

46. Seshiah V, Balaji V, Balaji MS, Paneerselvam A, Arthi T et al. 2008. Prevalence of gestational diabetes mellitus In South India – Tamil Nadu – a community-based study. *JAPI*. Vol 56. 329–333

47. Seshiah V, Das AK, Balaji V, Joshi SR. Parikh MN et al. 2006. Gestational diabetes mellitus-guidelines. *JAPI*. Vol 54. 622–28.

48. Sibai BM, Caritis SN, Hauth JC et al. 2000. Preterm delivery in women with pregestational diabetes mellitus or chronic hypertension relative to women with uncomplicated pregnancies. The National institute of Child health and Human Development Maternal-Fetal Medicine Units Network. *Am J Obstet Gynecol*. 183:1520.

49. Vandorsten JP, Dodson WC, Espeland MA et al. 2013. NIH consensus development conference: Diagnosing gestational diabetes mellitus. *NIH Consens State Sci Statements*. 29:1–31.

50. World Health Organization. 2018. WHO recommendation on the diagnosis of gestational diabetes in pregnancy. WHO, Geneva.

51. Yamamoto JM, Kellett JE, Balsells M et al. 2018. Gestational diabetes mellitus and diet: a systematic review and meta-analysis of randomized controlled trials examining the impact of modified dietary interventions on maternal glucose control and neonatal birth weight. *Diabetes Care*. 41 (7) 1346–1361.

52. Yogev, Chen, Hod et al. 2010. Hyperglycemia and Adverse Pregnancy Outcome (HAPO) study: Preeclampsia. *Am J Obstet Gynecol*. 202:255.e1.

Chapter 41

Thyroid Disorders in Pregnancy

INTRODUCTION

- Both hypothyroidism and uncontrolled thyrotoxicosis during pregnancy are associated with adverse outcomes.
- The fetal brain requires transplacental transfer of maternal thyroxine (T4) throughout pregnancy for normal neurocognitive development.

 Thyroxine (T4) is important for normal fetal brain development, especially before fetal thyroid hormone production begins, which happens at approximately 12 weeks of gestation.

PHYSIOLOGIC ADAPTATION DURING PREGNANCY

Changes in size and function

- The thyroid gland undergoes significant changes in size and function during pregnancy.
- By the third trimester, the gland increases in size by 30 per cent (Fister et al., 2009).
- Along with physical enlargement, several physiologic adaptive changes also occur.

Effect of human chorionic gonadotropin (hCG)

- Since hCG has structural homology to thyroid stimulating hormone (TSH), with a common alpha subunit and a distinctive beta subunit, it stimulates TSH receptors.
- This results in the following changes (Ross, 2021):
  - Increased thyroxine production
  - Suppression of TSH during the first trimester
  - Slight increase in TSH levels by the second trimester
  - Progressive increase in TSH levels in the third trimester
- These changes necessitate the use of **trimester-specific cut-offs** while interpreting TSH values. Thyroid tests show significant geographic and ethnic diversity in TSH concentrations during pregnancy (Alexander et al., Guidelines of the American Thyroid Association, 2017). It has been recommended that population-based trimester-specific reference ranges for serum TSH should be defined through assessment of local population data. The American Thyroid Association changed its 2011 recommendations in 2017, based on population studies from across the world.
- If population-specific data are not available, the ATA suggests 4 mIU/L as the upper limit of normal for TSH in pregnancy.

 Trimester-specific changes in TSH levels
Due to the effect of high levels of hCG, TSH levels decrease in the first trimester. In the second trimester, TSH levels return to baseline values and progressively increase in the third trimester (ACOG, 2015).

Trimester-specific cut-offs of TSH values for pregnant Indian women

- Marwaha and colleagues (2008), in a cross-sectional study, attempted to determine trimester-specific reference ranges for free triiodothyronine (FT3), free thyroxine (FT4) and TSH for healthy pregnant Indian women. They used the 5th to 95th percentile as the normal reference range for TSH, and arrived at the following values:
  - 0.6–5.0 mIU/L in the first trimester
  - 0.44–5.78 mIU/L in the second trimester
  - 0.74–5.7 mIU/L in the third trimester
- Kalra et al., (2018) in an editorial on the Indian perspective for trimester-specific TSH values, reviewed 19 Indian studies. Based on their analysis, they concluded that 4.0 mIU/L, as recommended by the ATA (Alexander et al., 2017), may be too high for pregnant Indian women, and suggested using the following values:
  - **3.0 mIU/L in the first trimester**
  - **3.5 mIU/L in the second and third trimesters**
- The Ministry of Health and Family Welfare, Government of India (2014), while formulating guidelines for screening for hypothyroidism in pregnant women, recommends the following cut-offs:
  - **2.5 mIU/L in the first trimester**
  - **3.0 mIU/L in the second and third trimesters**

Effect of estrogen on thyroid binding globulin

- Estrogen increases thyroid-binding globulin level. This results in an elevation of the total T3 and T4 levels.

 The diagnosis of thyroid dysfunction in pregnancy is based on **TSH** and **free T4** estimations.

- However, free (unbound) hormone levels are usually normal or at the upper limits of normal. Therefore, it is advisable to check **free thyroxine levels**, along with TSH, to evaluate thyroid function during pregnancy. Free T3 measurements are not generally used.

Iodine metabolism

The requirement of iodine increases from 150 μg/day to 250 μg/day during pregnancy due both to increased production by the thyroid gland to maintain euthyroid status as well as increased renal iodide clearance.

- Iodine requirement is increased during pregnancy and lactation.
- Women should be advised to consume only iodised salt during pregnancy and lactation to meet the demands of the fetus.

Placental transfer of thyroid hormones

- Maternal T4 crosses the placenta and is an important source of thyroid hormone for the fetus in the first trimester. It is particularly important for fetal brain growth before the fetal thyroid starts synthesising thyroid hormone at approximately 12 weeks of gestation.

- TSH does not cross the placenta.
- Thyroid antibodies cross the placenta and can cause fetal/neonatal hypothyroidism.

HYPOTHYROIDISM

Definition

- **Overt hypothyroidism** is defined as an elevated TSH (above the trimester-specific reference range) with decreased free T4 (below the reference range).

 There is a firm association between overt hypothyroidism in pregnancy and adverse maternal and fetal outcomes.

  – Overt hypothyroidism complicating pregnancy has been reported to be low (0.3–0.5 per cent of screened women) because hypothyroid women are anovulatory and have an increased rate of first-trimester spontaneous miscarriage (Ross, 2021). The prevalence of overt hypothyroidism is much higher in pregnant Indian women. Dhanwal et al. (2016) found a prevalence of 13.1 per cent in women from nine Indian states, with a cut-off of 4.5 mIU/L as upper limit of normal.
- **Subclinical hypothyroidism** is defined as an elevated TSH (above the trimester-specific reference range) and a normal free T4 concentration.
  – Subclinical hypothyroidism is more common than overt hypothyroidism. The incidence is higher in India, which is not an iodine-sufficient nation. Using an upper limit of 3.0 mIU/L as the cut-off, Murty et al. (2015) reported a prevalence rate of 16.1 per cent in a large South Indian population.

> **Diagnostic criteria for hypothyroidism in pregnancy**
> - **Overt hypothyroidism:**
>   – Elevated trimester-specific TSH concentration or >4 mIU/L
>   – Decreased free T4 concentration
> - **Subclinical hypothyroidism**
>   – Elevated trimester-specific serum TSH concentration or >4 mIU/L
>   – Normal free T4 concentration

Causes of hypothyroidism

- Iodine deficiency
- Autoimmune thyroiditis (Hashimoto thyroiditis), the diagnosis of which is based on elevated titres of thyroid peroxidase antibody (TPO Ab)
- Radioiodine treatment, hemithyroidectomy, exposure of the head and neck to high-dose irradiation (prior to pregnancy)

Screening for hypothyroidism

- India is not an iodine-sufficient nation. Iodine deficiency continues to exist despite the widespread use of iodine supplemented salt.

- **Universal screening for hypothyroidism is recommended** by the National Guidelines for Screening of Hypothyroidism during Pregnancy by the Maternal Health Division, Ministry of Health and Family Welfare, Government of India (2014).

Overt hypothyroidism

- Overt hypothyroidism is **hypothyroidism with clinical symptoms** that has been confirmed with blood tests for thyroid function.
- Women usually present in pregnancy with pre-existing hypothyroidism for which they are on replacement therapy.

Effects of untreated, overt hypothyroidism on pregnancy

- Studies have clearly demonstrated an association between adverse maternal and neonatal outcomes in untreated maternal hypothyroidism (LaFranchi et al., 2005; Männistö et al., 2013).
- **Maternal effects:**
  - Spontaneous miscarriage
  - Preterm delivery
  - Anemia
  - Gestational hypertension
  - Placental abruption
  - Postpartum hemorrhage
- **Effect on the fetus and neonate:**
  - Low birth weight
  - Neonatal respiratory distress
  - Perinatal death
  - Neurocognitive abnormalities (Willoughby et al., 2014)

Thyroxine is critically essential for neurological development of the fetus. Overt hypothyroidism in the mother is associated with neurocognitive abnormalities in the offspring (Willoughby et al., 2014).

Diagnosis of overt hypothyroidism

- **Symptoms:** The classic symptoms of overt hypothyroidism like tiredness and lethargy may not be present and if present, may be attributed to pregnancy itself.
- **Laboratory tests:**
  - TSH
    - An elevated serum TSH concentration, defined using population- and trimester-specific TSH reference ranges for pregnant women, is diagnostic of hypothyroidism.
    - If population- and trimester-specific TSH reference ranges are not available, then TSH >4.0 mIU/L is considered elevated.
  - **Free T4:** A decreased free T4 concentration, in the presence of elevated TSH levels, confirms hypothyroidism.
  - **Total T4:** If a trimester-specific reference range for free T4 is not provided by the lab, then a decreased total T4 is diagnostic.

TSH is the best parameter for monitoring hypothyroidism during pregnancy. The goal of therapy is to keep TSH between 0.1–2.5 mIU/L in the first half of pregnancy.

Treatment of overt hypothyroidism in pregnancy

- *Hypothyroidism diagnosed in pregnancy:* Levothyroxine is the treatment of choice for hypothyroidism in pregnancy. The recommended dose is 1–2 µg/kg body weight or approximately 50–100 µg daily to begin with (Ross, 2021).

 Levothyroxine should be taken on an empty stomach, ideally an hour before breakfast.

- *Hypothyroidism prior to pregnancy:* In a hypothyroid woman who is already on replacement therapy, the dose of levothyroxine should be increased by 25 per cent (25–50 µg) as soon as pregnancy is confirmed, and TSH levels should be monitored.
- The requirement of thyroxine increases as early as 4 weeks of pregnancy.
- Further adjustment of dosage by increments of 12.5–25 µg should aim at keeping the TSH levels within the normal range (<2.5 mIU/L in the first half of pregnancy).

Monitoring

- TSH is the best parameter to monitor therapy, and the currently recommended goal is to keep it below 2.5 mIU/L, especially during the first trimester.
- The frequency of monitoring is usually every four weeks in the first half of pregnancy and later, every two months.

 **The measurement of thyroid peroxidase antibodies (TPO)**
Currently there is no evidence to support routine testing for these antibodies (ACOG, 2015).

Postpartum follow-up

- Thyroid function may be assessed after the completion of breastfeeding.
- If the woman has a history of overt hypothyroidism prior to pregnancy, her requirements should be based on postpartum TSH values.

Subclinical hypothyroidism

Subclinical hypothyroidism (SCH) has no clinical symptoms but is diagnosed because of abnormalities in the thyroid function tests. **The TSH will be elevated, with a normal free T4**. TPO antibodies may be present or absent.

Effect of subclinical hypothyroidism on pregnancy

- The association between adverse pregnancy outcomes and SCH is not clear cut. Some authors have found an increased risk of adverse outcomes in women with SCH:
  - Spontaneous miscarriage (Negro et al., 2010)
  - Preterm birth (Schneuer et al., 2012)
  - Placental abruption (Breathnach et al., 2013)
  - Severe preeclampsia (Wilson et al., 2012)

However, Cleary-Goldman et al. (2008) failed to find a consistent pattern of adverse obstetric outcomes with subclinical hypothyroidism.

- **Cognitive impairment:** There is as yet inconclusive proof that the children of women with subclinical hypothyroidism are at risk for cognitive impairment. The Avon Longitudinal Study of Parents and Children (Nelson et al., 2018) concluded that 'maternal thyroid dysfunction in early pregnancy does not have a clinically important association with impaired child performance at school or educational achievement'. Similarly, a large study by Lazarus et al. (2012) failed to show any difference between neurocognitive development in the offspring of women who were screened and treated for subclinical hypothyroidism and those who were not.

 Current evidence does not show a direct correlation of subclinical hypothyroidism with cognitive impairment (Nelson et al., 2018; Lazarus et al., 2012).

Screening for subclinical hypothyroidism

- At present, there is no evidence that identification and treatment of subclinical hypothyroidism during pregnancy improve adverse pregnancy outcomes (ACOG, 2015).
- The Society for Maternal Fetal Medicine (2019) recommends against screening asymptomatic pregnant women for SCH.
- However, India is not an iodine-sufficient nation, and all women may not have access to iodised salt. The National Guidelines by the Government of India (2014) recommend universal screening for hypothyroidism.

Diagnosis of subclinical hypothyroidism

SCH is defined as **elevated TSH** (for the trimester) with **normal free T4** and no clinical signs or symptoms.

Treatment of subclinical hypothyroidism in pregnancy

- At present, there is contradictory evidence that identification and treatment of SCH during pregnancy improve adverse pregnancy outcomes.
  - Treatment of pregnant women with subclinical hyperthyroidism is not warranted (ACOG 2015, reaffirmed 2019).
  - However, other guidelines (Ross, 2021; De Groot et al., 2012) suggest treatment of pregnant women with subclinical hypothyroidism (with or without positive TPO antibodies).
- Levothyroxine is the treatment of choice.
- Treatment and monitoring recommendations for SCH are the same as those for overt hypothyroidism with the main goal being to normalise TSH to trimester-specific ranges.

Thyroid autoantibodies and pregnancy complications

- The thyroid antibodies are thyroid peroxidase (TPO) and thyroglobulin (Tg) thyroid autoantibodies. These are present in 2–17 per cent of unselected pregnant women. They are used to diagnose thyroid autoimmunity. Measurement of Tg antibody is not easily available.

- The presence of TPO has been associated with the following:
  - Adverse pregnancy outcomes (in the presence of SCH)
    - Fetal loss
    - Preterm delivery
    - Perinatal mortality
    - Large-for-gestational age infants
  - Developing subclinical hypothyroidism in the first trimester
  - Developing thyroiditis and hypothyroidism in the postpartum period
- Though universal screening for TPO in pregnancy is not recommended, it is useful in the following situations:
  - Subclinical hypothyroidism
  - Euthyroid women with thyroid enlargement
- Currently, treatment with levothyroxine is not recommended for euthyroid women (normal TSH) who are TPO antibody-positive.

HYPERTHYROIDISM

- Hyperthyroidism, as characterised by low TSH and elevated free T4 and/or free T3, is a relatively uncommon condition in pregnancy, occurring in 0.1–0.4 per cent of all pregnancies (Krassas et al., 2010; Lo et al., 2015).
- Pregnancy itself is an hCG-mediated mild hyperthyroid state during the first trimester of pregnancy and hence the free T3 and free T4 levels may occasionally go higher than the cut-offs.
- High serum hCG concentrations during early pregnancy may result in transient subclinical, or rarely, overt hyperthyroidism.

Definition

Overt hyperthyroidism is defined as a **decreased (<0.1 mIU/L) or undetectable (<0.01 mIU/L) TSH** value and an **increased free T4 and/or free T3** (or total T4 and/or total T3) measurement that exceeds the normal range for pregnancy.

Causes of hyperthyroidism in pregnancy

- **Autoimmune hyperthyroidism (Graves' disease)** is the most common cause of hyperthyroidism in pregnancy and occurs in 0.1–1 per cent of pregnancies (Ross, 2018). Graves' disease consists of hyperthyroidism, goiter, proptosis, and occasionally, pretibial or localised myxedema.
- **hCG-mediated hyperthyroidism** occurs because there is significant homology between the beta-subunits of hCG and TSH. As a result, hCG has weak thyroid-stimulating activity and may cause transient hyperthyroidism during the period of highest serum hCG concentrations (the first trimester).

- **Conditions that are associated with high hCG levels** may also present with thyrotoxicosis:
  - Hyperemesis gravidarum
  - Multiple pregnancy
  - Gestational trophoblastic disease
- **Toxic multinodular goitre** and **toxic adenoma** may present with hyperthyroidism.
- Other uncommon causes include drug-induced thyrotoxicosis, subacute thyroiditis, and thyroid carcinoma.

Maternal effects of hyperthyroidism

- The effect of thyrotoxicosis on pregnancy might be due to the disease itself or the anti-thyroid medications used.
- Before planning pregnancy, it is recommended that a woman with thyrotoxicosis undergo treatment until she is euthyroid. Inadequately controlled thyrotoxicosis is associated with the following:
  - Miscarriage
  - Placental abruption
  - Preterm labour
  - Preeclampsia

Fetal effects of hyperthyroidism

- Over-treatment of the mother may result in fetal hypothyroidism and goitre.
- Fetal hyperthyroidism and goitre may also be caused by transplacental transfer of TSH-stimulating antibodies. This may lead to the fetal complications listed below:
  - Growth restriction
  - Tachycardia
  - Advanced bone age, craniosynostosis
  - Hydrops
  - Intrauterine demise
  - Increase in perinatal mortality

 Overt hyperthyroidism has been implicated in adverse maternal and fetal outcomes.

Diagnosis

- **Clinical diagnosis** is difficult in pregnancy.
  - Clinical features of thyrotoxicosis like weight loss, tremors, sweating, heat intolerance, palpitation, and weakness are non-specific and may be attributed to pregnancy per se.

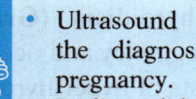
- Ultrasound has very little role in the diagnosis of thyrotoxicosis in pregnancy.
- Radionuclide scans are absolutely contraindicated in pregnancy.

  - Onset of symptoms prior to pregnancy, or persisting beyond the first trimester, diffuse goitre, significant infiltrative ophthalmopathy or dermopathy, and prior history of autoimmune problems may be a strong indicator of Graves' disease.

- **Laboratory tests**
  - TSH may be **suppressed (<0.1 mIU/L)** or **undetectable (<0.01 mIU/L)**; this confirms hyperthyroidism.
  - Free T4 and/free T3 will be **increased** above normal pregnancy levels.

Management of hyperthyroidism in pregnancy

- Women with symptomatic, *moderate to severe*, overt hyperthyroidism require treatment. Mild hyperthyroidism does not require treatment.
- The goal of therapy is to maintain mild hyperthyroidism in the mother in an attempt to prevent fetal hypothyroidism. To achieve this goal, the mother's serum free thyroxine (T4) concentration should be maintained at or just above the trimester-specific normal range for pregnancy (Ross et al., 2016).
- Thioamides are the most commonly prescribed drugs. Available thioamides include propylthiouracil (PTU), carbimazole (CBZ, which is completely metabolized to MMI), and methimazole (MMI).
- In the past, PTU was considered the drug of choice throughout pregnancy for women with hyperthyroidism. This is because of concerns about the possible teratogenic effects such as choanal atresia, tracheoesophageal fistula, and aplasia cutis with CBZ and MMI.
- However, there have been reports of severe PTU-related liver failure, though this is rare. This has led to a change in the recommendations. **Currently, PTU is used only in the first trimester and CBZ and MMI in the second and third trimesters**.
- Beta-blockers, such as metoprolol or propranolol (but not atenolol), may be required for the management of tachycardia and tremor. However, beta-blockers cannot be used for longer than two to six weeks because of concerns regarding fetal growth restriction and hypoglycemia.
- Radioiodine for ablating the thyroid gland may cause ablation of the fetal thyroid tissue, which is present by 10–12 weeks. It is therefore **absolutely contraindicated** during pregnancy.

> **Recommendations for the use of antithyroid drugs in pregnancy (Ross et al., 2016)**
> *Propylthiouracil* (PTU 50 mg 2–3 times daily)
> - **Recommended in first trimester**
> - Crosses placenta less readily than carbimazole
> - Can cause agranulocytosis and rarely hepatic failure
>
> *Carbimazole* (5–15 mg daily)
> - **Recommended in second and third trimesters**
> - Crosses placenta readily
> - Can be teratogenic (choanal atresia and aplasia cutis)
> - Can cause agranulocytosis

Monitoring of dosage

- Thyroid function tests should be performed every four weeks and more frequently immediately after switching antithyroid drugs.
- TSH and free T4 are measured and maintained within the trimester-specific range.
- Free T4 concentrations are maintained at or just above the upper limit of normal.

- Monitoring throughout pregnancy is essential because maternal hyperthyroidism in the third trimester may increase the risk of low birth weight.

 In the rare patient with a very large goitre, poor response to anti-thyroid medications and significant fetal effects, surgery may be offered in the second trimester.

Breastfeeding

- Antithyroid medications may be used safely during lactation up to a dose of 30 mg/day for carbimazole and 300 mg/day for propylthiouracil in divided doses.
- The medication should preferably be given after feeding.

POSTPARTUM THYROID DYSFUNCTION

Postpartum thyroiditis

- Postpartum thyroiditis is a destructive thyroiditis induced by an autoimmune mechanism within one year after pregnancy loss (miscarriage, induced abortion, ectopic pregnancy) or delivery.
- Approximately 5–10 per cent of women are affected by transient autoimmune thyroiditis after childbirth.
- Most women recover spontaneously. Permanent hypothyroidism may result in approximately 30 per cent of women with thyroiditis.
- The diagnosis of postpartum thyroiditis is based on clinical manifestations and thyroid function tests. The two recognised clinical phases are as follows:
  - **Phase 1:** *Hyperthyroidism (thyrotoxicosis)*, which usually begins abruptly 1–4 months after delivery
    - Associated with a small, painless goiter
    - Lasts 2–8 weeks
    - Symptoms of thyrotoxicosis may be controlled with β-blockers
  - **Phase 2:** *Hypothyroidism*, which usually begins 4–8 months after delivery
    - Lasts from about 2 weeks to 6 months
    - Associated with fatigue, constipation, or depression

Treatment

- The hyperthyroid phase is usually mild and may not require treatment.
- During the hypothyroid phase of postpartum thyroiditis, symptomatic women require treatment with thyroxine.

THYROID CANCER AND PREGNANCY

- Thyroid nodules are not an uncommon problem, especially with the routine use of ultrasonogram.
- Nodules greater than 1 cm should be subjected to FNAC (fine needle aspiration cytology). Nodules <1 cm may also need to be aspirated if they show any suspicious features sonologically like hypoechogenicity, microcalcifications, or increased vascularity.

- If the nodule is confirmed to be malignant very early in pregnancy and is rapidly growing as demonstrated clinically or by ultrasonogram, total thyroidectomy may be offered in the second trimester, followed by a suppressive dose of thyroxine.
- If detected in the second half of pregnancy, surgery may be deferred until the postpartum period as most well-differentiated thyroid cancers are slow-growing. In the latter scenario, thyroxine therapy may be started to keep the TSH low.
- Radioiodine therapy and scans are **absolutely contraindicated** in pregnancy and lactation.

 Well-differentiated thyroid cancers like papillary and follicular carcinoma are usually slow-growing. Unless rapid growth is demonstrated, surgery may be deferred till after delivery.

References

1. Alexander EK, Pearce EN, Brent GA et al. 2017. Guidelines of the American Thyroid Association for the Diagnosis and Management of Thyroid Disease During Pregnancy and the Postpartum. *Thyroid.* 27:315.

2. American College of Obstetricians and Gynecologists. 2015 (reaffirmed, 2019). ACOG Practice Bulletin No. 148. Thyroid disease in pregnancy. *Obstet Gynecol.* 125:996–1005.

3. Breathnach FM, Donnelly J, Cooley SM et al. 2013. Subclinical hypothyroidism as a risk factor for placental abruption: Evidence from a low-risk primigravid population. *Aust N Z J Obstet Gynaecol.* 53:553.

4. Cleary-Goldman J, Malone FD, Lambert-Messerlian G et al. 2008. Maternal thyroid hypofunction and pregnancy outcome. *Obstet Gynecol.* 112:85.

5. De Groot L, Abalovich M, Alexander EK et al. 2012. Management of thyroid dysfunction during pregnancy and postpartum: An Endocrine Society clinical practice guideline. *J Clin Endocrinol Metab.* 97:2543.

6. Dhanwal DK, Bajaj S, Rajput R et al. 2016. Prevalence of hypothyroidism in pregnancy: An epidemiological study from 11 cities in 9 states of India. *Indian J Endocrinol Metab.* 20(3):387–390. s

7. Fister P, Gaberscek S, Zaletel K et al. 2009. Thyroid volume changes during pregnancy and after delivery in an iodine-sufficient Republic of Slovenia. *Eur J Obstet Gynecol Reprod Biol.* 145:45–8.

8. Kalra S, Agarwal S, Aggarwal R et al. 2018. Trimester-specific thyroid-stimulating hormone: An Indian perspective. *Indian J Endocrinol Metab.* 22(1):1–4.

9. Krassas GE, Poppe K, Glinoer D. 2010. Thyroid function and human reproductive health. *Endocr Rev.* 31:702.

10. LaFranchi SH, Haddow JE, Hollowell JG. 2005. Is thyroid inadequacy during gestation a risk factor for adverse pregnancy and developmental outcomes? *Thyroid.* 15:60.

11. Lazarus JH, Bestwick JP, Channon S, Paradice R, Maina A, Rees R et al. 2012. Antenatal thyroid screening and childhood cognitive function. *N Engl J Med.* 366:493–501.

12. Lo JC, Rivkees SA, Chandra M et al. 2015. Gestational thyrotoxicosis, antithyroid drug use and neonatal outcomes within an integrated healthcare delivery system. *Thyroid.* 25:698.

13. Männistö T, Mendola P, Grewal J et al. 2013. Thyroid diseases and adverse pregnancy outcomes in a contemporary US cohort. *J Clin Endocrinol Metab.* 98:2725.

14. Marwaha R, Chopra S, Gopalakrishnan S, Sharma B, Kanwar R, Sastry A, Singh S. 2008. Establishment of reference range for thyroid hormones in normal pregnant Indian women. *BJOG.* 115: 602–606.

15. Murty NVR, Uma B, Rao JM et al. 2015. High prevalence of subclinical hypothyroidism in pregnant women in South India. *Int J Reprod Contracept Obstet Gynecol.* 4(2):453–456.

16. National Guidelines for Screening of Hypothyroidism during Pregnancy by the Maternal Health Division, Ministry of Health and Family Welfare, Government of India. 2014.

17. Negro R, Schwartz A, Gismondi R et al. 2010. Increased pregnancy loss rate in thyroid antibody negative women with TSH levels between 2.5 and 5.0 in the first trimester of pregnancy. *J Clin Endocrinol Metab.* 95:e44.

18. Nelson SM, Haig C, McConnachie A et al. 2018. Maternal thyroid function and child educational attainment: Prospective cohort study. *BMJ.* 360:k452.

19. Ross DS, Burch HB, Cooper DS et al. 2016. American Thyroid Association Guidelines for Diagnosis and Management of Hyperthyroidism and Other Causes of Thyrotoxicosis. *Thyroid.* 26:1343.

20. Ross DS. 2018. Hyperthyroidism during pregnancy: Clinical manifestations, diagnosis, and causes. Cooper DS, Lockwood CJ (Eds). *UpToDate.* Waltham, MA.

21. Ross DS. 2021. Overview of thyroid disease and pregnancy. Cooper DS, Lockwood CJ (Eds). *UpToDate.* Waltham, MA.

22. Schneuer FJ, Nassar N, Tasevski V et al. 2012. Association and predictive accuracy of high TSH serum levels in first trimester and adverse pregnancy outcomes. *J Clin Endocrinol Metab.* 97:3115.

23. Society for Maternal Fetal Medicine. 2019.

24. Willoughby KA, McAndrews MP, Rovet JF. 2014. Effects of maternal hypothyroidism on offspring hippocampus and memory. *Thyroid.* 24:576.

25. Wilson KL, Casey BM, McIntire DD et al. 2012. Subclinical thyroid disease and the incidence of hypertension in pregnancy. *Obstet Gynecol.* 119:315.

Chapter 42

Antiphospholipid Syndrome and its Impact on Pregnancy

INTRODUCTION

- Antiphospholipid syndrome (APS) is an autoimmune disorder characterised by circulating levels of antiphospholipid antibodies.
- The antiphospholipid antibodies (aPLA) are acquired antibodies against a phospholipid, and have been associated with slow, progressive thrombosis and infarction in the placenta.
- The syndrome is associated with thrombotic events and specific obstetric complications.
- Diagnosis requires that at least one clinical and one laboratory criterion be met (ACOG, 2012).
- Given that 70 per cent of individuals affected by antiphospholipid syndrome are women, it is not surprising to that APS is prevalent among women in the reproductive age group (Lockshin, 1997).

 When the antiphospholipid syndrome occurs in isolation, it is called **primary antiphospholipid syndrome**. When it occurs in association with connective tissue diseases, particularly systemic lupus erythematosus (SLE), it is called **secondary antiphospholipid syndrome**.

WHEN SHOULD ANTIPHOSPHOLIPID SYNDROME BE SUSPECTED?

Clinical suspicion for APS is raised when a woman presents with the following:
- One or more specific **adverse outcomes related to pregnancy**
  - Fetal death after 10 weeks' gestation
  - Multiple embryonic losses (<10 weeks' gestation)
  - Early-onset severe preeclampsia, fetal growth restriction, and placental insufficiency, leading to preterm birth
- Occurrence of one or more otherwise unexplained venous or arterial **thrombotic events**, especially in young women.

HOW IS ANTIPHOSPHOLIPID SYNDROME DIAGNOSED?

The diagnosis of APS is based on the revised Sapporo (or Sydney) criteria that includes both clinical and laboratory criteria (see box below). The revised criteria are an update of the classification criteria for definitive antiphospholipid syndrome by Miyakis et al., 2006. Though the Sapporo criteria are commonly accepted, they have their limitations. The adverse pregnancy outcomes that are associated with aPLA do occur commonly, and an association between these outcomes and aPLA is not always proven. A revision of these criteria is underway by an international consortium to provide more a precise interpretation of test results.

The revised Sapporo (or Sydney) criteria for the definitive diagnosis of APS
At least one of the following clinical criteria and at least one of the following laboratory criteria must be present.

- **Clinical criteria**
  - *Pregnancy morbidity*
    - Otherwise unexplained fetal death at ≥10 weeks' gestation of a morphologically normal fetus, or
    - One or more preterm births of a morphologically normal fetus before 34 weeks of gestation because of eclampsia, preeclampsia, or placental insufficiency* or
    - Three or more embryonic (<10 weeks' gestation) pregnancy losses unexplained by maternal or paternal chromosomal abnormalities or by maternal anatomic or hormonal causes
  - *Vascular thrombosis*
    - One or more clinical episodes of arterial, venous, or small vessel thrombosis in any tissue or organ
- **Laboratory criteria**
  The presence of aPLA on two or more occasions at least 12 weeks apart and no more than five years prior to clinical manifestations, as demonstrated by one or more of the following:
  - aCL IgG and/or IgM in moderate or high titer (>40 units GPL or MPL or >99th percentile for the testing laboratory)
  - Antibodies to β_2-glycoprotein I (anti-β_2GPI) of IgG or IgM isotype at a titer >99th percentile for the testing laboratory when tested according to recommended procedures
  - Lupus anticoagulant (LA) activity detected

APS, antiphospholipid syndrome; *aPLA*, antiphospholipid antibodies; *IgG*, immunoglobulin G; *IgM*, immunoglobulin M; *aCL*, anticardiolipin; *GPL*, IgG phospholipid; *MPL*, IgM phospholipid
*Features of placental insufficiency include:
1. Abnormal or non-reassuring fetal surveillance tests (e.g., non-reactive non-stress test, low score on a biophysical profile); 2. Abnormal Doppler waveform (e.g., absent or reversed end-diastolic flow in the umbilical artery); 3. Oligohydramnios (i.e., low amniotic fluid volume); 4. Birth weight <10th percentile for the gestational age (fetal growth restriction/small-for-gestational age infant)

ANTIPHOSPHOLIPID ANTIBODIES (aPLA)

An international consensus statement on the classification criteria for definitive antiphospholipid syndrome (Miyakis et al., 2006) states that only the following three antiphospholipid antibodies should be used to establish the diagnosis of APS:

- Anticardiolipin (IgG and IgM)
- Anti-β_2-glycoprotein I
- Lupus anticoagulant

 Some laboratories include other antiphospholipid antibodies (e.g., antiphosphatidylserine or anti-phosphatidylinositol) and antinuclear antibody (ANA) in their panel for aPLA screening. **These antibodies play no role in the diagnosis of APS**; testing for such antibodies is not recommended (Tebo et al., 2008; ACOG, 2012; Erkan and Ortel, 2019).

Timing of testing

- The initial testing is usually done following an adverse obstetric outcome that raises suspicion of APS (see above).
- Women who test positive for aPLA should have a repeat testing **after at least 12 weeks** to confirm the persistence of aCL, anti-β_2-GPI, or LA.

 If the clinical scenario is suggestive of APS, but the test for aPLA is negative, there is no reason to keep repeating the tests. A negative test clearly indicates that APS is not the cause of the obstetric complication.

- In India, if the cost of repeat testing after a positive test is an issue, a repeat test may be avoided if there is a high clinical suspicion and clinical diagnostic criteria are clearly met.
- However, in women in whom the clinical criteria are not sharply defined, a repeat test is mandatory. This is to avoid unnecessary treatment in the next pregnancy.

Anticardiolipin (ACL) antibodies

- Anticardiolipin antibodies are diagnosed using enzyme-linked immunosorbent assays (ELISA).
- Tests are done for both IgG and IgM ACL antibodies.
- Results are reported in international standard units, designated GPL for IgG phospholipid and MPL for IgM phospholipid.
- The result is considered positive if either serum or plasma IgG or IgM isotype are present in medium or high titre (i.e., >40 GPL or MPL or >the 99th percentile).

Anti-β_2-glycoprotein I antibodies

- Anti-β_2-glycoprotein I antibodies are most commonly detected using ELISA.
- Both IgG and IgM antibodies are measured.
- Reported in standard units known as SGU (for IgG) and SMU (for IgM), the antibodies are considered positive if they are >40 units or greater than the 99th percentile (Miyakis et al., 2006).

Lupus anticoagulant (LA)

- The term 'lupus anticoagulant' is a misnomer. The presence of LA is generally associated with a thrombotic tendency rather than an anticoagulant effect.
- The presence of lupus anticoagulant is assessed indirectly using a two-step process.

  > Lupus anticoagulant cannot be quantified. It is only reported as being *present* or *absent*.

- The initial laboratory screening test for lupus anticoagulant is **activated partial thromboplastin time (aPTT)**.
- If the aPTT is prolonged, confirmation for the presence of LA can be obtained by using the dilute Russell's viper venom time (dRVVT) or the kaolin clotting time.

> Lupus anticoagulant is a more specific but far less sensitive test than anticardiolipin (by ELISA) for the diagnosis of APS (Lockshin, 2008).

The confirmatory values for aPLA are presented in Table 42.1. The presence of any or all of the antiphospholipid antibodies confirms antipospholipid syndrome in the presence of at least one clinical criterion

Triple positivity

- The presence of all three antiphospholipid antibodies (LA, aCL, and anti-β_2-glycoprotein I antibody) is a very poor prognostic factor. Despite treatment with low-dose aspirin

Table 42.1　Confirmatory values for aPLA

Serum test	Positive for antiphospholipid syndrome
Anticardiolipin (aCL) antibody of IgG and/or IgM	>40 units of GPL or MPL or >the 99th percentile
Anti-β_2-glycoprotein-I antibody of IgG and/or IgM	>40 units of GPL or MPL or >the 99th percentile
Lupus anticoagulant (LA)	Present

and prophylactic low-molecular-weight heparin from the first trimester, only 30 per cent of women positive for all three aPL antibodies had a live birth (Saccone et al., 2017).

- In comparison, women positive for a single antibody had live birth rates ranging from 48–80 per cent, depending on the antibody.

Effect of antiphospholipid antibodies on pregnancy

- The pathogenic mechanisms by which aPL antibodies cause adverse events in APS are manifold. This leads to the varied clinical presentations in pregnant women.
- aPL antibodies are believed to cause obstetrical complications both by thrombotic and non-thrombotic mechanisms.

Thrombotic mechanisms

- Due to the thrombus-inducing actions of aPLA, thrombus formation in the uteroplacental vasculature leading to the impairment of maternal–fetal blood exchange was thought to be the main pathogenic mechanism underlying pregnancy morbidity.
- The most commonly proposed mechanisms of antiphospholipid antibody–induced thrombosis (Kutteh, 1997) include:
  - Decreased prostacyclin production by endothelial cells
  - Increased thromboxane production by platelets
  - Decreased protein C activation
- However, histological evidence of thrombosis in the uteroplacental circulation cannot be demonstrated in the majority of placentas from APS patients (Out et al., 1991).

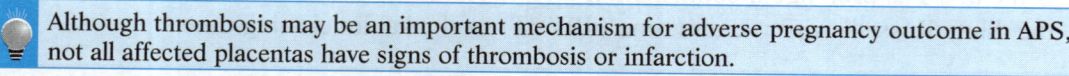

Although thrombosis may be an important mechanism for adverse pregnancy outcome in APS, not all affected placentas have signs of thrombosis or infarction.

Non-thrombotic mechanisms

- Obstetrical adverse events have been linked to a direct effect of the aPLA on the trophoblast, leading to defective placentation that is not necessarily associated with thrombotic phenomena (Abrahams et al., 2017).
- There is evidence (Di Simone et al., 2007) that aPLA has a direct effect on trophoblasts, resulting in increased:
  - Apoptosis and
  - Abnormal proliferation.

OBSTETRIC COMPLICATIONS DUE TO APS

The obstetric complications associated with the antiphospholipid antibody syndrome are:
- Fetal loss at ≥10 weeks' gestation
- Recurrent pregnancy loss (RPL)
- Hypertensive disorders (especially early-onset preeclampsia)
- Fetal growth restriction (FGR)
- Maternal thrombosis

Fetal loss

- Antiphospholipid antibodies are associated with late fetal loss (≥10 weeks' gestation) which is in contrast to pregnancy loss in women without aPLA, in whom it usually occurs before 10 weeks of gestation.
- Oshiro et al. (1996) found that 84 per cent of women with aPLA had at least one fetal death as compared to 24 per cent of women without aPLA.

 Fetal loss at ≥10 weeks' gestation occurs in 50 per cent of women with APS and only in 10 per cent in women without APS.

Recurrent pregnancy loss (RPL)

- A larger proportion of women with recurrent spontaneous pregnancy loss have a documented presence of antiphospholipid antibodies than controls (Yetman et al., 1996; Parazzini et al., 1991).
- RPL may occur both in the embryonic (<10 weeks) or in the fetal (≥10 weeks) stage.

 5–20 per cent of women with RPL will test positive for the presence of aPLA.

Preeclampsia

- There is a significant association between the development of preeclampsia and the presence of ACL antibodies and possibly, LA (Moodley et al., 1995; Sletnes et al., 1992; Robertson et al., 2006).

 Moderate-to-high levels of anticardiolipin antibodies are associated with preeclampsia, but there is insufficient evidence to use anticardiolipin antibodies as predictors of preeclampsia in clinical practice (do Prado et al., 2010).

- However, mild or near term/term preeclampsia does not appear to be strongly associated with APS.
- The association is strongest in women with severe preterm preeclampsia (onset before 34 weeks) and those who develop HELLP syndrome (hemolysis, elevated liver function enzymes, and low platelet count) (Yasuda et al., 1995; do Prado et al., 2010).

Fetal growth restriction (FGR)

- 15–30 per cent of pregnancies associated with antiphospholipid antibodies are complicated by fetal growth restriction (Caruso et al., 1993; Kutteh, 1996).

- In a prospective study, Yasuda and colleagues (1995) found that women with antiphospholipid antibodies had a significantly higher rate of FGR as compared to women without antiphospholipid antibodies.

Maternal thrombosis

- APS is associated with a significantly increased risk of pregnancy-related thromboses. Venous thromboses are more common than arterial thromboses (Lockwood and Lockshin, 2020).

 Women with APS in pregnancy must be educated regarding the signs and symptoms of thrombotic disease.

- Venous thrombosis most commonly occurs in the deep veins of the lower limbs. The most common site for arterial thrombosis is the cerebral vasculature, leading to transient ischemic attack or even stroke.
- Branch et al. (1992) found that the risk of thrombosis during pregnancy was 5 per cent among women with known APS, whereas it was 0.025–0.10 per cent in the general obstetrical population.

MANAGEMENT OF PREGNANCY WITH APS

- The aim of treatment of APS in pregnant women is to decrease maternal, fetal, and neonatal risks and to improve pregnancy outcome.
- The treatment of APS remains the same regardless of whether the syndrome is primary or secondary to SLE.
- Empson et al. (2002), in a systematic review, concluded that combination therapy with aspirin and heparin may reduce pregnancy loss in women with antiphospholipid antibodies by 54 per cent.
- Medical therapy includes the following:
  - Low-dose aspirin
  - Heparin
    - Unfractionated heparin
    - Low-molecular-weight heparin

 In a woman with **a history of a thrombotic event**, therapy is directed towards avoiding another thrombotic complication. In women with such a history, anticoagulation should be resumed after delivery and continued for six weeks postpartum.

Low-dose aspirin

- Low-dose aspirin reduces platelet aggregation and vasoconstriction by decreasing the synthesis of thromboxane A2.
- It also has a beneficial effect on implantation.
- The exact dosage of low-dose aspirin in APS has not been determined. The recommended daily dose ranges from 50–150 mg. It is commonly given as a dose of 75 mg/day as this dose is readily available in India.

- **Indications:**
  - *APS and recurrent pregnancy loss or fetal loss after >10 weeks:* Low-dose aspirin is used in combination with heparin. In a meta-analysis, Mak et al. (2010) showed that low-dose aspirin in combination with heparin is superior to aspirin alone for this indication and can increase the live birth rate to 71–84 per cent. A recent meta-analysis (Chang et al., 2019) confirmed this.
  - *APS and early-onset preeclampsia with severe features, fetal growth restriction, or other findings consistent with placental insufficiency:* In these situations, low-dose aspirin alone seems to be superior to a combination of aspirin and heparin. In a recent study, van Hoorn et al. (2016) found that in women with APS who had previously had an early delivery for preeclampsia and/or growth restriction before completing 34 weeks' gestation, aspirin treatment started before 12 weeks' gestation in a subsequent pregnancy reduced the incidence of recurrent preeclampsia. **It was also found that the addition of heparin did not improve outcome**.
- **Initiation of treatment:**
  - *RPL:* Aspirin may be started as soon as pregnancy is confirmed with a pregnancy test. Lockwood and Lockshin (2020) suggest starting low-dose aspirin when conception is being attempted.
  - *Previous hypertensive disorders, fetal growth restriction:* Aspirin may be started at the completion of 12 weeks' gestation.
- **Stopping treatment:**
  - Aspirin can be stopped any time after 36 weeks and definitely must be stopped 7–10 days before planned delivery to avoid minor perioperative bleeding.

Heparin (unfractionated or low-molecular-weight heparin)

- Both unfractionated heparin and low-molecular-weight heparin (LMWH) have been used in the treatment of obstetric adverse outcomes due to APS.
- In low-resource countries like India, unfractionated heparin is an acceptable and cheaper alternative.
- **Heparin acts by:**
  - Potentiating the antithrombin effects of antithrombin and other endogenous antithrombin effectors, increasing levels of factor Xa inhibitor, and inhibiting platelet aggregation
  - Binding to aPLAs and rendering them inactive
  - Inhibiting complement activation
  - Blocking tissue factor-mediated placental bed immunopathology
- **Indications:**
  - *APS and recurrent pregnancy loss or fetal loss after >10 weeks:* Both unfractionated and low-molecular-weight heparin have been effective when used for this indication. Ziakas et al. (2010) found a significant improvement in live birth rates in women with APS and recurrent pregnancy loss who were treated with unfractionated heparin and low-dose aspirin.

- **APS and early-onset preeclampsia with severe features, fetal growth restriction, or other findings consistent with placental insufficiency:** Heparin does not seem to have a therapeutic role for this indication.
- **Previous thrombotic event:** Women who have had an earlier thrombotic event must be started on heparin at confirmation of intrauterine pregnancy. The heparin should be continued throughout pregnancy and for six weeks postpartum (ACOG, 2012).

- **Initiation of treatment:**
  - Heparin is started after ultrasound confirmation of a viable intrauterine pregnancy.
- **Monitoring treatment:**
  - Platelet counts should be monitored since heparin-induced thrombocytopenia (HIT) may occur, and is not related to the dose of heparin. However, the incidence of HIT is very low in pregnancy (Greer and Nelson-Piercy, 2005).
  - aPTT does not need to be monitored while administering prophylactic heparin.
- **Stopping treatment:**
  - Subcutaneous LMWH or unfractionated heparin is discontinued for most patients in the following situations:
    - When spontaneous labour begins
    - 12–24 hours before planned induction of labour or cesarean delivery

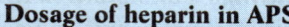

> **Dosage of heparin in APS**
> - Unfractionated heparin 5000 units subcutaneously *every 12 hours*
> - LMWH
>   - Dalteparin sodium 5000 units subcutaneously *once daily*
>   - Enoxaparin 40 mg subcutaneously *once daily*

> **Unfractionated heparin or LMWH?**
> - Most studies of heparin in pregnancy complicated by APS have used unfractionated heparin (Rosove et al., 1990; Rai et al., 1997; Kutteh, 1996). Ziakas et al. (2010) confirmed the effectiveness of unfractionated heparin when combined with aspirin.
> - Both are equally effective in reducing complications due to APS in pregnancy (Lockwood and Lockshin, 2020).
> - Unfractionated heparin is less expensive than LMWH.
> - LMWH has the advantage of once-daily dosing and lower risks of hemorrhage, thrombocytopenia, and osteoporosis.

MONITORING OF PREGNANCY

- A pregnancy complicated by APS is at high-risk and must be monitored appropriately.
- In women with a prior history of two or more fetal losses, there is a 70–80 per cent live birth rate when they are treated with some combination of the above modalities (Branch et al., 1992; Rai, 1997; Kutteh, 1996).
- However, even among women with live births, there is an increased risk of complications relating to the pregnancy, including preeclampsia, preterm birth, fetal distress. and fetal growth restriction. Careful monitoring is required to identify these complications.

Monitoring of pregnancy complicated by APS
- Weekly assessment of the mother's platelet count during the first three weeks of heparin therapy and monthly thereafter because of the risk of heparin-induced thrombocytopenia
- Frequent assessment of maternal weight, blood pressure, and urine protein to rule out preeclampsia
- Renal and liver function tests and platelet count in patients with signs or symptoms suggesting preeclampsia or HELLP syndrome
- Early sonography to establish a definitive due date followed by serial sonograms (every four to six weeks starting at 18–20 weeks' gestation) to evaluate fetal growth
- Umbilical artery Doppler flow analyses in the presence of FGR as an adjunct to fetal assessment
- Fetal heart rate and biophysical profile testing beginning at 32–34 weeks' gestation or earlier if fetal or maternal complications are diagnosed prior to 34 weeks
- Early delivery for deteriorating maternal or fetal condition

FGR, fetal growth restriction; *HELLP*, hemolysis, elevated liver function enzymes, and low platelet count

LABOUR AND DELIVERY

- In women in whom there have been no maternal or fetal complications as a consequence of APS, scheduled delivery is recommended at 38 weeks.
- In women who have maternal or fetal complications, delivery is dictated by obstetric indications.
- Heparin is stopped 12–24 hours before scheduled induction or elective cesarean section and resumed 12 hours after a cesarean and 6 hours after a vaginal birth, and continued for six weeks postpartum (ACOG, 2012).
- Epidural or spinal anesthesia is safe if unfractionated heparin has been stopped for a minimum of 24 hours or LMWH has been stopped for a minimum of 12 hours before the procedure.

References

1. Abrahams VM, Chamley LW, Salmon JE. 2017. Emerging treatment models in rheumatology: Antiphospholipid syndrome and pregnancy: Pathogenesis to Translation. *Arthritis Rheumatol.* 69:1710.

2. American College of Obstetricians and Gynecologists. 2012 (reaffirmed 2019). ACOG Practice Bulletin No. 132. Antiphospholipid syndrome. *Obstet Gynecol.*120:1514–21.

3. Branch DW, Silver RM, Blackwell JL et al. 1992. Outcome of treated pregnancies in women with antiphospholipid syndrome: An update of the Utah experience. *Obstet Gynecol.* 80:614.

4. Caruso A, De Carolis S, Ferrazzani S, Valesini G, Caforio L, Mancuso S. 1993. Pregnancy outcome in relation to uterine artery flow velocity waveforms and clinical characteristics in women with antiphospholipid syndrome. *Obstet Gynecol.* 82:970–7.

5. Chang Lu, Yong Liu, Hai-Li Jiang. 2019. Aspirin or heparin or both in the treatment of recurrent spontaneous abortion in women with antiphospholipid antibody syndrome: A meta-analysis of randomized controlled trials. *The Journal of Maternal-Fetal & Neonatal Medicine.* 32:8, 1299-1311.

6. Di Simone N, Luigi MP, Marco D et al. 2007. Pregnancies complicated with antiphospholipid syndrome: the pathogenic mechanism of antiphospholipid antibodies: A review of the literature. *Ann N Y Acad Sci.* 1108:505–514.

7. do Prado AD, Piovesan DM, Staub HL, Horta BL. 2010. Association of anticardiolipin antibodies with preeclampsia: A systematic review and meta-analysis. *Obstet Gynecol.* 116:1433.

8. Empson M, Lassere M, Craig JC, Scott JR. 2002. Recurrent pregnancy loss with antiphospholipid antibody: A systematic review of therapeutic trials. *Obstet Gynecol.* 99:135–44.

9. Erkan E, Ortel TL. 2019. Diagnosis of antiphospholipid syndrome. Pisetsky DS (Ed). *UpToDate.* Waltham, MA.

10. Greer IA, Nelson-Piercy C. 2005. Low-molecular-weight heparins for throm-boprophylaxis and treatment of venous thromboembolism in pregnancy:a systematic review of safety and efficacy. *Blood.* 106:401-7.

11. Kutteh WH. 1996. Antiphospholipid antibody-associated recurrent pregnancy loss: Treatment with heparin and low-dose aspirin is superior to low-dose aspirin alone. *Am J Obstet Gynecol.* 174:1584.

12. Kutteh WH. 1997. Antiphospholipid antibodies and reproduction. *J Reprod Immunol.* 35(2):151.

13. Lockshin MD. 1997. Antiphospholipid antibody. Babies, blood clots, biology. *JAMA.* 277: 1549–51.

14. Lockshin MD. 2008. Update on Antiphospholipid Syndrome. Bulletin of the NYU Hospital for Joint Diseases. 66(3):195-7

15. Lockwood CJ, Lockshin MD. 2020. Antiphospholipid syndrome: Pregnancy implications and management in pregnant women. Berghella V, Pisetsky DS (Eds). *UpToDate.* Waltham, MA.

16. Mak A, Cheung MW, Cheak AA, Ho RC. 2010. Combination of heparin and aspirin is superior to aspirin alone in enhancing live births in patients with recurrent pregnancy loss and positive anti-phospholipid antibodies: A meta-analysis of randomized controlled trials and meta-regression. *Rheumatology* (Oxford). 49:281.

17. Miyakis S, Lockshin MD, Atsumi T, Branch DW, Brey RL, Cervera R et al. 2006. International consensus statement on an update of the classification criteria for definite antiphospholipid syndrome (APS). *J Thromb Haemost.* 4:295–306.

18. Moodley J, Bhoola V, Duursma J, Pudifin D, Byrne S, Kenoyer DG. 1995. The association of antiphospholipid antibodies with severe early-onset pre-eclampsia. *S Afr Med J.* 85:105-7.

19. Oshiro BT, Silver RM, Scott JR et al. 1996. Antiphospholipid antibodies and fetal death. *Obstet Gynecol.* 87:489.

21. Out HJ, Kooijman CD, Bruinse HW, Derksen RH. 1991. Histopathological findings in placentae from patients with intra-uterine fetal death and anti-phospholipid antibodies. *Eur J Obstet Gynecol Reprod Biol.* 41(3):179–186.

22. Parazzini F, Acaia B, Faden D, Lovotti M, Marelli G, Cortelazzo S. 1991. Antiphospholipid antibodies and recurrent abortion. *Obstet Gynecol.* 77:854–8.

23. Rai R, Cohen H, Dave M, Regan L. 1997. Randomised controlled trial of aspirin and aspirin plus heparin in pregnant women with recurrent miscarriage associated with phospholipid antibodies (or antiphospholipid antibodies). *BMJ.* 314:253.

24. Robertson L, Wu O, Langhorne P et al. 2006. Thrombophilia in pregnancy: A systematic review. *Br J Haematol.* 132:171.

25. Rosove MH, Tabsh K, Wasserstrum N et al. 1990. Heparin therapy for pregnant women with lupus anticoagulant or anticardiolipin antibodies. *Obstet Gynecol.* 75:630.

26. Saccone G, Berghella V, Maruotti GM et al. 2017. Antiphospholipid antibody profile based obstetric outcomes of primary antiphospholipid syndrome: The PREGNANTS study. *Am J Obstet Gynecol.* 216:525.e1.

27. Sletnes KE, Wisloff F, Moe N, Dale PO. 1992. Antiphospholipid antibodies in pre-eclamptic women: relation to growth retardation and neonatal outcome. *Acta Obstet Gynecol Scand.* 71:112–7.

28. Tebo AE, Jaskowski TD, Phansalkar AR, Litwin CM, Branch DW, Hill HR. 2008. Diagnostic performance of phospholipid-specific assays for the evaluation of antiphospholipid syndrome. *Am J Clin Pathol.* 129:870–5.

29. van Hoorn ME, Hague WM, van Pampus MG et al. 2016. Low-molecular-weight heparin and aspirin in the prevention of recurrent early-onset pre-eclampsia in women with antiphospholipid antibodies: The FRUIT-RCT. *Eur J Obstet Gynecol Reprod Biol.* 197:168.

30. Yasuda M, Takakuwa K, Tokunaga A, Tanaka K. 1995. Prospective studies of the association between anticardiolipin antibody and outcome of pregnancy. *Obstet Gynecol.* 86:555.

31. Yetman DL, Kutteh WH. 1996. Antiphospholipid antibody panels and recurrent pregnancy loss: prevalence of anticardiolipin antibodies compared with other antiphospholipid antibodies. *Fertil Steril.* 66:540–6.

32. Ziakas PD, Pavlou M, Voulgarelis M. 2010. Heparin treatment in antiphospholipid syndrome with recurrent pregnancy loss: A systematic review and meta-analysis. *Obstet Gynecol.* 115:1256.

Chapter 43

Management of Rh Alloimmunisation in Pregnancy

INTRODUCTION

- Rh alloimmunisation is a condition that affects Rh-negative women when they are exposed to Rh-positive red blood cells in the following situations:
  - During a pregnancy with an Rh-positive fetus or
  - Through inadvertent transfusion of Rh-positive blood.
- An Rh-negative mother mounts an immune response when exposed to a blood group factor (red cell antigen) inherited from the father that is not present in her blood. The immune response results in the production of immunoglobulin G (IgG) antibodies. This is called *red cell alloimmunisation*.
- The IgG antibodies cross the placenta and attack the fetal red blood cells (RBCs) that are positive for these surface antigens, resulting in hemolytic disease of the fetus and newborn (HDFN). Therefore, Rh-positive fetuses/infants born to Rh-negative mothers are at risk and may face serious morbidity or mortality.
- Prior to the availability of anti-D immunoglobulin, the outcome for the fetus/neonate was uniformly poor. However, the prognosis is markedly improved when Rh-negative mothers routinely receive the immunoglobulin after the birth of an Rh-positive baby.
- However, hemolytic disease of the fetus and newborn due to maternal RhD alloimmunisation continues to occur worldwide, especially in low-income countries like India.
- Over the past three decades, advances in maternal–fetal medicine have enabled therapeutic options that can successfully treat this condition.

Causes of Rh alloimmunisation
- Transplacental fetal-to-maternal hemorrhage is the most common cause of alloimmunisation.
- Inadvertent transfusion with Rh-positive blood is the second most common cause.

RH BLOOD GROUP SYSTEM AND NOMENCLATURE

- The pregnant mother's blood group is identified using the ABO blood type and the presence ('positive') or absence ('negative') of the Rh antigen.

It is the presence or absence of RhD that defines a person as being Rh-positive (antigen present) or negative (antigen absent).

- The Rh system is known to be one of the most complex blood group systems, with over 50 different Rh antigens identified. Most of these are too rare to be of clinical relevance, but a few are immunologically and genetically significant.

- The nomenclature of the Rh (CDE) system is complicated and can be confusing.
- The Rh antigens are collectively called the 'Rhesus factor' and comprise five antigens—C, c, D, E and e. **No 'd' antigen has been identified and so 'd' indicates the absence of the D antigen**. The most immunogenic of these is D followed by c, E, e, and C.

Inheritance of the Rh factor

- The Rhesus antigens are encoded by three sets of allelomorphic genes—Dd, Cc, and Ee—in all humans. Every individual inherits one of each set (three each) from each parent, following Mendelian laws.
- If at least one D antigen is present, the individual becomes Rh-positive (Table 43.1). If D is inherited from only one parent, the individual is Rh-positive heterozygous (e.g., Cde/cDe). On the other hand, if D is inherited from both parents, the individual is Rh-positive homozygous (e.g., cDe/CDe).
- 60 per cent of Rh-positive individuals are heterozygous while approximately 40 per cent are homozygous. If d is inherited from both parents, the individual becomes Rh-negative (cde/cdE). Rh-negative individuals are always homozygous.
- If the woman is Rh-negative and her partner is a homozygous Rh-positive, she will have an Rh-positive baby. If, on the other hand, the partner is heterozygous, she has equal chances of having an Rh-positive or an Rh-negative child. An Rh-negative mother who has conceived with an Rh-negative partner cannot have an Rh-positive child (Table 43.2).

> Approximately 40 per cent of Rh-positive individuals are homozygous. 100 per cent of Rh-negative individuals are homozygous (cde/cdE).

OTHER MINOR ANTIBODIES

- Other than D, the most frequently encountered antibodies are Lewis antibodies (Le^a and Le^b) and I antibodies. However, these are not implicated in hemolytic disease of the fetus and newborn (HDFN).

Table 43.1 Inheritance patterns of the Rh factor

Sets of allelomorphic genes	How many inherited	Rh-positive: Homozygous (40% of Rh-positive population)	Rh-positive: Heterozygous (60% of Rh-positive population)	Rh-negative: Always homozygous
D (d), Cc, Ee	1 of each set (e.g., CDe or cDe)	DD	D (d)	dd

Table 43.2 Chances of Rh-negative mother having an Rh-positive fetus

	Father homozygous Rh-positive (DD)	Father heterozygous Rh-positive (Dd)	Father Rh-negative (dd)
Chance of baby being Rh-positive	100%	• 50% Dd: Rh-positive • 50% dd: Rh-negative	0%

- **Kell antibodies** (anti-K) can produce HDFN. Kell alloimmunisation is frequently caused by prior transfusion in cases where Kell compatibility was not checked for when the blood was cross-matched.
- **Anti-c** and **anti-E** antibodies can also cause hemolytic disease. Women with sensitisation to antigens other than D that are known to cause hemolytic disease are uncommon and are managed in the same way as women with D alloimmunisation.

INCIDENCE OF RH-NEGATIVE INDIVIDUALS

- The incidence of Rh-negative individuals varies by race, with a low of 0.3 per cent in the Chinese and Japanese to a high of 30–35 per cent in the Basques (Spain), in whom the mutation likely originated. In Caucasians, the incidence of the Rh-negative genotype is 15 per cent.
- In India, the incidence has been reported to vary between approximately 4 per cent in Kashmir (Latoo et al., 2006) and 10 per cent in Lucknow (Chandra and Gupta, 2012). Other studies from other parts of the country have shown prevalence rates between 4 and 10 per cent (Giri et al., 2011; Koram et al., 2014; Patel et al., 2012).

CAUSES OF RH ALLOIMMUNISATION IN PREGNANCY

- Rh alloimmunisation occurs as a result of exposure of the maternal immune system to Rh-positive RBCs. In pregnancy, this occurs in response to the fetal Rh antigen when a sufficient number of fetal RBCs gain access to the maternal circulation.

 Rh alloimmunisation does not occur if the partner is also Rh-negative, or if the fetus is Rh-negative.

- Just as the incidence of Rh-negative individuals varies with race, the incidence of alloimmunisation also varies greatly among populations.
- The overall incidence of alloimmunisation has declined dramatically since the late 1990s owing in part to immunoprophylaxis with anti-D immunoglobulin and couples opting for smaller families. From 12–13 per cent earlier, the overall incidence of Rh alloimmunisation has reduced to about 1–2 per cent worldwide.

 A study from New Delhi reported the incidence of alloimmunisation in their population to be 1.25 per cent (Pahuja et al., 2011).

Fetomaternal hemorrhage (FMH)

- Fetal RBCs may gain access to the maternal circulation any time during pregnancy, delivery, or in the immediate postpartum period. Using the sensitive Kleihauer-Betke acid elution test, Bowman and colleagues (1986) found 0.01 mL of fetal cells in 3 per cent, 12 per cent, and 46 per cent of women respectively, in each of the three successive trimesters (Table 43.3).
- In the majority of cases, FMH sufficient to incite alloimmunisation occurs only at the time of delivery. FMH occurs in as many as 75 per cent of women during delivery.

- The risk of sensitisation increases with the volume of fetal blood that crosses over into the maternal circulation (Table 43.4). Hemorrhage volumes sufficient to cause alloimmunisation are produced in 15–50 per cent of births. However, <1 per cent of women will have FMH of >15 mL. This is an important fact since the usual dose of anti-D immunoglobulin (see section on *Prophylactic anti-D immunoglobulin*) will cover 15 mL of fetal blood. Fetomaternal hemorrhage of 15 mL is usually not predictable but can occur in severe placental abruption, manual removal of placenta and rarely, instrumental delivery.

 During delivery, 99 per cent of women will have FMH of ≤3 mL. Less than 1 per cent of women will have FMH of >15 mL.

The causes of fetomaternal hemorrhage that may result in Rh alloimmunisation are listed in Table 43.5.

- Antibody response to FMH varies considerably in individuals and depends on the following factors:
  - Gestational age
  - Volume of hemorrhage
  - Antigenicity of fetal RBCs
  - Maternal capacity for immunogenic response
  - ABO incompatibility (protects against primary Rh immune response)

Table 43.3 Increasing risk of fetomaternal hemorrhage (FMH) with advancing pregnancy (Bowman et al., 1986)

Trimester	Risk of spontaneous FMH (%)
First	3%
Second	12%
Third	46%

Table 43.4 Volume of fetomaternal hemorrhage (FMH) and risk of sensitisation

Volume of FMH	Risk of sensitisation
0.1 mL	3%
0.2–1 mL	25%
>5 mL	65%

Table 43.5 Conditions in which transplacental leakage of blood may occur that may result in Rh alloimmunisation

Fetomaternal hemorrhage	Early pregnancy loss	Obstetric procedures
• Intrapartum – Uncomplicated vaginal delivery – Cesarean delivery • Antepartum – Multifetal gestation – Bleeding placenta previa or abruption – Abdominal trauma	• Miscarriage • Elective abortion • Ectopic pregnancy >7 weeks • Molar pregnancy	• External cephalic version • Manual removal of the placenta • Intrauterine manipulation • Amniocentesis • Chorionic villus sampling (CVS) • Fetal blood sampling (FBS)

PATHOGENESIS OF RH ALLOIMMUNISATION

- In an Rh-negative mother, if the fetal RBCs that enter the maternal circulation are Rh-positive, an alloimmune response may be stimulated against the fetal Rh antigen, which is paternally derived.

- A similar response may occur in response to non-self antigens if the mother has been inadvertently transfused with Rh-positive blood in her lifetime.
- Once sensitised, future pregnancies may be at risk for HDFN.

Natural progression of red cell alloimmunisation

In an Rh-negative mother, if the fetal RBCs that enter the maternal circulation are Rh-positive, an alloimmune response may be stimulated against the fetal Rh antigen, which is paternally derived. When this happens, the mother is said to be sensitised.

The first pregnancy

- The first pregnancy is referred to as the **primary sensitising pregnancy.**
- The primary immune response to the D antigen may occur over 6 weeks to 12 months (average of 12–16 weeks). It is usually weak, consisting predominantly of immunoglobulin M (IgM) that does not cross the placenta. This, combined with the fact that most of the significant FMH occurs during delivery, ensures that the first pregnancy is not typically at great risk.
- IgG antibodies are also formed but are not seen until at least six months from the time of sensitisation.
- Exceptions to this are as follows:
  - A woman who has developed antibodies following a blood transfusion and is pregnant for the first time
  - An Rh-negative woman whose mother was Rh-positive, as a result of which, she was exposed to maternal Rh antigens in utero—this is known as the *grandmother theory*

The second and subsequent pregnancies

- **Subsequent pregnancies are considered sensitised pregnancies.** A second antigen challenge (as in her next pregnancy with an Rh-positive fetus) generates an amnestic response from the previously primed red blood cells. Such a response is both rapid and almost exclusively immunoglobulin G (IgG). IgG crosses the placenta, destroys the fetal RhD-positive red cells and causes the following complications:
  - Fetal anemia
  - Hydrops in the fetus/newborn
  - Hyperbilirubinemia in the newborn
- After the delivery of the first Rh-positive baby, antibodies can be detected in up to 8 per cent of mothers at six months postpartum.
- By the end of the second Rh-positive pregnancy, in the absence of anti-D prophylaxis, 17 per cent of the mothers will have detectable antibodies.

MANAGEMENT OF THE RH-NEGATIVE MOTHER IN PREGNANCY

- On the first prenatal visit, all pregnant women should be tested for ABO blood group and RhD type. If the woman is Rh-negative and her husband/partner is Rh-positive, she should be tested for the presence of Rh antibodies.

- Further management of the Rh-negative mother depends on whether she has established alloimmunisation or not. If antibodies are not present at the first antenatal visit, they are checked again serially.
- The presence of anti-D antibodies in the maternal serum is diagnostic of maternal alloimmunisation. After the first alloimmunised pregnancy:
  - The fetal hemolytic disease will be more severe in each subsequent pregnancy with an Rh-positive fetus due to repeated maternal antibody production with each pregnancy.
  - Severe anemia will occur earlier in gestation than in the prior pregnancy.

Rh-negative mother with no alloimmunisation (antibodies absent)

The steps for managing an Rh-negative mother in her first pregnancy are as follows:
- Establishment of husband/partner's blood group and Rh type
- Screening for the presence of Rh antibodies initially and serially using indirect Coombs test (ICT), currently also known as indirect antiglobulin test (IAT)
- Prevention of Rh alloimmunisation in subsequent pregnancies

Establishment of husband/partner's blood group and Rh type

- **If the father is Rh-negative**, the fetus will also be Rh-negative. No further screening or management is indicated.
- **If the father is Rh-positive**, the fetus may or may not be Rh-positive, depending on the zygosity of the father.
  - If the father is homozygous (DD), the fetus will be Rh-positive.
  - If the father is heterozygous (Dd), the fetus has a 50 per cent chance of being Rh-positive.
- **Zygosity testing** of the father is recommended in Western guidelines (Moise, 2019). However, these tests are not available and not feasible in India (Agarwal et al., 2014).
- **Cell-free DNA testing for fetal Rh type** is possible using maternal blood. This test is available freely in the UK, Europe, and the USA (Moise, 2019). However, it is neither available nor affordable in India.

 Paternal zygosity testing is not available in India, neither is cell-free DNA testing for fetal Rh type (as of 2021).

Screening for the presence of Rh antibodies initially and serially

Indirect Coombs test (indirect antiglobulin test)

- The **indirect Coombs test** (ICT), currently called indirect antiglobulin test (IAT), is the most accurate test used to detect antibody titres in maternal serum.
- It should be offered to **every Rh-negative woman in each pregnancy**, even if she has received RhD immunoglobulin in a previous pregnancy (ACOG, 2018).
- ICT detects antibodies against RBCs that are present unbound in the mother's serum.
- Once the presence of anti-D antibodies has been established in the mother by ICT, the concentration of these antibodies has to be estimated by a titration procedure. Titre values

are reported as the integer of the greatest tube dilution with a positive agglutination reaction, for example, 1:8, 1:16, and 1:32.

- In most first sensitised pregnancies, the concentration of antibodies is very low and can be detected only in undiluted serum or after enzyme pre-treatment.
- If the ICT value is ≤1:8, serial titres are performed, typically every four weeks until 28 weeks' gestation and every two weeks thereafter (Moise, 2008).
- If the titre continues to be stable, the woman can be delivered at term. The blood group and Rh type of the newborn should be documented soon after birth.

 There is no direct relationship between the antibody titre and the severity of disease.

Critical titre

- Titres may continue to rise till a **critical titre** is reached. This is defined as the titre associated with a significant risk for fetal hydrops. These values vary between laboratories, as does the critical titre level associated with hydrops. Therefore, the same laboratory should be used when repeat titres are done. For most centres, critical titre values vary between 1:16 and 1:32 (Moise, 2019).
- When ICT is repeated, a change of more than one dilution is significant (ACOG, 2018).

Frequency of screening for Rh antibodies
In the first pregnancy
- At first booking
- At 20 weeks
- At 28 weeks
In subsequent pregnancies
- Previous pregnancy with no or mild hemolytic disease
  - At first booking
  - Every 4–6 weeks subsequently
- Previous pregnancy with severe hemolytic disease
  - Titre not required
  - Testing for fetal anemia beginning from 16–18 weeks

Prevention of Rh alloimmunisation in subsequent pregnancies

- Anti-D prophylaxis should be offered to all Rh-negative women after the delivery of the first Rh-positive infant if the ICT showed no antibodies (see section on *Prophylactic anti-D immunoglobulin*).
- There is robust evidence over many decades that administering anti-D immunoglobulin to Rh-negative women within 72 hours of giving birth to an Rh-positive baby is an effective way of preventing RhD alloimmunisation and HDFN (Crowther and Middleton, 1997).

 Administration of anti-D immunoglobulin to a sensitised woman will not prevent a rise in antibody titre and should be avoided.

Alloimmunised mother (antibodies present)

- If the previous baby was only mildly affected and antibody titres are below the critical titre, serial screening with ICT is recommended once in 3–4 weeks till 28 weeks and more frequently thereafter.
  - If the titres remain low, she may be delivered at term.
  - If the titers rise, management is as described below.
- The steps for managing an Rh-negative mother with rising antibody titres, established presence of Rh antibodies (above the critical titre), and/or previous severely affected baby are as follows:
  - Screening for fetal anemia using middle cerebral artery peak systolic velocity (MCA-PSV)
  - Management of fetal anemia, if present
  - Delivery and follow-up

Screening for fetal anemia using middle cerebral artery peak systolic velocity (MCA-PSV)

- Once it has been established that a woman has a critical antibody titre in a pregnancy, there is no necessity to repeat the antibody titre serially or in subsequent pregnancies.
- In the past, amniocentesis (for plotting Liley's curve) and direct fetal blood sampling were used to determine the extent of fetal hemolytic disease due to Rh alloimmunisation.
- In 2000, Mari et al. revolutionised the management of the alloimmunised pregnancy by introducing the non-invasive diagnosis of fetal anemia using Doppler measurement of the middle cerebral artery peak systolic velocity (MCA-PSV). This is based on the fact that hemolysis of fetal RBCs caused by Rh antibodies results in fetal anemia.
- Under physiologic circumstances, fetal hemoglobin, and not fetal oxygenation, is the primary determinant of the middle cerebral artery peak systolic velocity (Picklesimer et al., 2007).
- Consequently, MCA-PSV increases as the fetal hemoglobin level falls (Figure 43.1).

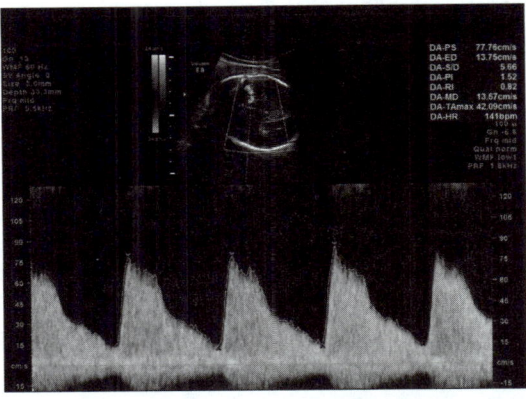

Figure 43.1   Doppler wave-form of the middle cerebral artery showing increased peak systolic velocity (MCA-PSV) (*Image courtesy:* Mediscan Systems, Chennai).

The proper technique for MCA-PSV evaluation includes assessment of the middle cerebral artery close to its origin, ideally at a zero degree angle without angle correction (SMFM, 2015).

Initiation of MCA-PSV screening

- When clinically indicated, MCA-PSV is performed at ≥20 weeks in the first affected pregnancy.
- In a woman whose previous pregnancy was complicated by severe hemolytic disease of the fetus, the screening with MCA-PSV should begin at 16 weeks.

 MCA-PSV values are best obtained when the fetus is in a quiet behavioural state. Results may be inaccurate when the fetus is active.

Interval between MCA-PSV testing

- The optimal interval between MCA-PSV testing has not been determined.
- However, it is usually repeated at 1–2 week intervals, depending on the degree of anemia detected and the natural progression of disease (Mari et al., 2000).

Interpretation of MCA-PSV values

- Conversion calculators are used to convert the actual MCA-PSV in cm/sec to multiple of medians (MoMs) to correct for gestational age. An online calculator is available at *www.perinatology.com.*
- The risk of anemia is high in fetuses with a peak systolic velocity of ≥1.50 times the median (MoM). Fetuses with values <1.50 MoM may not have anemia or will have only mild anemia.
- The sensitivity of the MCA-PSV for the prediction of moderate and severe anemia in fetuses without hydrops is 100 per cent, with a false positive rate of 12 per cent (Mari et al., 2000).

Other ultrasound parameters for identifying fetal anemia
- The first manifestation of hydrops secondary to fetal anemia is always ascites, followed by placental thickening (Figure 43.2) and hepatomegaly. Associated pleural or pericardial effusions are uncommon but may be present (Abbasi et al., 2017).
- When hydrops develops, it indicates severe anemia. However, the severity of anemia can only be assessed by direct fetal sampling.

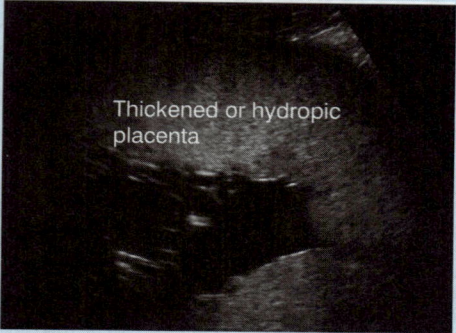

Thickened or hydropic placenta

Figure 43.2   Increased placental thickness in an alloimmunised fetus (*Image courtesy:* Mediscan Systems, Chennai).

Management of fetal anemia

- If the MCA-PSV value is >1.5 MoM, the risk of moderate to severe anemia is high, and anemia must be confirmed with an invasive procedure.
- A fetal blood sampling is performed, and fetal anemia is confirmed by assessing hemoglobin and hematocrit.
- The fetal hemoglobin and hematocrit values are compared to nomograms for the gestational age.
- If the fetal Hb is not lower than two standard deviations (SD) below the mean for that gestational age, or if the hematocrit is ≥30 per cent, the fetus is followed-up with a repeat blood sampling after 1–2 weeks.

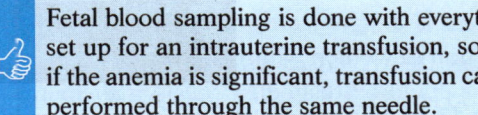 Fetal blood sampling is done with everything set up for an intrauterine transfusion, so that if the anemia is significant, transfusion can be performed through the same needle.

- If the fetal Hgb is lower than two standard deviations (SD) below the mean for that gestational age, or if the hematocrit is <30 per cent, the fetus requires serial intrauterine transfusions.

Intrauterine transfusions (IUT) of red cells

- Intrauterine transfusion of RBCs is indicated to prevent fetal death from severe anemia and is the only available therapeutic option in severe RhD alloimmunisation.
- Pregnancies with severe fetal anemia between 18 and 35 weeks of gestation are optimally suited for IUT (Moise, 2019a).
- If the gestational age is ≥35 weeks, delivery can be considered, since the risks of IUT outweigh the risk of preterm

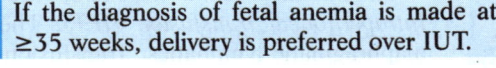 If the diagnosis of fetal anemia is made at ≥35 weeks, delivery is preferred over IUT.

birth. The postnatal management of the baby must be planned with a neonatal team.
- **Blood used for IUT**
  - Type O RhD-negative donor blood is used.
  - It is cross-matched with the mother's blood.
  - Units are washed and packed to a final hematocrit of 75–85 per cent to reduce the volume administered to the fetus.

Procedure

- IUT is performed under aseptic precautions in an operating theatre so that an emergency cesarean section can be performed if the need arises.
- The mother may be given mild intravenous sedation.
- The IUT is usually performed by accessing the fetal umbilical vein.

The umbilical vein may be accessed at the placental end of the cord insertion or at the intrahepatic portion of the umbilical vein (Figure 43.3).

- An initial sample of fetal blood is tested for a complete blood count and reticulocyte count.
- Packed RBCs are administered through the same needle to achieve a final fetal hematocrit of 35–40 per cent before 24 weeks and 40–50 per cent after 24 weeks.

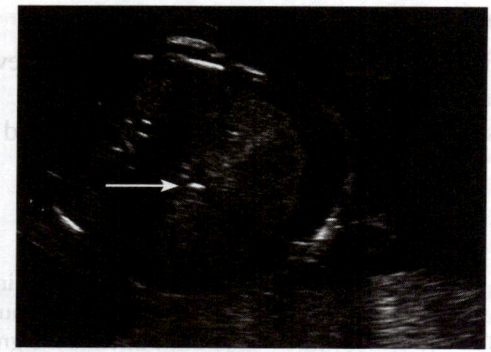

Figure 43.3 Intravascular intrauterine transfusion in a hydropic fetus; the needle tip (arrow) is seen in the intrahepatic portion of the umbilical vein.

- An additional intraperitoneal transfusion (IPT) may be done to delay the drop in hematocrit between procedures. The intraperitoneal reservoir of blood is absorbed more slowly.
- After the transfusion is completed, a second sample of fetal blood is obtained to confirm that the planned hematocrit level has been achieved.

> **Sites of transfusion**
> - *Intravascular transfusion (IVT):* This is much more effective than intraperitoneal transfusion, particularly in hydropic fetuses. The two sites used for direct vascular access are as follows:
>   – The intrahepatic portion of the umbilical vein (Figure 43.3)
>   – The umbilical vein at the site of cord insertion into the placenta
> - *Intraperitoneal transfusion (IPT):* The transfused blood cells are absorbed through the diaphragmatic lymphatics. Transfusion into the peritoneal cavity is not effective in fetuses with severe anemia and hydrops.
> - *Combined IPT and IVT:* The combined direct intravascular/intraperitoneal approach produces a stable hematocrit between procedures and offers the possibility of performing intrauterine transfusions at less frequent intervals (Moise, 2019a).

- *Calculating the transfusion volume*
  – There are charts and formulas available to calculate the volume of blood to be transfused.
  – The volume of blood required for IUT depends upon the following:
    ◆ The initial fetal hematocrit
    ◆ The hematocrit of the transfused RBCs
    ◆ The target hematocrit
- *Subsequent transfusions*
  – The subsequent transfusions are based on the predicted decline in fetal hematocrit between procedures.
  – The second transfusion is usually after 7–10 days. The subsequent transfusions are done at greater intervals for the following reasons:
    ◆ The circulating blood in the fetus is Rh-negative and cannot be hemolysed
    ◆ Fetal hematopoiesis is suppressed
  – No further IUTs are performed after 35 weeks.

The management of the Rh-negative mother in pregnancy is summarised in Figure 43.4.

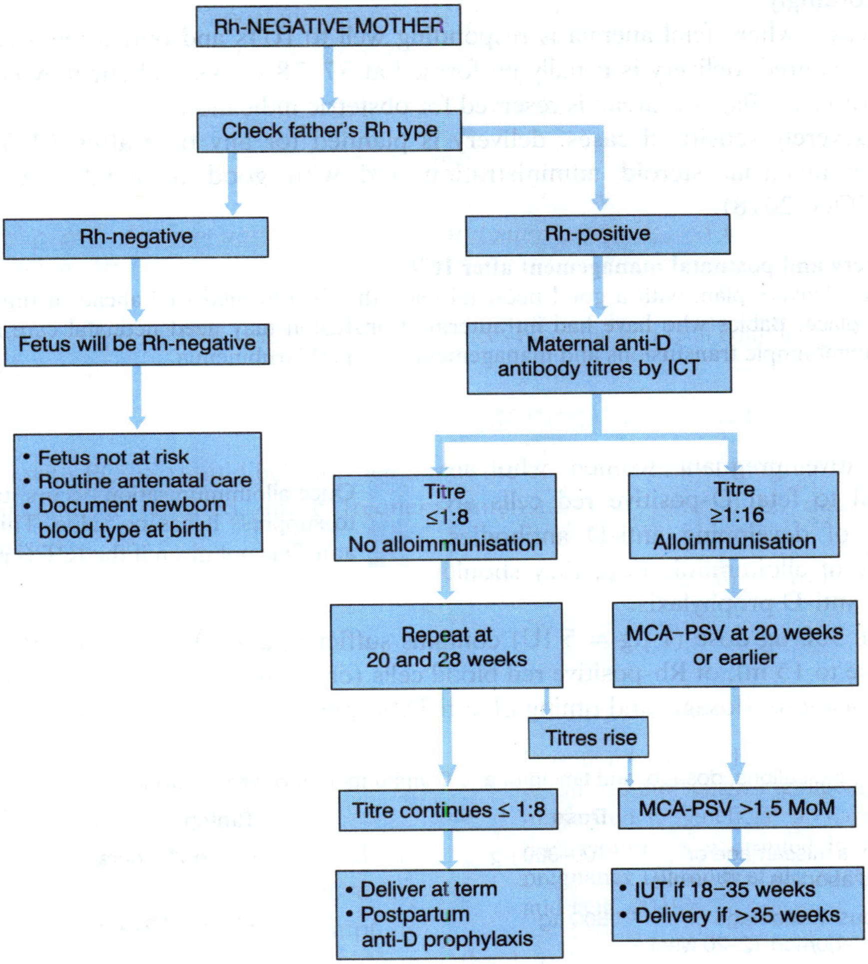

```
                    ┌─────────────────────┐
                    │  Rh-NEGATIVE MOTHER │
                    └─────────────────────┘
                               │
                    ┌─────────────────────┐
                    │ Check father's Rh type │
                    └─────────────────────┘
                      │                   │
            ┌──────────────┐       ┌──────────────┐
            │  Rh-negative │       │  Rh-positive │
            └──────────────┘       └──────────────┘
                   │                       │
        ┌─────────────────────┐   ┌─────────────────────┐
        │ Fetus will be Rh-negative │   │   Maternal anti-D   │
        └─────────────────────┘   │ antibody titres by ICT │
                   │               └─────────────────────┘
        ┌─────────────────────┐         │           │
        │ • Fetus not at risk │   ┌──────────┐ ┌──────────┐
        │ • Routine antenatal │   │  Titre   │ │  Titre   │
        │   care              │   │   ≤1:8   │ │  ≥1:16   │
        │ • Document newborn  │   │No alloim-│ │ Alloim-  │
        │   blood type at birth│  │munisation│ │munisation│
        └─────────────────────┘   └──────────┘ └──────────┘
                                        │           │
                                 ┌──────────┐ ┌─────────────┐
                                 │ Repeat at│ │MCA–PSV at 20│
                                 │20 and 28 │ │weeks or     │
                                 │  weeks   │ │earlier      │
                                 └──────────┘ └─────────────┘
                                        │           │
                                  ┌───────────┐     │
                                  │Titres rise│     │
                                  └───────────┘     │
                                        │           │
                              ┌──────────────┐ ┌─────────────┐
                              │Titre continues│ │MCA-PSV >1.5 │
                              │   ≤ 1:8      │ │    MoM      │
                              └──────────────┘ └─────────────┘
                                        │           │
                              ┌──────────────┐ ┌─────────────┐
                              │• Deliver at  │ │• IUT if 18–35│
                              │  term        │ │  weeks      │
                              │• Postpartum  │ │• Delivery if │
                              │  anti-D      │ │  >35 weeks  │
                              │  prophylaxis │ │             │
                              └──────────────┘ └─────────────┘
```

Figure 43.4   Algorithm for the management of Rh-negative women with and without Rh alloimmunisation; the critical titre level varies with laboratories and the value used should be standardised for the institution. (*ICT*, indirect Coombs test; *IUT*, intrauterine transfusion; *MCA-PSV*, middle cerebral artery peak systolic velocity)

 The overall survival after IUT can be as high as 95 per cent (Zwiers et al., 2018). The survival rate drops if severe anemia develops at <20 weeks' gestation.

Delivery and follow-up

- Delivery of the infant of an alloimmunised mother depends on several factors.
  - Treatment is usually prolonged until the fetus reaches a gestational age at which survival is ensured.
  - The maternal-fetal medicine specialist usually balances the risk of repeated invasive procedures against preterm birth.

- It is acceptable to time the last transfusion between 32 and 35 weeks and deliver accordingly.
- In cases where fetal anemia is responding well to IUTs and only a few transfusions are required, delivery is usually performed at 37–38 weeks. Labour may be induced (Moise, 2019a). Cesarean is reserved for obstetric indications.
- In severely sensitised cases, delivery is planned for any time after 32–34 weeks, after maternal steroid administration and with good neonatal care available (ACOG, 2018).

> **Delivery and postnatal management after IUT**
> A clear delivery plan, with a good neonatal team that is informed well ahead of time, should be in place. Babies who have had intrauterine transfusion may need neonatal care including exchange/simple transfusions and management of hyperbilirubinemia.

PROPHYLACTIC ANTI-D IMMUNOGLOBULIN

- Rh-negative pregnant women who are exposed to fetal D-positive red cells are at risk of developing anti-D antibodies. To prevent alloimmunisation, they should receive anti-D prophylaxis.

> Once alloimmunisation occurs, treatment to suppress it has no value. This is why anti-D is not given if the ICT is positive.

- A single 300 µg dose (1 µg = 5 IU) contains sufficient anti-D to suppress the immune response to 15 mL of Rh-positive red blood cells (or 30 mL Rh-positive whole blood).
- The indications, dosage, and timing of anti-D prophylaxis are presented in Table 43.6.

Table 43.6 Indications, dosage, and timing of anti-D immunoglobulin prophylaxis

Indication	Dose	Timing
Spontaneous miscarriage or therapeutic abortion <12 weeks	100–300 µg	Within 72 hours
Spontaneous miscarriage or therapeutic abortion 12–20 weeks	300 µg	Within 72 hours
Ectopic pregnancy	100–300 µg	Within 72 hours
Molar pregnancy	300 µg	Within 72 hours
Repeated, heavy bleeding in pregnancy <20 weeks	300 µg	At 6 weeks intervals, if bleeding persists
Intrauterine fetal death	300 µg	Within 72 hours of diagnosis, irrespective of the time of delivery
Invasive prenatal diagnostic or therapeutic procedures	300 µg	Within 72 hours
Postpartum	300 µg	• Within 72 hours • If inadvertently missed, it should be given as soon as possible
Postpartum, with sterilisation	Anti-D may be avoided, especially when cost is a concern	

- Postnatal administration of 300 μg of anti-D should be given to all Rh-negative non-sensitised women within 72 hours of delivery.
- If anti-D is not given within 72 hours of delivery or another potentially sensitising event, anti-D should be given as soon as the need is recognised for up to 28 days after delivery or another potentially sensitising event.
- If a woman has no plans to have children in the future and has undergone postpartum sterilisation, anti–D immunoglobulin may be avoided, especially when cost is a concern. This must be discussed with the couple.

Ensuring adequate dose of anti-D immunoglobulin

- 300 μg of anti-D immunoglobulin will neutralise only 30 mL of fetal whole blood.
- Fetomaternal bleeding >20–30 mL at delivery is estimated to occur in approximately 1 in 200–300 deliveries (Rubod et al., 2007).
- In suspected cases of fetomaternal hemorrhage exceeding 30 mL, the volume of fetal blood transfused into the maternal circulation can be calculated using the following investigations:
  - The rosette test
  - The Kleihauer–Betke test
  - Flow cytometry
- The **rosette test** is a qualitative test for fetomaternal bleeding. This may be performed as an initial screen. If the test is negative, it confirms that <2 mL of fetal blood was transfused. A standard dose of anti-D immunoglobulin is given to women with a negative test.
- The **Kleihauer–Betke acid elution assay** is the diagnostic test most often used for the detection and quantification of fetomaternal hemorrhage. It is performed if the rosette test is positive. A maternal blood sample is fixed to a slide, which is then exposed to an acidic pH solution. Adult red blood cells become 'ghost' cells since hemoglobin A is soluble at a low pH. Fetal red blood cells remain pink because hemoglobin F is stable at an acidic pH.
- **Flow cytometry** is another assay for detecting and quantitating fetomaternal hemorrhage. It is more accurate than the Kleihauer–Betke acid elution assay.
- These tests help determine if more than the standard dose of anti-D immunoglobulin needs to be given to a woman with a suspected fetomaternal hemorrhage.

Antenatal anti-D prophylaxis

- Western guidelines (ACOG, 2017; British Committee for Standards in Hematology, 2014) advise antenatal anti-D given as a single dose at 34 weeks or two doses at 28 and 34 weeks.
- The effects of antenatal anti-D (given at 28 weeks and/or 34 weeks) were assessed in a systematic review of the Cochrane Database (McBain et al., 2015). **There was no conclusive evidence that the use of anti-D during pregnancy benefits either mother or baby in terms of incidence of Rhesus D alloimmunisation during the pregnancy or postpartum or the incidence of neonatal morbidity.**

- The WHO (2016) does not recommend routine antenatal prophylaxis with anti-D immunoglobulin in non-sensitised Rh-negative pregnant women at 28 and 34 weeks of gestation to prevent RhD

> The WHO (2016) does not recommend routine antenatal prophylaxis with anti-D immunoglobulin at 28 and 34 weeks of gestation.

alloimmunisation. This recommendation is based on the following:
  - Postpartum anti-D is very effective in preventing sensitisation.
  - The cost of antenatal anti-D immunoglobulin adds to the cost of antenatal care, especially in low-income countries like India.
  - Approximately 40 per cent of women who receive antenatal anti-D immunoglobulin will deliver Rh-negative infants (Runkel et al., 2020), and would have incurred an unnecessary expense if given antenatal anti-D immunoglobulin.

References

1. Abbasi N, Johnson JA, Ryan G. 2017. Fetal anemia. *Ultrasound Obstet Gynecol.* 50: 145-153.

2. Agarwal K, Rana A, Ravi AK. 2014. Treatment and Prevention of Rh Isoimmunization. *J. Fetal Med.* 1, 81–88.

3. American College of Obstetricians and Gynecologists. 2017. ACOG Practice Bulletin No. 181. Prevention of Rh D alloimmunization. *Obstet Gynecol.* 2017;130:e57–70.

4. American College of Obstetricians and Gynecologists. 2018. ACOG Practice Bulletin No. 192. Management of alloimmunization during pregnancy. *Obstet Gynecol.* 131:e82–90.

5. Bowman JM, Pollock JM, Penston LE. 1986. Fetomaternal transplacental hemorrhage during pregnancy and after delivery. *Vox Sang.* 51:117.

6. Chandra T, Gupta A. 2012. Prevalence of ABO and Rhesus blood groups in Northern India. *J Blood Disord Transfus.* 3:132.

7. Crowther C, Middleton P. 1997. Anti-D administration after childbirth for preventing rhesus alloimmunization. *Cochrane Database Syst Rev.* Issue 2. Art. no.: CD000021.

8. Giri PA, Yadav S, Parhar GS et al. 2011. Frequency of ABO and rhesus blood groups: A study from a rural tertiary care teaching hospital in India. *Int J Biol Med Res.* 2(4):988–90.

9. Koram SK, Sadula M, Veldurthy VS. 2014. Distribution of ABO and Rh-blood groups in blood donors at a tertiary care centre. *Int J of Res in Health Sci.* 2:326–30.

10. Latoo JA, Masoodi NA, Bhat NA et al. 2006. The ABO and Rh blood groups in Kashmiri population. *Indian J Pract Doctor.* 3(2):2.

11. Mari G, Deter RL, Carpenter RL, Rahman F, Zimmerman R, Moise KJ Jr et al. 2000. Non-invasive diagnosis by Doppler ultrasonography of fetal anemia due to maternal red-cell alloimmunization. Collaborative Group for Doppler Assessment of the Blood Velocity of Anemic Fetuses. *N Engl J Med.* 342:9–14.

12. Mari G, Norton ME et al. 2015. Society for Maternal-Fetal Medicine (SMFM) Clinical Guideline No. 8. The fetus at risk for anemia—diagnosis and management. *Am J Obstet Gynecol.* 212:697.

13. McBain RD, Crowther CA, Middleton P. 2015. Anti-D administration in pregnancy for preventing Rhesus alloimmunisation. *Cochrane Database Syst Rev.* Issue 9. Art. no: CD000020.

14. Moise KJ. 2008. Fetal anemia due to non-Rhesus-D red-cell alloimmunization. *Semin Fetal Neonatal Med.* 13: 207–214.

15. Moise KJ. 2019. Management of pregnancy complicated by RhD alloimmunization. Lockwood CJ, Kleinman S (Eds). *UpToDate.* Waltham, MA.

16. Moise KJ. 2019a. Intrauterine fetal transfusion of red cells. Lockwood CJ, Kleinman S (Eds.). *UpToDate.* Waltham, MA.

17. Pahuja S, Gupta SK, Pujani M et al. 2011. The prevalence of irregular erythrocyte antibodies among antenatal women in Delhi. *Blood Transfus.* 9:388–93.

18. Patel P, Patel S, Shah J et al. 2012. Frequency and distribution of blood groups in blood donors in western Ahmedabad—a hospital-based study. *Natl J Med Res.* 2:202–6.

19. Picklesimer AH, Oepkes D, Moise KJ Jr et al. 2007. Determinants of the middle cerebral artery peak systolic velocity in the human fetus. *Am J Obstet Gynecol.* 197:526.e1.

20. Qureshi H, Massey E, Kirwan D et al. 2014. British Committee for Standards in Haematology guideline for the use of anti-D immunoglobulin for the prevention of haemolytic disease of the fetus and newborn. *Transfusion Med.* 24: 8-20.

21. Rubod C, Deruelle P, Le Goueff F et al. 2007. Long-term prognosis for infants after massive fetomaternal hemorrhage. *Obstet Gynecol.* 110:256.

22. Runkel B, Bein G, Sieben W et al. 2020. Targeted antenatal anti-D prophylaxis for RhD-negative pregnant women: A systematic review. *BMC Pregnancy Childbirth.* 20, 83.

23. WHO Reproductive Health Library. 2016. WHO recommendation on antenatal anti-D immunoglobulin prophylaxis. The WHO Reproductive Health Library. WHO, Geneva.

24. Zwiers C, Oepkes D, Lopriore E et al. 2018. The near disappearance of fetal hydrops in relation to current state-of-the-art management of red cell alloimmunization. *Prenat Diagn.* 38:943.

Chapter 44

High Maternal BMI: Obstetric Implications

INTRODUCTION

- The World Health Organization (WHO, 2004) defines overweight and obesity in Asians as presented in Table 44.1.

Table 44.1 Categories of overweight and obesity based on body mass index (BMI) for Asians

Category	Body mass index (BMI) kg/m²
Overweight	23–27.5
Obesity class I	27.5–31
Obesity class II	31–35
Obesity class III	35 or greater

- In the past two decades, overweight and obesity and their attendant morbidity have become a major public health problem in India.
- In a study done to estimate the global and country-level burden of overweight and obesity in pregnancy, Chen et al. (2018) looked at data from 20 countries between 2005 and 2014. In 2014, the percentage of overweight and obese women in India was 21.7 per cent, i.e., one out of every five women.
- This reflects on the number of overweight and obese women who are pregnant. Consequently, India has the the largest proportion in the world of pregnant women with this issue.

> There has been a sharp increase in the number of overweight and obese pregnant women in lower and middle income countries like India. India has the **largest number of overweight and obese pregnant women** (4.3 million), which accounts for the largest proportion (11.1%) in the world (Chen et al., 2018).

ADIPOSE TISSUE: AN ENDOCRINE ORGAN

- Earlier views of adipose tissue as a passive reservoir for energy storage do not hold good any longer. Adipose tissue acts as an endocrine and immune organ that has wide-reaching effects on the physiology of the body (Kershaw and Flier, 2004).
- An excess of adipose tissue leads to adverse metabolic consequences. Adipose tissue, particularly central deposition (intra-abdominal and subcutaneous tissue over the abdomen), is associated with features of the metabolic syndrome (Grundy et al., 2004):
  - Insulin resistance
  - Hyperglycemia

- Dyslipidemia
- Hypertension
- Prothrombotic and proinflammatory states
- Though it is difficult to accurately assess central obesity in pregnant women, measurement of maternal abdominal subcutaneous fat thickness (SFT) by ultrasound has been recommended as a surrogate measure for central obesity and is a predictor for pregnancy complications in overweight and obese women (Kennedy et al., 2016). Suresh et al. (2012), in a retrospective study, concluded that abdominal SFT between 18 and 22 weeks' gestation is superior to BMI in identifying risk for obesity-related complications.
- Though it may not be practical to measure SFT in pregnant women, these studies provide proof that excess adipose tissue is a significant predictor of complications in pregnancy.

EFFECTS OF OBESITY ON PREGNANCY

When overweight and obese women are compared to women with a normal BMI, there is a small but statistically significant increase in antenatal, intrapartum, and postpartum events, including severe maternal morbidity and mortality.

Early pregnancy loss

- In a systematic review (Boots and Stephenson, 2011), there appeared to be a mild increase in the risk of spontaneous miscarriage in obese women (16.6 per cent) as compared to 10.7 per cent in women with normal weight.
- Similarly, Cavalcante et al., in a meta-analysis (2019) found that obese women with recurrent pregnancy loss (RPL) had a greater risk of having a future miscarriage. This risk did not apply to overweight women.

Antenatal complications

Gestational hypertension and preeclampsia

- Most studies have shown a consistently strong positive association between maternal pre-pregnancy BMI and the risk of gestational hypertension and preeclampsia (O'Brien et al., 2003; Weiss et al., 2004; Anderson et al., 2012). As obesity becomes a public health issue in developing countries, the incidence of preeclampsia continues to rise.
- The risk of preeclampsia has been shown to double with each 5 to 7 kg/m^2 increase in pre-pregnancy BMI (O'Brien et al., 2003). Pre-pregnancy weight loss has been shown to have a positive impact on decreasing the risk of hypertensive disorders (Maggard et al., 2008).
- The insulin resistance, hyperlipidemia, and subclinical inflammation associated with excess adipose tissue may explain the risk for hypertension and preeclampsia.

Congenital anomalies and aneuploidy (ACOG, 2015)
Detection of congenital anomalies by ultrasound scanning is decreased with increasing maternal BMI by at least 20 per cent in obese women compared to women within the normal weight range.
Maternal obesity decreases the detection rate of Down syndrome because of the effect of increased plasma volume on the measurement of serum analytes.

Diabetes

- Compared with pregnant women who are within the normal weight range, the risk of developing gestational diabetes mellitus is as follows (Chu et al., 2007):
  - Two times higher in overweight women
  - Four times higher in obese women
  - Eight times higher in severely obese women
- Screening at the first visit is mandatory for obese women who have not been screened for diabetes recently and who do not know their diabetes status. Early screening may reveal the presence of pre-gestational diabetes (see **Chapter 40**, *Gestational and pre-gestational diabetes*).
- The increased insulin resistance associated with obesity is the underlying cause for GDM.

Preterm birth

- Maternal overweight and obesity have been correlated to medically indicated preterm delivery for indications such as hypertension, preeclampsia, and diabetes (McDonald, 2010).
- Though obesity seems to be associated with spontaneous extremely preterm delivery, it does not seem to have any correlation with spontaneous preterm births (Ramsey and Schenken, 2019).

Postterm pregnancy

Obesity is associated with postterm pregnancies, but the exact cause is not known.

Macrososomic fetus and large-for-gestational-age (LGA) infant

- The obese gravida is at an increased risk of delivering a large-for-gestational age (LGA) infant.
- Fetal macrosomia is due to fetal and maternal hyperinsulinemia. The consequence of macrosomia is shoulder dystocia leading to maternal/neonatal injury, and increased risk of cesarean delivery.

Cesarean delivery

- Cesarean delivery risk is increased by 50 per cent in overweight women. In obese women, the risk is more than double that in women with normal BMI (Poobalan et al., 2009).
- Obese women are also at a higher risk for endometritis and wound rupture or dehiscence following a cesarean delivery (ACOG, 2015).

Stillbirth

- Obese gravidas have a 40 per cent greater risk of having a stillbirth than non-obese gravidas (Catalano, 2007). This is particularly true in class II and class III obese women.
- There is no evidence that antepartum surveillance with obesity as the sole indication improves pregnancy outcomes. A recommendation cannot be made for or against routine fetal surveillance (ACOG, 2015).

Non-obstetric complications

- **Obstructive sleep apnea** is more common in obese pregnant women. This condition is associated with increased risk of the following complications:
  - Preeclampsia and eclampsia
  - Cardiomyopathy
  - Delayed recovery from opiates given during cesarean section
  - Pulmonary embolism
  - In-hospital mortality
- **Carpal tunnel syndrome** may develop in a pregnancy in a non-obese woman, but the risk is higher in obese women.

ANTENATAL MANAGEMENT

Recommended gestational weight gain for overweight and obese pregnant women

- Overweight and obese women should be educated on optimal weight gain in pregnancy. The recommended weight gain for such women is less than it is for women with normal BMI at the first visit (see **Chapter 3**, *Dietary advice and nutritional supplements*).
- However, severely restricted weight gain or gestational weight loss in class II and III obese pregnant women is not recommended since it is associated with small-for-gestational age infants (Kapadia et al., 2015).

 All women presenting for their first antenatal visit should have their height and weight measured and their BMI calculated (see **Chapter 2**, *Antenatal care: Initial assessment*).

Screening for gestational diabetes and hypertension

Since the risks of gestational diabetes and hypertension are higher in overweight and obese women, routine screening is mandatory for them.

Assessment of fetal growth

- Assessment of fetal size by palpation may be a challenge in obese women.
- Serial ultrasound examination is recommended for fetal growth and estimated fetal weight.

INTRAPARTUM MANAGEMENT OF VAGINAL DELIVERY

Appropriate equipment

Class II and III obesity present a need for appropriate equipment: larger blood pressure cuffs, labour beds and stirrups capable of supporting the woman's weight, and wheelchairs that are wide enough.

Induction at term

- Induction of labour at term is recommended in obese pregnant women for the following indications (Schuster et al., 2016):

- Pre-pregnancy class III obesity
- Pre-pregnancy class II obesity with gestational diabetes or macrosomia
- Pre-pregnancy class I obesity with gestational diabetes and macrosomia
- Induction at term has not been found to increase the cesarean section rate in this protocol.

Epidural analgesia

- The use of epidural for intrapartum pain relief may present a challenge in an obese parturient because of the loss of anatomical landmarks.
- In a study on the influence of BMI on the performance of epidural analgesia in labour, Dresner et al. (2006) found that the risk of epidural analgesic failure is greater in obese women when compared with women who have normal weight and those who are overweight.

Management of third stage of labour

Obese pregnant women are at an increased risk of PPH (Sebire et al., 2001) and hence active management of the third stage of labour should be routinely recommended for these women.

OPERATIVE AND INTRAOPERATIVE ISSUES WITH CESAREAN DELIVERY

Anesthesia

- Spinal and epidural anesthesia may be a challenge in obese women due to the loss of anatomical landmarks and the increase in the thickness of the subcutaneous layer.
- Epidural analgesia in women with class III obesity is associated with a greater degree of hypotension and significant fetal heart rate decelerations than in pregnant women with normal weight.
- Spinal anesthesia is associated with significant respiratory impairment for a prolonged period after a cesarean section.
- General anesthesia may be administered to obese pregnant women but may pose a problem due to excess tissue, edema, and difficulty in positioning of the neck. Special precautions include the following:
  - Preoxygenation
  - Proper patient positioning
  - Availability of fiberoptic equipment for intubation

Prophylactic antibiotics

For obese women undergoing cesarean delivery, consideration may be given to using a higher preoperative antibiotic dose for surgical prophylaxis.

Skin incision

There is not enough evidence to recommend one incision over another, but vertical skin incisions may be associated with a greater risk of complications.

Subcutaneous drains

- The routine use of subcutaneous drains to reduce the risk of wound infection after cesarean sections in obese women is not recommended because of the lack of good-quality evidence (RCOG, 2018).
- Ramsey et al. (2005) found that not only is the use of a subcutaneous drain in obese women not effective in preventing wound complications, it may actually worsen the risk of post-cesarean wound infection.

Prophylaxis for venous thromboembolism (VTE)

- Class II and III obesity in pregnancy increases the risk of VTE.
- These women should receive VTE prophylaxis 6–12 hours postoperatively, after the risk of hemorrhage has decreased. It should be continued until the woman is fully ambulating (ACOG, 2015).

Vaginal birth after cesarean section (VBAC)

Obese gravidas undergoing a trial of labour after a previous cesarean delivery have an almost two-fold increase in composite maternal morbidity and a five-fold increased risk of neonatal injury (Hibbard, 2006).

POSTPARTUM MANAGEMENT

- Breastfeeding is less likely to be initiated and maintained by obese mothers (Li et al., 2003).
- Symptoms of depression and anxiety are more commonly encountered in the puerperium (Carter, 2000).
- Women should be counselled regarding interventions employing both diet and exercise to improve postpartum weight reduction as opposed to regimens that prescribe exercise alone.
- Intrauterine contraception is safe and effective. It may be preferred over combined contraceptive pills, which may increase the risk of VTE in obese women.
- Overweight and obese women must be routinely monitored for diabetes and hypertension.

References

1. American College of Obstetricians and Gynecologists. 2015. ACOG Practice Bulletin No. 156. Obesity in pregnancy. *Obstet Gynecol*. 126:e112–26.

2. Anderson NH, McCowan LM, Fyfe EM, Chan EH, Taylor RS, Stewart AW et al. 2012. The impact of maternal body mass index on the phenotype of pre-eclampsia: A prospective cohort study. *SCOPE Consortium*. 19:589–95.

3. Boots C, Stephenson MD. 2011. Does obesity increase the risk of miscarriage in spontaneous conception? A systematic review. *Semin Reprod Med*. 29:507.

4. Carter AS, Baker CW, Brownell KD. 2000. Body mass index, eating attitudes, and symptoms of anxiety and depression in pregnancy and the postpartum period. *Psychosom Med.* 62: 264-70.

5. Catalano PM. 2007. Management of obesity in pregnancy. *Obstet Gynecol.* 109:419–33.

6. Cavalcante MB, Sarno M, Peixoto AB et al. 2019. Obesity and recurrent miscarriage: A systematic review and meta-analysis. *J Obstet Gynaecol Res.* 45:30.

7. Chen C, Xu X, Yan Y. 2018. Estimated global overweight and obesity burden in pregnant women based on panel data model. *PLoSONE.* 13(8): e0202183.

8. Chu SY, Callaghan WM, Kim SY et al. 2007. Maternal obesity and risk of gestational diabetes mellitus. *Diabetes Care.* 30(8):2070–6.

9. Dresner M, Brocklesby J, Bamber J. 2006. Audit of the influence of body mass index on the performance of epidural analgesia in labour and the subsequent mode of delivery. *BJOG.* 113:1178–81.

10. Grundy SM, Brewer Jr HB, Cleeman JI et al. 2004. Definition of metabolic syndrome: Report of the National Heart, Lung, and Blood Institute/American Heart Association conference on scientific issues related to definition. Circulation 109: 433–438.

11. Hibbard JU, Gilbert S, Landon MB et al. 2006. Trial of labor or repeat cesarean delivery in women with morbid obesity and previous cesarean delivery. National Institute of Child Health and Human Development Maternal-Fetal Medicine Units Network. *Obstet Gynecol.* 108:125–33.

12. Kapadia MZ, Park CK, Beyene J et al. 2015. Weight loss instead of weight gain within the guidelines in obese women during pregnancy: A systematic review and meta-analyses of maternal and infant outcomes. *PLoS ONE.* 10(7): e0132650.

13. Kennedy N, Peek MJ, Quinton AE, Lanzarone V, Martin A, Nanan R, Benzie R. 2016. Maternal abdominal subcutaneous fat thickness as a predictor for adverse pregnancy outcome: A longitudinal cohort study. *BJOG.*

14. Kershaw EE, Flier JS. 2004. Adipose tissue as an endocrine organ. *J Clin Endocrinol Metab.* 89:2548–56.

15. Li R, Jewell S, Grummer-Strawn L. 2003. Maternal obesity and breast-feeding practices. *Am J Clin Nutr.* 3: 77, 931–6.

16. Maggard MA, Yermilov I, Li Z et al. 2008. Pregnancy and fertility following bariatric surgery: A systematic review. *JAMA.* 300:2286.

17. McDonald SD, Han Z, Mulla S et al. 2010. Overweight and obesity in mothers and risk of preterm birth and low birth weight infants: Systematic review and meta-analyses. *BMJ.* 341:c3428.

18. O'Brien TE, Ray JG, Chan WS. 2003. Maternal body mass index and the risk of preeclampsia: A systematic overview. *Epidemiology.* 14:368.

19. Poobalan AS, Aucott LS, Gurung T et al. 2009. Obesity as an independent risk factor for elective and emergency caesarean delivery in nulliparous women—A systematic review and meta-analysis of cohort studies. *Obes Rev.* 10:28.

20. Ramsey PS, Schenken RS. 2019. Obesity in pregnancy: Complications and maternal management. Lockwood CJ, Pi-Sunyer X (Eds). *UpToDate.* Waltham, MA.

21. Ramsey PS, White AM, Guinn DA et al. 2005. Subcutaneous tissue reapproximation, alone or in combination with drain, in obese women undergoing cesarean delivery. *Obstet Gynecol.* 105:967–73.

22. RCOG Green-top Guideline No. 72. Denison FC, Aedla NR, Keag O, Hor K, Reynolds RM, Milne A, Diamond A, on behalf of the Royal College of Obstetricians and Gynaecologists. 2018. Care of Women with Obesity in Pregnancy. *BJOG.*

23. Schuster M, Madueke-Laveaux OS, Mackeen AD et al. 2016. The effect of the MFM obesity protocol on cesarean delivery rates. *Am J Obstet Gynecol.* 215:492.e1.

24. Sebire NJ, Jolly M, Harris JP et al. 2001. Maternal obesity and pregnancy outcome: A study of 287,213 pregnancies in London. *Int J Obes Relat Metab Disord.* 25:1175–82.

26. Suresh A, Liu A, Poulton A, Quinton A, Amer Z, Mongelli M et al. 2012. Comparison of maternal abdominal subcutaneous fat thickness and body mass index as markers for pregnancy outcomes: Astratified cohort study. *Aust N Z J Obstet Gynaecol.* 52:420–6.

26. Weiss JL, Malone FD, Emig D et al. 2004. Obesity, obstetric complications and cesarean delivery rate—A population-based screening study. *Am J Obstet Gynecol.* 190:1091.

27. World Health Organization. 2004. Appropriate Body Mass Index for Asian populations and its implications for policy and intervention strategies. *Lancet.* 363:157–63.

Chapter 45

Pregnancy in Women with Polycystic Ovary Syndrome

INTRODUCTION

- Polycystic ovary syndrome (PCOS) is one of the most common endocrinopathies in women of reproductive age, affecting between 6 and 10 per cent of women globally (Bozdag et al., 2016).
- With the advent of assisted reproductive techniques, it has become possible for many women with PCOS to achieve pregnancy.
- Pregnancy in these women may be associated with several complications: increased risk of miscarriage, gestational diabetes mellitus, hypertensive disorders of pregnancy, preterm delivery, and the birth of small-for-gestational age (SGA) infants.
- Women with PCOS have associated metabolic syndrome, which is characterised by the following:
  - Insulin resistance/diabetes
  - Dyslipidemia
  - Hypertension

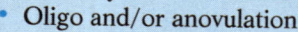

> **Criteria for the diagnosis of PCOS**
> According to the ASRM/ESHRE consensus group opinion (The Rotterdam ESHRE/ASRM consensus workshop group, 2004), the criteria for diagnosis of polycystic ovary syndrome include any two of the following:
> - Oligo and/or anovulation
> - Clinical and/or biochemical evidence of hyperandrogenism
> - Polycystic ovaries on ultrasonography

CONCEIVING WITH PCOS

Most women with PCOS conceive with ovulation induction or assisted reproductive techniques (ART) although spontaneous conception can occur in a few.

PREGNANCY OUTCOMES IN WOMEN WITH PCOS

- Pregnancy in women with PCOS is associated with several complications due to the endocrinological changes associated with the syndrome.
- The risk is further increased by obesity, which is an associated finding in 50 per cent of women with PCOS (Boomsma et al., 2006).
- Advanced maternal age may also have a bearing on the outcomes of pregnancy since many women with PCOS conceive late (Roos et al., 2011).

- Low-grade, chronic inflammation is commonly seen in women with PCOS, as evidenced by high serum concentrations of C-reactive protein (CRP). This worsens during pregnancy and may explain the excess risk of adverse pregnancy outcomes in women with PCOS (Palomba et al., 2014).

 Pregnancy in PCOS is associated with a high risk of complications due to the associated metabolic syndrome, obesity, and the use of ovulation induction and ART.

Spontaneous miscarriage

- The miscarriage rate in women with PCOS has been reported to be 20–40 per cent (Glueck et al., 2002), which is higher than the 10–20 per cent risk in the general obstetric population.
- Though the pathophysiology of excess pregnancy loss in these patients is unknown, it may be related to the following factors (Tulandi and Al-Fozan, 2019):
  - Elevated serum luteinising hormone (LH) levels
  - High testosterone and androstenedione concentrations (which may adversely affect the endometrium)
  - Insulin resistance
- Løvvik et al., in the PregMet2 study (2019), concluded that in pregnant women with PCOS, metformin treatment from the late first trimester until delivery might reduce the risk of late miscarriage and preterm birth but that it does not prevent gestational diabetes.

Gestational diabetes

- Women with PCOS demonstrate a significantly higher chance of developing gestational diabetes. This risk is independent of obesity (Boomsma et al., 2006).
- Gestational diabetes occurs in 5–40 per cent of women with PCOS.

Hypertensive disease

- The incidence of hypertensive disease in pregnancy is higher among women who have PCOS than those who do not (Radon et al., 1999; Boomsma et al., 2006).
- Roos and colleagues (2011), in a population-based cohort study, observed a strong association between polycystic ovary syndrome and preeclampsia.
- Women with PCOS have increased levels of androgens, which may be linked to the development of preeclampsia (Troisi et al., 2003).

Preterm birth

- Women with PCOS have a significant risk of delivering prematurely (Boomsma et al., 2006; Roos et al., 2011).
- There is a correlation between ART, polycystic ovary syndrome, and preterm birth (Schieve et al., 2002; Cnattingius et al., 1998; Roos et al., 2011).
- As the risk of multiple gestation increases with ART, the risk of preterm birth increases in women with PCOS who have conceived with ART.

- The risk of preterm birth among women with polycystic ovary syndrome does not seem to be related to maternal characteristics such as advanced age, smoking, or obesity (Roos et al., 2011).

 The strongest predictor for preterm birth in women with polycystic ovary syndrome is multiple gestation.

Increase in cesarean section and operative vaginal deliveries

- There is a significant increase in the risk of both operative vaginal deliveries and cesarean section in women with PCOS.
- This could be related to obesity (Sheiner et al., 2004) or other obstetric complications that may arise due to the underlying PCOS.

Macrosomia and SGA infants

- There is no consensus about the effect of PCOS on birth weight.
- Roos and colleagues (2011) found an increased rate of macrosomia even after adjusting for maternal obesity and gestational diabetes.
- In other studies, women with PCOS were not found to be at risk of having macrosomic or SGA babies (Turhan et al., 2003; Sir-Petermann et al., 2005).

Increase in admission to neonatal intensive care unit and increased perinatal mortality

- Infants born to women with PCOS have a higher incidence of low Apgar scores at five minutes and meconium aspiration. There are also more instances of fetal distress during labour (Roos et al., 2011).
- Infants born to women with PCOS have a significantly higher rate of admission to NICU and also have increased perinatal mortality (Boomsma et al., 2006).
- These adverse outcomes might be related to maternal complications like gestational diabetes, hypertension, and preeclampsia.

Fetal programming and long-term complications in the offspring

The Barker hypothesis of fetal programming suggests that excess fetal nutrition and hyperinsulinemia in utero may affect neuroendocrine systems regulating body weight, food intake, and metabolism, with consequences for long-term health (especially coronary heart disease) in the offspring of mothers with PCOS and gestational diabetes (Barker, 2004).

PRECONCEPTIONAL MANAGEMENT

Women with PCOS should be counselled prior to conception regarding the following:
- Lifestyle changes and weight reduction
- Increased risk of maternal and fetal complications
- Continuation of medications

Lifestyle changes and weight reduction

- Weight reduction is an important component of preconceptional management and should be achieved through diet and exercise. Women should be advised about regular exercises and a balanced diet.
- In addition to reducing complications due to obesity, weight reduction also helps in reducing insulin resistance and the risk of gestational diabetes.
- The optimum weight gain in pregnancy should be calculated based on the woman's BMI (see **Chapter 3**, *Dietary advice and nutritional supplements*), and a diet plan should be made for her.

 Achieving an optimal BMI before pregnancy reduces maternal and fetal complications.

Increased risk of maternal and fetal complications

- Women with PCOS should be informed about the complications of pregnancy.
- Regular and, if required, more frequent antenatal visits should be discussed and emphasised.
- The mother should be advised to have her delivery in a tertiary centre with neonatal care facilities.

METFORMIN IN PREGNANCY WITH PCOS

- Women with PCOS may be on metformin for weight reduction as part of an ovulation induction protocol.

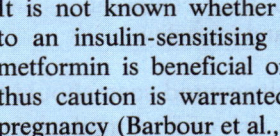 It is not known whether fetal exposure to an insulin-sensitising agent such as metformin is beneficial or harmful, and thus caution is warranted in its use in pregnancy (Barbour et al., 2018; Barbour and Feig, 2019).

- Metformin is widely prescribed to pregnant women with polycystic ovary syndrome (PCOS) in an attempt to reduce pregnancy complications. However, the drug is not approved for this indication, and evidence for this practice is lacking. Vanky et al., in a randomised, controlled multicentre study (2010), found no difference in the prevalence of preeclampsia, gestational diabetes mellitus, or preterm delivery in women with PCOS who received metformin treatment from the first trimester to delivery.
- Overall weight gain during pregnancy was found to be less in women on metformin than in those who were not on the drug (Vanky et al., 2010).
- The ACOG and the American Diabetes Association do not recommend that metformin be continued in women with PCOS and glucose intolerance. Such women should be switched to insulin once pregnancy is confirmed. However, the Government of India (2018) recommends metformin for GDM after 20 weeks of gestation as an alternative to insulin in low-resource areas where access to insulin is not always available.

Metformin treatment from the late first trimester until delivery might reduce the risk of late miscarriage and preterm birth but does not prevent gestational diabetes (Løvvik et al., 2019).

ANTENATAL MANAGEMENT

First trimester

- Ultrasonography is advisable for the following reasons:
  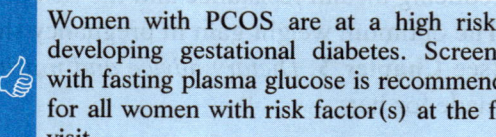 Women with PCOS are at a high risk of developing gestational diabetes. Screening with fasting plasma glucose is recommended for all women with risk factor(s) at the first visit.
  - Most women with PCOS have irregular cycles, which makes ultrasonography necessary to accurately date the pregnancy.
  - Induction of labour may be required before term for preeclampsia or gestational diabetes and hence it is important to know the correct EDD.
  - Multiple pregnancy is a possibility, especially if ovulation was induced.
- A fasting plasma sugar test should be performed and if ≥92 mg/dL, a diagnosis of gestational diabetes is made (Metzger et al., 2010).

Second trimester

- Blood pressure must be monitored regularly since women with PCOS have a higher risk of hypertension and preeclampsia.

 There are no preventive measures against hypertension, preeclampsia, or preterm labour. Early diagnosis of these complications and appropriate management can, however, reduce perinatal morbidity and mortality.

- A detailed ultrasound scan should be performed at 18–20 weeks. PCOS per se does not increase the risk of fetal malformations (Boomsma et al., 2006), but the risk increases if the woman has pre-gestational diabetes.
- Since women with PCOS are at a high risk of preterm birth, cervical length by ultrasonography may be considered between 18 and 24 weeks.
- Oral glucose tolerance test (GTT) should be done at 24 weeks if fasting plasma glucose is normal in the first trimester.
- Maternal weight gain must be closely monitored, and the woman should be advised on the optimum weight gain in pregnancy based on her pre-pregnancy BMI.

Third trimester

- Clinical evaluation must be done for macrosomia and fetal growth restriction (FGR).
   Routine elective cesarean section is not recommended in women with PCOS without an obstetric indication.
- Ultrasonography is indicated if macrosomia/FGR is suspected or if the woman is obese.
- Close monitoring of blood pressure must be continued.

- If there are no complications, the baby may be delivered at term.
- PCOS is not an indication for elective cesarean section. Cesarean section should be performed only for obstetric indications.

POSTNATAL MANAGEMENT

- PCOS is a lifelong metabolic disorder. Hence lifestyle modifications should be maintained, and optimal weight sustained.
- Since many women continue to be anovulatory, low-dose oral contraceptives may be used to regularise cycles and serve as a temporary method of contraception. An intrauterine device may also be used.

 Since women with PCOS are at high risk for metabolic syndrome and endometrial cancer, long-term follow-up and monitoring are mandatory.

References

1. Barker DJ. 2004. The developmental origins of adult disease. *J Am Coll Nutr.* 23:588S95S.
2. Boomsma CM, Eijkemans MJC, Hughes EG, Visser GHA et al. 2006. A meta-analysis of pregnancy outcomes in women with polycystic ovary syndrome. *Human Rep Update.* 12: 673–683.
3. Bozdag G, Mumusoglu S, Zengin D et al. 2016. The prevalence and phenotypic features of polycystic ovary syndrome: A systematic review and meta-analysis. *Hum Reprod.* 31:2841.
4. Barbour LA, Scifres C, Valent AM et al. 2013. A cautionary response to SMFM statement: Pharmacological treatment of gestational diabetes. *Am J Obstet Gynecol.* 219:367.e1.
5. Barbour LA, Feig DS. 2019. Metformin for gestational diabetes mellitus: Progeny, perspective, and a personalized approach. *Diabetes Care.* 42:396.
6. Cnattingius S, Bergstrom R, Lipworth L, Kramer MS. 1998. Pre-pregnancy weight and the risk of adverse pregnancy outcomes. *N Engl J Med.* 338:147–52.
7. Glueck CJ, Wang P, Goldenberg N, Sieve-Smith L. 2002. Pregnancy outcomes among women with polycystic ovary syndrome treated with metformin. *Hum Reprod.* 17:2858.
8. Government of India. 2018. Maternal and Health Division, Diagnosis and Management of Gestational Diabetes Mellitus. Technical and Operational Guidelines. Ministry of Health & Family Welfare, New Concept Information Systems. New Delhi, India.
9. Løvvik TS, Carlsen SM, Salvesen Ø et al. 2019. Use of metformin to treat pregnant women with polycystic ovary syndrome (PregMet2): A randomised, double-blind, placebo-controlled trial. *Lancet Diabetes Endocrinol.* 7(4):256–266.
10. Metzger BE, Gabbe SG et al. 2010. International Association of Diabetes and Pregnancy Study Groups Consensus Panel. International association of diabetes and pregnancy study groups recommendations on the diagnosis and classification of hyperglycemia in pregnancy. *Diabetes Care.* 33:676.
11 Palomba S, Falbo A, Chiossi G et al. 2014. Low-grade chronic inflammation in pregnant women with polycystic ovary syndrome: A prospective controlled clinical study. *J Clin Endocrinol Metab.* 99:2942.

12. Roos N, Kieler H, Sahlin L, Ekman-Ordeberg et al. 2011. Risk of adverse pregnancy outcomes in women with polycystic ovary syndrome: Population-based cohort study. *BMJ.* 343:d6309.

13. Radon PA, McMahon MJ, Meyer WR. 1999. Impaired glucose tolerance in pregnant women with polycystic ovary syndrome. *Obstet Gynecol.* 94:194–7.

14. Schieve LA, Meikle SF, Ferre C, Peterson HB, Jeng G, Wilcox LS. 2002. Low and very low birth weight in infants conceived with use of assisted reproductive technology. *N Engl J Med.* 346:731–7.

15. Sheiner E, Levy A, Menes TS, Silverberg D, Katz M, Mazor M. 2004. Maternal obesity as an independent risk factor for caesarean delivery. *Paediatr Perinat Epidemiol.* 18:196–201.

16. Sir-Petermann T, Hitchsfeld C, Maliqueo M, Codner E, Echiburu B, Gazitua R, Recabarren S, Cassorla F. 2005. Birth weight in offspring of mothers with polycystic ovarian syndrome. *Hum Reprod.* 2122–2126.

17. Troisi R, Potischman N, Johnson CN, Roberts JM, Lykins D, Harger G et al. 2003. Estrogen and androgen concentrations are not lower in the umbilical cord serum of pre-eclamptic pregnancies. *Cancer Epidemiol Biomarkers Prev.* 12(11 Pt 1):1268–70.

18. The Rotterdam ESHRE/ASRM – Sponsored PCOS Consensus Workshop Group. 2004. Revised 2003 consensus on diagnostic criteria and long-term health risks related to polycystic ovary syndrome. *Fertil Steril.* 81:19–25.

19. Tulandi T, Al-Fozan HM. 2019. Definition and etiology of recurrent pregnancy loss. Lockwood CJ (Ed). *UpToDate.* Waltham, MA.

20. Turhan NO, Seckin NC, Aybar F, Inegol I. 2003. Assessment of glucose tolerance and pregnancy outcome of polycystic ovary patients. *Int J Gynaecol Obstet.* 81,163–168.

21. Vanky E, Stridsklev S, Heimstad R et al. 2010. Metformin versus placebo from first trimester to delivery in polycystic ovary syndrome: A randomized, controlled multicenter study. *J Clin Endocrinol Metab.* 95:E448.

Chapter 46

Management of Pregnancy After Assisted Reproductive Technology

INTRODUCTION

- Assisted reproductive technology (ART) is defined as treatments and procedures which involve the handling of human oocytes, sperm, or embryos outside the human body with the intent of establishing a pregnancy.
- ART includes in vitro fertilisation-embryo transfer (IVF-ET), gamete intrafallopian transfer (GIFT), zygote intrafallopian transfer (ZIFT), and frozen embryo transfer (FET).
- This term also applies to oocyte donation, gestational carriers (surrogates), and related procedures such as intracytoplasmic sperm injection (ICSI), blastocyst culture, and assisted hatching.
- After four decades of clinical experience, ART is now considered part of routine medical practice.

 ART does NOT include intrauterine insemination (IUI) with unstimulated cycles, or with ovarian stimulation using gonadotropins or clomiphene.

PREGNANCY OUTCOME AFTER ART

- The outcomes of ART pregnancies, both short- and long-term, have been studied extensively; the results of these studies have been generally reassuring (Wilson et al., 2011; Allen et al., 2006).
- However, ART pregnancies do seem to have a higher risk of certain obstetric and perinatal complications. These are often related to the higher number of multiple pregnancies after ART and also to fact that it is generally older women who get pregnant with ART.
- The risk of adverse outcomes is related to the following factors (Paulson, 2020):
    - Maternal and paternal characteristics
    - Baseline medical conditions leading to subfertility and infertility
    - Sperm factors
    - Use of gonadotropins
    - Extraneous factors such as laboratory conditions during embryo culture, culture medium, cryopreservation, and thawing
    - Increased incidence of multiple gestations and vanishing twins
    - Obstetric management

THE EFFECT OF ART ON ADVERSE MATERNAL OUTCOMES

These will be discussed under the following three headings:
- ART-associated adverse outcomes in early pregnancy
- ART-associated obstetric complications
- ART-associated adverse outcomes in late pregnancy

ART-associated adverse outcomes in early pregnancy

Early spontaneous pregnancy loss

- The rate of early spontaneous pregnancy loss is similar for both natural and ART conceptions (Schieve et al., 2003; Pezeshki et al., 2000).
- If multiple sacs are identified by ultrasound before 6 weeks, spontaneous loss of at least one gestation ('vanishing twin') occurs in 35 per cent of twin pregnancies, and 55 per cent of triplet pregnancies (La Sala et al., 2004).
- The number of gestational sacs has an impact on the rate of spontaneous miscarriage, with 53 per cent of women with triplet pregnancies and 65 per cent of quadruplet pregnancies having spontaneous reduction before 12 weeks (Dickey et al., 2002).

 After spontaneous reduction, the surviving fetuses weigh less at birth and are born earlier than those from unreduced pregnancies with the same initial number of fetuses (Dickey et al., 2002; Luke et al., 2009).

- Greater maternal age resulting in an older egg, and consequent chromosomal aberrations in the fetus are important contributory factors.
- Spontaneous miscarriage rates are higher with the use of thawed embryos as compared to fresh fertilised embryos (Paulson, 2020).

Ectopic pregnancy

- The risk of ectopic pregnancy after IVF-ET has been reported to be 2.2 per cent of all clinical pregnancies (Clayton et al., 2006).
- The rate of ectopic pregnancy is higher in women with the following:
  - Tubal factor infertility
  - Zygote intrafallopian transfer (ZIFT)
  - Endometriosis
  - History of ectopic pregnancy
- The higher risk of heterotopic pregnancy in ART is mainly due to the transfer of multiple embryos resulting in multiple gestations after IVF (Paulson, 2020).

 Heterotopic pregnancy is more common in pregnancies conceived by ART (1/100 vs. 1/30,000 in natural conceptions).

Ovarian hyperstimulation syndrome (OHSS)

- Ovarian hyperstimulation syndrome is a potentially life-threatening iatrogenic complication of ART. It is a complex pathology with multi-organ impairment in its severe form.

- There are two distinct patterns of OHSS: the early type that occurs 3–7 days after ovulation is triggered by hCG, and the late type that occurs 12–17 days after hCG (Lyons et al., 1994).

 Late OHSS is induced by endogenous hCG of pregnancy and is observed in women who become pregnant, especially in those with more than one initial gestational sac (Navot et al., 1992).

- Once a clinical pregnancy has been established in a patient with OHSS (both early and late), there is a normal risk of miscarriage.
- In a large study, Abramov and colleagues (1998) found an association between miscarriage and severe OHSS, with a total clinical miscarriage rate of about 30 per cent, of which 25 per cent were early (7–13 weeks) and almost 5 per cent were late miscarriages (13–20 weeks).

ART-associated obstetric complications

Multiple conceptions and multiple births

- Multiple pregnancy is the commonest treatment-related adverse outcome of in vitro fertilisation (IVF) and is caused by the practice of transferring more than one embryo into the uterus.
- The alarming rise in the multiple pregnancy rate resulting from the use of assisted reproductive technology (ART) has raised concerns globally because of the significant maternal, fetal, and neonatal risks associated with these pregnancies (Wen et al., 2004; El-Toukhy et al., 2006).
- Maternal complications include increased risk of pregnancy-induced hypertension, gestational diabetes, peripartum hemorrhage, operative delivery, postpartum depression and anxiety, and parenting stress from having to bring up twins, triplets or more (see **Chapter 35**, *Multiple pregnancy*).
- Multiple pregnancy is also associated with a six-fold increase in the risk of preterm birth, which is a leading cause of infant mortality and long-term mental and physical disabilities, including cerebral palsy, learning difficulties, and chronic lung disease (Chambers and Ledger, 2014).
- Despite the significant risks associated with multiple pregnancy, double embryo transfer (DET) during IVF treatment continues to be widely practiced (Maheshwari et al., 2011).
- Clinicians as well as patients harbour the misconception that the success rate of IVF treatment is higher with the transfer of two embryos than it is with the transfer of one embryo, and ignore the risks involved with multiple pregnancy. However, a systematic review of the Cochrane Database (Pandian et al., 2013) showed that in women with good prognosis, the cumulative live birth rate after single embryo transfer (SET), followed by the transfer of a thawed embryo in a subsequent frozen embryo transfer cycle is comparable to that after DET but with a significantly lower risk of multiple pregnancy.

Though single embryo transfer is strongly recommended to avoid multiple pregnancy, the cost of undergoing two or three IVF cycles is prohibitive and drives couples to demand multiple embryo transfer.

Preterm birth (PTB), low-birth-weight (LBW) and small-for-gestational age (SGA) infants

- Singleton pregnancies resulting from ART are associated with a two-fold risk of preterm birth (McGovern et al., 2004) and a three-fold risk of low birth weight ≤2500 g (McDonald et al., 2009).
- A meta-analysis of 15 studies which compared 12,283 singleton ART babies to 1.9 million spontaneously conceived singletons has shown significantly higher rates for perinatal mortality, preterm delivery, low-birth-weight, very-low-birth-weight, and small-for-gestational age infants (Jackson et al., 2004) .
- A systematic review and meta-analysis of twins conceived after IVF showed small but significantly increased risks of PTB, LBW, and lower mean birth weight compared to spontaneously conceived twins after matching or controlling for at least maternal age (McDonald et al., 2010).

 It has been hypothesised that an increase in adverse outcomes among singletons resulting from ART is due to the 'vanishing twin' phenomenon (Paulson, 2020).

ART-associated adverse outcomes in late pregnancy

Placenta previa

- Romundstad and colleagues (2006) found a six-fold higher risk of placenta previa in singleton pregnancies conceived by ART than naturally conceived pregnancies.
- A systematic review and meta-analysis by Vermey and colleagues (2019) found that the risk of placenta previa, placental abruption, and morbidly adherent placenta was higher in ART than in spontaneously conceived pregnancies.
- The placement of embryos in the lower half of the uterine cavity and the myometrial movements arising from the fundus towards the cervix during the early secretory phase could account for the implantation of the embryo in the lower part of the uterus.

 The risk of placenta previa, placental abruption, and morbidly adherent placenta increases with ART (Vermey et al., 2019).

Gestational hypertension, preeclampsia, and placental abruption

- The use of IVF is associated with a statistically significant increase in preeclampsia, gestational hypertension, and placental abruption (Shevell et al., 2005).
- IVF in primiparous women is an independent risk factor for preeclampsia (Erez et al., 2006). Assisted conceptions are associated with more severe preeclampsia with a suggestion of end-organ damage (Calhoun et al., 2011).

Gestational diabetes

- After controlling for maternal age and nulliparity, twin pregnancies conceived with the assistance of IVF and ovulation induction are at an increased risk of gestational diabetes mellitus (GDM) (Adler-Levy et al., 2007).
- Jackson and colleagues (2004) found significant prevalence of gestational diabetes in singleton pregnancies resulting from IVF.

 The high prevalence of PCOS in women who conceive with IVF may contribute to the risk of GDM in pregnancy.

Stillbirth and perinatal mortality

Stillbirth and perinatal mortality rates are much higher in ART pregnancies (Bay et al., 2019), due partly to hypertensive disorders, gestational diabetes, LBW, and multiple gestation.

THE EFFECT OF ART ON FETAL AND NEONATAL OUTCOMES

Congenital abnormalities

- Women who undergo ART appear to be at an increased risk of delivering babies with congenital malformations when compared with fertile women who conceive naturally. The reason for this increase is unclear.
- However, patients can be reassured that the absolute risk of having a child with a congenital anomaly is low.
- A meta-analysis that included 124,468 infants (Wen et al., 2012) showed that the increased risk of birth defects was observed for all major organ systems, and was highest for the nervous system.

Chromosomal abnormalities

- Studies have not shown a higher prevalence of karyotype abnormalities (including mosaicism) in infants of IVF-conceived pregnancies than in naturally conceived pregnancies. Prenatal diagnosis is not typically offered for this indication alone.
- However, subfertile men and women may themselves have aneuploidies, structural abnormalities, gene mutations, and microdeletions that may be contributing to their subfertility. There is a risk of these abnormalities being passed on to their offspring (Paulson, 2020).

Cerebral palsy

- It is difficult to pinpoint ART as an independent risk factor for the development of cerebral palsy.
- A meta-analysis done to identify the incidence of cerebral palsy, autism spectrum disorders, and developmental delay in children born after assisted conception showed that children born after IVF had an increased risk of cerebral palsy associated with preterm delivery (Hvidtjørn et al., 2009).

The increased risk of cerebral palsy in the IVF group is strongly related to the high incidence of low birth weight, preterm birth, and multiple gestation.

Cognitive and motor development

- In a large European study, no differences were identified among ICSI, IVF, and naturally conceived children with respect to verbal and performance IQ (Ponjaert-Kristoffersen et al., 2005).
- Similarly, Leunens et al. (2008) followed up children at 8 years and 10 years after birth and found that both ICSI and naturally conceived children show comparable cognitive and motor development until the age of 10.

LONG-TERM OUTCOMES FOR ART BABIES

- Singleton babies conceived with IVF–ICSI may have slower postnatal growth as compared to naturally conceived babies (Koivurova et al., 2003). This effect is seen upto 3 years of age. This has not been observed in twins born after IVF–ICSI.
- IVF and IVF–ICSI children followed-up for 5 years (Bonduelle et al., 2005) were found to be more likely than spontaneously conceived children to have had the following:
  - A significant childhood illness
  - A surgical operation
  - Requirement for medical therapies
  - An admission to hospital
- Basatemur and colleagues (2010) found reassuring information regarding the growth of IVF and ICSI children upto 12 years. No significant differences were observed with respect to head circumference, height, and weight between the IVF, ICSI, and naturally conceived groups during the period of study.

OVARIAN AND BREAST CANCER RISK AFTER ART

Ovarian cancer

- The use of clomiphene and gonadotropin therapy has been implicated in the development of ovarian tumours, especially borderline ovarian tumours (Shushan et al., 1996). This was particularly so in women who had taken clomiphene for more than 12 months and not conceived. Based on this, prescribing clomiphene for more than 6–12 months is discouraged.
- However, in a pooled analysis of case–control studies, Ness et al. (2002) found that:
  - Among nulliparous, subfertile women, neither the use of any particular fertility drug nor its use for more than 12 months was associated with ovarian cancer.
  - Fertility drug use in nulligravid women was associated with borderline serous tumours but not with any invasive histologic subtypes.
  - Endometriosis and unknown cause of infertility increased the risk of cancer.
  - These data suggest a role of specific biologic causes of infertility, but not that of fertility drugs in the overall risk for ovarian cancer.

Infertility per se, not fertility drugs, plays a role in the risk for ovarian cancer (Ness et al., 2002).

Breast cancer

- An increased risk of breast cancer has not been demonstrated in women treated with fertility drugs (Doyle et al., 2002).
- There is evidence that the use of clomiphene and exogenous FSH in infertile women with anovulation might actually decrease the risk of breast cancer (Terry et al., 2006).

OBSTETRIC MANAGEMENT OF PREGNANCIES FOLLOWING ART

Luteal phase support

- Endometrial receptivity plays a major role in the success or failure of embryo implantation after IVF. Progesterone is administered in the luteal phase to optimise endometrial receptivity (ASRM Practice Bulletin, 2008).
- Progesterone supplementation is generally initiated on the day of oocyte retrieval or at the time of embryo transfer. However, a systematic review (Connell et al., 2015) could not establish what timing was the most optimal.
- The optimum duration of supplementation has not been established; progesterone is usually administered until a positive or negative pregnancy test is obtained or until the end of the first trimester.
- A systematic review of the Cochrane Database (van der Linden et al., 2015) concluded that hCG or progesterone given during the luteal phase may be associated with higher rates of live birth or ongoing pregnancy than placebo or no treatment, but the evidence is not conclusive.

 hCG for luteal phase support is associated with a greater risk of ovarian hyperstimulation syndrome (OHSS).

Surveillance for maternal complications

- Maternal blood pressure must be monitored regularly, and more frequently after 30 weeks' gestation.
- Screening for gestational diabetes must start at the first antenatal visit and must be repeated at 24 and 32 weeks.
- During the second trimester ultrasound examination, placenta previa must be specifically looked for and if present, followed up in the third trimester.

Antenatal counselling

- After conceiving with IVF or IVF–ICSI, couples tend to be extra careful during pregnancy. However, the woman must be made to understand that she does not require complete bed rest and can carry on with her normal activities.
- Reassurance must be given to the couple that the pregnancy will be monitored vigilantly.

Surveillance for fetal complications

Singleton pregnancy

- Compared to spontaneous conceptions, IVF and IVF–ICSI singleton pregnancies are at an increased risk of the following complications:
  - Stillbirth or neonatal death   2-fold
  - Preterm delivery (<37 weeks)   1- to 2-fold
  - Low birth weight (<2500 g)   2-fold
  - Very low birth weight (<1500 g)   2- to 3-fold
  - Small for gestational age (<10th percentile)   1- to 2-fold
  - NICU admission   1- to 2-fold
- These pregnancies must have close surveillance for growth restriction. If growth restriction is suspected, serial scans must be obtained and appropriate intervention used (see **Chapter 36**, *Fetal growth disorders: growth restriction and macrosomia*).

Multiple pregnancy

- The risk of morbidity and mortality increases with each additional fetus in a multiple gestation.
- Since there is a 1- to 2-fold increase in the risk of preterm delivery, close surveillance is required.

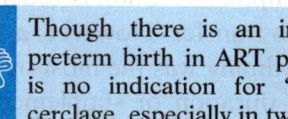

Though there is an increased risk of preterm birth in ART pregnancies, there is no indication for 'routine' cervical cerclage, especially in twin pregnancy.

Monitoring with ultrasonography

- Early ultrasound examination is required to establish the following:
  - Number of fetuses
  - Viability
  - Chorionicity in the case of multiple gestation
- First-trimester screening for Down syndrome should be done at $11–13^{+6}$ weeks' gestation.
- A complete obstetric scan should be done between 18–22 weeks' gestation.
- Serial scans should be done to monitor fetal growth and rule out placenta previa.

Mode of delivery

- There is no doubt that obstetricians have a lower threshold for performing cesarean section for ART pregnancies.
- Minkoff and Berkowitz (2005) have labelled this practice the 'precious baby' effect, which in essence postulates that obstetricians change their practice and deliver by cesarean section based on the knowledge that the pregnancy is the result of ART.
- There is enough evidence to show that pregnancies achieved by fertility treatment have a higher risk of obstetric and perinatal complications and obstetric interventions compared with spontaneous pregnancies.

- Sullivan and colleagues (2010) make a strong argument for allowing women to have a vaginal birth after conceiving with ART. However, the cesarean section rate for women who have conceived after IVF or IVF–ICSI has been reported to be as high as 75 per cent.
- In younger women with no obstetric morbidity, vaginal delivery may be attempted under intensive monitoring. Labour may be induced to ensure the availability of staff.
- Older women who have conceived after several years of fertility treatment may request an elective pre-labour cesarean.
- Gillet et al. (2011) found that IVF and ICSI pregnancies in older nulliparous women more often end in a pre-labour cesarean. They also found that a large number of obstetricians tend to go along with a mother's request for an elective cesarean section. However, the authors recommend that obstetricians should continue to support vaginal delivery as the optimal mode of birth until evidence clearly proves that prelabour cesarean section optimises outcomes for mothers and their infants.

References

1. Allen VM, Wilson RD, Cheung A et al. 2006. Pregnancy outcomes after assisted reproductive technology. *J Obstet Gynaecol Can.* 28:220.

2. ASRM Guidelines. 2008. Practice Committee of the American Society for Reproductive Medicine. Progesterone supplementation during the luteal phase and in early pregnancy in the treatment of infertility: An educational bulletin. *Fertil Steril.* 89:789.

3. Abramov Y, Elchalal U, Schenker JG. 1998. Obstetric outcome of in vitro fertilized pregnancies complicated by severe ovarian hyperstimulation syndrome: A multicenter study. *Fertil Steril.* 70,1070–1076.

4. Adler-Levy Y, Lunenfeld E, Levy A. 2007. Obstetric outcome of twin pregnancies conceived by in vitro fertilization and ovulation induction compared with those conceived spontaneously. *Eur J Obstet Gynecol Reprod Biol.* 133(2):173–8.

5. Basatemur E, Shevlin M, Sutcliffe A. 2010. Growth of children conceived by IVF and ICSI up to 12 years of age. *Reprod Biomed Online.* 20:144–9.

6. Sullivan EA, Chapman MG, Wang YA, Adamson GD. 2010. Population-based study of caesarean section after in vitro fertilization in Australia. *Birth.* 37:3; p184–191.

7. Bay B, Boie S, Kesmodel US. 2019. Risk of stillbirth in low-risk singleton term pregnancies following fertility treatment: A national cohort study. *BJOG.* 126:253.

8. Bonduelle M, Wennerholm UB, Loft A, Tarlatzis BC, Peters C, Henriet S et al. 2005. A multicentre cohort study on the physical health of 5-year-old children conceived after intracytoplasmic sperm injection, in vitro fertilization and natural conception. *Hum Reprod.* 20:413–9.

9. Calhoun KC, Barnhart KT, Elovitz MA, Srinivas S. 2011. Evaluating the Association between assisted conception and the severity of preeclampsia. *ISRN Obstet Gynecol.* 928592.

10. Chambers GM, Ledger W. 2014. The economic implications of multiple pregnancy following ART. *Semin Fetal Neonatal Med.* 19:254–61.

11. Clayton HB, Schieve LA, Peterson HB et al. 2006. Ectopic pregnancy risk with assisted reproductive technology procedures. *Obstet Gynecol.* 107:595–604.

12. Connell MT, Szatkowski JM, Terry N et al. 2015. Timing luteal support in assisted reproductive technology: A systematic review. *Fertil Steril.* 103:939.

13. Doyle P, Maconochie N, Beral V et al. 2002. Cancer incidence following treatment for infertility at a clinic in the UK. *Hum Reprod.* 17:2209.

14. Dickey RP, Taylor SN, Lu PY et al. 2002. Spontaneous reduction of multiple pregnancy: Incidence and effect on outcome. *Am J Obstet Gynecol.* 186:77.

15. El-Toukhy T, Khalaf Y, Braude P. 2006. IVF results: Optimize not maximize. *Am J Obstet Gynecol.* 194:322–31.

16. Erez O, Vardi IS, Hallak M, Hershkovitz R, Dukler D, Mazor M. 2006. Preeclampsia in twin gestations: Association with IVF treatments, parity and maternal age. *Journal of Maternal-Fetal and Neonatal Medicine.* 19(3):141–146.

17. Gillet E, Martens E, Martens G, Cammu H. 2011. Prelabour caesarean section following IVF/ICSI in older-term nulliparous women: Too precious to push? *Journal of Pregnancy.* Article ID 362518.

18. Hvidtjørn D, Schieve L, Schendel D, Jacobsson B, Svaerke C, Thorsen P. 2009. Cerebral palsy, autism spectrum disorders, and developmental delay in children born after assisted conception: A systematic review and meta-analysis. *Arch Pediatr Adolesc Med.* 163:72–83.

19. Jackson RA, Gibson KA, Wu YW, Croughan MS. 2004. Perinatal outcomes in singletons following in vitro fertilization: A meta-analysis. *Obstet Gynecol.* 103:551–63.

20. Koivurova S, Hartikainen A-L, Sovio U, Gissler M, Hemminki E, Järvelin M-R. 2003. Growth, psychomotor development and morbidity up to 3 years of age in children born after IVF. *Hum Reprod.* 18:2328–36.

21. La Sala GB, Nucera G, Gallinelli A et al. 2004. Spontaneous embryonic loss following in vitro fertilization: incidence and effect on outcomes. *Am J Obstet Gynecol.* 191:741.

22. Leunens L, Celestin-Westreich S, Bonduelle M, Liebaers I, Ponjaert-Kristoffersen I. 2008. Follow-up of cognitive and motor development of 10-year-old singleton children born after ICSI compared with spontaneously conceived children. *Hum Reprod.* 23:105–11.

23. Luke B, Brown MB, Grainger DA et al. 2009. The effect of early fetal losses on twin assisted-conception pregnancy outcomes. *Fertil Steril.* 91:2586.

24. Lyons D, Wheeler CA, Frishman GN, Hackett RJ, Seifer DB, Haning RV. 1994. Early and late presentation of the ovarian hyperstimulation syndrome: Two distinct entities with different risk factors. *Hum Reprod.* 9(5):792–9.

25. Maheshwari A, Griffiths S, Bhattacharya S. 2011. Global variations in the uptake of single embryo transfer. *Hum Reprod Update.* 17:107–20.

26. McGovern PG, Llorens AJ, Skurnick JH et al. 2004. Increased risk of preterm birth in singleton pregnancies resulting from in vitro fertilization-embryo transfer or gamete intrafallopian transfer: A meta-analysis. *Fertil Steril.* 82:1514.

27. McDonald SD, Han Z, Mulla S, Murphy KE, Beyene J, Ohlsson A. 2009. Preterm birth and low birth weight among in vitro fertilization singletons: A systematic review and meta-analyses. *Eur J Obstet Gynecol Reprod Biol.* 146:138–48.

28. McDonald SD, Han Z, Mulla S, Ohlsson A, Beyene J, Murphy KE. 2010. Preterm birth and low birth weight among in vitro fertilization twins: A systematic review and meta-analyses. *Eur J Obstet Gynecol Reprod Biol.* 148:105–13.

29. Minkoff HL, Berkowitz R. 2005. The myth of the precious baby. *Obstet Gynecol.* 106:607–609.

30. Navot D, Bergh PA, Laufer N. 1992. Ovarian hyperstimulation syndrome in novel reproductive technologies: Prevention and treatment. *Fertil Steril.* 58,249–261.

31. Ness RB, Cramer DW, Goodman MT et al. 2002. Infertility, fertility drugs, and ovarian cancer: A pooled analysis of case-control studies. *Am J Epidemiol.* 155:217.

32. Pandian Z, Marjoribanks J, Ozturk O, Serour G, Bhattacharya S. 2013. Number of embryos for transfer following in vitro fertilisation or intra-cytoplasmic sperm injection. *Cochrane Database Syst Rev.* Issue 7. Art. no.: CD003416.

33. Ponjaert-Kristoffersen I, Bonduelle M, Barnes J et al. 2005. International collaborative study of intracytoplasmic sperm injection-conceived, in vitro fertilization-conceived, and naturally conceived 5-year-old child outcomes: Cognitive and motor assessments. *Pediatrics.* 115:e283.

34. Paulson R. 2020. Pregnancy outcome after assisted reproductive technology. Lockwood CJ (Ed). *UpToDate.* Waltham, MA.

36. Pezeshki K, Feldman J, Stein DE et al. 2000. Bleeding and spontaneous abortion after therapy for infertility. *Fertil Steril.* 74:504.

36. Romundstad LB, Romundstad PR, Sunde A et al. 2006. Increased risk of placenta previa in pregnancies following IVF/ICSI: A comparison of ART and non-ART pregnancies in the same mother. *Hum Reprod.* 21:2353–2358.

37. Schieve LA, Tatham L, Peterson HB et al. 2003. Spontaneous abortion among pregnancies conceived using assisted reproductive technology in the United States. *Obstet Gynecol.* 101:959.

38. Shevell T, Malone FD, Vidaver J et al. 2005. Assisted reproductive technology and pregnancy outcome. *Obstet Gynecol.* 106:1039–1045.

39. Sullivan EA, Chapman MG, Wang YA, Adamson GD. 2010. Population-based study of caesarean section after in vitro fertilization in Australia. *Birth.* 37:3; p184–191.

40. Shushan A, Paltiel O, Iscovich J et al. 1996. Human menopausal gonadotropin and the risk of epithelial ovarian cancer. *Fertil Steril.* 65:13.

41. Terry KL, Willett WC, Rich-Edwards JW, Michels KB. 2006. A prospective study of infertility due to ovulatory disorders, ovulation induction, and incidence of breast cancer. *Arch Intern Med.* 166:2484.

42. van der Linden M, Buckingham K, Farquhar C, Kremer JAM, Metwally M. 2015. Luteal phase support for assisted reproduction cycles. *Cochrane Database Syst Rev.* Issue 7. Art. no.: CD009154.

43. Vermey BG, Buchanan A, Chambers GM, Kolibianakis EM, Bosdou J, Chapman MG, Venetis CA. 2019. Are singleton pregnancies after assisted reproduction technology (ART) associated with a higher risk of placental anomalies compared with non-ART singleton pregnancies? A systematic review and meta-analysis. *BJOG.* 126: 209– 218.

44. Wen SW, Demissie K, Yang Q, Walker MC. 2004. Maternal morbidity and obstetric complications in triplet pregnancies and quadruplet and higher-order multiple pregnancies. *Am J Obstet Gynecol.* 191:254–8.

45. Wen J, Jiang J, Ding C et al. 2012. Birth defects in children conceived by in vitro fertilization and intracytoplasmic sperm injection: A meta-analysis. *Fertil Steril.* 97:1331.

46. Wilson CL, Fisher JR, Hammarberg K et al. 2011. Looking downstream: A review of the literature on physical and psychosocial health outcomes in adolescents and young adults who were conceived by ART. *Hum Reprod.* 26:1209.

Chapter 47

Anemia and Hemoglobinopathies in Pregnancy: (Nutritional Anemia, Sickle Cell Disease, Thalassemia)

INTRODUCTION

- **Nutritional anemia** is the late manifestation of nutrient deficiency that impacts hemoglobin synthesis. Most nutritional anemias are due to inadequate supply of iron, folic acid, and/or vitamin B12. Iron deficiency is the commonest cause of anemia in pregnancy.

> In India, anemia antedates pregnancy, is worsened by the increased demand of pregnancy and blood loss at the time of delivery, and perpetuated by the early occurrence of the next pregnancy (Sharma, 2003).

- India has the dubious honour of being the country with the highest prevalence of anemia in the world (WHO, 2015; Ramachandran and Kalaivani, 2018). With a population of more than a billion, India has the largest number of anemic people in the world, and consequently, the largest number of pregnant anemic women.
- The National Family Health Survey statistics (NFHS-4, 2016) showed that the prevalence of anemia in pregnant women in India was 50 per cent, though other studies have found a prevalence of 80–90 per cent (Agarwal et al., 2006).
- It is estimated that about 20–40 per cent of maternal deaths in India are due to anemia (Upadhyay et al., 2012).
- **Sickle cell disease (SCD)** is the most common hemoglobinopathy in pregnancy and is associated with chronic compensated anemia.
- **Thalassemias** are hemoglobinopathies caused by abnormal globin chain synthesis resulting in a microcytic, hypochromic anemia.

DEFINITION OF ANEMIA IN PREGNANCY

- Anemia is defined by the World Health Organization (WHO, 2015) and ACOG (2008) as follows:
  - Hemoglobin levels of <11 g/dL and hematocrit of <33% in the **first** and **third trimesters**
  - Hemoglobin levels of <10.5 g/dL and hematocrit of <32% in the **second trimester**
  - Hemoglobin levels of <11 g/dL at **1 week postpartum**
  - Hemoglobin levels of <12 g/dL at **8 weeks postpartum**

- The lower value of the definition of anemia in the second trimester is due to the hemodilution of pregnancy. During pregnancy, there is a greater increase in plasma volume than red cell mass. This results in a modest fall in hemoglobin level, causing **physiological anemia** in healthy pregnant women.

Physiological anemia: The biggest discrepancy between plasma and red cell mass happens in the late second and early third trimester, resulting in physiological anemia. This is most common at 28–36 weeks.

CATEGORIES AND TYPES OF ANEMIA

Categories of anemia in pregnancy

The World Health Organization (2011) has defined four categories of anemia in pregnant women as presented in Table 47.1.

Table 47.1   Categories of anemia in pregnant women (WHO, 2011)

Category	Severity of anemia	Hemoglobin level (g/dL)
1	Mild	10.0–10.9
2	Moderate	7.0 – 9.9
3	Severe	<7.0
4	Very severe, decompensated	<4

Types of anemia in pregnancy

The types of anemia in pregnancy are categorised in the box below.

Types of anemia in pregnancy
Nutritional deficiency
- Iron deficiency
- Folic acid deficiency
- Vitamin B12 deficiency
- Dimorphic

Decreased red cell production (non-nutritional causes)
- Bone marrow disorders (aplastic anemia, marrow infiltration)
- Chronic diseases: Tuberculosis, HIV, renal failure, hypothyroidism

Hemorrhagic (due to blood loss)
- Acute (antepartum hemorrhage, postpartum hemorrhage)
- Chronic (hemorrhoids, worm infestation)

Hemolytic (red cell destruction)
- Hereditary hemoglobinopathies
  - Sickle cell disease
  - Thalassemia major
  - Hb variants
- Acquired: Malaria, chronic renal failure

IRON DEFICIENCY ANEMIA (IDA)

- Iron deficiency anemia is the most common type of anemia in pregnancy (Auerbach and Landy, 2020). It develops when dietary iron intake cannot meet iron needs over a period of time, especially during pregnancy, when iron requirements are particularly high.

> **Iron deficiency and anemia**
> Iron deficiency evolves in the following three stages:
> 1. Depletion of stored iron
> 2. Iron-deficient erythropoiesis
> 3. Anemia

- Causes of IDA that are especially pertinent to India are as follows:
  - Insufficient dietary iron due to:
    - Limited resources
    - Vegetarian/vegan diet
  - Defective absorption due to:
    - High levels of phytates (cereals and legumes) in the Indian diet
    - Hyperemesis of pregnancy
  - Increased loss due to:
    - Frequent pregnancies
    - Postpartum blood loss
    - Hookworm infestation
    - Chronic malaria
    - Untreated hemorrhoids

IRON REQUIREMENT IN PREGNANCY

- In pregnancy, iron is mobilised from maternal iron stores. These stores may be already depleted in women living in developing countries. For this reason, **in addition to dietary iron, supplemental iron should be mandatory in pregnant Indian women.**
- A systematic review of the Cochrane Database (Peña-Rosas et al., 2015) supports daily iron and folic acid supplementation and shows that it reduces the risk of maternal anemia and iron deficiency in pregnancy.

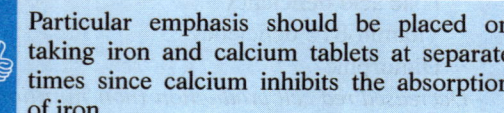
Particular emphasis should be placed on taking iron and calcium tablets at separate times since calcium inhibits the absorption of iron.

- In a singleton pregnancy, the average iron requirement is about 1000 mg for the entire pregnancy of which about 500 mg is used for the expansion of the RBC mass and roughly 300 mg is used for the fetus and placenta. An additional 200 mg of iron is conserved due to amenorrhea of pregnancy. This amount would have otherwise been lost with menstruation.
- The requirement of iron increases mainly in the second half of pregnancy. The requirement becomes 6 mg/day after mid-pregnancy, whereas the requirement is only 1–2 mg/day in the non-pregnant state. Since only 10 per cent of ingested iron is absorbed, the daily intake should be at least 60 mg of elemental iron, especially after 20 weeks' gestation.

- Inhibitors of iron absorption are calcium, milk, phytates (cereals and legumes) and tannins in tea and coffee, while enhancers of iron absorption are ascorbic acid, citric juices, and ferrous iron (Abel et al., 1999).

> **Iron requirement in pregnancy**
> - 0.8 mg/day in the initial 10 weeks of gestation
> - 6 mg/day after mid-pregnancy
>   - 10 per cent of ingested iron is absorbed
>   - Daily intake should be at least 60 mg of elemental iron per day
> - 10 mg/day in the last 10 weeks of gestation (provided by 100 mg of elemental iron per day)
> - Since diet alone cannot provide such large amounts of iron, supplemental iron is a must in pregnancy

EFFECTS OF ANEMIA ON PREGNANCY

Maternal effects

- Mild to moderate anemia is associated with weakness, fatigue, exercise intolerance, palpitations, irritability, and breathlessness. These symptoms respond well to iron supplementation. Severe anemia ($<7\,g/dL$) may be associated with cardiac decompensation and failure.
- Iron deficiency anemia at delivery is associated with an increased risk of adverse maternal and neonatal outcomes. It is important to monitor hemoglobin levels in the third trimester. Correction of anemia, even in late pregnancy, helps prevent these adverse events.
- Adverse maternal outcomes include the following (Scholl, 2005; Drukker et al., 2015):
  - Preterm birth
  - Hypertensive disorders
  - Cesarean section
  - Susceptibility to infection
- Corwin et al. (2003) correlated anemia to an increased risk of postpartum depression.
- Severe anemia (hemoglobin $<7\ g/dL$) increases the risk of maternal mortality (Brabin et al., 2001). A recent study by the WHO (Daru et al., 2018) confirmed that severe antenatal or postnatal maternal anemia (of any type) is associated with **a two-fold increase in mortality** in low- and middle-income countries.

Fetal and neonatal effects

- Iron is required for fetal growth and development (Scholl, 2005).
- Maternal anemia is associated with an increased risk of the following fetal complications (Tunkyi and Moodley, 2018; Rahman et al., 2016):
  - Low birth weight
  - Small-for-gestational age neonates
  - Low iron stores at birth
- Even before anemia manifests itself, iron deficiency, i.e., depletion of iron stores may lead to low birth weight (Pratt and Khan, 2016).

- Nair et al. (2016), in a study from North India, found an association between severe antenatal anemia and **stillbirth** and **perinatal death**.
- Anemia before 30 weeks of pregnancy is also associated with the following conditions in the offspring (Wiegersma et al., 2019):
  - Autism spectrum disorder
  - Attention deficit hyperactivity disorder
  - Intellectual disability

DIAGNOSIS OF IRON DEFICIENCY ANEMIA IN PREGNANCY

Screening for iron deficiency anemia

- **Hemoglobin** estimation is easily performed and is a cost-effective, rapid test. The most accurate method is the cyanomethemoglobin method.

 Every woman should be screened for anemia at the first antenatal visit and again at 28 weeks (NICE, 2016).

- **Peripheral blood smear** is an easy, rapid, and informative investigation that helps to differentiate between iron deficiency and vitamin B12/folate deficiency anemia. Classically, iron deficiency anemia (IDA) exhibits smaller RBCs, which is why it is called *microcytic anemia*. With vitamin B12 or folate deficiency, the RBCs are much larger and hence it is called *macrocytic anemia*.
- **Red cell indices** help identify the type of anemia, and therefore, it is important to test for these indices in anemic women as part of the complete blood count (CBC) (Table 47.2).
  - Mean corpuscular volume (MCV), mean corpuscular hemoglobin (MCH), and mean corpuscular hemoglobin concentration (MCHC) are all decreased in IDA. Red cell distribution width (RDW) is an index of anisocytosis and is generally high in IDA.

 Among the RBC indices, MCV is the first to get reduced and is the most sensitive indicator of IDA.

Table 47.2 Red cell indices in iron deficiency anemia

Red cell indices	Formula	Normal range	Iron deficiency anemia (IDA)
MCV (fL)	Hct/RBC	75–96	Decreased (<80)
MCH (pg)	Hb/RBC	27–33	Decreased
MCHC (g/dL)	Hb/Hct	32–35	Decreased (<30)
RDW			High

Hb, hemoglobin; *Hct*, hematocrit; *MCH*, mean corpuscular hemoglobin; *MCHC*, mean corpuscular hemoglobin concentration; *MCV*, mean corpuscular volume; *RDW*, red cell distribution width

Screening for iron deficiency

- Women who have iron deficiency *without* anemia may benefit from screening for deficiency of iron stores. Women with low iron reserves should be advised measures to replete iron stores. The same factors that can result in iron deficiency anemia also cause low iron stores.

Non-anemic iron deficiency in pregnancy is associated with low birth weight (Pratt and Khan, 2016).

- **Serum ferritin:** Measurement of serum ferritin is considered to be a sensitive test for the diagnosis of iron deficiency with or without anemia. The levels do not change with recent iron intake. Ferritin levels <15 µg/L are diagnostic of iron deficiency, but treatment should only be initiated when levels are <30 µg/L.
- **Serum iron and total iron-binding capacity:** Serum iron (<30 µg/dL) and total iron-binding capacity (TIBC >400 µg/dL) are indicative of iron deficiency but are not as sensitive or specific as ferritin levels.

PREVENTION OF IRON DEFICIENCY ANEMIA IN PREGNANCY

Pre-pregnancy strategies

- In India, the prevalence of low iron stores and iron deficiency anemia in women in the reproductive age group and pregnant women is significant.
- Starting oral supplementation in the pre-pregnancy period is an effective strategy to combat IDA.

 Encouraging adolescent girls and women in the reproductive age group to consume iron supplements for at least three months in a year (60 mg of elemental iron/day) helps reduce the risk of iron deficiency before pregnancy.

Increase in dietary iron

- The Indian diet is packed with grains, legumes, nuts, and seeds. These are high in phytates, which prevent the absorption of minerals like iron, calcium, and vitamin D. The bio-availability of iron from phytate and fibre-rich vegetarian Indian diets is only 5–8 per cent, whereas bio-availability of heme iron from animal food is over 40 per cent (Ramachandran and Kalaivani, 2018).
- Pregnant women should be advised to consume a diet rich in iron, such as green leafy vegetables, sprouts, jaggery, meats, and liver. Overcooking of food should be avoided.

Routine iron supplementation

- Supplementation during pregnancy decreases the prevalence of maternal anemia at delivery.
- WHO guidelines (2018) have recommended the following:
  - Iron supplements should be provided to pregnant women during antenatal visits.
  - Iron supplementation should be started at the first antenatal visit or as soon as the mother can starting tolerating the medication.
  - For countries such as India, where prevalence of anemia is 80–90 per cent in pregnancy, the WHO recommends **daily supplementation of 60 mg elemental iron in the form of ferrous salts along with 400 µg of folic acid** for the following durations:
    - At least six months during pregnancy
    - Three months postpartum

- The Government of India (Ministry of Health) recommends **100 mg of elemental iron (335 mg of ferrous sulphate) and 500 μg of folic acid for at least 100 days from 14 weeks' gestation for all pregnant women.** The tablets of ferrous sulphate and folic acid are supplied free of cost by the Government of India.

> **Instructions for the administration of oral iron supplements**
> - The supplements should be taken early in the morning, on an empty stomach. However, women who may not be able to tolerate this may be asked to take the tablet at least two hours after a meal.
> - Citrus fruit juices (containing vitamin C) help in absorption.
> - Milk, coffee, tea, antacids, and eggs delay absorption.
> - They should not be taken with calcium tablets. Calcium can be taken after a different meal.
> - Nausea/stomach pain/diarrhea may occur, but ease up within two weeks.
> - Constipation may occur, but can be relieved with stool softeners/laxatives.

Other preventive strategies

- **Treating hookworm infestations:** In areas where hookworm infestation is **endemic** (prevalence of 20–30 per cent), deworming is recommended once in the second trimester. Where the

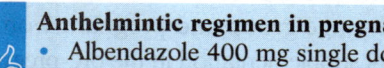

> **Anthelmintic regimen in pregnancy**
> - Albendazole 400 mg single dose
> - Mebendazole 500 mg single dose or 100 mg twice daily for three days

infestation is highly endemic (>50 per cent), deworming should be done once more in the third trimester (Stoltzfus and Dreyfuss, 1998).
- **Chemoprophylaxis of malaria:** In **endemic areas**, pregnant women in their first and second pregnancies should be given curative antimalarials at their first prenatal visit followed by antimalarial prophylaxis according to local recommendations.

TREATMENT OF IRON DEFICIENCY ANEMIA IN PREGNANCY

The choice of therapy depends upon the following factors:
- Severity of anemia
- Gestational age
- Tolerance and compliance

Oral iron therapy

- Treatment with oral iron may take as long as six to eight weeks to completely correct the anemia, and as long as six months to replenish iron stores.

> Women with established iron deficiency anemia should be given 120–200 mg elemental iron daily.

- Women with established iron deficiency anemia should have daily elemental iron increased to 120–200 mg until the Hb concentration rises to normal (Hb 11.0 g/dL or higher). This may require iron tablets/capsules to be taken two to three times daily.
- The mother should be advised on the correct method of intake to optimise absorption (see the box above on *Instructions for the administration of oral iron supplements*).

- A repeat Hb testing is recommended two weeks after commencing treatment for established anemia to:
  - Assess compliance
  - Correct administration
  - Assess response to treatment
- Once the hemoglobin concentration is in the normal range, replacement should continue for at least three more months and until at least six weeks postpartum to replenish iron stores (WHO, 2018; Pavord et al., UK guidelines on the management of iron deficiency in pregnancy, 2019).

 For nausea and epigastric discomfort, alternate day dosing or preparations with lower iron content should be tried. Slow release and enteric-coated forms should be avoided.

Response to therapy

- An increase in the reticulocyte count is used as an indicator of response to iron therapy. Reticulocyte count increases 7–10 days after the start of therapy.
- Hemoglobin level increases by 0.3–1 g/dL per week with adequate replacement.
- Failure to respond to iron therapy should prompt further investigation and may suggest an incorrect diagnosis, coexisting disease, malabsorption (sometimes caused by the use of enteric-coated tablets or concomitant use of antacids), non-compliance, or blood loss (ACOG, 2008).

Choice of preparation

- The most appropriate and effective oral iron therapy is a tablet/capsule containing ferrous salts (Pavord et al., 2019).
  - **Ferrous fumarate:** 210/300 mg (65/100 mg elemental iron) per tablet/capsule
  - **Ferrous sulphate:** 150 mg/200 mg (45 mg/60 mg elemental iron) per tablet/capsule
  - **Ferrous gluconate:** 300 mg (35 mg elemental iron) per tablet/capsule

A large number of other oral iron-containing preparations and nutritional supplements are available. Some enteric-coated, sustained-release preparations such as carbonyl iron, iron polymaltose complex, and ferrous glycine sulphate are also available. These are more expensive but poorly absorbed because they do not release the drug in the duodenum where iron is best absorbed. **These preparations are not superior to the ferrous salts mentioned in this section and are not recommended** (Mehta, 2003; Ruiz-Argüelles, 2007).

- The efficacy of all iron salts mentioned above is similar, and no one preparation is superior to the other.

Parenteral iron therapy

Intramuscular iron therapy

- For years, parenteral iron was administered only by the intramuscular (IM) route.
- Iron dextran or iron sorbitol citrate was given in a dose of 100 mg/day, deep IM in the gluteal region, using the 'Z' technique to avoid staining skin.

- Intramuscular iron is recommended by the Ministry of Health and Family Welfare, Government of India. However, the IM route is no longer preferred for the following reasons:

 **Intramuscular iron therapy** is no longer recommended because it is painful and significantly less effective than the intravenous route.

  – Mobilisation of iron from IM sites is slow.
  – Rise in the hemoglobin concentration is not appreciably faster with IM administration.
  – Intramuscular iron injection also has the following drawbacks:
    - It is poorly absorbed
    - It is painful
    - It stains the buttocks
    - It is associated with the development of gluteal sarcomas

Intravenous iron therapy

- Intravenous (IV) iron therapy has proved safe and effective for use in the second and third trimesters of pregnancy and the

 IV iron is contraindicated in the first trimester of pregnancy.

postpartum period. It should not be administered in the first trimester.
- In a systematic review and meta-analysis, Govindappagari and Burwick (2019) concluded that in pregnancy, IV iron achieved the target Hb more often, had an increased Hb after four weeks and had fewer side effects when compared to oral iron.
- Indications for IV iron include the following:
  – Absolute non-compliance with oral iron therapy
  – Intolerance of oral iron therapy
  – Proven malabsorption
  – Requirement for rapid Hb response (e.g., in the late third trimester)
- Contraindications to IV iron therapy include the following:
  – First trimester of pregnancy
  – History of anaphylactic reaction to parenteral iron
  – Sepsis
  – Abnormal liver function tests
- When compared to oral ferrous salt administration, IV iron raises the Hb faster in pregnant women (Khalafallah et al., 2018; Breymann et al., 2016).
- In calculating the dose of parenteral iron required, the hemoglobin deficit is calculated by subtracting the woman's hemoglobin from the normal level

 In clinical practice, there is no evidence that total doses above 1000 mg of elemental iron are useful (Auerbach, 2020).

(14 g/dL). The total dose is calculated, and 1000 mg is added to replenish the iron stores. The formula for calculating total dose of iron required is given as follows:

Total dose of iron required = 2.4 × pre-pregnancy weight (kg) × hemoglobin deficit (g/dL) + 1000 mg

Intravenous iron preparations

There are a number of intravenous iron formulations approved for use in pregnancy (Table 47.3).

Table 47.3 Intravenous iron dosage preparations, their therapeutic dosages and need for test dose

Drug	Elemental iron concentration (mg/mL)	Administration dose	Test dose
Iron dextran (low molecular weight)	50 mg of elemental iron/mL	• Repeated doses of 100 mg IV/day *or* • Total dose infusion of 1000 mg in 250 mL over 1 hour	• 25 mg given as slow IV push over 5 minutes • Observed for 15 minutes for reaction
Iron sucrose	20 mg iron/mL	Divided doses of 200 mg/day (over 60 minutes) as daily infusions	Only if history of drug allergies
Ferric gluconate complex	12.5 mg iron/mL	125 mg diluted in 100 mL of isotonic saline	Only if history of drug allergies
Iron isomaltoside	100 mg iron/mL	20 mg/kg infused over 15 minutes	Not required
Ferric carboxymaltose complex	50 mg iron/mL	• 20 mg/kg infused over 15 minutes. • Maximum dose of 1000 mg	Not required

IV, intravenous

Allergic and infusion reactions

- Serious adverse events with IV iron are extremely rare, with an estimated frequency of less than 1:200,000 (Wang et al., 2015).
- Women may experience fever, arthralgias, and myalgias, either during the infusion or within 24 hours of administration. This is not an allergic reaction and subsides spontaneously or with paracetamol (Auerbach, 2020).
- Treatment of minor reactions is by temporarily stopping the infusion until the symptoms subside.
- Methylprednisolone (25 mg IV) may be given to women with:
  - History of asthma
  - Persistent tachypnea, tachycardia, wheezing, stridor, or periorbital edema
- A true anaphylactic reaction is rare but must be treated as an emergency.

Blood transfusion

- Blood transfusions are very rarely required. If required, it is usually in situations where rapid improvement in hemoglobin is essential, e.g., women in labour or close to term.
- Indications for blood transfusion include the following:
  - Hemoglobin <5 g/dL at any gestational age
  - Hemoglobin <7 g/dL in the late third trimester
  - Women with severe anemia in labour
  - Severe anemia with decompensation
  - Acute hemorrhage

- Packed cells are used to avoid fluid overload. Transfusion should be given slowly at the rate of 80–100 mL/hour.

MANAGEMENT OF SEVERE ANEMIA DURING LABOUR

- The aim is to deliver the woman vaginally; cesarean section is only for obstetric indications.
- The woman must be in a comfortable position during the first stage of labour.
- Intrapartum management of severe iron deficiency anemia consists of the following:
  - Close monitoring for signs of fluid overload and congestive cardiac failure
  - Oxygen by mask
  - Restriction of IV fluids to decrease the risk of pulmonary edema
  - Sedation and pain relief
  - Delivery by forceps to avoid prolongation of the second stage of labour since the risk of cardiac failure is high in the second stage
  - Active management of the third stage in all cases to prevent excessive blood loss
  - Oxytocics to be administered to prevent third-stage hemorrhage
- Cross-matched blood units should be kept ready in case of emergencies.
- In case of preterm labour, steroids and betamimetics should be used as per standard indications. A patient with severe anemia must be carefully monitored for the risk of pulmonary edema.
- Cardiac failure should be managed with utmost caution as it carries a significant mortality.

 Women with severe anemia (Hb <7 g/dL) are at increased risk of mortality (from cardiac failure and thromboembolism) during the last trimester, during labour, immediately after labour, and during the puerperium.

MANAGEMENT OF SEVERE ANEMIA IN THE PUERPERIUM

- Adequate rest is necessary.
- Iron and folate therapy must be continued until the levels of hemoglobin return to normal and thereafter, for at least three more months to replenish iron stores.
- Prompt identification and energetic treatment of any infections is mandatory.
- The woman should be discouraged from getting pregnant for the next two years at least, and an effective means of contraception must be prescribed.

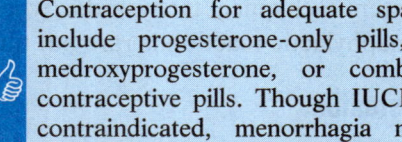 Contraception for adequate spacing may include progesterone-only pills, injection medroxyprogesterone, or combined oral contraceptive pills. Though IUCDs are not contraindicated, menorrhagia may be a problem and may worsen anemia.

- Special care of the newborn is warranted as these babies tend to have low iron stores, and are at increased risks of perinatal morbidity and mortality.

MEGALOBLASTIC ANEMIAS IN PREGNANCY

- Deficiency of folic acid and/or vitamin B12 affects DNA replication in red blood cells, causing derangement of red cell maturation with production of abnormal precursor cells called megaloblasts. The resulting anemia is termed *megaloblastic anemia*.

- Macrocytic anemia with an increased MCV (typically >100 fL) is suggestive of folic acid and/or vitamin B12 deficiency.
- The presence of hypersegmented neutrophils (even 1 neutrophil with ≥5 lobes) is diagnostic of vitamin B12/folic acid deficiency.
- Determining serum levels of vitamin B12 and folic acid helps differentiate between the two. Since the two deficiencies coexist often and the assays are expensive, megaloblastic anemia is usually treated with a combination of folic acid and vitamin B12.

FOLATE DEFICIENCY ANEMIA

- Folic acid, reduced first to dihydrofolic acid and then to tetrahydrofolic acid (folinic acid), is required for cell growth and division. Its requirement increases in pregnancy. Its deficiency affects upto one-third of all pregnancies in developing countries, and is more common in multiple pregnancies.
- Folate deficiency usually coexists with iron deficiency or vitamin B12 deficiency. Folate deficiency is much less common than iron deficiency. Most iron supplements contain folic acid.
- Unlike vitamin B12, folic acid reserves in the body are low, and deficiency is caused by factors such as:
    - Poor dietary intake
    - Prolonged cooking, which destroys vitamins
    - Malabsorption syndromes, worm infestations, and chronic blood-losing conditions such as hemorrhoids, malaria, and other infections
    - Antifolate medications such as anti-epileptics, pyremethamine, and trimethoprim
    - HIV infection

Presenting features of folate deficiency anemia

- Most women with folate deficiency anemia are asymptomatic, especially with milder forms of anemia.
- Pallor, bleeding spots on the skin, hepatosplenomegaly and polyneuropathy can be seen in severe folate deficiency.

Treatment of folic acid deficiency anemia

- **Prophylaxis**
    - 400–500 µg of folic acid/day during pregnancy
    - Diet rich in folic acid
        - Fresh leafy vegetables, legumes, animal proteins
- **Treatment**
    - Oral folic acid tablets 1–5 mg/day (along with iron)
    - Dietary advice
    - Correction of concurrent iron and B12 deficiency

B12 DEFICIENCY ANEMIA

- Vitamin B12 is found in food derived from animal sources such as meat, fish, eggs, and milk. It is not destroyed by cooking.
- The daily requirement of vitamin B12 is 3 μg, which is easily met in a normal diet. However, vegetarians and vegans should take supplementation during pregnancy.
- The causes of vitamin B12 deficiency include the following:
  - Inadequate dietary intake (vegetarians and vegans)
  - Pernicious anemia caused by lack of intrinsic factor
  - Gastrectomy and gastritis
  - Insufficient pancreatic protease (e.g., chronic pancreatitis, Zollinger–Ellison syndrome)
  - Malabsorption syndromes
  - HIV infection
  - Hereditary disorders

Presenting features of B12 deficiency anemia

- Most women with B12 deficiency anemia are asymptomatic, especially with milder forms of anemia.
- In severe vitamin B12 deficiency, the woman presents with profound anemia and macrocytic red cells (MCV >100 fL) with or without varying neurological disturbances. The signs and symptoms of peripheral neuropathy often can be used to differentiate between folic acid deficiency and vitamin B12 deficiency states. General features like loss of appetite, diarrhea, and vomiting are seen.
- Vitamin B12 stores are very large in the body, and it takes years to deplete them. Symptoms therefore take a long time to manifest. If there is iron deficiency anemia concomitantly, vitamin B12 deficiency anemia may get masked.

Treatment of vitamin B12 deficiency anemia

Parenteral B12 (cobalamin)
- Intramuscular or deep subcutaneous cobalamin is administered as follows:
  - 1000 μg (1 mg) every week for 4 weeks
  - Followed by 1000 μg (1 mg) every month for 4–6 months

Oral therapy
- If the anemia is diagnosed early in pregnancy, when there is sufficient time to correct the deficiency, oral B12 is equally effective in women with normal absorption.
- A dose of 1000 μg orally once a day is effective and may be continued for 6–12 months.

EFFECTS OF MEGALOBLASTIC ANEMIA ON PREGNANCY AND THE FETUS

- An association between B12/folate deficiency and miscarriage, preeclampsia, placental abruption, growth restriction, and premature births has been reported but not proven.
- Folate and B12 deficiency are associated with an increased incidence of **neural tube defects**.

DIAGNOSTIC CRITERIA

- Characteristically, in megaloblastic anemia, the Hb is <10 g/dL, the MCV is >100 fL, the MCH is >33 pg, and the MCHC is normal.
- The peripheral blood smear exhibits macrocytic anemia with hypersegmentation of neutrophils along with neutropenia and thrombocytopenia.
- Low serum folate (<3 ng/mL) along with red cell folate level of <150 ng/mL are diagnostic of folate deficiency.
- Vitamin B12 levels in blood of <90 µg/L are diagnostic of B12 deficiency.
- Serum lactic acid dehydrogenase (LDH) and homocysteine levels are elevated in folic acid deficiency.

DIMORPHIC ANEMIA

- Dimorphic anemia refers to anemia that has two different causes acting together, for example, iron deficiency as well as a vitamin B12 deficiency, or iron deficiency and folate deficiency.
- Dimorphic anemia can occur in pregnancy and is not uncommon in women with chronic malnutrition, multifetal pregnancy, or malabsorption.
- The peripheral smear shows macrocytic and microcytic, hypochromic red cells with anisocytosis.
- It is treated by correcting iron and vitamin B12/folate deficiencies.

HEMOGLOBINOPATHIES

SICKLE CELL DISEASE IN PREGNANCY

- Sickle cell disease (SCD) is the most common hemoglobinopathy in pregnancy. Deoxygenation of the abnormal RBCs results in sickling. These permanently damaged RBCs are then removed by the reticuloendothelial system, with the average RBC life span reduced to 17 days (as compared to the normal life span of 120 days). The result is a chronic compensated anemia, with hemoglobin level typically between 6.5 and 9.5 g/dL.
- **Anemia** and **acute painful episodes** (sickle cell crisis) are the most common maternal SCD complications associated with pregnancy, and occur in over 50 per cent of pregnant women with SCD (Vichinsky, 2020).
- Women with SCD are more likely to undergo cesarean delivery, and to experience pregnancy-related complications such as gestational hypertension/preeclampsia, eclampsia, abruption, antepartum bleeding, preterm labour, and fetal growth restriction (Villers et al., 2008).
- Preconceptional counselling and examination of the male partner is essential. If the father is a carrier of the sickle cell trait, then the risk of inheritance of the condition has to be discussed. Prenatal diagnosis must be offered early and pregnancy termination discussed in the event of an affected pregnancy.

- Folic acid supplementation of 5 mg must be initiated preconceptionally and continued throughout pregnancy.

 Iron supplementation should not be given to women with sickle cell disease unless laboratory evidence of iron deficiency is present.

Transfusions during pregnancy

- In a recent meta-analysis (Malinowski et al., 2015), prophylactic transfusions were associated with reduced maternal mortality, reduced painful episodes, and reduced pulmonary complications.
- Exchange or top-up transfusions may be needed in women with a history of perinatal mortality, severe anemia, acute complications, or in preparation for surgery.
- Transfusions should be given under the guidance of a hematologist.
- Blood should be matched for an extended phenotype including complete Rhesus typing (C, D and E) as well as Kell typing.

Monitoring of pregnancy

- Serial scans are recommended to monitor the fetal growth as there is a risk of growth restriction and increased perinatal morbidity.
- Very close observation is needed throughout pregnancy, labour, and the postnatal period, with special emphasis on identifying imminent sickle cell crisis, maintaining hydration, and diagnosing and treating bacteriuria and other infections.

Delivery

- There are no medical contraindications to vaginal delivery. It is clinically safe to await spontaneous labour in the absence of maternal or fetal complications.

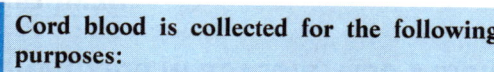 Cord blood is collected for the following purposes:
- Testing the newborn for hemoglobinopathy
- Storing stem cells (if negative for hemoglobinopathy) for future transplantation to a family member affected with SCD

- Induction of labour and cesarean delivery are performed only for obstetrical indications.
- Thromboprophylaxis, adequate hydration, and blood transfusion are recommended in the case of a cesarean delivery.

THALASSEMIA IN PREGNANCY

- Thalassemia is the commonest monogenetic disease in the world. **Thalassemias are hemoglobinopathies caused by abnormal globin chain synthesis resulting in a microcytic, hypochromic anemia.**
- There are two major types—α- and β-thalassemia—resulting from the decreased synthesis of the alpha and beta chains respectively.
  - α-thalassemia **major** is incompatible with extrauterine life.

- β-thalassemia **major** is associated with lifelong transfusion-dependent anemia. Women affected by this condition have an increased rate of infertility. Women with β-thalassemia major should only pursue pregnancy if they have normal cardiac function and have undergone chronic transfusion therapy with iron chelation (ACOG, 2007).
- α- or β-thalassemia **minor** or **trait**
  - Majority of affected adults are asymptomatic
  - Microcytic, hypochromic red cells
  - With or without minor degree of anemia
- The prevalance of thalassemia varies in different ethnic groups and is estimated to be 3–8 per cent in India.
- Within the Indian subcontinent, prevalence varies in different states. High-risk populations can be encountered in different geographical and ethnic groups because of intermarriage and migration.
- If given optimal therapy and care, women with thalassemia (including β-thalassemia major, hemoglobin H disease, and β-thalassemia intermedia, and others) may have a good outcome in pregnancy. In a study from North America and the United Kingdom, Thompson et al. (2013) found that over 70 per cent of pregnancies in women with thalassemia resulted in live births and 88 per cent of live births occurred at full term.

- α-Thalassemia or β-thalassemia minor or trait
  - Majority of affected adults are asymptomatic
  - Microcytic, hypochromic red cells
  - With or without minor degree of anemia
- Thalassemia intermedia
  - Common throughout the world
  - More than one hemoglobin mutation in the same woman
  - For example, sickle cell thalassemia, hemoglobin E (HbE)/β-thalassemia
- β-Thalassemia major
  - Lifelong transfusion-dependent anemia
- α-Thalassemia major
  - Incompatible with extrauterine life

β–Thalassemia minor or trait and pregnancy

- Fertility is not impaired in these women, and pregnancy outcomes are good.
- They may become disproportionately anemic in pregnancy and require iron and folate supplementation in pregnancy.

As both iron deficiency anemia and thalassemias may present as microcytic hypochromnic anemias, the latter may be missed and treated as IDA.

α–Thalassemia minor or trait and pregnancy

- These women may have mild-to-moderate hypochromic, microcytic anemia.
- Affected women tolerate pregnancy well.

Genetic counselling and prenatal diagnosis

- It is possible to identify the mutation in carriers and affected individuals by molecular genetics. These mutations are usually region-specific.
- At-risk couples and those in whom the carrier status is identified should be offered genetic counselling. Prior to prenatal diagnostic testing, the specific mutation in the family should be identified by a blood test.
- A couple who tests positive for the mutation should be offered chorionic villus sampling or amniocentesis for prenatal diagnosis during the pregnancy (see **Chapter 7**, *Prenatal diagnostic testing for genetic disorders*). Prenatal invasive testing is the gold standard for the detection of thalassemia. Although non-invasive prenatal diagnosis is being offered for both α- and β-thalassemia, it needs validation (Vrettou et al., 2018).

References

1. Abel R, Rajaratnam J, Sampathkumar V. 1999. Anemia in pregnancy. Impact of iron, deworming and IEC, RUSHA Dept. Tamil Nadu. CMC Vellore.
2. Agarwal KN, Agarwal DK, Sharma A et al. 2006. Prevalence of anemia in pregnant and lactating women in India. *Indian J Med Res*. 124(2):173-84.
3. American College of Obstetricians and Gynecologists. 2007 (reaffirmed 2018). ACOG Practice Bulletin No. 78. Hemoglobinopathies in pregnancy. *Obstet Gynecol*. 109:229.
4. American College of Obstetricians and Gynecologists. 2008 (reaffirmed 2019). ACOG Practice Bulletin No. 95. Anemia in pregnancy. *Obstet Gynecol*. 112: 201–7.
5. Auerbach M, Landy HJ. 2020. Anemia in pregnancy. Simpson LL (Ed). *UpToDate*. Waltham, MA.
6. Auerbach M. 2020. Treatment of iron deficiency anemia in adults. Mentzer WC (Ed). *UpToDate*. Waltham, MA.
7. Brabin BJ, Hakimi M, Pelletier D. 2001. An analysis of anemia and pregnancy-related maternal mortality. *J Nutr*. 131:604S.
8. Breymann C, Milman N, Mezzacasa A et al. 2016. Ferric carboxymaltose vs. oral iron in the treatment of pregnant women with iron deficiency anemia: An international, open-label, randomized controlled trial (FER-ASAP). *J Perinat Med*.
9. Corwin EJ, Murray-Kolb LE, Beard JL. 2003. Low hemoglobin level is a risk factor for postpartum depression. *Journal of Nutrition*. 133, 4139–4142.
10. Daru J, Zamora J, Fernández-Félix BM et al. 2018. Risk of maternal mortality in women with severe anemia during pregnancy and postpartum: A multilevel analysis. *Lancet Glob Health*. 6:e548.
11. Drukker L, Hants Y, Farkash R et al. 2015. Iron deficiency anemia at admission for labor and delivery is associated with an increased risk for cesarean section and adverse maternal and neonatal outcomes. *Transfusion*. 55:2799.
12. Govindappagari S, Burwick RM. 2019. Treatment of iron deficiency anemia in pregnancy with intravenous versus oral iron: Systematic review and meta-analysis. *Am J of Perinat*. 36, 366–376.
13. Khalafallah AA, Hyppa A, Chuang A et al. 2018. A prospective randomised controlled trial of a single intravenous infusion of ferric carboxymaltose vs. single intravenous iron polymaltose

or daily oral ferrous sulphate in the treatment of iron deficiency anemia in pregnancy. *Semin Hematol.* 55:223.

14. Malinowski AK, Shehata N, D'Souza R et al. 2015. Prophylactic transfusion for pregnant women with sickle cell disease: A systematic review and meta-analysis. *Blood.* 126:2424.

15. Mehta BC. 2003. Ineffectiveness of iron polymaltose treatment of iron deficiency anemia. *J of the Association of Physicians of India.* 51:419–421.

16. Nair M, Choudhury MK, Choudhury SS, Kakoty SD, Sarma UC, Webster P, Knight M. 2016. The IndOSS-Assam Steering Committee. Association between maternal anemia and pregnancy outcomes: A cohort study in Assam, India. *British Medical Journal Global Health.* 1, e000026.

17. NFHS-4. 2016. National Family Health Survey India 2015–2016. 1–8.

18. NICE. 2016. Antenatal care for uncomplicated pregnancies. Clinical Guideline [CG62]. National Institute for Health and Care Excellence. London, UK.

19. Pavord S, Daru J, Prasannan N, Robinson S, Stanworth S, Girling J. 2019. UK guidelines on the management of iron deficiency in pregnancy. *Br J Haematol.*

20. Peña-Rosas JP, De-Regil LM, Garcia-Casal MN, Dowswell T. 2015. Daily oral iron supplementation during pregnancy. *Cochrane Database Syst Rev.* Issue 7. Art. No.: CD004736.

21. Pratt JJ, Khan KS. 2016. Non-anemic iron deficiency – a disease looking for recognition of diagnosis: A systematic review. *European J of Haemat.* 96, 618–628.

22. Rahman M, Abe SK, Rahman MS, Kanda M, Narita S, Bilano V, Ota E, Gilmour S, Shibuya K. 2016. Maternal anemia and risk of adverse birth and health outcomes in low- and middle-income countries: Systematic review and meta-analysis. *Am J of Clinical Nutrition.* 103, 495–504.

23. Ramachandran P, Kalaivani K. 2018. Prevalence of anaemia in India and strategies for achieving sustainable development goals (SDG) target. *Proc Indian Natn Sci Acad.* 84 No. 4. pp. 899–912.

24. Ruiz-Argüelles GJ, Díaz-Hernández A, Manzano C, Ruiz-Delgado GJ. 2007. Ineffectiveness of oral iron hydroxide polymaltose in iron-deficiency anemia. *Hematology.* 12(3):255–256.

25. Scholl TO. 2005. Iron status during pregnancy: setting the stage for mother and infant. *Am J Clin Nutr.* 81: 1218S–22S.

26. Sharma JB. 2003. Nutritional anemia during pregnancy in non-industrialised countries. Studd J (Ed). *In Progress in Obstetrics and Gynecology,* Vol 15. 103–122. Edinburgh: Churchill Livingstone.

27. Stoltzfus R, Dreyfuss ML. 1998. Guidelines for the use of iron supplements to prevent and treat iron deficiency anemia. Geneva: INACG, WHO, UNICEF.

28. Thompson AA, Kim HY, Singer ST et al. 2013. Pregnancy outcomes in women with thalassemia in North America and the United Kingdom. *Am J Hematol.* 88:771.

29. Tunkyi K, Moodley J. 2018. Anemia and pregnancy outcomes: A longitudinal study. *J Matern Fetal Neonatal Med.* 31:2594.

30. Upadhyay RP, Palanivel C, Kulkarni V. 2012. Unrelenting burden of anemia in India: Highlighting possible prevention strategies. *Int J Med and Pub Health.* Vol. 2, Issue 4.

31. Vichinsky EP. 2020. Pregnancy in women with sickle cell disease. Simpson LL, Barss VA (Eds). *UpToDate.* Waltham, MA.

32. Villers MS, Jamison MG, De Castro LM, James AH. 2008. Morbidity associated with sickle cell disease in pregnancy. *Am J Obstet Gynecol.* 199:125.e1.

33. Vrettou C, Kakourou G, Mamas T, Traeger-Synodinos J. 2018. Prenatal and preimplantation diagnosis of hemoglobinopathies. *Int J Lab Hematol.* 40 Suppl 1:74.

34. Wang C, Graham DJ, Kane RC et al. 2015. Comparative risk of anaphylactic reactions associated with intravenous iron products. *JAMA*. 314:2062.

35. Wiegersma AM, Dalman C, Lee BK et al. 2019. Association of prenatal maternal anemia with neurodevelopmental disorders. JAMA Psychiatry.American College of Obstetricians and Gynecologists. 2015. ACOG Practice Bulletin No. 156. Obesity in pregnancy. *Obstet Gynecol*. 126:e112–26.

36. World Health Organization. 2011. Haemoglobin concentrations for the diagnosis of anemia and assessment of severity. Vitamin and Mineral Nutrition Information System. WHO, Geneva.

37. World Health Organization. 2015. The global prevalence of anemia in 2011. WHO, Geneva.

38. World Health Organization. 2018. WHO recommendations: Antenatal care for a positive childbirth experience. WHO, Geneva.

Chapter 48

Infections in Pregnancy

INTRODUCTION

- Pregnant women are as vulnerable to infections as non-pregnant women. However, infections during pregnancy may be associated with exaggerated maternal morbidity and mortality, which may not be seen in a non-pregnant woman.
- Infection in pregnancy is complicated by the fact that it may be transmitted to the fetus in utero or to the neonate during or after childbirth.
- The effect of the infection on the fetus depends on the gestational age at which the infection occurs. In general, infections that occur in the first trimester, when organogenesis is occurring, render the fetus susceptible to congenital anomalies. Some infections are transmitted transplacentally even at later periods of gestation.
- Therapy for antepartum infection is complicated by the concern regarding teratogenicity.
- Transmitted infections are an important cause of fetal and neonatal mortality and contribute significantly to early and later childhood morbidity. The infected neonate may be affected by abnormal growth, developmental anomalies, or multiple clinical and laboratory abnormalities.
- Transmission may occur through the transplacental route, as an ascending infection from the lower genital tract, direct contact after birth, or through breastfeeding (Table 48.1).

Table 48.1 Routes of transmission of infection from mother to fetus

Gestational period	Route of transmission
Antenatal period	• Transplacental • Ascending infection
Intrapartum	• Ascending infection
Neonatal period	• Direct contact • Breastfeeding

IMMUNE RESPONSE TO INFECTION

- **Acute phase of infection**
  - IgM antibodies are produced in response to a new infection.
  - They are produced within 1–2 weeks of the initial infection and eventually decline to undetectable levels.
  - They do not cross the placenta.
  - Diagnosis of current infection in the mother is made by testing for IgM antibodies.
- **Lifelong immunity**
  - IgG antibodies are produced a few weeks after the initial infection.
  - They provide lifelong protection against that specific infection.

- They cross the placenta and provide passive immunity to the fetus.
- The presence of IgG antibodies indicates past infection in the mother.
- **Fetal infection status** may also be confirmed by the presence of IgM antibodies in amniotic fluid or fetal blood. The presence of IgG antibodies in the amniotic fluid or fetal blood is inconclusive since maternal IgG antibodies can cross the placenta.

Interpretation of maternal antibody status

- The distinction between current, recent, and old infections is possible by comparing the absence or presence of IgG and IgM antibodies in the same sample. The interpretation of maternal antibody status is presented in Table 48.2.

Table 48.2   Interpretation of maternal antibody status

Antibody status	Interpretation of infection status
IgM-negative, IgG-negative	• No recent infection • Susceptible to future infection
Only IgM-positive	• Current infection
IgM-positive and IgG-positive	• Recent infection
Only IgG-positive	• Old infection (immune)

TYPES OF INFECTIONS

This chapter will deal with the following common infections that have an impact on maternal/fetal health:

Viral infections

- Herpes simplex virus (HSV)
- Cytomegalovirus (CMV)
- Varicella
- Zika
- Rubella
- H1N1 infection and seasonal influenza
- Parvovirus B19

Infection with SARS-CoV-2 is addressed in **Chapter 49**, *COVID-19 in Pregnancy*. Infection with human immunodeficiency virus (HIV) is dealt with separately in **Chapter 51**, *Management of pregnancy in a woman with HIV (human immunodeficiency virus)*.

Protozoal infection

- Toxoplasmosis
- Malaria

Bacterial infection

- Tuberculosis

VIRAL INFECTIONS

Genital herpes simplex in pregnancy

- Herpes simplex virus type 1 (HSV-1) and herpes simplex virus type 2 (HSV-2) can cause genital herpes in the mother. HSV-1 is responsible for 80 per cent of primary genital herpes infections (Lafferty et al., 2000).

- Herpes simplex infection is one of the most common sexually transmitted diseases.
- Transmission to the neonate depends on the following:
  - Whether the infection is a primary or a recurrent maternal infection
  - Duration of rupture of membranes before delivery
  - Mode of delivery

Maternal infection

Primary infection

- Primary genital infection refers to the first occurrence of HSV infection.
- The primary presentation of HSV infection can be severe, with painful genital ulcers, pruritus, and fever. The woman may develop severe 'splash' dysuria due to the presence of the ulcerated vesicles. The infection may be accompanied by tender inguinal lymphadenopathy and headache.

 Type-specific antibodies to HSV generally develop within the first 12 weeks of primary infection and persist indefinitely (Workowski and Bolan, 2015).

Recurrent infection

Most cases of recurrent infection are caused by HSV-2 (Workowski and Bolan, 2015). The symptoms are milder (due to pre-existing antibodies) and the lesions last for 3–10 days.

Diagnosis of HSV

Diagnosis of HSV infection is based on the following features:
- *Clinical examination reveals* painful vesicles that form ulcers.
- *Viral cultures of fluid from deroofed vesicles* have a sensitivity of approximately 80 per cent during primary HSV infection and 35 per cent during recurrent infection.
- *PCR* is a more sensitive test than viral culture (Wald et al., 2003) and is becoming the preferred test for diagnostic testing in symptomatic patients.
- *Type-specific serologic ELISA tests* are available that accurately distinguish between HSV-1 and HSV-2 antibodies and can be used for diagnosis (ACOG, 2007).

Implications for pregnancy

- *First and second trimester (up to 28 weeks of gestation)*
  - Primary infection in the first trimester is not associated with miscarriage or congenital anomalies (Foley et al., 2014).
- *Third trimester (after 28 completed weeks of gestation)*
  The major significance of herpes infection in the third trimester, especially if it occurs close to labour, is maternal–fetal transmission at the time of delivery.
  - Primary infection: The transmission rate can be up to 40 per cent with primary infection within 6 weeks of delivery (Brown et al., 1991).
  - Recurrent infection: The risk of neonatal transmission at delivery is 0–3 per cent (Prober et al., 1987).

- However, 80 per cent of infected infants are born to mothers with no reported history of HSV infection (ACOG, 2007).

 HSV infection in the third trimester can give rise to neonatal infection, with the risk of transmission greater with a primary rather than a recurrent infection.

Neonatal infection

- Neonatal HSV is a serious condition. It may present in one of the following ways:
  - Neonatal   : Due to intrapartum genital exposure (commonest)
  - Congenital : Due to vertical transmission by hematogenous spread
  - Postpartum : Due to contact with the infected mother
- The sequelae of neonatal HSV may include the following (Whitley et al., 1988):
  - **Mucocutaneous infection**: Skin, eye, and mouth (SEM) disease accounts for approximately 45 per cent of neonatal HSV.
  - **Central nervous system disease:** Approximately one-third of neonatal HSV disease involves the CNS. It may present with seizures (focal or generalised), lethargy, irritability, tremors, poor feeding, temperature instability, and a full anterior fontanel.
  - **Disseminated form:** Approximately 25 per cent of neonatal HSV disease is the disseminated form, which involves multiple organs, including the liver, lungs, adrenals, central nervous system, skin, eye, or mouth. This is fatal in 90 per cent of the cases.

 Neonates with disseminated HSV often present in the first week of life with non-specific signs and symptoms of neonatal sepsis.

Treatment of HSV infection

Primary infection

- Antiviral therapy can decrease the symptoms and consequences of primary infection in the mother.
  - Acyclovir, valacyclovir, and famciclovir are used for the treatment of maternal herpes.
  - Acyclovir is safe in pregnancy. There is no evidence of an increased risk of birth defects with acyclovir, famciclovir, or valacyclovir even if they are used in the first trimester (Pasternak and Hviid, 2010).
  - Recommended dosage schedule
    - Acyclovir 400 mg orally thrice daily for 7–10 days or
    - Valacyclovir 1 g orally twice daily for 7–10 days
- For symptom control
  - Analgesia with paracetamol can be considered along with Sitz baths.
  - Topical lidocaine 2% gel may be used for local pain relief.
  - An indwelling Foley catheter may be required in women with severe dysuria.

Recurrent infection

- Active lesions at the time of delivery have a 0–3 per cent risk of causing neonatal infection.

- If infections are recurrent in pregnancy, suppressive treatment with acyclovir from 36 weeks is recommended.

Prevention of mother-to-child transmission

- Maternal HSV infection transmitted to the infant during delivery can result in major neonatal morbidity and mortality.
- Neonatal infection results from fetal contact with virus shed from infected sites in the cervix, vagina, and the vulva.

Suppressive therapy

- Suppressive therapy given from 36 weeks' gestation reduces the risk of HSV lesions at term and thereby, the need for cesarean section.
- It is used in women with primary active infection in the first or second trimester and recurrent infections in any trimester.

> **Suppressive therapy for recurrent HSV infection in pregnancy**
> Acyclovir 400 mg taken orally three times daily from 36 weeks of gestation reduces HSV lesions at term and thereby, the need for delivery by cesarean section (Watts et al., 2003).

Management of obstetric procedures

- Transabdominal invasive procedures like amniocentesis and fetal blood sampling can be performed in the presence of active genital infection.
- Transvaginal procedures like artificial rupture of membranes and/or instrumental deliveries (Kohelet et al., 2004), and application of fetal scalp electrode should be avoided in women with active lesions.

Management of labour and delivery

Cesarean section

- Cesarean section should be recommended to all women presenting with a primary episode of genital herpes lesions at the time of delivery or within six weeks of the expected date of delivery (Brown et al., 2003).
- This reduces exposure of the fetus to HSV, which may be present in maternal genital secretions.
- Though the risk of neonatal infection increases if membranes have been ruptured for more than four hours, cesarean is still recommended in these cases.

Vaginal delivery

- Vaginal delivery should be avoided in the presence of primary herpes lesions at the time of delivery.
- Vacuum or forceps delivery is avoided to prevent neonatal transmission in asymptomatic women with a history of HSV infection.
- Vaginal delivery may be offered to women with a recurrent herpes infection due to the very small risk (0–3 per cent) of transmission to the neonate.

Care of the neonate

- If a cesarean section has been performed
  - The neonate is at low risk of infection
  - No active treatment is required, nor do swabs need to be collected
- If a vaginal delivery has occurred in the presence of a primary infection
  - Swabs should be sent for PCR
  - Empirical treatment with intravenous acyclovir (20 mg/kg every 8 hours) should be initiated until evidence of active infection is ruled out (Foley et al., 2014)

Postpartum management

- Thorough handwashing is recommended if the mother or anyone who handles the newborn has HSV lesions.
- Breastfeeding is contraindicated only if the woman has active lesions on her breast, which is quite rare.

Rubella

- Rubella (or German measles) is caused by an RNA virus that is transmitted through respiratory droplets.
- Infection usually occurs in school-going children living in crowded areas.
- The incubation period is 12–19 days.
- Although rubella is a mild infection in older children and adults, it can have potentially devastating effects on the developing fetus.

Maternal infection

- Approximately 25–50 per cent of infections with the rubella virus are asymptomatic and go unnoticed (Riley, 2019).
- Symptoms consist of fever, malaise, lymphadenopathy, and a rash.
- The rash starts on the face and extends to the trunk and extremities.
- Conjunctivitis, thrombocytopenia, and neuritis can occur.
- The affected woman is infectious during viremia, which starts a week prior to symptoms and lasts for 5–7 days after the onset of the rash.

Fetal infection: Congenital rubella syndrome (CRS)

- The rubella virus spreads through the vascular system of the developing fetus after infecting the placenta.
- Rubella infection can have devastating effects on the developing fetus, resulting in miscarriage, fetal infection, stillbirth, or fetal growth restriction.
- Congenital infection can affect almost all organs of the fetus, but infection rates among fetuses depend on the weeks of gestation (Table 48.3).
- The earlier the gestational age of infection, the more severe are the effects. The risk of fetal infection is highest in the first and third trimesters. **However, congenital defects are**

Table 48.3   Clinical features of congenital rubella syndrome

Clinical features	Comments
Sensorineural hearing loss	• Most common defect
Eye defects	• Cataract • Glaucoma • Retinitis • Microphthalmia

Cardiac lesions	• Most common
	  – Patent ductus arteriosus
	  – Branch pulmonary artery stenosis
	• Other lesions
	  – Pulmonary valvular stenosis
	  – Aortic valve stenosis
	  – Ventricular septal defect
	  – Tetralogy of Fallot
	  – Coarctation of the aorta

Neurological defects	• Microcephaly • Cerebral palsy • Intellectual disability
Hepatobiliary system	• Hepatosplenomegaly and jaundice
Growth disorder	• Fetal growth restriction
Extended rubella syndrome	• Type I diabetes or panencephalitis in the second decade of life

almost always restricted to infection that occurs before 16 weeks of gestation (Miller et al., 1982). After 20 weeks, there are no congenital defects due to rubella infection. Infection at ≥36 weeks may result in fetal growth restriction (Table 48.4).

• McIntosh and Menser (1992), in a fifty-year follow-up of CRS, found that some neonates may have no clinical features at birth but may develop type I diabetes or panencephalitis in the second decade of life. This is known as the **extended rubella syndrome**.

Diagnosis of rubella infection

Enzyme-linked immunoassays (ELISAs) are sensitive, easy to perform, and measure rubella-specific IgM and IgG.

Maternal infection

• Serum should be obtained within 7–10 days of the onset of the rash and repeated two to three weeks later.

Table 48.4   Risk of infection and congenital defects based on gestational age

Gestational age (weeks)	Risk of infection (%)	Risk of congenital defect (%)
<11	80	100
13–16	50	35 (sensorineural deafness only)
>16	25	0–1
>36	100	Only fetal growth restriction

- Acute rubella infection is diagnosed by the following features:
  - The presence of rubella-specific IgM
  - A four-fold rise in IgG titer between serum specimens obtained two weeks apart

Fetal infection (prenatal diagnosis)

- Polymerase chain reaction (PCR) has been shown to accurately diagnose infection in the fetus (Tanemura et al., 1996).
- The test can be used on chorionic villi samples (CVS), fetal blood, and amniotic fluid (amniocentesis). Though diagnosis made from fetal blood sampling is most accurate, CVS can be obtained much earlier in gestation (10–12 weeks).
- Ultrasound diagnosis of a rubella-affected fetus is difficult. Cardiac lesions and cataracts can potentially be identified. Fetal growth restriction may also be diagnosed in the third trimester.

Prevention of rubella infection

- To prevent the outbreak of rubella, it is currently recommended that all children be vaccinated with live attenuated rubella vaccine. The vaccination confers almost 95 per cent immunity.
- The first dose is given at 12–15 months and the second dose is given one month later.
- Antibody levels remain elevated for as long as 20 years after the vaccination.

Documentation of rubella immunity and immunisation of non-immune women

- Routine testing for the mother's immune status by testing for rubella IgG antibodies at the booking visit is good clinical practice. The interpretation of the immune status is presented in Table 48.5. A woman who is both IgM- and IgG-negative is susceptible to future infection and should receive **postpartum immunisation**.

 Inadvertent vaccination just prior to pregnancy or during pregnancy does not warrant termination of pregnancy since the risk of fetal infection is negligible (Keller–Stanislawski et al., 2014).

- All young women of reproductive age who are rubella IgG-negative should be vaccinated and should avoid pregnancy for 1–3 months after vaccination.
- Rubella vaccination **should not be administered to pregnant women** since it is a live attenuated vaccine. However, it may be administered in the postpartum period to a woman who is not immune.

Table 48.5   Interpretation of rubella immune status

Antibody status	Interpretation
IgM-negative, IgG-negative	• No recent infection • No immunity • Susceptible to future infection • Immunisation advised (prior to pregnancy or postpartum)
IgM-positive, IgG-negative or -positive	• Recent infection
IgM-negative, IgG-positive	• Past vaccination/infection • Immune to future infection

IgG, immunoglobulin G; *IgM*, immunoglobulin M

Management of rubella infection in pregnancy

- Maternal rubella infection does not require any specific treatment other than supportive therapy for the fever. Most women are not even aware that they had the infection.
- The main concern is the risk of congenital rubella syndrome and decision regarding termination of pregnancy.
- In the event of suspected exposure to rubella, IgG and IgM antibodies should be checked for (Table 48.5).
- If recent maternal infection is diagnosed by positive serology, further management depends on gestational age.
  - *Gestational age <16 weeks*
    - Risk of congenital rubella syndrome (CRS) is high
    - The mother should be counselled and offered termination of pregnancy
  - *Gestational age between 16–20 weeks*
    - Risk of sensorineural deafness present
    - Counsel for prenatal diagnosis of infection
    - Discuss termination of pregnancy
  - *If >20 weeks, risk of CRS very low*
    - The mother should be reassured
    - Serial scans for FGR are performed
    - The fetus is evaluated by ultrasonography
  - *If late third trimester or in labour*
    - Follow-up
    - No congenital defect expected in the neonate

Cytomegalovirus (CMV) infection in pregnancy

- Cytomegalovirus (CMV) is a commonly occurring DNA herpesvirus that presents with a wide variety of clinical manifestations. It is the most common congenital viral infection, with a prevalence of approximately 0.5 per cent in the newborn.
- Congenital human CMV infection is the leading infectious cause of intellectual disability and sensorineural deafness.
- CMV is transmitted by direct person-to-person contact, especially with children younger than 3 years of age.
- It may also be transmitted by contact with infected nasopharyngeal secretions, urine, saliva, semen, cervical and vaginal secretions, breast milk, tissue, or blood.
- CMV can be transmitted to infants via the transplacental route (most common), through contact with maternal genital secretions during delivery, or through breast milk.

 Congenital human CMV infection is the leading infectious cause of intellectual disability and sensorineural deafness.

Maternal infection

- Since it is a very common infection, seroprevalence of CMV increases with age, ranging from 50–100 per cent, depending upon geographic area and socioeconomic status (Sheffield and Bopanna, 2019).

- The infection persists in the latent form with periodic reactivation.
- **IgG antibodies do not protect against reinfection or reactivation of infection.**
- Infection in adults is asymptomatic in 90 per cent of individuals, though some may develop fever, lymphadenopathy, and pharyngitis.

> **Primary infection** during pregnancy is associated with a 40 per cent risk of fetal infection. **Recurrent infection/reactivation** is associated with a much lower risk of fetal infection (<1 per cent).

Diagnosis of maternal infection

- In clinical practice, screening for CMV is most often done in pregnancy when a fetal anomaly suggestive of congenital CMV infection is detected on routine ultrasound examination.
- Diagnosis of primary infection is established by looking for evidence of seroconversion in pregnancy as detailed in Table 48.6 (Lazzarotto. 2004).
- The **avidity index** helps to differentiate acute from chronic infection (Leruez–Ville et al., 2013). This is based on the fact that antibodies bind less avidly to antigens during the acute stages (*low avidity*) than in chronic stages of infection (*high avidity*).

Congenital infection

- Congenital human cytomegalovirus infection is the leading infectious cause of intellectual disability and sensorineural deafness (Revello and Gerna, 2004).
- Approximately 25 per cent of pregnant women with primary infection will transmit it to their fetus (Picone et al., 2013).

> The majority of women with primary CMV diagnosed before 20 weeks' gestation will deliver an unaffected infant.

- CMV is transmitted to infants most commonly via transplacental infection. Though the neonate can be infected by contact with maternal genital secretions during delivery or

Table 48.6   Interpretation of antibody status and avidity index in suspected CMV infection

Serum antibody	Timing of antibody response	Interpretation
CMV IgM	• Appears within 2 weeks of primary infection • Persists for 3–4 months after primary infection • **May persist at low levels for many years**	• Primary infection, reinfection or reactivation
CMV IgG	• Appears within 2–3 weeks of primary infection • Persists lifelong • 4-fold rise indicates infection	• Seroconversion confirms diagnosis • IgG levels may be boosted by reinfection or reactivation
CMV IgG avidity	• **Low avidity IgG** indicates infection within the past 2–4 months • **High avidity IgG** indicates infection more than 6 months ago	• Differentiates primary infection from reactivation or reinfection • Useful when there is low IgM and +ve IgG with no previous sample to compare with for seroconversion

through breast milk, the resulting infection is asymptomatic and not associated with severe sequelae.

- The risk of intrauterine transmission is **highest in the third trimester** (40 per cent). However, there is a significantly higher risk of ultrasound-detected abnormalities when maternal infection occurs during the preconceptional or periconceptional period and in the first trimester.
- 90 per cent of infants with congenital CMV infection will have no manifestations at birth.
- 10 per cent of infants will exhibit some or all of the following clinical manifestations of congenital CMV at birth:
    - Ventriculomegaly/hydrocephalus
    - Microcephaly
    - Periventricular leukomalacia
    - Cystic abnormalities in the brain
    - Sensorineural hearing loss
    - Chorioretinitis
    - Hepatosplenomegaly
    - Purpuric skin eruption
    - Jaundice
    - Petechiae
    - Fetal growth restriction
    - Inguinal hernia
- Blood tests help confirm hepatitis, hemolytic anemia, thrombocytopenia, and hyperbilirubinemia.

Diagnosis of congenital infection

- As maternal CMV infection is mostly asymptomatic, congenital CMV infection is suspected only when there are abnormal ultrasound findings during an antenatal scan.
- Ultrasound abnormalities (see box) predict symptomatic congenital infection in only 35 per cent of cases (Guerra et al., 2008).
- Though fetal magnetic resonance imaging (MRI) may be used as an adjunct to confirm the diagnosis, it is not routinely used.

Ultrasound findings in congenital CMV infection may include the following:

- Symmetric fetal growth restriction (FGR)
- Oligohydramnios/polyhydramnios
- Hydrops
- Pleural effusion
- Ventriculomegaly/microcephaly
- Hyperechogenic bowel
- Periventricular calcifications
- Placental enlargement

Prenatal diagnosis of congenital CMV infection

- Following a diagnosis of maternal infection, serial ultrasonography should be performed every two weeks to detect fetal abnormalities. Abnormal findings on ultrasound should prompt further testing with amniocentesis.
- Amniotic fluid is tested by polymerase chain reaction (PCR) for CMV DNA and is the preferred diagnostic approach for identifying an infected fetus.

- It takes 6–8 weeks for placental infection and replication, transmission to the fetus, and excretion into amniotic fluid. Therefore, amniocentesis is most sensitive when done after 20 weeks of gestation and at least six weeks after the suspected maternal infection (Enders et al., 2001).

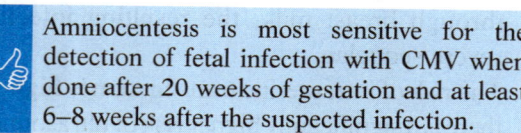 Amniocentesis is most sensitive for the detection of fetal infection with CMV when done after 20 weeks of gestation and at least 6–8 weeks after the suspected infection.

- Although infection before 20 weeks' gestation is associated with a minimal risk of the fetus being infected, women may choose to terminate the pregnancy if they find that the fetus is infected because of the concern about long-term sequelae.

Treatment of cytomegalovirus infection in pregnancy

- The use of antiviral drugs for treatment of CMV infections is rarely indicated in immunocompetent pregnant women since they do not decrease perinatal transmission (Sheffield and Boppanna, 2019).

 Treatment of symptomatic neonates with gancyclovir for 6 weeks has been proven to prevent late-onset hearing loss (Kimberlin, 2003).

- Pregnant couples must be counselled in depth about the extent of CMV infection and risk of neurological sequelae.

Neonatal management of suspected congenital CMV infection

- All neonates at risk of congenital CMV infection should be assessed and investigated by a neonatologist after delivery.
- Investigations to be done before three weeks of age are as follows:
  - CMV culture or PCR of urine or saliva samples for CMV IgM
  - Complete blood examination and liver function tests
  - Central nervous system imaging
  - Ocular examination and newborn hearing screen
- Treatment of symptomatic neonates with ganciclovir for 6 weeks has been proven to prevent late-onset hearing loss (Kimberlin, 2003).

 Role of routine antenatal screening for CMV
It is not currently possible to accurately determine which pregnancies are likely to result in the birth of an infected infant. There is also no way to determine which infected infants will have serious sequelae. Therefore, routine serologic screening of pregnant women for CMV is not recommended (ACOG, 2015).

Seasonal influenza and H1N1 infection

- Influenza, also known as 'the flu', is an infectious respiratory disease caused by an influenza virus. Commonly, influenza virus A (which includes H1N1 and H3N2) and influenza virus B are implicated in seasonal influenza and pandemics.

- Symptoms can be mild to severe and include high fever, runny nose, sore throat, muscle and joint pain, headache, coughing, and fatigue.
- Pneumonia may be the result of the primary viral infection or a superimposed bacterial infection. This complication of influenza may lead to respiratory distress. Diffuse bilateral infiltrates may be seen on chest X-ray. Signs of pneumonia include coarse rales and rhonchi, wheezing, dyspnea, and tachypnea.

 Superimposed bacterial pneumonia typically occurs up to 14 days after symptoms of influenza have resolved.

Maternal consequences of influenza

- Pregnant and postpartum women are at increased risk of influenza and its sequelae. The risk increases with increasing maternal age, exposure in the third trimester, and underlying medical condition (Ramakrishna et al., 2012; Koul et al., 2016).
- The greatest morbidity and mortality were observed with the H1N1 pandemic in 2009.
- Pregnant women are more susceptible to the infection due to the normal physiologic changes that occur during pregnancy including:
  - Increased heart rate
  - Increased oxygen consumption
  - Decreased lung capacity
  - Suppression of maternal cell-mediated immunity
- **Preterm birth:** The risk of preterm birth increases in severely ill pregnant women. Close to 65 per cent of severely affected women hospitalised for pandemic influenza A (H1N1) delivered preterm in a study conducted by Newsome et al. (2011).
- **Morbidity:** Influenza in pregnant women leads to a more severe clinical course compared with non-pregnant women. The need for ICU admission, mechanical ventilation, and dialysis for acute kidney injury is increased in pregnancy.
- **Mortality:**
  - Maternal mortality rates observed in most Indian studies are higher than those reported in other countries. In the 2009 H1N1 pandemic, mortality rates varied from 70 per cent in Rajasthan (Mathur et al., 2013) to 52.6 per cent in a study from South India (Ramakrishna et al., 2012). The mortality was found to be 25 per cent in a tertiary care centre in South India (Pramanick et al., 2011).
  - The mortality rate was reportedly higher in women in their third trimester (80 per cent) as compared to those admitted in early pregnancy (63 per cent) (Mathur et al., 2013).
  - Severity of disease, need for invasive ventilation, and dialysis were associated with a poor outcome.

Fetal consequences of influenza

- The fetal effects of influenza and influenza-like respiratory illness have not been well documented.

- Some studies have associated influenza with congenital anomalies. Maternal febrile hyperthermia may be the cause for the occurrence of certain anomalies like neural tube defects.
- Severely ill women who had the 2009 H1N1 influenza during pregnancy were found to be more likely to have preterm birth and low-birth-weight/growth-restricted babies (Newsome et al., 2011).

Prevention

- Vaccination with the **inactivated** influenza vaccine or quadrivalent recombinant influenza vaccine is strongly recommended for all pregnant women (ACOG Committee Opinion, 2018) during the influenza season.

 Influenza vaccination has been shown to decrease the risk of influenza and its complications among pregnant women and their infants up to six months of age (ACOG, 2018).

- Internationally available vaccines for the control of seasonal influenza are **safe and efficacious in pregnant women** (Vaccines against influenza – WHO position paper, 2012).
- In a randomised blinded trial conducted in Bangladesh among 340 pregnant women in the third trimester, maternal influenza vaccination was found to result in a 36 per cent reduction in febrile respiratory illness among mothers and a 63 per cent reduction in respiratory illness in their infants (Zaman et al., 2008).
- Influenza vaccine **may be given in any trimester** (Ding et al., 2017). Annually, a new batch of vaccines is released that is effective against the previous year's strains. Since influenza season usually starts in October, this is usually the time that the new vaccine becomes available.

 Quadrivalent inactivated influenza vaccine or recombinant influenza vaccine usually contains four killed influenza virus strains: two strains of influenza A (H1N1, H3N2) and two strains of influenza B.

Treatment

- Since pregnant and postpartum women are at a high risk of morbidity and mortality, the diagnosis of seasonal influenza should be made clinically without waiting for results of diagnostic testing.
- **Oseltamivir** is the antiviral drug of choice because of its systemic absorption and the greater clinical experience with using this drug in pregnancy.
- Dosage of oseltamivir
  - **Prophylaxis** for women who have been exposed to the infection
    - Oseltamivir 75 mg once daily orally for 7 days after exposure
  - **Treatment** of influenza
    - Oseltamivir 75 mg twice daily orally for 5 days
- Hyperthermia should be avoided with the administration of paracetamol as required.

Varicella (chickenpox) in pregnancy

- Chickenpox is caused by the varicella-zoster virus (VZV). VZV is a DNA virus from the herpesvirus family.
- It is transmitted as a droplet infection and by direct personal contact. The incubation period for varicella is 10–21 days.
- The primary infection is characterised by malaise, tiredness, fever, and an itchy rash. The rash evolves into a maculopapular rash which becomes vesicular and crusts over before healing. Adults are at risk of more severe disease and have a higher risk of complications as compared to children.
- The person is considered infectious 48 hours before the rash appears and until the vesicles crust over.
- Recovery from primary varicella infection usually provides immunity for life (SOGC, 2012).
- VZV stays dormant in the sensory nerve ganglia as a latent infection. Reactivation of latent infection causes herpes zoster (shingles).

Herpes zoster in pregnancy
Herpes zoster results from reactivation of VZV that has been dormant in sensory nerve ganglia. It presents as localised painful vesicles along a sensory nerve dermatome. Maternal herpes zoster infection is not associated with a significant risk of adverse effects on the fetus.

Maternal risks of varicella infection

- Varicella is a disease of children. Less than 2 per cent of reported cases of varicella infections occur among adults. However, 25 per cent of all VZV-related mortality occurs in adults, placing pregnant women at particular risk (Marin et al., 2007).
- In adults, varicella-related complications include pneumonia, hepatitis, encephalitis, and very rarely, death.
- **Varicella pneumonia** is the most common clinical manifestation of complicated varicella infection in pregnancy. Pneumonia occurs in up to 10–20 per cent of pregnant women with chickenpox (ACOG, 2015) and usually develops within one week of the rash. The clinical course is unpredictable and may rapidly progress to hypoxia and respiratory failure (Smego and Asperilla, 1991).

Pneumonia associated with chickenpox is more common in pregnancy and can lead to maternal mortality.

Diagnosis of maternal infection

- The diagnosis is clinical and is based on the classical appearance of the lesions. Laboratory testing is almost never required.
- In cases of doubt, varicella virus can be isolated from scrapings from the lesions by culture or fluorescent antibody testing.

Pregnant women who have chickenpox must be advised to avoid contact with other pregnant women and neonates until the lesions have crusted over. This is usually about five days after the onset of the rash.

Fetal and neonatal risks of varicella infection

- The risk of spontaneous miscarriage does not appear to be increased with varicella infection in the first trimester (RCOG, 2015).
- Women who contract chickenpox before 28 weeks have a small risk (0.5–1.5 per cent) of their fetus developing congenital varicella syndrome.
- **Congenital varicella syndrome (CVS)** has a mortality rate of 30 per cent in the first few months of life, and the infant has a 15 per cent risk of developing herpes zoster in the first four years of life (Lamont et al., 2011). It is characterised by one or more of the following:

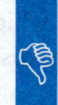

> Since the risk of congenital varicella syndrome is very low (0.5–1.5 per cent), termination of pregnancy is not warranted and need not be offered unless definitive ultrasound signs of CVS are seen.

  - Dermatomal skin scarring
  - Eye defects
    - Microphthalmia
    - Chorioretinitis
    - Cataracts
  - Limb hypoplasia
  - Neurological abnormalities
    - Microcephaly
    - Cortical atrophy
    - Intellectual disability
    - Dysfunction of bowel and bladder sphincters

> **Prenatal diagnosis of congenital varicella syndrome**
> Targeted ultrasound done at least five weeks after the maternal infection may identify microcephaly, limb hypoplasia, or fetal growth restriction. Amniotic fluid or a fetal blood sample may be used for PCR testing for VZV DNA.

- **Neonatal infection** results from maternal infection near or during the delivery (transplacental or ascending vaginal route) or immediately postpartum (direct contact).
  - Neonatal mortality is as high as 25 per cent.
  - **Severe neonatal chickenpox is most likely to occur if the infant is born within seven days of the onset of the mother's rash or if the mother develops the rash up to seven days after delivery, when cord blood VZV IgG is low.**
  - It is advisable to avoid elective delivery until seven days after the onset of maternal rash to allow for the fetus to develop immunity by passive transfer of antibodies from mother to child (ACOG, 2015).

Management of varicella in pregnancy

Management of varicella in pregnancy includes postexposure prophylaxis, treatment of active varicella, and treatment of the neonate.

Postexposure prophylaxis

- A pregnant woman with an unknown immune status is significantly exposed if she has a household contact, face-to-face contact with an index case for five minutes, or direct contact for an hour or longer with an infectious person inside an enclosed space (Riley, 2019a).

> Varicella vaccine is **not recommended** in pregnancy. However, no cases of CVS have been reported after inadvertent vaccination in pregnancy, and therefore, pregnancy termination should not be offered for that reason (SOGC, 2012).

- The woman should be offered serum testing for varicella IgM and IgG. If she is IgG-positive, it implies that she is already immune. If the IgG is negative or unavailable within 96 hours from exposure, varicella zoster immunoglobulin (VZIG) should be administered (SOGC, 2012).
- Passive immunisation with VZIG reduces the risk of varicella infection and also reduces the severity of infection in those who develop chickenpox.
- VZIG is effective when given up to 10 days after contact. However, due to the fact that VZIG is not manufactured in India, this option is not available to most women.

Management of active varicella infection

- Uncomplicated varicella infection is treated with oral acyclovir:
  - 800 mg five times a day for 7 days
  - Most effective if started within 24 hours of developing vesicles
  - Leads to faster healing of skin lesions and a shorter duration of fever
  - Appears to be safe in pregnancy (ACOG, 2015)
- Varicella pneumonia is associated with 40 per cent mortality if untreated. With **intravenous acyclovir**, the mortality rate reduces to 14 per cent (Smego and Asperilla, 1991).
- The recommended dosage of IV acyclovir is 10 mg/kg every eight hours.
- Though the drug crosses the placenta, there is no evidence that it reduces congenital varicella syndrome.

Treatment of the neonate

- Neonates born to mothers who contract chickenpox within five days before to two days after delivery have the greatest risk of developing severe disease and may have a poor outcome.
- Infants who develop varicella within the first two weeks of life should be treated with **intravenous acyclovir** (ACOG, 2015).
  - 30 mg/kg per day in 3 divided doses for 10 days
- Neonatal ophthalmic examination is essential.

Parvovirus B19 in pregnancy

- Parvovirus B19 causes *erythema infectiosum* in children. Most infections in immunocompetent adults are mild. The infection may present with a reticular rash on the trunk and arthralgia. Approximately 20 per cent of infected individuals are asymptomatic.

- Maternal parvovirus B19 infection may occur in 50 per cent of women who have an infected family member. The risk is lower (20–50 per cent) if the mother is in close contact with toddlers or children in a classroom.

Effect on pregnancy

- The rates of mother-to-fetus transmission after parvovirus B19 infection range from 17–33 per cent (Gratacos et al., 1995).
- Most cases of fetal infection resolve spontaneously with no adverse outcomes.
- However, there is a 15 per cent chance of pregnancy loss if the infection occurs before 20 weeks' gestation and 2.3 per cent risk after 20 weeks (Crane, 2002).
- Congenital anomalies (craniofacial/neurological/eye) are rarely reported.
- The most serious fetal outcome is **non-immune hydrops fetalis** due to fetal aplastic myocarditis, or chronic renal failure. Parvovirus B19 infection contributes to 18–27 per cent of non-immune hydrops in pregnancy (Markenson and Yancey, 1998).

 Parvovirus B19 infection is one of the leading infectious causes of non-immune hydrops. It usually manifests within eight weeks of maternal infection.

Diagnosis

- If there is clinical suspicion or recent known exposure, a maternal serological screening for IgM and IgG is essential (ACOG, 2015).
- An IgM-positive with IgG-positive or -negative test result is suggestive of recent infection. If only IgG immunoglobulin is present, it confirms established immunity, in which case, fetal infection will not occur.
- In the presence of fetal hydrops, infection by parvovirus B19 is confirmed or ruled out by testing for DNA in amniotic fluid obtained by amniocentesis.

Management of fetal hydrops due to parvovirus B19 infection

- Once fetal infection is diagnosed, the primary management consists of the following measures:
  - Middle cerebral artery (MCA) Doppler to assess for the presence of fetal anemia (Hernandez-Andrade et al., 2004)
  - Fetal blood sampling to assess fetal hemoglobin and reticulocyte count (usually just prior to intrauterine transfusion)
  - Intrauterine transfusion, if necessary
  - Delivery, if the fetus is term or near term
- Long-term prognosis is good after intrauterine transfusion.

Treatment of parvovirus B19 infection

- There is no known antiviral treatment for this condition.
- The infection is usually self-limiting, but a careful watch must be kept for the development of non-immune hydrops for 8–12 weeks after a confirmed acute infection.

Zika virus in pregnancy

- Zika virus (ZIKV) is a mosquito-borne flavivirus that was first identified in humans in 1952. The bite of the *Aedes* mosquito primarily transmits Zika virus.
- Zika virus is also known to be transmitted in the following ways:
  - From mother to fetus during pregnancy
  - Through sexual contact
  - Through transfusion of blood and blood products
  - Through organ transplantation

 Since Zika virus can be transmitted sexually, the use of condoms or abstinence is advised for three months in case either partner has been exposed to Zika virus (ACOG, 2019).

Maternal symptoms

- 20–25 per cent of women affected by Zika virus will have symptoms of the infection.
- Clinical infection is confirmed by the presence of two or three of the following symptoms and signs:
  - Low-grade fever (37.8–38.5°C)
  - Pruritic rash on the face, trunk, extremities, palms, and soles of the feet
  - Arthralgia (notably in the small joints of the hands and feet)
  - Non-purulent conjunctivitis
  - Myalgia, headache, retro-orbital pain
  - Extreme exhaustion
- Guillain-Barré syndrome has been associated with Zika virus infection. This was particularly noted during the recent epidemic in Brazil (de Oliveira et al., 2017).

Fetal risks

- Maternal infection affects the placenta, causing injury. After the Zika virus infects the placenta, it replicates there and disrupts the fetoplacental barrier.
- Vertical transmission may occur in any trimester and happens in both symptomatic and asymptomatic mothers.
- Though the risk for sequelae in the fetus and newborn is most with first- and second-trimester maternal infection, third-trimester infection has also been known to result in serious sequelae (Cauchemez et al., 2016).
- The congenital Zika syndrome (CZS) is caused by the neurotropic action of ZIKV. A recent systematic review (Krauer et al., 2017) confirmed ZIKV as a cause of congenital brain abnormalities.
- Even if the maternal symptoms are mild, ZIKV infection during pregnancy harms the fetus and is associated with fetal death, fetal growth restriction, and a spectrum of central nervous system abnormalities, the most prominent being **microcephaly**. More recent studies have described craniofacial disproportion, specific brain abnormalities, and neurological symptoms associated with confirmed ZIKV in pregnancy (Perry et al., 2017).

Percentage of adverse effects after ZIKV infection in each trimester
1st trimester : 55%
2nd trimester : 50%
3rd trimester : 30%
42% have severe neurological defects, including **microcephaly** (Brasil et al., 2016).

Diagnosis of Zika virus infection

Maternal infection

The diagnosis of symptomatic women is established with the following tests:
- Reverse-transcription polymerase chain reaction (RT-PCR) of serum (or whole blood) and urine for the detection of Zika virus RNA. If positive, this confirms infection.
- If negative, then Zika virus serologic testing (Zika virus IgM and plaque reduction neutralization test [PRNT]) are done.

Fetal evaluation

- In women with exposure to the Zika virus or with confirmed infection, the available data is not sufficient to define:
  - The optimal interval between exposure and initial ultrasonographic screening or
  - Frequency of ultrasonography in women with confirmed Zika virus infection
- A baseline ultrasound at 18–20 weeks followed by serial examinations every 4–6 weeks has been suggested.
- The most common Zika-associated abnormalities are as follows (Pereira et al., 2018):
  - CNS abnormalities including microcephaly, calcifications, and ventriculomegaly
  - Fetal growth restriction
  - Abnormal umbilical artery and MCA Doppler abnormalities that are sometimes transiently abnormal
- Pereira et al. (2018) found that major Zika virus-associated abnormalities seen on prenatal ultrasonography were associated with a 6-fold to 27-fold increase in adverse neonatal outcomes.
- However, normal prenatal ultrasonography does not guarantee good perinatal outcome. **Almost 50 per cent of women who have a normal ultrasound examination will have neonates with adverse outcomes.**

Treatment

- There is no specific treatment for infection with ZIKV.
- Women should be advised to rest and use paracetamol and antihistamines for symptomatic relief from fever and pruritus.
- Measures should be taken to reduce the risk of transmission to others during the viremic stage. This includes using barrier contraception methods or abstaining from sexual intercourse.
- Women with features of Guillain-Barré syndrome require urgent assessment and specialist management.

PROTOZOAL INFECTIONS

Toxoplasmosis in pregnancy

- *Toxoplasma gondii* is a common protozoan parasite that infects humans. It is usually an infection of children and adolescents.

Due to the relatively low prevalence of the disease in pregnancy, routine screening of all pregnant women for toxoplasmosis is not recommended (ACOG, 2015; SOGC, 2018).

- A pan-India study of serologic prevalence in Indian women of childbearing age (Singh et al., 2014) found that 66 per cent of women living in mud houses tested positive for *T. gondii* IgG antibodies. The region-wise distribution showed the highest prevalence in South India (37.3 per cent) and the lowest in West India (8.8 per cent). Prevalence was 21.2 per cent in East India and 19.7 per cent in North India.
- *T. gondii* infection is acquired through the ingestion of oocysts that may contaminate soil, water, and food. A recent outbreak in a South Indian city was attributed to contaminated municipal water (Palanisamy et al., 2006). **Undercooked meat is not a major source of infection in India** (Singh et al., 2014).
- When the initial toxoplasmic infection occurs in pregnancy, transmission to the fetus results in congenital toxoplasmosis with associated neurological and ocular manifestations.

Maternal risks

- Women with toxoplasmosis infection are usually asymptomatic but may experience a brief febrile illness.
- Transmission to the fetus resulting in congenital toxoplasmosis mostly happens in women who acquire their primary infection during gestation. However, preconceptional disease may be transmitted to the fetus in women with AIDS.

Fetal risks

- The incidence of acute toxoplasmosis in pregnancy is low in India. However, Singh (2016) estimated that cumulatively, child births (live birth or stillbirth) with risk of congenital toxoplasmosis would be approximately 387,904 per annum.
- The risk of fetal infection increases with advancing gestational age at the time of maternal infection (Cortina-Borja, 2010).

The frequency of congenital toxoplasmosis increases with increasing gestational age at maternal infection, but the earlier the gestational age at infection, the more severe the fetal sequelae.

- A systematic review of all available cohorts (SYROCOT Study Group, 2007) estimated the risk of transmission to be 15 per cent when the mother was infected at 13 weeks, 44 per cent at 26 weeks, and 71 per cent at 36 weeks.
- Most infected fetuses have no clinical manifestations.
- Clinical features in infected fetuses include:
  - Preterm birth and low birth weight (fetal growth restriction)

- Rash, hepatosplenomegaly, ascites, fever, periventricular calcifications, ventriculomegaly, and seizures
- Approximately 40 per cent of fetuses with abnormal intracranial findings on prenatal ultrasound will have serious neurological sequelae that include the following (Cortina-Borja, 2010):
  - Cerebral palsy
  - Microcephaly
  - Bilateral blindness
  - Hydrocephalus
  - Epilepsy requiring treatment

 Neonates that are infected in the first trimester of pregnancy have a good outcome if the fetal ultrasound findings are normal. Therefore, termination of pregnancy is not indicated unless ultrasonographic evidence of fetal abnormalities is seen (Berrebi et al., 2007).

Diagnosis

- The diagnosis of toxoplasmosis is usually made by the detection of *Toxoplasma*-specific IgG, IgM, or IgA antibodies using enzyme-linked immunosorbent assays (ELISA).

 Toxoplasma-specific IgM antibodies may persist for many months or years and hence their presence is not always diagnostic. IgM positivity with IgG negativity is suggestive of acute infection.

- IgM positivity indicates a recent infection, but since IgM persists for months to years, testing for IgM alone cannot be used for diagnosis. All three antibodies (IgG, IgM, and IgA) should be tested for.
- Repeat testing should be performed 2–3 weeks later if acute infection is suspected.
- An **avidity test** may be performed. *High avidity* for IgG is indicative of an infection at least >4 months old. *Low avidity* for IgG may indicate a recent infection. However, low avidity may persist for several months and is not as specific as high avidity.

Prenatal diagnosis

- If toxoplasmosis is suspected in pregnancy due to confirmed maternal infection or ultrasound findings suggestive of congenital infection, prenatal diagnosis is required.
- Abnormalities suggestive of toxoplasmosis on ultrasound examination include the following (ACOG, 2015):
  - Hydrocephalus
  - Brain or hepatic calcifications
  - Microcephaly
  - Fetal growth restriction
  - Hyperechoic bowel
- If these ultrasound features are seen, amniotic fluid (amniocentesis) or fetal blood sample is obtained for PCR/DNA amplification techniques after 18 weeks for confirmation of a

diagnosis of congenital infection (Gilbert and Petersen, 2020). Amniocentesis before 18 weeks has a high false-positive rate.
- Prenatal confirmation allows decision making for drug therapy. It also allows women to decide whether they want to continue or terminate the pregnancy.

Treatment

- Women who have confirmed infection but in whom fetal infection is not confirmed (<18 weeks of gestation):
  - **Spiramycin** is recommended to prevent the vertical transmission of the parasite.
- Women who have confirmed infection and in whom fetal infection has been confirmed with amniocentesis (>18 weeks of gestation):
  - **Pyrimethamine-sulfadiazine plus folinic acid** is recommended.
  - Treatment is continued until delivery.
- In a meta-analysis, the SYROCOT study group (2007) concluded that maternal treatment appears to carry a lower risk of mother-to-child transmission, but does not seem to decrease the risk of clinical manifestations in infected liveborn infants. However, it may reduce the severity of congenital disease.

Preventing congenital toxoplasmosis

- A systematic review of the Cochrane Database (Di Mario et al., 2015) was unable to find robust evidence to show that educating pregnant women prenatally about preventive strategies is effective in reducing congenital toxoplasmosis.
- Protecting water sources from contamination and wearing protective footwear when working in wet soil conditions could potentially be effective public health measures in India.

Malaria in pregnancy

- Each year, 50 million women living in malaria-endemic areas become pregnant and 75,000–200,000 infants die of malaria infection during pregnancy (Steketee et al., 2001).

 India reported the largest absolute reductions in malaria cases, with 2.6 million fewer cases in 2018 than in 2017 (WHO World Malaria Report, 2019).

- In India, over 90 per cent of the population lives in malaria transmission areas that follow a pattern of unstable transmission. Transmission is seasonal and the risk of contracting malaria is highest before the monsoon. This means that **the majority of Indians do not develop acquired immunity and are susceptible to infection with malaria**.
- Two-thirds of infections in India are caused by *Plasmodium falciparum* and one-third by *P. vivax* (Anvikar et al., 2016).
- An estimated 13 million cases and 24,000 maternal/infant deaths occur each year in India as a result of malaria (WHO, World Malaria Report, 2019). More than half of these deaths are due to severe maternal anemia, prematurity, and fetal growth restriction/low birth weight.

Most infections are due to either *Plasmodium falciparum* (2/3rd) or *P. vivax* (1/3rd), but mixed infections with more than one malarial species also occur. The majority of malaria-related deaths are due to *P. falciparum*.

Maternal effects

- Pregnant women are more susceptible to malaria than the general population and often have more complications. Pregnant women with no previous immunity to malaria have a two- to three-fold likelihood of developing severe malarial infection as compared with non-pregnant adults living in the same area.
- The increased risk of malaria in pregnancy is due to the following factors (Rogerson, 2017):
  - Immunological and hormonal changes
  - A unique ability of *P. falciparum*-infected erythrocytes to adhere to and sequester in the intervillous space on the maternal side of the placenta

Placental malaria infection helps the parasite avoid clearance by the immune system and especially, filtration by the spleen. *P. falciparum* parasites express a protein on the red cell surface called VAR2CSA. Currently, VAR2CSA is the leading vaccine candidate to protect malaria-exposed pregnant women against poor outcomes related to malaria in pregnancy (Doritchamou et al., 2021).

- In pregnancy, malaria is more common in:
  - Younger women
  - First or second pregnancy
  - First or second trimester
  - Women with HIV
- Maternal anemia is a common consequence of malaria in pregnancy. Severe anemia has been related to maternal mortality.
- Maternal mortality may also result from cerebral malaria, acidosis, and organ failure (pulmonary, renal, hepatic).

Fetal and neonatal consequences

- Systemic infection may result in:
  - Miscarriage
  - Preterm birth
  - Stillbirth
- Parasitemia may result in:
  - Severe fetal anemia
  - Fetal growth restriction and low birth weight
  - Susceptibility of the infant to malaria

Diagnosis

- **Microscopic examination:** The most preferred and reliable diagnosis of malaria is the microscopic examination of Giemsa-stained blood smears as all four major parasite species can be distinguished easily.

- **Malaria rapid diagnostic tests (RDT):**   These tests use a finger-stick and a drop of venous blood. They are accurate and easy to use. The reading can be assessed visually as the presence of coloured bands on the dipstick. It takes a total of 15–20 minutes to complete the procedure. RDTs for the detection of malaria parasite antigens are important diagnostic tools in low-resource endemic settings like India. They require no electricity or laboratory infrastructure, yield results within 15–20 minutes, and can be performed successfully even by health workers with limited training (WHO, 2017).

Prevention

- The National Portal of Health, India (2016), recommends the following preventive measures for pregnant women:
    - Use of treated nets (ITNs)/long-lasting insecticidal nets (LLINs)
    - General measures:
        - Prevention of mosquito breeding by ensuring all exposed water is emptied or covered
        - Use of mosquito repellent creams, liquids, coils, and mats
        - Use of indoor residual spray (IRS) with insecticides
        - Fitting homes with wire meshes
        - Covering the body properly to prevent mosquito bites
- *Chemoprophylaxis* is indicated in pregnant women travelling to endemic areas.
    - Mefloquine is safe in all trimesters.
        - 250 mg orally once a week
        - Started 2–3 weeks prior to travel
    - Chloroquine is used for chemoprophylaxis in areas where the disease is chloroquine-sensitive.
    - Atovaquone-proguanil and doxycycline are **contraindicated** in pregnancy.

Treatment

- Treatment regimens may be less efficacious in pregnancy due to lower concentrations of serum levels achieved in pregnancy. Repeated screening with blood tests may be needed to detect ineffective treatment and relapse.
- Antipyretics are necessary for pyrexia. Women with malaria are screened for anemia and treated with iron or blood transfusion appropriately.
- Malaria in pregnancy should be treated as an emergency.
- *P. falciparum* is chloroquine-resistant in India; primaquine is contraindicated in pregnancy.
- **Artesunate + sulfadoxine-pyrimethamine** and **artesunate + mefloquine** are the most commonly recommended   artemisinin combination therapy (ACTs) in India for the treatment of falciparum malaria in the second and third trimester of pregnancy (Anvikar et al., 2018).
- Compliance may be more with the shorter course with no difference in efficacy according a systematic review of the Cochrane Database (Milligan et al., 2019).
- Treatment regimens for malaria are listed in Table 48.7.

Table 48.7　Treatment regimens for malaria based on WHO Guidelines for the treatment of malaria (2015) and Govt. of India Guidelines for diagnosis and treatment of malaria (2011)

Type of infection	Trimester	Dose
Uncomplicated P. falciparum infection	First trimester	Quinine 600 mg orally t.i.d PLUS Clindamycin 20 mg base/kg/day (up to 1.8 grams) orally divided t.i.d x 7 days
	Second or third trimester	Artemisinin combination therapy (ACTs): Artesunate + sulfadoxine-pyrimethamine OR Artesunate + mefloquine 2 tabs b.i.d x 3 days OR Artemether + lumefantrine 2 tabs b.i.d x 3 days (after a meal) OR Dihydroartemisinin + piperaquine 3–4 tabs per day x 3 days OR Quinine plus clindamycin x 7 days
Uncomplicated P. vivax infection	First trimester	Chloroquine 600 mg base orally immediately followed by 300 mg base orally at 6, 24, and 48 hours OR Quinine 600 mg orally 3 times daily for 3 or 7 days
	Second or third trimester	Chloroquine OR Artemisinin combination therapy (as given above)
Prevention of relapse of P. vivax infection	During pregnancy and breastfeeding infants less than six months	Chloroquine prophylaxis: 300 mg base orally once weekly for the duration of the pregnancy; to be initiated following completion of antimalarial therapy
	After delivery and completion of breastfeeding	Primaquine 0.5 mg/kg/day for 7 days or 14 days
Treatment of severe P. falciparum/ P. vivax cases	First trimester	Parenteral artesunate OR Parenteral quinine
	Second or third trimester	Parenteral artesunate

Congenital malaria

- Vertical transmission to the fetus can occur particularly when there is infection at the time of birth and blood films of the placenta and cord are positive for malaria.
- Infection of the newborn can occur despite appropriate treatment in the mother during pregnancy.
- If the placenta is positive for parasites, weekly screening of the newborn for 28 days is useful to allow early detection and treatment of congenital malaria.

BACTERIAL INFECTIONS

Tuberculosis in pregnancy

- In India, tuberculosis (TB) continues to be a major public health issue despite a global fall in the incidence of TB.
- Tuberculosis during pregnancy is associated with poor outcomes including increased mortality in both the pregnant woman and the neonate. The disease is among the three leading causes of death among women aged 15–45 years.

- India contributes to nearly 21 per cent of the global burden of TB among pregnant women, and the estimated prevalence of TB stands at 2.3 per 1000 pregnant women, which translates to about 44,500 patients annually (Sugarman et al., 2014).
- The National Tuberculosis (TB) Programme in India (2016) recommends screening all pregnant women for TB, but this is rarely implemented. A study from South India that looked at routine screening for TB in pregnancy found that the yield of TB was extremely low (0.02%) and that 4203 women had to be screened to find one case of TB (Vijayageethaa et al., 2019).

Signs and symptoms

- Pulmonary tuberculosis with respiratory symptoms is more commonly seen in pregnancy than extrapulmonary TB.
- The signs and symptoms are the same as those in non-pregnant women, and include fever, cough lasting more than two weeks, weight loss, night sweats, and malaise.
- TB in pregnant women may be missed, since malaise and fatigue may be a normal physiological part of pregnancy.

Tuberculosis is intricately linked with human immunodeficiency virus (HIV).
- HIV infection increases the risk of TB reactivation.
- Maternal tuberculosis increases the vertical transmission of HIV.

Effect of tuberculosis on pregnancy

- Tuberculosis in pregnancy is associated with a two-fold increased risk of preterm birth, low birth weight, fetal growth restriction, and a six-fold increase in perinatal death (Adhikari, 2009).
- Outcome in pregnancy is unfavourably influenced by delays in diagnosis or treatment.

Tuberculosis and the newborn

- Postpartum transmission of pulmonary TB from mother to child is possible if the mother has active TB. The infant must be kept away from the mother until both have been evaluated and necessary preventive measures have been implemented.
- Congenital TB due to transplacental transmission has been described but is very rare.

Diagnosis

In a woman suspected of having pulmonary TB, the following diagnostic tests are recommended:
- Chest X-ray with abdominal shield
- Three sputum specimens for the following investigations:
  - Smear microscopy for acid-fast bacilli (AFB), which is the most rapid and inexpensive test
  - Culture and sensitivity for *Mycobacterium tuberculosis*
- Molecular DNA detection methods such as Xpert MTB/RIF.
  - The WHO endorsed the Xpert MTB/RIF assay in 2011. In 2017, the WHO recommended the use of Xpert Ultra as a replacement for Xpert in all settings (WHO,

2017). These are rapid tests that simultaneously detect tuberculosis and rifampicin resistance in persons with signs and symptoms of tuberculosis.

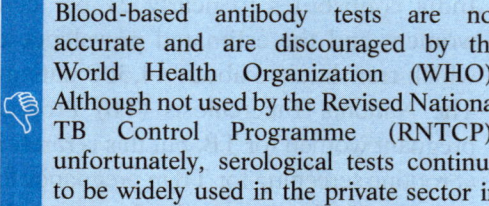

Blood-based antibody tests are not accurate and are discouraged by the World Health Organization (WHO). Although not used by the Revised National TB Control Programme (RNTCP), unfortunately, serological tests continue to be widely used in the private sector in India (Jaroslawski and Pai, 2012).

- The diagnostic accuracy and effectiveness of the Xpert MTB/RIF assay have been validated in high-incidence, resource-limited settings such as India.

- A systematic review of the Cochrane Database (Horne et al., 2019) concluded that Xpert MTB/RIF and Xpert Ultra provide accurate results and can allow rapid initiation of treatment for multidrug-resistant tuberculosis.

- The Xpert MTB/RIF assays are particularly useful in settings of high HIV burden.

• Lymph node biopsy may be required in women with extrapulmonary TB.

Treatment

• **Drug-susceptible tuberculosis**

- Untreated TB disease represents a greater hazard to a pregnant woman and her fetus than its treatment.

- Rifampicin, isoniazid, ethambutol, and pyrazinamide (Table 48.8) can be used safely during pregnancy (Czeizel et al., 2001).

- Streptomycin is contraindicated in pregnancy because it is associated with damage to the eighth cranial nerve, which results in ototoxicity with the risk of bilateral deafness in the fetus.

- Prophylactic pyridoxine in a dosage of 25–50 mg/day is recommended along with anti-tuberculosis treatment (ATT).

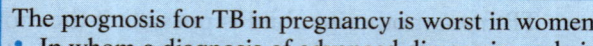

The prognosis for TB in pregnancy is worst in women:
• In whom a diagnosis of advanced disease is made in the puerperium
• Who have HIV coinfection
• Who fail to comply with treatment

Table 48.8 Treatment of tuberculosis in pregnancy (WHO, 2010)

Drugs	Frequency	Duration of treatment
Intensive phase Isoniazid AND Rifampicin, pyrazinamide, and ethambutol	Daily	2 months
Continuation phase Isoniazid AND Rifampicin	Daily	4 months

• **Multidrug-resistant tuberculosis (MDR-TB)**

- This is defined as disease caused by strains of *M. tuberculosis* with resistance to isoniazid and rifampicin. It is a global health crisis that also affects pregnant women.

- MDR-TB requires more aggressive treatment than does its pan-susceptible counterpart. Second-line agents are recommended in an individualised, oral regimen (Schluger et al., 2020) which is as follows:
  - An *intensive phase* of at least five effective drugs for at least 5–7 months after sputum culture conversion followed by
  - A *continuation phase* of at least four effective drugs for 15–21 months beyond sputum culture conversion.
- Though the safety of the second line of drugs is not established in pregnancy, several case reports have shown that the second-line drugs are safe and effective in pregnancy and elective termination of pregnancy need not be the only option offered to women with MDR-TB.

Treatment of tuberculosis in lactating women

- Although ATT drugs are excreted in milk, women can breastfeed their infants two weeks after starting the first-line drug therapy because none of them have been shown to harm the infant.
- Supplemental pyridoxine should be administered to an infant on isoniazid (INH) or if the breastfeeding mother is taking INH because pyridoxine deficiency may cause seizures in the newborn.

Follow-up of the newborn infant

- If the mother is not documented to be sputum-negative or if she is sputum-positive, the infant needs evaluation for active tuberculosis with a chest radiograph and examination of gastric aspirate or sputum for AFB.

 The infant needs evaluation for active tuberculosis and depending on the status, will require INH prophylaxis.

- If the infant shows no evidence of active tuberculosis, the infant should receive INH prophylaxis for three months until after the mother's sputum becomes negative for AFB and the baby is tuberculin-negative.
- If the infant is tuberculin-positive, INH prophylaxis should be given for a period of six months after ruling out active tuberculosis.
- If the newborn does not have evidence of active or latent infection, routine BCG vaccination at birth is warranted in countries like India where tuberculosis is endemic.

References

1. Adhikari M. 2009. Tuberculosis and tuberculosis/HIV co-infection in pregnancy. *Semin Fetal Neonatal Med.* 14: 234–240.

2. American College of Obstetricians and Gynecologists. 2007 (reaffirmed 2019). ACOG Practice Bulletin No. 82. Management of herpes in pregnancy. *Obstet Gynecol.* 109:1489–98.

3. American College of Obstetricians and Gynecologists. 2015. ACOG Practice Bulletin No. 151. Cytomegalovirus, parvovirus B19, varicella zoster, and toxoplasmosis in pregnancy. *Obstet Gynecol.* 125:1510–25.

4. American College of Obstetricians and Gynecologists. 2018. ACOG Committee Opinion No. 732. Influenza vaccination during pregnancy. *Obstetrics & Gynecology*. Volume 131, Issue 4, e109–e114.

5. American College of Obstetricians and Gynecologists. 2019. ACOG Committee Opinion No. 784. Management of patients in the context of Zika virus. *Obstet Gynecol.* 134:e64–70.

6. Anvikar AR, Kuepfer I, Mishra V et al. 2018. Efficacy of two artemisinin-based combinations for the treatment of malaria in pregnancy in India: A randomized controlled trial. *Malaria Journal.* 17, 246.

7. Anvikar AR, Shah N, Dhariwal AC et al. 2016. *Am J Trop Med Hyg.* 95 (Suppl 6). pp. 108–120.

8. Berrebi A, Bardou M, Bessieres MH et al. 2007. Outcome for children infected with congenital toxoplasmosis in the first trimester and with normal ultrasound findings: A study of 36 cases. *Eur J Obstet Gynecol Reprod Biol.* Vol. 135. 53–7.

9. Brasil P, Pereira JP Jr, Moreira ME et al. 2016. Zika virus infection in pregnant women in Rio de Janeiro. *N Engl J Med.* 375:2321.

10. Brown ZA, Benedetti J, Ashley R et al. 1991. Neonatal herpes simplex virus infection in relation to asymptomatic maternal infection at the time of labor. *N Engl J Med.* 324:1247.

11. Brown ZA, Wald A, Morrow RA, Selke S, Zeh J, Corey L. 2003. Effect of serologic status and cesarean delivery on transmission rates of herpes simplex virus from mother to infant. *JAMA.* 289:203–9.

12. Cauchemez S, Besnard M, Bompard P et al. 2016. Association between Zika virus and microcephaly in French Polynesia, 2013-15: A retrospective study. *Lancet.* 387:2125.

13. Central Tuberculosis Division, Government of India. 2016. Technical and operational guidelines for tuberculosis control in India. Ministry of Health & Family Welfare. New Delhi.

14. Cortina-Borja M, Tan HK, Wallon M et al. 2010. Prenatal treatment for serious neurological sequelae of congenital toxoplasmosis: An observational prospective cohort study. *PLoS Med.* 7.

15. Crane J. 2002. Parvovirus B19 infection in pregnancy. *J Obstet Gynaecol Can.* 24:727.

16. Czeizel AE, Rockenbauer M, Olsen J et al. 2001. A population-based case-control study of the safety of oral anti-tuberculosis drug treatment during pregnancy. *Int J Tuberculosis Lung Dis.* Vol. 5. 564–8.

17. de Oliveira WK, Carmo EH, Henriques CM et al. 2017. Zika virus infection and associated neurologic disorders in Brazil. *N Engl J Med.* 376:1591.

18. Di Mario S, Basevi V, Gagliotti C, Spettoli D, Gori G, D'Amico R, Magrini N. 2015. Prenatal education for congenital toxoplasmosis. *Cochrane Database Syst Rev.* Issue 10. Art. no.: CD006171.

19. Ding H, Black CL, Ball S, Fink RV, Williams WW, Fiebelkorn AP et al. 2017. Influenza vaccination coverage among pregnant women – United States, 2016–17 influenza season. *MMWR Morb Mortal Wkly Rep.* 66:1016–22.

20. Doritchamou, JYA, Suurbaar J, Ndam NT. 2021. Progress and new horizons toward a VAR2CSA-based placental malaria vaccine. *Expert Review of Vaccines.* 20:2, 215-226.

21. Enders G, Bäder U, Lindemann L, Schalasta G, Daiminger A. 2001. Prenatal diagnosis of congenital cytomegalovirus infection in 189 pregnancies with known outcome. *Prenat Diagn.* 21(5):362–77.

22. Foley E, Clarke E, Beckett VA et al. 2014. RCOG Guideline. Management of Genital Herpes in Pregnancy.

23. Gilbert R, Petersen E. 2020. Toxoplasmosis and pregnancy. Simpson LL, Weller PF (Eds). *UpToDate.* Waltham, MA.

24. Gratacos E, Torres PJ, Vidal J, Antolin E, Costa J, Jimenez de Anta MT et al. 1995. The incidence of human parvovirus B19 infection during pregnancy and its impact on perinatal outcome. *J Infect Dis.* 171:1360–3.

25. Guerra B, Simonazzi G, Puccetti C et al. 2008. Ultrasound prediction of symptomatic congenital cytomegalovirus infection. *Am J Obstet Gynecol.* 198:380.e1–380.e7.

26. Guidelines for Diagnosis and Treatment of Malaria in India 2011 (2nd edition). Government of India, National Institute of Malaria Research, New Delhi.

27. Hernandez-Andrade E, Scheier M, Dezerega V, Carmo A, Nicolaides KH. 2004. Fetal middle cerebral artery peak systolic velocity in the investigation of non-immune hydrops. *Ultrasound Obstet Gynecol.* 23:442–5.

28. Horne DJ, Kohli M, Zifodya JS et al. 2019. Xpert MTB/RIF and Xpert MTB/RIF Ultra for pulmonary tuberculosis and rifampicin resistance in adults. *Cochrane Database Syst Rev.* Issue 6. Art. no.: CD009593.

29. Jaroslawski S, Pai M. 2012. Why are inaccurate tuberculosis serological tests widely used in the Indian private healthcare sector? A root-cause analysis. *J Epidem and global health.* 2. 39-50.

30. Keller-Stanislawski B, Englund JA, Kang G et al. 2014. Safety of immunization during pregnancy: A review of the evidence of selected inactivated and live attenuated vaccines. *Vaccine.* 32:7057.

31. Kimberlin DW, Lin CY, Sánchez PJ et al. 2003. Effect of ganciclovir therapy on hearing in symptomatic congenital cytomegalovirus disease involving the central nervous system: A randomized, controlled trial. *J Pediatr.* 143:16.

32. Kohelet D, Katz N, Sadan O, Somekh E. 2004. Herpes simplex virus infection after vacuum-assisted vaginally delivered infants of asymptomatic mothers. *J Perinatol.* 24:147–9.

33. Koul PA, Bali NK, Mir H, Jabeen F, Ahmad A. 2016. Influenza illness in pregnant Indian women: A cross-sectional study. *Infectious Diseases in Obstetrics and Gynecology.* 2016:1248470.

34. Krauer F, Riesen M, Reveiz L et al. 2017. Zika virus infection as a cause of congenital brain abnormalities and Guillain–Barré Syndrome: Systematic review. *PLoS Med.* 14:e1002203.

35. Lafferty WE, Downey L, Celum C, Wald A. 2000. Herpes simplex virus type 1 as a cause of genital herpes: Impact on surveillance and prevention. *J Infect Dis.* 181: 1454–7.

36. Lamont RF, Sobel JD, Carrington D et al. 2011. Varicella-zoster virus (chickenpox) infection in pregnancy. *BJOG.* 118:1155.

37. Lazzarotto T, Gabrielli L, Lanari M et al. 2004. Congenital cytomegalovirus infection: Recent advances in the diagnosis of maternal infection. *Hum Immunol.* 65:410.

38. Leruez-Ville, Sellier Y, Salomon LJ et al. 2013. Prediction of fetal infection in cases with cytomegalovirus immunoglobulin in the first trimester of pregnancy: A retrospective cohort. *Clinical Infectious Diseases.* Volume 56, Issue 10. p1428–1435.

39. Marin M, Güris D, Chaves SS et al. 2007. Prevention of varicella: Recommendations of the Advisory Committee on Immunization Practices (ACIP). *MMWR Recomm Rep.* 56:1.

40. Markenson GR, Yancey MK. 1998. Parvovirus B19 infections in pregnancy. *Semin Perinatol.* 22:309–17.

41. Mathur S, Dubey T, Kulshrestha M et al. 2013. Clinical profile and mortality among novel influenza A (H1N1) infected patients: 2009–2010, Jodhpur, Rajasthan pandemic. *Journal of Association of Physicians of India.* Vol. 61, No.9, p627–632.

42. McIntosh ED, Menser MA. 1992. A fifty-year follow-up of congenital rubella. *Lancet.* 340:414.

43. Miller E, Cradock-Watson JE, Pollock TM. 1982. Consequences of confirmed maternal rubella at successive stages of pregnancy. *Lancet.* 2:781.

44. Milligan R, Daher A, Graves PM. 2019. Primaquine at alternative dosing schedules for preventing relapse in people with *Plasmodium vivax* malaria. *Cochrane Database Syst Rev.* Issue 7. Art. no.: CD012656.

45. National Portal of Health/Malaria. 2016.

46. Newsome K, Williams J, Way S et al. 2011. Maternal and infant outcomes among severely ill pregnant and postpartum women with 2009 pandemic influenza A (H1N1)—United States, April 2009–August 2010. *Morbidity and Mortality Weekly Report.* 60(35):1193–1196.

47. Palanisamy M, Madhavan B, Balasundaram MB, Andavar R, Venkatapathy N. 2006. Outbreak of ocular toxoplasmosis in Coimbatore, India. *Indian J Ophthalmol.* 54:129–131.

48. Paquet C, Yudin MH. SOGC Clinical Practice Guideline No. 285. 2018. Toxoplasmosis in pregnancy: Prevention, screening, and treatment. *J Obstet Gynaecol Can.* 40(8):e687–e693

49. Pasternak B, Hviid A. 2010. Use of acyclovir, valacyclovir, and famciclovir in the first trimester of pregnancy and the risk of birth defects. *JAMA.* 304:859–66.

50. Pereira JP, Nielsen-Saines K, Sperling J et al. 2018. Association of prenatal ultrasonographic findings with adverse neonatal outcomes among pregnant women with Zika virus infection in Brazil. *JAMA Netw Open.* 1(8):e186529.

51. Perry H, Khalil A, Aarons E et al. 2017. Management of Zika virus in pregnancy: A review, *British Medical Bulletin.* Vol. 124, Issue 1, p157–169.

52. Picone O, Vauloup-Fellous C, Cordier AG et al. 2013. A series of 238 cytomegalovirus primary infections during pregnancy: Description and outcome. *Prenat Diagn.* 33:751.

53. Pramanick A, Rathore S, Peter JV, Moorthy M, Lionel J. 2011. Pandemic (H1N1) 2009 virus infection during pregnancy in South India. *Int J Gynaecol Obstet.* 113(1):32–35.

54. Prober CG, Sullender WM, Yasukawa LL et al. 1987. Low risk of herpes simplex virus infections in neonates exposed to the virus at the time of vaginal delivery to mothers with recurrent genital herpes simplex virus infections. *N Engl J Med.* 316:240–4.

55. Ramakrishna K, Sampath S, Chacko J et al. 2012. Clinical profile and predictors of mortality of severe pandemic (H1N1) 2009 virus infection needing intensive care: A multi-centre prospective study from South India. *Journal of Global Infectious Diseases.* Vol. 4, no. 3, p45–152.

56. RCOG Green-top Guideline No. 13. 2015. Royal College of Obstetricians and Gynaecologists, UK.

57. Revello MG, Gerna G. 2004. Pathogenesis and prenatal diagnosis of human cytomegalovirus infection. *J Clin Virol.* 29:71.

59. Riley LE. 2019. Rubella in pregnancy. Hirsch MS, Lockwood CJ (Eds). *UpToDate.* Waltham, MA.

60. Riley LE. 2019a. Varicella-zoster virus infection in pregnancy. Hirsch MS, Lockwood CJ (Eds). *UpToDate.* Waltham, MA.

61. Rogerson SJ. 2017. Management of malaria in pregnancy. *Ind J of Med Research.* Vol. 146, Issue 3, 328–333.

62. Schluger NW, Heysell SK, Friedland G. 2020. Treatment of drug-resistant pulmonary tuberculosis in adults. Bernardo J (Ed). *UpToDate.* Waltham, MA.

63. Sheffield JS, Boppanna SB. 2019. Cytomegalovirus infection in pregnancy. Wilkins-Haug L, Hirsch MS, (Eds). *UpToDate.* Waltham, MA.

64. Shrim A, Koren G, Yudin MH, Farine D. SOGC Clinical Practice Guideline No. 274. 2012. Management of varicella infection (chickenpox) in pregnancy. *J Obstet Gynaecol Can.* 34(3):287–292.

65. Singh S, Munawwar A, Rao S et al. 2014. Serologic prevalence of Toxoplasma gondii in Indian women of child bearing age and effects of social and environmental factors. *PLoS Negl Trop Dis.* 8:e2737.

66. Singh S. 2016. Symposium. Congenital toxoplasmosis: Clinical features, outcomes, treatment, and prevention. *Tropical parasitology.* Vol. 6, Issue 2, p113–122.

67. Smego RA Jr, Asperilla MO. Use of acyclovir for varicella pneumonia during pregnancy. *Obstet Gynecol.* 1991; 78:1112.

68. Steketee RW, Nahlen BL, Parise ME, Menendez C. 2001. The burden of malaria in pregnancy in malaria-endemic areas. *Am J Trop Med Hyg.* 64:28–35.

69. Sugarman J, Colvin C, Moran AC et al. 2014. Tuberculosis in pregnancy: An estimate of the global burden of disease. *Lancet Glob Heal.* 2:e710–716.

70. Tanemura M, Suzumori K, Yagami Y et al. 1996. Diagnosis of fetal rubella infection with reverse transcription and nested polymerase chain reaction: A study of 34 cases diagnosed in fetuses. *Am J Obstet Gynecol.* 174:578.

71. The National Tuberculosis (TB) Programme, Central Tuberculosis Division, Government of India. 2016. Technical and operational guidelines for tuberculosis control in India. New Delhi: Ministry of Health & Family Welfare.

72. Thiebaut R, Leproust S, Chene G, Gilbert R. 2007. SYROCOT (Systematic Review on Congenital Toxoplasmosis) study group. Effectiveness of prenatal treatment for congenital toxoplasmosis: A meta-analysis of individual patients' data. *Lancet.* 369:115–22.

73. Vijayageethaa M, AMV Kumar, Ramakrishnan J et al. 2019. Tuberculosis screening among pregnant women attending a tertiary care hospital in Puducherry, South India: Is it worth the effort? *Global Health Action.* Vol. 12, 1564488.

74. Wald A, Huang ML, Carrell D, Selke S, Corey L. 2003. Polymerase chain reaction for detection of herpes simplex virus (HSV) DNA on mucosal surfaces: Comparison with HSV isolation in cell culture. *J Infect Dis.* 188: 1345–51.

75. Watts DH, Brown ZA, Money D et al. 2003. A double-blind, randomized, placebo-controlled trial of acyclovir in late pregnancy for the reduction of herpes simplex virus shedding and cesarean delivery. *Am J Obstet Gynecol.* 188:836–43.

76. Whitley RJ, Corey L, Arvin A, Lakeman FD, Sumaya CV, Wright PF et al. 1988. Changing presentation of herpes simplex virus infection in neonates. *J Infect Dis.* 158: 109–116.

77. Workowski KA, Bolan GA. 2015. Centers for Disease Control and Prevention (CDC). Sexually transmitted diseases treatment guidelines. *MMWR Recomm Rep.* 64 (No. 3).

78. World Health Organization. 2010. WHO guidelines for treatment of tuberculosis, 4th edition. WHO, Geneva.

79. World Health Organization. 2015. Guidelines for the treatment of malaria – 3rd edition. WHO Press, Geneva.

80. World Health Organization. 2017. Malaria rapid diagnostic test performance: Summary results of WHO product testing of malaria RDTs: Round 1–7 (2008–2016). WHO, Geneva.

81. World Health Organization. 2017. Next-generation Xpert MTB/RIF Ultra assay recommended by WHO. WHO, Geneva.

82. World Health Organization. 2019. World malaria report 2019. WHO, Geneva.

83. World Health Organization. WHO position paper. 2012. Vaccines against influenza – November 2012. No. 47, 87, 461–476.

84. Zaman K, Roy E, Arifeen SE et al. 2008. Effectiveness of maternal influenza immunization in mothers and infants. *N Engl J Med.* 359:1555–1564.

Chapter 49

COVID-19 Infection in Pregnancy

INTRODUCTION

- The World Health Organization (WHO) declared coronavirus disease (COVID-19) a pandemic on 11 March 2020.
- COVID-19 infection is a severe acute respiratory syndrome caused by the RNA virus SARS-CoV-2. Like any virus, it has continued to mutate and has resulted in 'variants of concern' that have clinical and public health implications. The first outbreak was caused by the Alpha variant; the Delta variant caused the second wave and had more serious consequences on pregnancy outcomes. The Omicron variant is responsible for the third wave and is more infectious. However, it seems to have a lesser impact on pregnancy outcomes.
- Since this is a new virus, information about its effects on pregnancy is still being accumulated. However, it is clear that symptomatic pregnant women are at an increased risk for developing severe sequelae of COVID-19 compared to non-pregnant women of reproductive age.
- Vaccination against COVID-19 not only reduces the risk of infection but also reduces the severity of disease in women who contract an infection despite being immunised. The safety of currently available SARS-CoV-2 vaccines before, during, and after pregnancy has been established (see the section on *Vaccination against COVID-19*).
- Emerging data have confirmed that the COVID-19 pandemic has increased maternal and perinatal morbidity and mortality, not only caused directly by the disease itself, but also due to the inability to access healthcare facilities (Chmielewska et al., 2021). Nationwide lockdowns, disruption of healthcare services, and fear of contracting the disease in a hospital have negatively impacted pregnant mothers and their babies. This is especially true of low- and middle-income countries (LMICs).
- Managing a pregnant woman who has a COVID-19 infection requires a multidisciplinary approach.

> **Is it safe to plan for pregnancy during the COVID-19 pandemic?**
> Evidence accumulated during the pandemic shows that the absolute pregnancy-related risks of SARS-CoV-2 infection are not higher than with other infectious exposures among pregnant women. Though there appears to be an increase in preterm birth compared with uninfected or asymptomatic pregnant women, there seems to be no substantial increase in the rates of miscarriage and congenital anomalies. In utero transmission is rare and neonatal outcome is largely good (Berghella and Hughes, 2022).
>
> It has been reported that infection after 20 weeks increases the risk for adverse obstetric outcomes, and that infection after 26 weeks increases the risk for adverse neonatal outcomes (Badr et al., 2021). It is strongly recommended that vaccination be administered as soon as possible for women planning to conceive and for pregnant women.

CLINICAL MANIFESTATIONS AND COURSE OF DISEASE

- Though pregnant women *without comorbidities* are not more susceptible to infection with SARS-CoV-2 than non-pregnant women, pregnancy does appear to worsen the clinical course of COVID-19 infection (Berghella and Hughes, 2022).
- Pregnant women *with comorbidities* such as pre-existing diabetes, BMI > 25 kg/m^2, and gestational diabetes being managed with insulin are at an **increased risk** of contracting SARS-CoV-2 infection (RCOG, 2022).
- Approximately 70 per cent of infected pregnant women are asymptomatic.
- When pregnant women are symptomatic, they manifest signs and symptoms similar to those that non-pregnant women present with. These include fever with/without cough, headache, sore throat, breathlessness, body ache, recent loss of taste or smell, fatigue, and diarrhea.
- Some of the signs and symptoms of infection such as fatigue, shortness of breath, nasal congestion, and nausea/vomiting, are very similar to those of normal pregnancy.

> Pregnant women are less likely to present with symptoms such as fever, dyspnea, and myalgia. However, they are at risk of rapid progression of disease and are more likely to be admitted to the intensive care unit or to require invasive ventilation than non-pregnant women of reproductive age (Allotey et al., 2021).

Diagnosis of COVID-19 infection

- **Antigen-detecting rapid diagnostic tests (Ag-RDTs)**
  - Direct detection of SARS-CoV-2 viral proteins (antigens) in nasal swabs and other respiratory secretions using lateral flow immunoassays offers a faster and less expensive method to test for SARS-CoV-2 (WHO, 2021). They are good for point-of-care tests since it takes <1 hour to perform these tests.
  - The RDT is best performed within 5–7 days of the onset of symptoms.
  - These tests are used for primary case detection in symptomatic individuals suspected to be infected, for asymptomatic individuals at a high risk of COVID-19, or for contact tracing (Figure 49.1).
- **Nucleic acid amplification tests (NAATs)**
  - The RT-PCR (real-time reverse transcription polymerase chain reaction) test is performed on a combined anterior nasal/oropharyngeal swab. This is the gold standard for the diagnosis of a current infection.
  - RT-PCR has high sensitivity and specificity with a low false-negative rate. The results are usually available within 24 hours.

Classification of disease severity

The National Institutes of Health (2021) classifies COVID-19 disease severity as follows:
- **Asymptomatic or pre-symptomatic infection**: Positive test for SARS-CoV-2 but no symptoms.

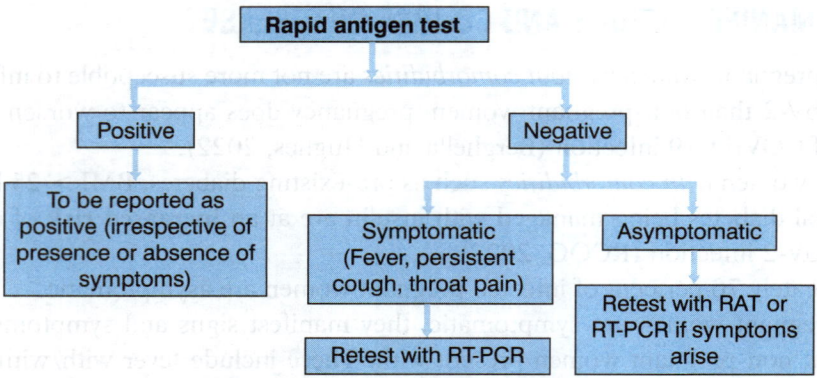

Figure 49.1   Algorithm for testing with point-of-care rapid antigen test (RAT).
RT-PCR, real-time reverse transcription polymerase chain reaction

- **Mild illness:** Any signs and symptoms (e.g., fever, cough, sore throat, malaise, headache, muscle pain) without shortness of breath, dyspnea, or abnormal chest imaging.
- **Moderate illness:** Evidence of lower respiratory disease gathered by clinical assessment or imaging, and oxygenation (SpO_2) ≥94 per cent on room air at sea level.
- **Severe illness:** Respiratory frequency >30 breaths per minute, SpO_2 <94 per cent on room air at sea level, ratio of arterial partial pressure of oxygen to fraction of inspired oxygen (PaO_2/FiO_2) <300, or lung infiltrates >50 per cent.
- **Critical illness:** Respiratory failure, septic shock, and/or multiple organ dysfunction.

The World Health Organization classification (2022) of COVID-19 disease severity in adults is as follows:
- **Non-severe:** Absence of signs of severe or critical disease
- **Severe:** Oxygen saturation <90 per cent on room air, signs of pneumonia, signs of severe respiratory distress
- **Critical:** Requires life-sustaining treatment; acute respiratory distress syndrome, sepsis, septic shock

MATERNAL CONSEQUENCES OF INFECTION WITH SARS-COV-2

Risk of miscarriage

- The data collected since the start of the pandemic clearly show that women with COVID-19 are **NOT** at a greater risk for early pregnancy loss (Elshafeey et al., 2020; Juan et al., 2020; Cosma et al., 2021; Rotshenker-Olshinka et al., 2021).
- This is true for both symptomatic and asymptomatic pregnant women.

Risk of congenital malformations

- Observational studies since the beginning of the pandemic have failed to show an increase in congenital anomalies above the baseline (Berghella and Hughes, 2022).

- Unlike other viruses that can cause specific congenital anomalies, SARS-CoV-2 has not been associated with any anomalies unique to it.

Preterm birth (PTB)

- Fever and hypoxemia may increase the risks of preterm labour and prelabour rupture of membranes.
- Symptomatic COVID-19 seems to almost double the rate of PTB in pregnant women as compared to those without infection. Asymptomatic infection and resolved prenatal infection are not associated with increased risk.
- In a study comprising almost 2500 women, Blitz et al. (2021) found that 19 per cent of symptomatic women with COVID-19 had preterm birth as opposed to 8.8 per cent of asymptomatic and 7.1 per cent of uninfected women.
- The increase in preterm birth was more pronounced during the second wave with the Delta variant. Mahajan et al. (2022) reported that spontaneous PTB in Mumbai, India, was higher during the second wave than in the first wave (12.5 per cent vs. 8.3 per cent).
- Interestingly, Mahajan et al. also reported that iatrogenic PTB decreased in the second wave in their cohort. This differs from other studies that show an increase in medically-indicated preterm deliveries, including cesarean births (Martinez-Perez et al., 2021; Blitz et al., 2021).

Risk of preeclampsia

- COVID-19 during pregnancy is strongly associated with preeclampsia, preeclampsia with severe features, eclampsia, and hemolysis, elevated liver enzymes, and low platelets (HELLP) syndrome, especially among nulliparous women. Papageorghiou et al. (INTERCOVID prospective longitudinal study, 2021) reported that as a consequence, these women are at very high risk for PTB, severe perinatal morbidity and mortality, and adverse maternal outcomes.
- **Both symptomatic and asymptomatic women are at an increased risk, with the risk being higher among symptomatic mothers.**

Risk of stillbirth

- The risk of stillbirth has been reported to be 1.9 times higher among women admitted with a diagnosis of COVID-19 compared to those without (DeSisto et al., 2021). The risk was further elevated from July–September 2021, when the Delta variant caused the majority of infections.
- The inability to access institutional care due to lockdowns resulted in an increase in stillbirths in many LMICs.
- In India too, the pandemic resulted in a spike in stillbirths. Mahajan et al. (2021) reported a doubling of the stillbirth rate in the second wave of the COVID-19 pandemic (34 per 1000 births between February 2021 and May 2021).
- COVID-19 has decimated the progress that was being made in reducing the national stillbirth rate. This has also been attributed to the fact that women could not access

medical facilities for delivery since medical care and transportation were disrupted by the pandemic.

- Hospital births decreased by 43 per cent (Kumari et al., 2020) and 45 per cent (Goyal et al., 2021) respectively in two tertiary centres during the first lockdown.
- Many hospitals refused to accept a woman for delivery without a negative test for COVID-19 (Srivastava, 2021). This is despite the MoHFW, GOI issuing a guideline (2021) that 'although testing should be done wherever indicated and feasible, no emergency procedure (including deliveries) should be delayed for lack of a COVID test report'.

Maternal morbidity

- More than 90 per cent of infected pregnant women recover without the need for hospitalisation.
- However, pregnant and recently pregnant women with COVID-19 are at a higher risk of rapid progression of disease, admission to the intensive care unit, and requiring invasive ventilation than non-pregnant women of reproductive age (Berghella and Hughes, 2022).
- Comorbidities that increase the risk of hospitalisation, intubation and mechanical ventilation, and admission to the critical care unit include asthma, chronic hypertension, type 2 diabetes mellitus, autoimmune disease, and high body mass index (Allotey et al., 2021; Lokken et al., 2021).

Maternal mortality

- In the United States, Zambrano et al. (2020) found increased mortality in pregnant women with COVID-19 disease as compared to non-pregnant women in the reproductive age group (1.5 vs. 1.2 per 1000 cases). Similarly, Lokken et al. (2021) found a higher case fatality rate in women admitted with severe COVID-19.
- In comparison, the risk of maternal mortality was reported to be **22 times higher** (1.6 per cent) in institutions in less developed regions, where comprehensive ICU services are not fully available (Villar et al., The INTERCOVID Multinational Cohort Study, 2021).
- In India, maternal mortality from the SARS-CoV-2 virus has been high. Asalkar et al. (2021) reported a mortality rate of 1.03 per cent in their cohort of pregnant women in a dedicated COVID hospital during the pandemic. The PregCovid registry analysed data from 19 medical colleges relating to pregnant women with COVID-19 across the State of Maharashtra (Gajbhiye et al., 2021). The authors reported a case fatality rate of 0.8–1.1 per cent. Maternal deaths were increased in the presence of comorbidities such as anemia, tuberculosis, and diabetes mellitus.
- The overall maternal mortality in India also increased because of the inability of women to access institutional care. Nair (2021), in a study of 202,000 hospital births in India, found that institutional births decreased by more than 30 per cent at the start of the first wave of the pandemic and by 35 per cent in May 2021, as compared with May 2020.

NEONATAL CONSEQUENCES OF INFECTION WITH SARS-COV-2

- More than 95 per cent of babies born to infected mothers show no signs of infection and are healthy at birth (Berghella and Hughes, 2022).
- When newborns of infected mothers develop symptoms of infection postnatally, it is a result of droplet transmission from the mother or a caregiver infected with COVID-19.
- Neonatal morbidity is usually the result of preterm birth. The risk of neonatal mortality is not increased unless the mother has a severe infection in the third trimester.
- Neonatal outcome is affected by the following factors:
  - **Severity of maternal disease** affects pregnancy outcomes. The risk of preterm birth is higher in women with severe and critical disease because delivery is often indicated due to worsening maternal status.
  - **Gestational age at the time of infection** is important since infection after 26 weeks increases the risk of poor neonatal outcome (Badr et al., 2021). Villar et al. (2021) reported severe neonatal complications, including NICU stay for seven days or longer, to be substantially higher in women with COVID-19 diagnosed in the third trimester.
- Infants born to mothers with suspected or confirmed infection should be tested with RT-PCR for the SARS-CoV-2 virus. The test should be performed 24 hours after birth and if negative, repeated at 48 hours.

ANTENATAL CARE

Several professional bodies have released guidelines for the management of antenatal visits during the COVID-19 pandemic (MoHFW, GOI, 2021; FOGSI, 2020; ACOG, 2020; RCOG 2022).

Uninfected mother

- Most guidelines have modified the traditional number of antenatal visits to avoid exposing the uninfected pregnant mother to the risk of infection. The number of visits also depends on the prevalence of disease in the community at the time.
- Each in-person visit is maximised for efficiency by grouping laboratory tests and imaging when required.
- Telehealth consultations by telephone or video calls have replaced some in-person visits when physical examination or laboratory test/ultrasound imaging is not required.
- The risk of infection is further reduced by restricting the number of accompanying individuals and maintaining physical distancing.
- Uninfected and unvaccinated mothers and their families should receive vaccination against COVID-19 as soon as possible.

Asymptomatic infected mother

- The mother is advised self-monitoring for the development of COVID-19 symptoms.
- Self-isolation is recommended for the known duration of infectivity for the variant, e.g., 14 days for the Delta variant and 5–7 days for the Omicron variant.

- A negative RAT or RT-PCR is not required for discontinuation of isolation and precautions.
- Since asymptomatic infected women are at equally high risk for the development of preeclampsia, they should be educated about self-monitoring of blood pressure and also be tested during in-person visits.

Symptomatic infected mother

- Pregnant mothers with suspected or documented COVID-19 should be evaluated for the following indicators of severe disease (Table 49.1):
  - Laboratory indicators of severe illness
  - Signs of severe illness
  - Comorbidities that may worsen disease

Table 49.1   Laboratory, clinical, and CT scan indicators of severe COVID-19

Laboratory findings	Clinical findings	CT scan findings
D-dimer >1000 ng/mL (normal range: <500 ng/mL)	Oxygen saturation (SpO$_2$) <94 per cent on room air at sea level	Lung infiltrates >50 per cent
CRP >100 mg/L (normal range: <8.0 mg/L)	Respiratory rate >30 breaths/minute	
LDH >245 units/L (normal range: 110–210 units/L)	Pressure of oxygen (PaO$_2$)/fraction of inspired oxygen (FiO$_2$) <300 mmHg	
Ferritin > 500 mg/L (normal range for females: 10–200 mg/L		
CPK >2 × the upper limit of normal (normal range: 40–150 units/L)		
Absolute lymphocyte count <800/mL (normal range for age ≥21 years: 1800–7700/mL)		

INTRAPARTUM CARE

- Universal screening should be performed prior to or at the time of admission, particularly at times when there is a surge of cases in the community.
- If a woman has not been tested, she should be treated as infected, and all necessary precautions taken.
- During spikes of COVID-19 cases in the community, the approach to the care of a woman in labour is three-pronged:
  - Protection of the uninfected mother against acquiring COVID-19 in the hospital
  - Availability of facilities to take care of the infected woman in labour
  - Protection of healthcare workers involved in the care of the woman in labour

Protection of the uninfected pregnant woman against acquiring infection

- Universal masking should be mandated for the mother, her support person (if hospital policy allows one during the pandemic), and healthcare workers.
- Limiting the time spent in the labour room may reduce the woman's risk of exposure. She may be allowed to labour at home (if it is close to the hospital), or in a separate

hospital room (if available) until she needs to be shifted to the labour room for delivery.

- Reducing the number of attendants or visitors that the labouring mother may have decreases her risk of getting infected.

Infected woman in labour

Availability of facilities to take care of the infected woman in labour

- Since pregnant women are at a much higher risk of deterioration of disease, labour and delivery should ideally happen in a hospital that can handle the complications that can arise, both in labour and as a consequence of COVID-19.
- If such facilities are not available, the mother should be transferred to a tertiary care unit when complications arise. During surges in the pandemic, with healthcare facilities strained to maximum capacity, this is not always possible.

Protection of healthcare workers involved in the care of the infected woman in labour

- It is important that contact and droplet precautions be taken with the use of the following:
  - Gown and gloves
  - N95, surgical, or medical procedure mask
  - Face shield or goggles
- When the labouring woman is making deep respiratory efforts in the active phase and while pushing in the second stage, the risk of droplet infection is greatly increased. Healthcare workers should be aware of this and should be well protected.

 Ideally, women with COVID-19 should wear a mask while pushing. However, many women find it hard to breathe with a mask, especially during expulsive efforts. It is reasonable to allow them to remove the mask at this time (Berghella and Hughes, 2022).

Timing of birth

- When the infection occurred earlier in pregnancy and the mother has completely recovered, there is no indication to alter the timing of delivery (ACOG, 2020).
- In women who develop the infection in the third trimester, it is recommended that delivery be delayed until the woman is out of the suggested quarantine period. This recommendation does not apply if there is a medical indication to deliver the mother.

Route of birth

- COVID-19 infection by and of itself is not an indication for cesarean delivery (ACOG, 2020). However, a higher prevalence of cesarean birth in pregnant women with COVID-19 has been reported globally. This may stem from the fact that healthcare staff are reluctant to spend time with an infected labouring woman during the pandemic.
- Cesarean delivery should be based on obstetric (fetal or maternal) indications and not COVID-19 status alone. Omar et al. (2022), in a meta-analysis that included 42 studies,

concluded that vaginal delivery was not associated with worse maternal or neonatal outcomes when compared with cesarean birth.

POSTPARTUM CARE

- **Postpartum hemorrhage (PPH)**
  - Methergin is contraindicated in women receiving nirmatrelvir–ritonavir because of the risk of ergot toxicity.
  - The increased risk of thrombosis with COVID-19 and its pulmonary manifestations have raised some questions.
    - *Tranexamic acid* may need to be given with caution due to the increased risk of clotting.
    - *Carboprost tromethamine (PGF$_{2a}$)* is known to cause bronchial spasm in asthmatics and is withheld for them. It is not clear yet whether the viral pneumonia in COVID-19 should be considered a contraindication to the use of PGF$_{2a}$.
- **Breastfeeding**
  - Though breastfeeding by itself does not transmit the SARS-CoV-2 virus to the neonate, droplet transmission from the mother can cause infection in the newborn.
  - Expressed breastmilk may be used to feed the infant until the mother is able to resume direct breastfeeding. If the mother is very particular about breastfeeding the infant, she must use precautions like hand washing, wearing a mask/face covering and keeping the infant at a distance of two metres (six feet) between feeds.
  - Temporary separation of the child from the mother may be indicated in the following circumstances (ACOG, 2020):
    - It is <10 days since symptoms first appeared; in women with more severe to critical illness, and in severely immunocompromised women, 20 days of isolation is recommended
    - <24 hours have passed since her last fever without the use of antipyretics
    - Symptoms such as cough and breathlessness persist
    - The mother is critically ill and is unable to take care of the infant

THERAPEUTICS FOR THE MANAGEMENT OF COVID-19

As therapy is rapidly evolving for the management of COVID-19 in adults, it is best to follow live updates released by several professional bodies such as WHO (2022), ACOG (2020), RCOG (2022) and the MoHFW, GOI (2021).

VACCINATION AGAINST COVID-19

- Immunisation against COVID-19 is recommended for all pregnant women who have not been vaccinated earlier (WHO, 2021; ACOG, 2020; RCOG, 2021).
- The Government of India, Ministry of Health and Family Welfare (MoHFW), Immunization Division, based on the recommendations from the National Technical Advisory Group on Immunization (NTAGI), has approved the vaccination of pregnant women against COVID-19 (2021a).

- Pregnant women at a high risk of exposure to COVID-19 and pregnant women with comorbidities that place them in a high-risk group for severe COVID-19 should definitely be vaccinated (WHO, 2021).
- The benefits of vaccination of pregnant women outweigh the potential risks of the same. A recent study from Scotland of over 18,000 pregnant women (Stock et al., 2022) clearly demonstrated the advantage of vaccination. Of the women hospitalised for COVID-19 infection, 77 per cent were unvaccinated. **98 per cent of critical care admissions and 100 per cent of perinatal deaths occurred in unvaccinated women**.
- Pregnant women should be informed about the risks of exposure to COVID-19 infection along with the risks and benefits associated with the COVID-19 vaccines available in the country.
- A pregnant woman who opts for vaccination can be vaccinated at any time during pregnancy.

- COVID-19 vaccination should be carried out regardless of pregnancy status. There is no need to perform a pregnancy test for a woman before vaccinating her for COVID-19 since vaccination does not increase the risk of miscarriage. Though the majority of the available data at present are for mRNA vaccines (Zauche et al., 2021, Kharbanda et al., 2021), studies that included the AstraZeneca vaccine have also shown no increase in miscarriages (Vaccine surveillance report, UK Health Security Agency, 2022).
- It is important to reassure women that they cannot contract COVID-19 infection from the vaccine.

- The three vaccines available in India are Covishield, Sputnik V (non-replicating viral vector platforms), and Covaxin (inactivated vaccine). Since these three vaccines are not live vaccines, all three have been approved by the GOI for use in pregnancy. The WHO has approved both Covishield and Covaxin for use in pregnancy.
- The ACOG and the CDC have approved mRNA vaccines for use in pregnancy because of the extensive safety studies conducted. Though the majority of pregnant women in the UK have received mRNA vaccines, 10 per cent have received the AstraZeneca vaccine (Covishield).
- Vaccination in lactating women is recommended as in other adults. The mother should not discontinue breastfeeding because of vaccination (WHO, 2021).

Vaccination with the AstraZeneca vaccine (Covishield) has resulted in an extremely rare syndrome—vaccine-induced immune thrombotic thrombocytopenia (VITT). The incidence of this syndrome has been reported to be 1 in 26,000 (Schultz et al., 2021). The benefits of vaccination greatly outweigh the risk of VITT. In comparison to the extremely low rate of VITT following vaccination, the mortality rate for COVID-19 is as high as 1 in 100.

REFERENCES

1. Allotey, J, Stallings, E, Bonet, M et al. 2021. PregCOV-19 Living Systematic Review Consortium. Clinical manifestations, risk factors, and maternal and perinatal outcomes of coronavirus disease 2019 in pregnancy: Living systematic review and meta-analysis. *BMJ*. 370.

2. American College of Obstetricians and Gynecologists. 2020. COVID-19 FAQs for obstetricians, gynecologists and obstetricians. Washington DC.

3. American College of Obstetricians and Gynecologists. 2020 (updated 2022). ACOG Practice Advisory. COVID-19 vaccination considerations for obstetric–gynecologic care.

4. Asalkar M, Thakkarwad S, Rumani I, Sharma N. 2021. Prevalence of maternal mortality and clinical course of maternal deaths in COVID-19 pneumonia: A cross-sectional study. *J Obstet Gynaecol India*. 6:1-10.

5. Badr DA, Picone O, Bevilacqua E et al. 2021. Severe acute respiratory syndrome of coronavirus-2 and pregnancy outcomes according to gestational age at time of infection. *Emerg Infect Dis*. 27(10):2535.

6. Berghella V, Hughes BL. 2022. COVID-19: Overview of pregnancy issues. Lockwood CJ (Ed). *UpToDate*. Waltham, MA.

7. Blitz MJ, Gerber RP, Gulersen M et al. 2021. Preterm birth among women with and without severe acute respiratory syndrome coronavirus-2 infection. *Acta Obstet Gynecol Scand*. 100(12):2253-2259.

8. Chmielewska B, Barratt I, Townsend R et al. 2021. Effects of the COVID-19 pandemic on maternal and perinatal outcomes: A systematic review and meta-analysis. *Lancet Glob Health*. pp. e759-e772.

9. Cosma S, Carosso AR, Cusato J et al. 2021. Coronavirus disease 2019 and first-trimester spontaneous abortion: A case-control study of 225 pregnant patients. *Am J Obstet Gynecol*. 224:391.e1.

10. COVID-19 vaccine surveillance report—week 6. London: UK Health Security Agency; 2022. https://assets.publishing.service.gov.uk/government/uploads/system/uploads/attachment_data/file/1054071/vaccine-surveillance-report-week-6.pdf).

11. DeSisto CL, Wallace B, Simeone RM et al. 2021. Risk for stillbirth among women with and without COVID-19 at delivery hospitalization, United States, March 2020–September 2021.

12. Elshafeey F, Magdi R, Hindi N et al. 2020. A systematic scoping review of COVID-19 during pregnancy and childbirth. *Int J Gynaecol Obstet*. 150:47.

13. Federation of Obstetric and Gynaecological Societies of India (FOGSI) Good Clinical Practice Recommendation on Pregnancy with COVID-19. 2020.

14. Gajbhiye RK, Mahajan NN, Waghmare RB et al. 2021. PregCovid Registry Network. Clinical characteristics, outcomes and mortality in pregnant women with COVID-19 in Maharashtra, India. *Ind J Med Res*. Vol. 153. Issue 5–6. pp 629–636.

15. Government of India Ministry of Health and Family Welfare (MoHFW), Immunization Division Operational Guidance for COVID-19 Vaccination of Pregnant Women. 2021a. https://www.mohfw.gov.in/pdf/OperationalGuidanceforCOVID19vaccinationofPregnantWoman.pdf (last accessed March 2022).

16. Government of India, Ministry of Health and Family Welfare (MoHFW), Maternal Health Division, Guidelines on operationalization of maternal health services during Covid-19 pandemic. 2021. https://www.nhm.gov.in/New_Updates_2018/Guidelines_on_Operationalization_of_Maternal_Health_Services_during_the_Covid-19_Pandemic.pdf. Retrieved March 24 2022.

17. Goyal M, Singh P, Singh K et al. 2021. The effect of the COVID 19 pandemic on maternal health due to delay in seeking health care: Experience from a tertiary center. *Int Journal Gyn & Obstet.* 152(2), 231–235.

18. Juan J, Gil MM, Rong Z et al. 2020. Effect of coronavirus disease 2019 (COVID-19) on maternal, perinatal and neonatal outcome: A systematic review. *Ultrasound Obstet Gynecol.* 56:15.

19. Kharbanda EO, Haapala J, DeSilva M et al. 2021. Spontaneous abortion following COVID-19 vaccination during pregnancy. *JAMA.* 326(16):1629–1631.

20. Kumari V, Mehta K, Choudhary R. 2020. COVID-19 outbreak and decreased hospitalisation of pregnant women in labour. *Lancet Glob Health.* 8 (e1116-e7).

21. Lokken EM, Huebner EM, Taylor GG et al. 2021. Disease severity, pregnancy outcomes, and maternal deaths among pregnant patients with severe acute respiratory syndrome coronavirus-2 infection in Washington State. *Am J Obstet Gynecol.* 225:77.e1.

22. Mahajan NN, Pednekar R, Gaikwad C et al. 2022. Increased spontaneous preterm births during the second wave of the coronavirus disease 2019 pandemic in India. *Int J Gynaecol Obstet.* 157(1):115-120.

23. Mahajan NN, Pophalkar M, Patil S, Yewale B et al. 2021. Pregnancy outcomes and maternal complications during the second wave of coronavirus disease 2019 (COVID-19) in India. *Obstet Gynecol.* 138: 660–662.

24. Martinez-Perez O, Prats Rodriguez P, Muner Hernandez M et al. 2021. The association between SARS-CoV-2 infection and preterm delivery: A prospective study with a multivariable analysis. *BMC Pregnancy Childbirth.* 21, 273.

25. MMWR Morb Mortal Wkly Rep. 2021. 70(47):1640.

26. Nair M. MaatHRI writing group. 2021. Reproductive health crisis during waves one and two of the COVID-19 pandemic in India: Incidence and deaths from severe maternal complications in more than 202,000 hospital births. *The Lancet.* Vol. 39, 101063.

27. National Institutes of Health. 2021. COVID-19 Treatment Guidelines Panel. Coronavirus Disease 2019 (COVID-19) Treatment Guidelines. https://www.covid19treatmentguidelines.nih.gov/. Accessed March 2022.

28. Omar M, Youssef MR, Trinh LN et al. 2022. Excess of cesarean births in pregnant women with COVID-19: A meta-analysis. *Birth.* 00:1– 0.

29. Papageorghiou AT, Deruelle P, Gunier RB et al. 2021. Preeclampsia and COVID-19: Results from the INTERCOVID prospective longitudinal study. *Am J Obstet Gynecol.* 225(3):289.e1-289.e17.

30. RCOG guidance on Coronavirus (COVID-19) infection in pregnancy. 2022. Version 15. https://www.rcog.org.uk/guidance/coronavirus-covid-19-pregnancy-and-women-s-health/coronavirus-covid-19-infection-in-pregnancy.

31. Rotshenker-Olshinka K, Volodarsky-Perel A, Steiner N et al. 2021. COVID-19 pandemic effect on early pregnancy: Are miscarriage rates altered in asymptomatic women? *Arch Gynecol Obstet.* 303:839.

32. Royal College of Obstetricians and Gynaecologists. 2021. Guidance on COVID-19 vaccines, pregnancy and breastfeeding FAQs. https://www.rcog.org.uk/guidance/coronavirus-covid-19-pregnancy-and-women-s-health/vaccination/covid-19-vaccines-pregnancy-and-breastfeeding-faqs.

33. Schultz NH, Sørvoll IH, Michelsen AE et al. 2021. Thrombosis and thrombocytopenia after ChAdOx1 nCoV-19 vaccination. *N Engl J Med.* 384:2124.

34. Srivastava K. 2021. Covid-19: Why has India had a spike in stillbirths? *BMJ.* 374:n2133.

35. Stock SJ, Carruthers J, Calvert C et al. 2022. SARS–CoV-2 infection and COVID-19 vaccination rates in pregnant women in Scotland. *Nat Med.*

36. Villar J, Ariff S, Gunier RB et al. 2021. Maternal and neonatal morbidity and mortality among pregnant women with and without COVID-19 infection: The INTERCOVID multinational cohort study. *JAMA Pediatr.* 175(8):817–826.

37. World Health Organization.2022. Therapeutics and COVID-19: Living guideline. https://apps.who.int/iris/bitstream/handle/10665/352285/WHO-2019-nCoV-therapeutics-2022.2-eng.pdf.

38. World Health Organization. 2021. Antigen-detection in the diagnosis of SARS-CoV-2 infection. Interim guidance. https://www.who.int/publications/i/item/antigen-detection-in-the-diagnosis-of-sars-cov-2infection-using-rapid-immunoassays.

39. World Health Organization. 2021.Update on WHO Interim recommendations on COVID-19 vaccination of pregnant and lactating women. https://cdn.who.int/media/docs/default-source/2021-dha-docs/update-on-who-interim-recommendations-on-c-19-vaccination-for-pregnant-and-lactating-women-70-.pdf.

40. Zambrano LD, Ellington S, Strid P et al. 2020. Update: Characteristics of symptomatic women of reproductive age with laboratory-confirmed SARS-CoV-2 infection by pregnancy status - United States. *MMWR Morb Mortal Wkly Rep.* 69:1641.

41. Zauche LH, Wallace B, Smoots AN et al. 2021. Receipt of mRNA COVID-19 vaccines and risk of spontaneous abortion. *N Engl J Med.* 385(16):1533.

Chapter 50

Immunisations During Pregnancy

INTRODUCTION

- It is not just children but also adults who require immunisations to ensure protection against many infections.
- Pregnant women are susceptible to certain infections that may increase the risk of morbidity and mortality, not only for themselves, but also for their fetus and newborn.
- Fetal morbidity from maternal infection may result in congenital anomalies, spontaneous miscarriage, preterm birth, and fetal growth restriction/low birth weight (see **Chapter 48,** *Infections during pregnancy*).

> Vaccinating pregnant women is essential and safe (ACOG, 2018) when:
> - The likelihood of disease exposure is high
> - The infection would pose a risk to the mother or her fetus

- Obstetrician–gynecologists are primary care physicians who should routinely assess their adult patients for susceptibility to infection and should document their immunisation status (ACOG, 2018). This is particularly important in pregnant women.
- The safety in pregnancy for several vaccines containing inactivated viruses and bacterial vaccines or toxoids has been firmly established (WHO, 2014).

IMMUNISATIONS RECOMMENDED IN PREGNANCY

The Centers for Disease Control and Prevention (CDC, 2016) recommends the following vaccines in pregnancy:
- Essential in pregnancy
  - Td/Tdap
  - Influenza
- Specifically recommended during the postpartum period in non-immune women
  - Varicella
  - MMR
- Recommended in pregnancy based on additional risk factors
  - Hepatitis B
  - Pneumococcal vaccine
  - Meningococcal vaccine
  - Travel-related
    - Yellow fever
    - Japanese encephalitis

> **How are vaccines made?**
> Disease-causing pathogens are manipulated in the laboratory through multiple rounds of tissue culture or animal embryos, mutagenesis, or targeted genetic alterations to specifically select strains with very low virulence that can only provoke an immune response but not cause disease.
>
> Vaccines may contain *live viruses* that have been attenuated (weakened or altered so as not to cause illness); *inactivated or killed organisms or viruses; inactivated toxins* (for bacterial diseases in which toxins generated by the bacteria, and not the bacteria themselves, cause illness); or merely *segments of the pathogen*, including both subunit and conjugate vaccines (The College of Physicians of Philadelphia, 2020).

TYPES OF VACCINES

The types of vaccines available are as follows (Swamy and Heine, 2015).

- **Inactivated or killed vaccine:** Inactivated or killed vaccines are created by inactivating the infectious pathogen using heat or chemicals like formalin or formaldehyde. The inactivation prevents replication and clinical infection but still provokes the body to mount an immune response. Vaccines against influenza, diphtheria, and pertussis are inactivated or killed vaccines (Table 50.1).

- **Live attenuated vaccine:** Live attenuated vaccines contain living disease-causing pathogens that have 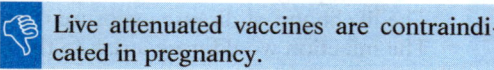 Live attenuated vaccines are contraindicated in pregnancy.
been weakened or altered in the laboratory so as not to cause infection. The resulting strains have very low virulence. However, they are contraindicated in pregnancy. The vaccines against measles, mumps, and rubella (MMR), and varicella are live attenuated vaccines.

- **Toxoid vaccines:** Certain bacteria like *Clostridium tetani* cause disease by producing a toxin rather than by direct bacterial action. Tetanus is prevented by a toxoid vaccine which is created by inactivating this neurotoxin using heat or chemicals. Toxoid immunisations include the tetanus and diphtheria vaccines, which are available in a combined form.

- **Subunit and conjugate vaccines:** Both subunit and conjugate vaccines contain fragments of the pathogens they protect against, which subsequently provoke a protective immune response. The acellular pertussis vaccine and injectable influenza vaccine are subunit vaccines. Subunit vaccines may also be produced using recombinant technology; the hepatitis B vaccine is an example of this. The pediatric pneumococcal vaccine is an example of a conjugate vaccine.

DURATION OF PROTECTION OR IMMUNITY

- Inactivated and toxoid vaccines elicit an immune response that is less robust than that elicited by live attenuated vaccines.
- Protection provided by a live attenuated vaccine typically lasts longer.
- Protection provided by an inactivated vaccine is short-lasting, and therefore, booster doses are required.

Table 50.1   Types of vaccines and their use in relation to pregnancy

Type of vaccine	Given during pregnancy	Given postpartum or 1–3 months before attempting conception (in non-immune women)	Recommended in pregnancy based on additional risk factors
Inactivated or killed	• Influenza (injectable) • Diphtheria and pertussis (part of Tdap, Td)	–	–
Toxoid (inactivated toxin)	• Tetanus • Diphtheria	–	–
Subunit/conjugate	• Influenza (injectable) • Pertussis (part of Tdap)	–	• Pneumococcal • Meningococcal
Live attenuated	–	• Measles, mumps, rubella (MMR combined vaccine) • Varicella (chickenpox)	–

 When a vaccine virus is given to a human, it is unable to replicate enough to cause illness but still provokes an immune response that can protect against future infection.

IMMUNISATION AGAINST TETANUS, DIPHTHERIA, AND PERTUSSIS

- Worldwide, tetanus kills an estimated 180,000 neonates per year. Five per cent of all maternal deaths (up to 30,000 women each year) are due to tetanus. In 2015, 45 per cent of neonatal deaths due to tetanus were in South Asian countries (Kyu et al., 2017).
- A tetanus and diphtheria toxoid (Td) is recommended every 10 years for all adults to provide immunity against both tetanus and diphtheria.
- In 2018, the Ministry of Health and Family Welfare, India, recommended the replacement of tetanus toxoid (TT) vaccine with tetanus–diphtheria (Td) vaccine in India's immunisation programme for all age groups including pregnant women (Ministry of Health and Family Welfare, Operational Guidelines, 2018). This was based on a recent WHO/UNICEF joint communique (2018) urging countries to switch from TT to Td vaccine.

Rationale for switch from TT to Td

- Globally, there has been a resurgence of diphtheria. It has also been documented from surveillance data in India that the majority of the cases of diphtheria are occurring in the age group of 5 years and above (approximately 70 per cent in 2018). In the 2016 diphtheria outbreak in Kerala, nearly 80 per cent of cases occurred in the >10 years age group (MoHFW, Operational Guidelines, 2018).

 Since 2005, the global incidence of **diphtheria** has increased dramatically. India contributes to nearly three-fourth of all cases in South-East Asia.

- The use of Td rather than TT during pregnancy is recommended because not only does it protect the mother and the newborn against tetanus, it also protects the mother against adult diphtheria. Td also protects the neonate against diphtheria before he/she receives the diphtheria, tetanus, and pertussis vaccine (DTP) as part of childhood immunisation.

 Tetanus and adult diphtheria (Td) vaccine is a combination of tetanus and diphtheria with lower concentration of diphtheria antigen (d), as recommended for older children and adults. It is currently being used in 133 countries.

- It has been shown that immunity to diphtheria subsides following the primary series of DTP infant immunisation. Vaccination during pregnancy serves to boost immunity and increase the duration of protection in those pregnant women who had not received the full set of recommended booster doses.
- Td also helps to limit diphtheria outbreaks in the community.

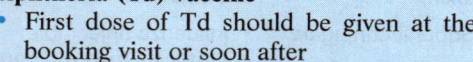
Recommended dosage of tetanus–diphtheria (Td) vaccine
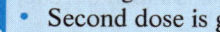
- First dose of Td should be given at the booking visit or soon after
- Second dose is given after 4 weeks
- Third dose given 6–12 months later provides immunity for 10 years
- Booster dose—if pregnancy occurs within three years of the last pregnancy and two Td doses were received beforehand

Tetanus–diphtheria–pertussis vaccination (Tdap)

- Vaccination with the tetanus toxoid, reduced diphtheria toxoid, and acellular pertussis (Tdap) is also recommended during pregnancy.
- Pertussis ('whooping cough') has seen a resurgence globally, especially in adolescents and adults, possibly due to the waning of protection from DTP given as part of childhood immunisation.
- The CDC recommends that at least one Tdap vaccine be given between 27 and 36 weeks in each pregnancy to protect the new-born against pertussis (Liang et al., 2018).
- In under-resourced areas, Tdap may not be feasible because of the cost. In such cases, Td alone may suffice.

IMMUNISATION AGAINST SEASONAL INFLUENZA AND H1N1 INFECTION

- Pregnant women infected with flu have increased rates of hospitalisation, cardiopulmonary complications, and mortality than the general population (see **Chapter 48**, *Infections in pregnancy*).
- Vaccination with the quadrivalent inactivated influenza vaccine or recombinant influenza vaccine is strongly recommended for all pregnant women (ACOG Committee Opinion, 2018a). It is recommended that all pregnant women be immunised during the influenza season.
- Internationally available vaccines for the control of seasonal influenza are safe and efficacious in pregnant women (WHO position paper, 2012).
- In a randomised blinded trial conducted in Bangladesh on 340 pregnant women in their third trimester, maternal influenza vaccination was found to result in a 36 per cent reduction in febrile respiratory illness among mothers and a 63 per cent reduction

in respiratory illness in their infants (Zaman et al., 2008).

 Influenza vaccination has been shown to decrease the risk of influenza and its complications among pregnant women and their infants up to six months of age (ACOG, 2018).

- Influenza vaccine may be given in any trimester (Ding et al., 2017). Annually, a new batch of vaccines is released that is effective against the previous year's strains. Since influenza season usually starts in October, this is usually the time that the new vaccine is available.

 Quadrivalent inactivated influenza vaccine or recombinant influenza vaccine usually contains four killed influenza virus strains: two strains of influenza A (H1N1, H3N2) and two strains of influenza B.

IMMUNISATION AGAINST COVID-19

- Coronavirus disease (COVID-19) is an infectious disease caused by the SARS-CoV-2 virus.
- Immunisation against COVID-19 is recommended for all pregnant women who have not been vaccinated earlier. See **Chapter 49**, *COVID-19 infection in pregnancy*, for details.

IMMUNISATION AGAINST MEASLES-MUMPS-RUBELLA (MMR)

- **Measles** is a viral infection that may present with a rash, diarrhea, and otitis media along with bronchopneumonia or encephalitis in severe cases. Infection during pregnancy increases the risk of spontaneous miscarriage, preterm birth, and low-birth-weight newborns.
- **Mumps** is a viral infection that presents with flu-like symptoms and bilateral parotitis and is associated with spontaneous miscarriage.
- **Rubella** is a virus that may present with non-specific symptoms including lymphadenopathy, arthralgias, fever, and a rash (see **Chapter 48**, *Infections in pregnancy*). Infection during pregnancy, especially in the first trimester, can have devastating consequences for the fetus. Serious sequelae of congenital rubella syndrome include deafness, cataracts, cardiac defects, neurologic damage, and death.
- Before administering MMR to an adult woman, pregnancy status should be documented to avoid conception for four weeks post-vaccination.

 MMR is a live attenuated vaccine and contraindicated in pregnancy.

- **However, inadvertent measles–mumps–rubella vaccination during pregnancy should not be considered grounds for pregnancy termination** (CDC, 2001).
- All pregnant women should be screened for rubella immunity at the booking visit, and the decision for postpartum MMR vaccination made based on the results.
- Non-immune women should be vaccinated immediately after delivery. Breastfeeding is not a contraindication to the MMR vaccine.

IMMUNISATION AGAINST VARICELLA

- Varicella zoster virus, a member of the herpes virus family, causes chickenpox (see **Chapter 48**, *Infections in pregnancy*).
- Vaccination is the most effective means of preventing varicella infection and congenital varicella syndrome.
- Since the vaccine is a live attenuated virus, it is contraindicated in pregnancy.

  > Varicella is a live attenuated vaccine and contraindicated in pregnancy.

- **However, inadvertent varicella vaccination during pregnancy does not imply a need for pregnancy termination** (Marin et al., 2007).
- The decision for the need for postpartum varicella vaccine should be based on whether the woman is immune to varicella. Varicella immunity should be established for all pregnant women during early pregnancy by self-reported history of infection, history of vaccination, or documented serologic immunity.
- Susceptible women should receive two doses of vaccine postpartum—the first immediately postpartum and the second 4–8 weeks later (Swamy and Heine, 2015).

IMMUNISATION WITH HEPATITIS B VACCINE

- Hepatitis B virus causes acute liver infection characterised by jaundice accompanied by nausea and vomiting. It can be transmitted through close contact with infected blood and bodily fluids.
- Hepatitis B virus is usually self-limiting but some individuals achieve a *chronic carrier state* associated with long-term consequences including cirrhosis, liver cancer, liver failure, and death.
- All pregnant women should be screened for hepatitis B surface antigen status as part of standard prenatal laboratory testing (see **Chapter 2**, *Antenatal care: initial assessment*).
- Neonates born to women positive for hepatitis B surface antigen are at risk of acquiring the infection and should receive hepatitis B immunoglobulin prophylaxis and be given the first hepatitis B virus vaccine dose within the first hours of life.
- The hepatitis B virus vaccine is a recombinant DNA formulation based on the hepatitis B surface antigen envelope protein. A three-vaccine course is highly effective for disease prevention, providing an indefinite protective antibody response in greater than 90 per cent of vaccinated individuals.

Indications and schedule of hepatitis B vaccine

- Non-immune pregnant women who have not been vaccinated previously may be at high risk of acquiring hepatitis B if they have a hepatitis B virus-positive sexual partner or household contact. A pregnant healthcare worker who has not been vaccinated may also receive the course.
- The three-dose hepatitis B virus vaccine course should be initiated for these pregnant women.
- **Vaccination schedule**
  - 1st dose (0): As soon as the decision is made
  - 2nd dose (1): 1 month (or 28 days) after the first dose
  - 3rd dose (6): 6 months after the first dose

– **Accelerated course:**   If a woman is at a high risk of acquiring the infection (e.g., when her partner is infected), an accelerated course may be given at 0, 1 and 2 months, followed by a booster dose 1 year after the first dose.

IMMUNISATION AGAINST PNEUMOCOCCAL AND MENINGOCOCCAL DISEASE

- *Streptococcus pneumoniae* (pneumococcus) is a gram-positive bacterium associated with significant morbidity and mortality related to pneumonia, bacteremia, and meningitis.
- An encapsulated bacterium called *Neisseria meningitidis* can cause meningococcal disease (meningitis and sepsis).
- Currently, there is no recommendation for routine vaccination of pregnant women for these two infections (CDC, 2016).
- However, in high risk women, vaccines against these two bacteria may be given. There seems to be no risk to the fetus or neonate from these vaccines (Makris et al., 2012).
- Women at high-risk for these infections are those with:
  - Chronic lung disease including asthma
  - Pre-existing diabetes
  - Chronic liver disease
  - Sickle cell disease and other hemoglobinopathies
  - Complement deficiencies
  - Asplenia

VACCINATIONS SPECIFIC TO TRAVEL

Yellow fever

- Yellow fever is a mosquito-borne disease caused by an RNA flavivirus. Though it is commonly an asymptomatic infection, severe infection may result in multisystem organ failure, hemorrhage, and death.
- Vaccination for yellow fever is mandatory for the issuance of travel visas to some tropical areas in South America and sub-Saharan Africa. It is recommended for individuals planning to travel to endemic areas.
- Though the yellow fever vaccine is a live attenuated vaccine, the CDC (Staples et al., 2010) recommends yellow fever vaccine during pregnancy if a woman is travelling to endemic areas and the risks of exposure and infection are high.
- Suzano et al. (2006) documented no association between the vaccination given during pregnancy and teratogenesis, spontaneous miscarriage, or preterm birth.

Japanese encephalitis

- Japanese encephalitis is a mosquito-borne virus that represents the most common vaccine-preventable disease cause of encephalitis in Asia (CDC, 2014).
- Though the data is limited, there is some evidence that Japanese encephalitis virus may cause miscarriages in pregnant women.
- Women travelling to endemic areas may be given the vaccine if necessary.

References

1. American College of Obstetricians and Gynecologists. 2018. ACOG Committee Opinion No. 741. Maternal immunization. *Obstet Gynecol.* 131:e214–7.

2. American College of Obstetricians and Gynecologists. 2018a. ACOG Committee Opinion No. 732. Influenza vaccination during pregnancy. *Obstet Gynecol.* 131:e109–14.

3. Centers for Disease Control and Prevention (CDC). 2001. Revised ACIP recommendation for avoiding pregnancy after receiving a rubella-containing vaccine. *MMWR Morb Mortal Wkly Rep.* 50:1117.

4. Centers for Disease Control and Prevention (CDC). 2014. CDC health information for international travel. Oxford University Press, New York (NY).

5. Centers for Disease Control and Prevention (CDC). 2016. Guidelines for vaccinating pregnant women.

6. Ding H, Black CL, Ball S, Fink RV, Williams WW, Fiebelkorn AP et al. 2017. Influenza vaccination coverage among pregnant women, United States, 2016–17 influenza season. *MMWR Morb Mortal Wkly Rep.* 66:1016–22.

7. Kyu HH, Mumford JE, Stanaway JD. 2017. Mortality from tetanus between 1990 and 2015: Findings from the global burden of disease study 2015. *BMC Public Health.* 17:179.

8. Liang JL, Tiwari T, Moro P et al. 2018. Prevention of pertussis, tetanus, and diphtheria with vaccines in the United States: Recommendations of the Advisory Committee on Immunization Practices (ACIP). MMWR Recomm Rep. 67:1.

9. Makris MC, Polyzos KA, Mavros MN, Athanasiou S, Rafailidis PI, Falagas ME. 2012. Safety of hepatitis B, pneumococcal polysaccharide and meningococcal polysaccharide vaccines in pregnancy: A systematic review. *Drug Saf.* 35:1–14.

10. Marin M, Güris D, Chaves SS et al. 2007. Prevention of varicella: Recommendations of the Advisory Committee on Immunization Practices (ACIP), Centers for Disease Control and Prevention (CDC). *MMWR Recomm Rep.* 56:1–40.

11. Ministry of Health and Family Welfare, Government of India. 2018. Updates on tetanus and adult diphtheria. Operational Guidelines.

12. Staples JE, Gershman M, Fischer M. 2010. Centers for Disease Control and Prevention (CDC). Yellow fever vaccine: Recommendations of the advisory committee on immunization practices (ACIP). *MMWR Recomm Rep.* 59:1–27.

13. Suzano CE, Amaral E, Sato HK, Papaiordanou PM. 2006. Campinas Group on Yellow Fever Immunization during Pregnancy. The effects of yellow fever immunization (17DD) inadvertently used in early pregnancy during a mass campaign in Brazil. *Vaccine.* 24:1421–6.

14. Swamy GK, Heine RP. 2015. Vaccinations for Pregnant Women. *Obstet Gynecol.* 125 (1).

15. The College of Physicians of Philadelphia. 2020. The history of vaccines–different types of vaccines. An educational resource.

16. WHO position paper. 2012. Vaccines against influenza. No. 47, 2012, 87, 461–476.

17. WHO/UNICEF joint communique. 2018. Replacement of TT with Td vaccine for dual protection.

18. World Health Organization. 2014. Safety of immunization during pregnancy: A review of the evidence. Global Advisory Committee on Vaccine Safety. WHO Press, Geneva.

19. Zaman K, Roy E, Arifeen Se et al. 2008. Effectiveness of maternal influenza immunization in mothers and infants. *N Engl J Med.* 359:1555–1564.

Chapter 51

Management of Pregnancy in a Woman With HIV (Human Immunodeficiency Virus)

INTRODUCTION

- The human immunodeficiency virus (HIV) is a lentivirus (a subgroup of retrovirus) that causes **acquired immunodeficiency syndrome** (AIDS). In AIDS, there is a progressive failure of the immune system. Life-threatening opportunistic infections and cancers flourish in this immunosuppressed state. Without treatment, life expectancy after infection with HIV is estimated to be 9–11 years.
- There are two types of HIV: HIV-1 and HIV-2. **HIV-1 is responsible for the vast majority of HIV infections globally**.
- Infection with HIV occurs by the transfer of blood, semen, vaginal fluid, or breast milk. HIV is present both as free virus particles and virus within infected immune cells in these bodily fluids.
- India has the third largest HIV epidemic in the world, with 2.1 million people reported to be living with HIV in 2017. However, between 2010 and 2017, new infections declined by 27 per cent and AIDS-related deaths decreased by more than half, falling by 56 per cent (UNAIDS data, 2018). Unfortunately, despite free antiretroviral treatment being available, uptake remains low, as many people face difficulty in accessing clinics.

 Since 2010, there has been a steady decline in the number of new HIV cases in India, with AIDS-related deaths decreasing by more than half.

- The prevalence of HIV in adults (15–49 years) in India has been estimated as 0.25 per cent in the male population and 0.19 per cent in the female population (National AIDS Control Organization [NACO], 2019).
- Public health interventions in preventing the transmission of HIV and AIDS are most effective when targeted at the detection and treatment of sexually transmitted diseases, and prevention of mother-to-child transmission (MTCT) of HIV.

 Managing a pregnant woman with HIV is a team effort involving the obstetrician, pediatrician, HIV specialist, health advisor, and the primary care provider.

HIV AND PREGNANCY

- India is estimated to have had approximately 23,000 HIV-positive women who gave birth in 2017.

- The UNAIDS data (2018) showed that 60 per cent of pregnant women living with HIV in India accessed antiretroviral medicine to prevent transmission of the virus to their baby, thereby preventing 3500 new HIV infections among newborns.
- Early infant diagnosis, i.e., the percentage of HIV-exposed infants tested for HIV before eight weeks of age, stood at 23 per cent in 2017.

MANAGEMENT OF PREGNANCY IN HIV-POSITIVE WOMEN

- Women who are HIV-positive may become pregnant. Alternately, pregnant women may be found to be HIV-positive when they are tested during antenatal check-ups.

 Pregnancy does not appear to worsen HIV or increase the risk of death from HIV. It is not clear if it is HIV or the treatment for HIV that increases the risk of pregnancy complications such as prematurity, low birth weight, or stillbirth.

- The management of the HIV-positive pregnant woman has evolved significantly over the past four decades due to advancements in drug development and a better understanding of the prevention of mother-to-child transmission (MTCT) of HIV.
- This success has been brought about by the following measures.
  - Universal testing of pregnant women for HIV infection
  - Use of cesarean section, when appropriate
  - Avoidance of breastfeeding, when feasible
  - Lifelong combination ART for women living with HIV
- Perinatal HIV infection can occur during pregnancy, labour and delivery, or during the breastfeeding period.
- With appropriate antiretroviral therapy (ART) and effective viral suppression, the risk of an infant becoming infected via perinatal transmission is now estimated to be <2 per cent.

Sequelae of maternal HIV infection

- Untreated HIV itself is associated with low birth weight and neonatal death (Ndirangu et al., 2012). There is also evidence that HIV-positive pregnant women have a higher risk of fetal malformations if they do not receive ART during pregnancy (Bérard et al., 2017).
- The most significant sequela of maternal HIV infection in pregnancy is **mother-to-child transmission (MTCT)** of HIV. Without intervention, rates of MTCT range from 15–30 per cent without breastfeeding and rise to 30–45 per cent with prolonged breastfeeding (John and Kreiss, 1996).
- MTCT is responsible for 90 per cent of HIV infections in children worldwide. It is estimated that 5–10 per cent of MTCT of HIV results from intrauterine transmission, 10–20 per cent takes place during delivery, while post-delivery transmission accounts for 5–20 per cent (Ogundele et al., 2003).
- To prevent MTCT, mothers should receive combination antiretroviral therapy (ART) in pregnancy. See further details of the effects of ART on pregnancy in the section on *Safety of ART in pregnancy*.

Screening for HIV in pregnancy

- All pregnant women should be given pre-test counselling regarding screening for HIV.
- All pregnant women (except those who opt out of/decline testing) should undergo HIV screening early in each pregnancy.
- Repeat testing in the third trimester is recommended for those who are at a high risk for infection.
- Women who present in labour without prior HIV testing should undergo rapid HIV testing. Rapid tests can be performed anywhere and do not require laboratory facilities for highly trained staff. Results are obtained in as little as 20 minutes.
- A pregnant woman with a positive rapid HIV test result should be managed as if HIV-infected to prevent perinatal HIV transmission.
- If no rapid testing is available, the untested woman should also be managed as if HIV-infected to prevent perinatal HIV transmission.

It is strongly recommended that all pregnant women undergo screening for HIV infection at their booking antenatal visit in every pregnancy.

Care before pregnancy

- Any HIV-positive woman planning conception should be educated and counselled.
- A detailed discussion should be carried out with the couple on the medications required, their side effects, compliance issues, risks of vertical transmission, monitoring tests, mode of delivery, and postpartum care. All treatment should be documented, and strict confidentiality maintained.

Care during pregnancy

- A thorough history should be obtained in HIV-infected pregnant women to identify health concerns that may also affect fetal well-being.
- A detailed history of opportunistic infections, sexually transmitted infections (STI), medication use, immunisation status, and substance abuse should be obtained.
- The physical examination should focus on signs of advanced HIV infection and concomitant STIs.
- Counselling should be provided to modify high-risk behaviour pertaining to HIV transmission, smoking, and illicit drug use.
- **Immunisations:** Tetanus/diphtheria booster (Td) is indicated if the woman has not had one in the previous ten years. One dose of tetanus/diphtheria/acellular pertussis (Tdap) vaccine should be given in the second trimester. Hepatitis B and pneumococcal vaccine are indicated for all HIV-positive women during pregnancy if not given earlier. Inactivated influenza vaccine is also strongly advised, as it is for all pregnant women.
- **Chemoprophylaxis for pneumocystis pneumonia:** This is recommended for all pregnant women with a CD4 count of <200 cells/mL. The preferred dosage is one double-strength trimethoprim-sulfamethoxazole tablet once a day after the first trimester (due to teratogenicity concerns).

- **Antiretroviral therapy (ART) regimen:** If the mother is already on antiretroviral therapy, she should continue it. If she is not, a combination ART regimen should be initiated as early

 Pre-conceptional combination ART has the highest impact on reducing MTCT. If the mother is not on ART, it should be initiated as early as possible in pregnancy to maximise its effects.

in pregnancy as possible because earlier initiation of ART is associated with lower rates of transmission (Dinh et al., 2018). ART regimens are explained in detail in the section on *General principles of ART during pregnancy*.

Investigations

- Hemoglobin and hematocrit should be tested for—anemia is associated with an increased risk of adverse pregnancy outcomes as well as increased mother-to-child transmission (Mehta et al., 2008)
- CD4 counts (pregnancy itself is associated with a decline in CD4 counts)
- Viral load measurement (especially at 34–36 weeks to decide on the mode of delivery)
- Viral hepatitis markers (HBsAg, HCV antibodies)
- Screening for gestational diabetes
- Screening for sexually transmitted infections (STIs)
- Testing for tuberculosis
- Screening for genital infections
- Screening for fetal anomalies

Ultrasound imaging and invasive procedures
- Accurate determination of gestational age by early ultrasound scan is important as early delivery may be necessary to decrease the risk of HIV transmission.
- In addition to the first-trimester ultrasound for gestational age, a detailed second-trimester ultrasound evaluation is advised to detect fetal anomalies in women on combination antiretrovirals.
- Invasive diagnostic procedures are preferably avoided in HIV-infected pregnant women. However, in a person with viral suppression who is on combination antiretrovirals, such procedures do not appear to pose any extra risk of HIV transmission in utero.

GENERAL PRINCIPLES OF ART DURING PREGNANCY

The goals of antiretroviral therapy (ART) are as follows:
- To treat maternal HIV disease
- To reduce mother-to-child transmission (MTCT)

 Without antiretroviral preventive interventions, the risk of perinatal HIV transmission is between 15 and 45 per cent. Breastfeeding increases this risk.

- The World Health Organization, in its consolidated guideline on when to start antiretroviral therapy and on pre-exposure prophylaxis for HIV (2016), strongly recommends that ART should be initiated as follows:
  - In all pregnant and breastfeeding women living with HIV

- Regardless of WHO clinical stage
- At any CD4 cell count
It should be continued lifelong.
- A woman must be counselled regarding antiretroviral therapy so that she is able to make an informed decision.
- There is a direct positive correlation between maternal plasma viral load at the time of delivery and risk of transmission to the infant. Townsend and colleagues (2014) demonstrated that MTCT rates were lower among women who had a viral load <50 copies/mL near delivery than women who had higher viral loads.
- Factors associated with an increased risk of MTCT include the following:
  - Low CD4 cell counts
  - Anemia
  - More advanced WHO clinical disease stage
  - Maternal mastitis
  - Acute maternal seroconversion during pregnancy or breastfeeding

Initiating and maintaining maternal ART

- The following recommendations are for women in *resource-limited settings* like India and are based on WHO guidelines (2016).
  - ART is recommended for all pregnant and breastfeeding women with HIV, regardless of their CD4 cell count or disease stage. This not only benefits the mother but also reduces the risk of transmission to their infants.
  - Women already on ART should continue it.
- The goal of ART is to reduce the viral load to undetectable levels. As mentioned above, MTCT decreases with lowering of viral load.

Delay in the initiation of ART may increase the risk of MTCT, especially if delayed beyond 28 weeks.

Treatment regimens

- The World Health Organization's 2019 guidance recommends tenofovir, lamivudine (or emtricitabine), and dolutegravir as the preferred first-line regimen for the treatment of HIV (Table 51.1). As of 2019, 75 countries have incorporated dolutegravir in their first-line regimens.
- The advantages and benefits of the use of dolutegravir in pregnant women include the following:
  - Fewer potential drug interactions
  - A high barrier to drug resistance development
  - More rapid viral suppression

> The advantages of dolutegravir outweigh the possible small increase in the risk of neural tube defects with peri-conception dolutegravir exposure.

Table 51.1 Preferred and alternative first-line combination antiretroviral therapy (ART) during pregnancy and breastfeeding (based on WHO updated recommendations on first- and second-line antiretroviral regimens, 2019)

First-line ART regimens		Second-line ART regimens	
Preferred	Tenofovir (TDF) + lamivudine (3TC) (or emtricitabine, FTC) + dolutegravir (DTG)	Preferred	Zidovudine (AZT) + lamivudine (3TC) + atazanavir/ritonavir (ATV/r) or lopinavir/ritonavir (LPV/r)
Alternative	Tenofovir TDF + lamivudine (3TC) + efavirenz (EFV)	Alternative	Zidovudine (AZT) + lamivudine (3TC) + darunavir/ritonavir DRV/r

Monitoring of disease progression and response to ART

HIV disease progression and response to ART are monitored using the following two surrogate markers:

- *CD4 T lymphocyte (CD4) cell count*
  - Defines overall immune function of an HIV-infected patient
  - Determines the urgency to initiate ART
  - Progression to AIDS signified by a count of <200 cells/μL
- *HIV RNA (viral load)*
  - Marker of response to ART
  - Helps monitor the effectiveness of therapy

PREVENTING MOTHER-TO-CHILD TRANSMISSION

Modes of transmission from mother to child

Transmission of HIV from mother to child may occur:

- In utero
- Intrapartum
- During breastfeeding

In utero

- A significant proportion of in utero transmission is thought to occur between 28 and 36 weeks of gestation (Lallemant et al., 2000).
- Maternal blood carrying the virus reaches the fetus by crossing the placenta due to a breakdown of the intrinsic integrity of the placenta (Kourtis et al., 2001).
- Genital tract infections and placental inflammation, especially chorioamnionitis, can increase in utero HIV transmission.

Intrapartum

- As the infant passes through the vagina, its mucous membranes come into contact with the HIV virus present in the blood and secretions associated with birth.
- In a woman who is not on ART, duration of membrane rupture >4 hours before delivery has been associated with increased risk of transmission (Landesman et al., 1996).

However, it is now accepted that the duration of membrane rupture of 4 or more hours is not a risk factor for the perinatal transmission of HIV in women with a viral load <1000 copies/mL receiving combination ART (Cotter et al., 2012). **A viral load of >10,000 copies/mL is now considered a risk factor for perinatal transmission if membranes have been ruptured for >4 hours**.

- During labour contractions, maternal infected blood is transfused across the placenta into the fetus.

Breastfeeding

- Though it is clear that HIV is transmitted from mother to child during breastfeeding, the exact mechanism has not been clearly understood.
- HIV-infected cells within breast milk may play an important role in transmission to the infant. Infected breast milk cells may have a greater role in transmission than cell-free virus (Rousseau et al., 2004).
- The virus may then enter the child's circulation through the tonsillar or intestinal tissues.

Drug regimens for the prevention of MTCT

- Early initiation of combination antiretroviral drug regimens during or before pregnancy (rather than at delivery) is associated with a lower risk of infant transmission.

 MTCT rates at birth and in the early postpartum period are <5 per cent with combination ART (Flynn et al., 2020).

- Earlier, treatment in resource-limited settings focused on and demonstrated the efficacy of one- or two-drug regimens (zidovudine, zidovudine/lamivudine, nevirapine) given in the last trimester and around labour/delivery because they were less expensive and more deliverable in resource-limited settings.
- However, a recent study from Africa and India (Fowler et al., 2016) that compared the one- or two-drug regimens with immediate three-drug ART initiated at diagnosis showed that combination ART is much more effective in preventing MTCT.

Duration of treatment

- The WHO guidance (2016) recommends lifelong ART.
- The advantages of lifelong ART include the following:
  - Clinical benefit of ART even at high CD4 cell counts
  - Prevention of HIV transmission to uninfected sexual partners with successful ART
  - Prevention of MTCT in future pregnancies with no interruption in therapy
  - Overall decreasing costs of HIV therapy in many low-income countries

Safety of ART in pregnancy

- ART is associated with an increase in the risk for preterm birth, small-for-gestational age babies and stillbirth (Chen et al., 2012). However, a recent study from South Africa

(Chetty et al., 2018) demonstrated decreased rates of preterm births and SGA infants by changing the ART regimens.

- Overall, first-trimester antiretroviral exposure is not associated with an increased risk of birth defects (Abrams, 2021).

MANAGEMENT OF LABOUR AND DELIVERY

Choice of route of delivery

The decision about the mode of delivery depends on the mother's viral load near the time of delivery since the risk of HIV transmission can be predicted by the viral load.

 Viral load measurement at 34–36 weeks is important for making a decision regarding the mode of delivery.

- **Lowest risk:** Undetectable viral load (<50 copies/mL)
  - May be delivered by the vaginal route. A cesarean section is determined by obstetric indications. IV zidovudine (AZT) is not recommended.
- **Low-to-moderate risk:** Detectable (≥50 copies/mL but ≤1000 copies/mL)
  - Should be delivered based on the obstetric indication and may be given intrapartum IV AZT.
- **High risk:** >1000 copies/mL near time of delivery or no ART during pregnancy
  - Should be delivered by an elective cesarean section at 38 weeks' gestation. The mother should receive intrapartum IV AZT.
  - In low-resource settings, where cesarean section is not easily available, the presence and status of HIV infection in the mother does not affect decisions on the mode of delivery.
  - In settings where testing for viral load is not available, decisions regarding the mode of delivery should be based on antenatal ART, the combination of ART used, and adherence to therapy. Risks and benefits of a cesarean section should be considered.
  - In some resource-poor settings, a vaginal delivery may be the only option, considering the non-availability of surgical facilities and also the associated increased morbidity in low-resource settings.
- These guidelines are summarised in Table 51.2.

Vaginal delivery

- When a woman presents in labour, her recent viral load results should be confirmed as <50 copies/mL. Planned vaginal delivery can be offered to women

 The risk of HIV acquisition in babies born vaginally to women who have a viral load <50 copies/mL is <1%.

taking combination ART who have an undetectable viral load (< 50 copies/mL). The risk of HIV acquisition in babies born to these women is <1 per cent.
- If the viral load is undetectable, the woman should continue her baseline ART. No additional drug is required.

Table 51.2 Intrapartum management and infant prophylaxis for pregnant women with HIV (based on WHO's consolidated guidelines on the use of antiretroviral drugs for treating and preventing HIV infection, 2016)

Treatment based on maternal viral load (VL)	Mother on antepartum ART			No antepartum ART
	Undetectable VL (<50 copies/mL) near time of delivery	Detectable (≥50 copies/mL) but ≤1000 copies/mL near time of delivery	>1000 copies/mL near time of delivery	
Risk of HIV transmission	Lowest risk	Low–moderate risk	High risk	High risk
Mode of delivery	Vaginal delivery or cesarean section based on obstetric indication	Cesarean section based on obstetric indication	Elective cesarean delivery* at 38 weeks	Cesarean delivery*
Intrapartum ART	Continue ART mother was on	In addition, consider IV AZT	In addition, administer IV AZT	IV AZT
Infant prophylaxis	4 weeks of NVP/AZT	Combination prophylaxis	Combination prophylaxis	Combination prophylaxis

IV AZT, intravenous zidovudine; *NVP*, nevirapine; *VL*, viral load
*In low-resource settings, vaginal delivery may be the only option available. In such situations, the presence and status of HIV infection in the mother does not affect decisions regarding route of delivery.

- Intrapartum zidovudine is given to women with detectable viral loads.
- Invasive procedures such as fetal scalp blood sampling and fetal scalp electrodes are contraindicated.
- If labour progress is normal, amniotomy should be avoided unless delivery is imminent.
- Amniotomy and possible use of oxytocin may be considered for augmentation of labour.

Elective cesarean section

- Elective cesarean section is associated with reduced rates of mother-to-child transmission among women who have received either no antiretroviral drugs or zidovudine alone.
- It is therefore recommended for women who have a viral load of >1000 copies/mL at or near delivery (ACOG, 2018).
- However, this recommendation may not be feasible in resource-limited regions and may increase maternal morbidity.

Precautions during elective cesarean section

- The surgical field should be kept as hemostatic as possible to reduce the exposure of the infant to the virus in the maternal blood.
- Care should be taken to avoid rupturing the membranes until the head is delivered through the surgical incision.
- In elective cesarean, intravenous AZT infusion should be started three hours before the cesarean section is performed and should continue until the umbilical cord has been clamped.

Intrapartum ART

- Women with an undetectable viral load (<50 copies/mL) should continue their baseline ART regimen.
- Intrapartum intravenous zidovudine should be given to the following women:
  - Those who have a detectable viral load
  - Those who have not received antepartum ART and are diagnosed when they present in labour

Special situations

Preterm premature rupture of membranes

- In the case of preterm premature rupture of membranes before 37 weeks, the decision to deliver should be based on best obstetric practices.
- Antenatal corticosteroids for fetal lung maturation may be given according to obstetric norms. There is no evidence that the recommendations for mothers with HIV need to be different from those who do not have the infection.

Postdated pregnancy

- For women on combination ART with plasma viral load of <50 copies/mL, the decision regarding the induction of labour for prolonged pregnancy should be individualised.
- There is no contraindication to membrane sweep or the use of prostaglandins.

Vaginal birth after cesarean section (VBAC)

VBAC may be considered for women on combination ART whose plasma viral load is <50 copies/mL.

HIV diagnosed in labour

- For women diagnosed as HIV-positive during labour, intrapartum zidovudine should be given intravenously.
- Delivery should be by cesarean section if possible, and IV AZT should be started three hours before the cesarean (if time permits).
- Postpartum combination ART for the infant for six weeks is strongly recommended.

Postpartum care

- Decisions regarding the continuation of ART in the postpartum period are based on the CD4 count, just as in non-pregnant individuals.
- Women may find it difficult to adhere to an antiretroviral regimen in the postpartum period. The whole family should be educated on the necessity for lifelong ART.

INFANT PROPHYLAXIS AT BIRTH

The WHO updates for infant prophylaxis (2019) strongly recommend the following:
- **Low-risk infants:** Infants born to mothers on combination ART during pregnancy, low viral load, and compliant with therapy should receive the following treatment:
  - Zidovudine (AZT) for 4 weeks

- **High-risk infants:** Infants born to mothers with HIV and who are at a high risk of acquiring HIV should receive prophylaxis (whether they are breastfed or formula-fed) with the following first-line regimen:
  - Zidovudine (AZT) + lamivudine (3TC) + raltegravir (RAL) for 6 weeks
    The alternative first-line regimen is:
  - Zidovudine (AZT) + lamivudine (3TC) + nevirapine (NVP) for 6 weeks
- **Breastfed infants** who are at a high risk of acquiring HIV, including those first identified as exposed to HIV during the postpartum period, should continue to receive infant prophylaxis for an additional 6 weeks (total of 12 weeks of infant prophylaxis).
- **Infants receiving replacement feeds** should be given 4–6 weeks of infant prophylaxis.

Breastfeeding and prevention of MTCT

- The portal of entry of HIV in the breastfed infant has not been defined but may include the intestine or tonsillar tissues.
- Breaches in intestinal epithelial integrity or compromise in intestinal cellular tight junctions (e.g., between epithelial or dendritic cells) may allow the entry of infectious virions.
- Mastitis and breast abscesses have been associated with an increased risk of HIV transmission, which may be due to the increased recruitment of HIV-infected inflammatory cells in an area of infection.
- **All breastfeeding women should be on a combination ART** as recommended by the WHO 2019 guidelines.
- Both maternal ART and infant prophylaxis are associated with very low breastfeeding transmission and high infant HIV-free survival (Flynn et al., 2018).

 In low-resource settings like India, where replacement feeds may not be affordable, mothers known to be infected with HIV should be encouraged to exclusively breastfeed their infants for the first six months of life. At that stage, other foods can be introduced and breastfeeding may continue for the first 12 months of life (WHO, 2016).

THE NATIONAL AIDS CONTROL ORGANISATION GUIDELINES AND PPTCT PROGRAMME

- The National AIDS Control Organisation (NACO), under the Ministry of Health, Government of India, launched the Prevention of Parent to Child Transmission (PPTCT) of HIV programme in 2001–2002.
- In 2012, the policy of multidrug regimen, as recommended by the WHO, has also been adopted by the PPTCT programme. The PPTCT services are provided through integrated counselling and testing centers (ICTCs).
- With effect from 1 January 2014, pregnant women who are found to be HIV-positive are initiated on lifelong ART, irrespective of CD4 count and WHO clinical stage.
- The newborn (HIV-exposed) babies are initiated on 6 weeks of syrup NVP immediately after birth so as to prevent transmission of HIV from mother to child; this is extended to 12 weeks of syrup NVP if the duration of the ART of the mother is <24 weeks.

References

1. Abrams EJ. 2021. Safety and dosing of antiretroviral medications in pregnancy. Mofenson LM (Ed). *UpToDate*. Waltham, MA.

2. American College of Obstetricians and Gynecologists. 2018. ACOG Committee Opinion No. 751. Labor and delivery management of women with human immunodeficiency virus infection. *Obstet Gynecol*. 132(3):e131–137.

3. Bérard A, Sheehy O, Zhao JP et al. 2017. Antiretroviral combination use during pregnancy and the risk of major congenital malformations. *AIDS*. 31:2267.

4. Chen JY, Ribaudo HJ, Souda S et al. 2012. Highly active antiretroviral therapy and adverse birth outcomes among HIV-infected women in Botswana. *J Infect Dis*. 206:1695.

5. Chetty T, Thorne C, Coutsoudis A. 2018. Preterm delivery and small-for-gestation outcomes in HIV-infected pregnant women on antiretroviral therapy in rural South Africa: Results from a cohort study, 2010–2015. *PLoSONE*. 13(2):e0192805

6. Cotter AM, Brookfield KF, Duthely LM et al. 2012. Duration of membrane rupture and risk of perinatal transmission of HIV-1 in the era of combination antiretroviral therapy. *Am J Obstet Gynecol*. 207:482.e1.

7. Dinh TH, Mushavi A, Shiraishi RW et al. 2018. Impact of timing of antiretroviral treatment and birth weight on mother-to-child human immunodeficiency virus transmission: Findings from an 18-month prospective cohort of a nationally representative sample of mother-infant pairs during the transition from option A to option B+ in Zimbabwe. *Clin Infect Dis*. 66:576.

8. Flynn PM, Abrams EJ, Fowler MG. 2020. Prevention of mother-to-child HIV transmission in resource-limited settings. Mofenson LM, Paul ME (Eds). *UpToDate*. Waltham, MA.

9. Flynn PM, Taha TE, Cababasay M et al. 2018. Prevention of HIV-1 transmission through breastfeeding: Efficacy and safety of maternal antiretroviral therapy versus infant nevirapine prophylaxis for duration of breastfeeding in HIV-1-infected women with high CD4 cell count (IMPAACT PROMISE): A randomized, open-label, clinical trial. *J Acquir Immune Defic Syndr*. 77:383.

10. Fowler MG, Qin M, Fiscus SA et al. 2016. Benefits and risks of antiretroviral therapy for perinatal HIV prevention. *N Engl J Med*. 375:1726.

11. John GC, Kreiss J. 1996. Mother-to-child transmission of human immunodeficiency virus type 1. *Epidemiol Rev*. 18:149.

12. Kourtis AP, Bulterys M, Nesheim SR, Lee FK. 2001. Understanding the timing of HIV transmission from mother to infant. *JAMA*. 285:709.

13. Lallemant M, Jourdain G, Le Coeur S et al. 2000. A trial of shortened zidovudine regimens to prevent mother-to-child transmission of human immunodeficiency virus type 1. Perinatal HIV Prevention Trial (Thailand) Investigators. *N Engl J Med*. 343:982.

14. Landesman SH, Kalish LA, Burns DN et al. 1996. Obstetrical factors and the transmission of human immunodeficiency virus type 1 from mother to child. The Women and Infants Transmission Study. *N Engl J Med*. 334:1617.

15. Mehta S, Manji KP, Young AM et al. 2008. Nutritional indicators of adverse pregnancy outcomes and mother-to-child transmission of HIV among HIV-infected women. *Am J Clin Nutr*. 87:1639.

16. National AIDS Control Organization (NACO) – Ministry of Health and Family Welfare, Government of India. 2019. https://mohfw.gov.in.

17. Ndirangu J, Newell ML, Bland RM, Thorne C. 2012. Maternal HIV infection associated with small-for-gestational age infants but not preterm births: Evidence from rural South Africa. *Hum Reprod.* 27:1846.

18. Ogundele MO, Coulter JBS. 2003. HIV transmission through breastfeeding: Problems and prevention. *Ann Trop Paediatr.* 23:91–106.

19. Rousseau CM, Nduati RW, Richardson BA et al. 2004. Association of levels of HIV-1-infected breast milk cells and risk of mother-to-child transmission. *J Infect Dis.* 190:1880.

20. Townsend CL, Byrne L, Cortina-Borja M et al. 2014. Earlier initiation of ART and further decline in mother-to-child HIV transmission rates, 2000–2011. *AIDS.* 28:1049.

21. UNAIDS data 2018. https://www.unaids.org/en/regionscountries/countries/india.

22. World Health Organization. 2016. WHO consolidated guidelines on the use of antiretroviral drugs for treating and preventing HIV infection: Recommendations for a public health approach, 2nd ed. WHO Press, Geneva.

23. World Health Organization. 2019. Update of recommendations on first- and second-line antiretroviral regimens. WHO, Geneva.

Chapter 52

Intrahepatic Cholestasis of Pregnancy

INTRODUCTION

- Intrahepatic cholestasis of pregnancy (ICP) is the most common pregnancy-specific liver disorder (ACOG, 2017). It is a reversible type of cholestasis thought to be caused primarily by a genetic predisposition that makes the mother sensitive to estrogen.
- Since estrogen levels are higher in the third trimester, cholestasis usually manifests later in pregnancy. It is for the same reason that cholestasis is more common in multiple gestation, where the estrogen levels are higher than with a singleton pregnancy.
- It is characterised by maternal pruritus and altered liver functions. The pruritus resolves, and serum bile acid levels return to normal with delivery.
- ICP is associated with increased risk of spontaneous preterm birth, fetal hypoxia, stillbirth, meconium-stained amniotic fluid, admission to the neonatal unit, and perinatal death.

INCIDENCE

- The incidence of this disorder varies with the genetic and ethnic background of the population. Dang et al. (2010) found an incidence of 0.7 per cent in pregnant women attending a hospital in Delhi.
- In a multi-ethnic population in the United Kingdom, cholestasis was found to affect 1.2–1.5 per cent of women from the Indian subcontinent (Abedin et al., 1999).
- In Europe, the incidence varies between 0.5 and 1.5 per cent. In the United States, the incidence is very low among Caucasians but is as high as 5 per cent among Hispanic women. The incidence of ICP worldwide is highest among the Araucanos Indians in Chile—27.6 per cent (Lindor and Lee, 2019).

ETIOLOGY

The exact etiology of cholestasis of pregnancy is unknown but seems to be multifactorial in origin. A combination of the following factors is considered to result in this disease.

- **Genetic susceptibility:** Cholestasis in pregnancy occurs in genetically susceptible women. At least some cases are related to the gene mutations that control hepatocellular transport systems (Hay, 2008). The genetic predisposition is suggested by familial clustering, increased risk in first-degree relatives, increased risk in some ethnic groups, and a recurrence rate of up to 60–70 per cent (Pataia et al., 2017).
- **Gestational hormonal milieu:** Since women who develop ICP have no symptoms outside the pregnant state, it is obvious that hormonal changes of pregnancy play an important role in disease etiology.

- *Estrogen* is implicated for the following reasons:
  - ICP occurs in late pregnancy when estrogen levels are highest
  - ICP is more common in multiple pregnancy which is associated with higher levels of estrogen
  - Estrogen-containing contraceptive pills can precipitate cholestasis
- *Progesterone* may also play a role in ICP. Pregnancy is associated with large amounts of sulphated progesterone metabolites. This may result in saturation of the hepatic transport systems utilised for biliary excretion of these compounds (Abu-Hayyeh et al., 2016). Sulphated progesterone metabolites are a prognostic indicator of ICP and can help distinguish it from benign pruritus gravidarum.
- **Environmental factors** may play a role and are implicated because of the geographical and seasonal variation of ICP.

CLINICAL FEATURES

- Pruritus is the primary clinical symptom of ICP.
  - It usually manifests in the third trimester of pregnancy, commonly after 30 weeks of gestation, though occasionally it may be seen in the second trimester.
  - It often commences on the palms of the hands and soles of the feet, and then spreads to the torso and face, with no other skin manifestations.
  - It may be mild and tolerable for some women, but may be very severe and disabling for others. A woman's quality of life may be severely affected, with it having an adverse psychological impact on some women.
  - It is most severe in the evening and at night, leading to a distressing lack of sleep.
  - It resolves with delivery along with a return of serum bile acid levels to normal (Geenes and Williamson, 2015).
- **Physical examination:** ICP is not associated with any specific skin lesions. However, there may be scratch marks which may be quite severe. These should be differentiated from other common conditions such as eczema and benign pruritus gravidarum.
- **Other symptoms:** ICP may also be associated with right upper quadrant pain, nausea, poor appetite, or steatorrhea (Lindor and Lee, 2019).
- **Mild jaundice** with only moderately elevated serum levels of conjugated bilirubin occurs in 10–15 per cent of cases (Kondrackiene and Kupcinskas, 2008). Jaundice may occasionally be the initial symptom but in the majority of cases, develops 1–4 weeks after the onset of pruritus.
- **Vitamin K deficiency** leading to prolonged prothrombin time (PT) results from subclinical steatorrhea and fat malabsorption. The risk of postpartum hemorrhage may increase due to this.
- Symptoms and laboratory abnormalities generally resolve within hours to days after delivery (Geenes et al., 2015).

> Pruritus, which may be intolerable and disabling, is usually generalised but may be prominent on the palms and the soles of the feet. It is characteristically worse at night (Hay, 2008).

LABORATORY CONFIRMATION

- **Elevated serum bile acids:**   The main biochemical alteration is elevation of serum bile acids >10 μmol/L. This may be the first and only laboratory abnormality (Lindor and Lee, 2019). Pruritus may precede the elevation of bile acids.
- **Elevated serum aminotransferases:**   Serum aminotransferases (alanine aminotransferase and aspartate aminotransferase) are elevated in 60 per cent of cases. Though they are usually less than two times the upper limit of normal, they may reach values greater than 1000 units/L. In the presence of such high levels, it is important to differentiate the condition from viral hepatitis.
- **Elevated serum bilirubin:**   Total and direct bilirubin concentrations may be elevated in 25 per cent of cases, although total bilirubin levels rarely exceed 6 mg/dL.
- **Elevated alkaline phosphatase:**   There may be a four-fold elevation of alkaline phosphatase in ICP but it is not specific for cholestasis.
- **Prothrombin time (PT):**   The prothrombin time is usually normal. However, it may be prolonged secondary to vitamin K deficiency. Vitamin K deficiency may result from:
  - Severe steatorrhea leading to fat malabsorption or
  - Use of bile acid sequestrants such as cholestyramine

 Biochemical changes may lag behind pruritus by days or weeks.

DIFFERENTIAL DIAGNOSIS

- In the third trimester of pregnancy, the common condition to be excluded is viral hepatitis.
- Acute fatty liver of pregnancy and the HELLP syndrome should be ruled out.

EFFECTS OF CHOLESTASIS ON PREGNANCY

Maternal

- The maternal prognosis in ICP is good.
- Pruritus rapidly disappears in the first few days after delivery.
- Liver function tests return to normal; affected women do not have any hepatic sequelae.

Fetal

- ICP carries a significant risk for the fetus. The accumulation of maternal bile acids in the fetus results in adverse outcomes.
- A recent meta-analysis (Ovadia et al., 2019) found that the risk of **stillbirth** in ICP is similar to that of pregnant women in the general population. However, the risk of stillbirth is increased when serum bile acids concentrations are 100 μmol/L or more. It is recommended that frequent bile acid testing be done until delivery.

The risk of stillbirth increases when serum bile acids concentrations are 100 μmol/L or more. Stillbirth is due to acute anoxia that may be caused by:
- Vasoconstrictive effect of bile acids in placental veins or
- Vasoconstrictive effect of meconium on the umbilical vein

- Other adverse fetal outcomes include the following:
  - Spontaneous preterm birth
  - Iatrogenic preterm birth
  - Meconium-stained amniotic fluid
  - NICU admission

MANAGEMENT OF ICP

The management of ICP includes the following measures:
- Symptomatic relief of pruritus
- Follow-up of pregnancy
- Timing of delivery of the baby
- Postnatal follow-up

Symptomatic relief for pruritus

- **Ursodeoxycholic acid (UDCA)** is a naturally-occurring bile acid that performs several actions which result in the improvement of cholestasis, including increasing biliary bile acid excretion.
  - UDCA is the recommended treatment for the management of the pruritus that accompanies ICP.
  - In a meta-analysis, Bacq and colleagues (2012) found that patients who received UDCA had better outcomes than those who received S-adenosyl-methionine, cholestyramine, or dexamethasone, placebo, or no specific treatment.
  - Earlier small studies concluded that UDCA not only decreases maternal pruritus, it also decreases adverse outcomes. However, a recent study (Chappell et al., 2019) found that though women given UDCA had less itching compared with placebo, there was no difference in adverse outcomes such as perinatal death, preterm delivery, or neonatal unit admission.
  - The dose of UDCA is 300 mg twice daily and can be increased to 500 mg twice daily if the itching does not decrease in 1–2 weeks.
  - Weekly estimation of bile acid levels is recommended.

 The dose of UDCA is 300 mg twice daily and can be increased to 500 mg twice daily if there is no significant decrease in 1–2 weeks.

- **Rifampicin** is an antibiotic with choleretic properties that can alleviate pruritus and lower serum bile acids in other cholestatic conditions by enhancing their excretion. In women who do not respond to UDCA, combined UDCA and rifampicin therapy can be effective as a second-line treatment (Geenes et al., 2015).
- **Cholestyramine** increases the fecal excretion of bile salts. However, it also increases vitamin K deficiency and hence its role in ICP is limited.
- **S-adenosyl methionine (SAMe)**—a meta-analysis (Zhang et al., 2016) that compared UDCA with SAMe concluded that UDCA decreased the pruritus score, bile acids, and aminotransferase levels more effectively than SAMe.

- **Chlorpheniramine** may provide some relief at night to help the mother sleep but does not help in controlling pruritus.
- **Dexamethasone** 12 mg per day has not been shown to improve pruritus or reduce the serum aminotransferase levels.

 A systematic review of the Cochrane Database for interventions in ICP (Gurung et al., 2013) found insufficient evidence to recommend the use of cholestyramine, SAMe, chlorpheniramine, or dexamethasone for cholestasis of pregnancy.

Follow-up of pregnancy

- **Laboratory evaluation:** Weekly measurement of maternal total serum bile acid concentrations is recommended due to the significantly increased risk of stillbirth in women with total bile acid concentrations ≥100 μmol/L (Ovadia et al., 2019). This, along with severity of maternal symptoms, contributes to clinical decision-making for delivery.
- **Fetal surveillance:** No ideal method of fetal surveillance has been determined for cholestasis of pregnancy; fetal antenatal testing has had limited predictability in this disorder (Zimmerman et al., 1991; Fisk and Storey, 1988). In an analysis of fetal deaths in cholestasis, it has been shown that there are no valid indicators in fetal monitoring that can predict fetal death (He et al., 2011).

Timing of delivery

- **Elective delivery at 36 weeks:** In a retrospective cohort study, Puljic and colleagues (2015) found that among women with ICP, delivery at 36 weeks' gestation reduced the risk of stillbirth as compared to expectant management. If the diagnosis is made after 36 weeks, immediate delivery is suggested.
- **Indications for delivery before 36 weeks:** In some cases of ICP, delivery prior to 36 weeks may be indicated if:
  - Maternal pruritus is extremely distressing and is not responding to medication
  - Jaundice is present
  - Fetal demise before 36 weeks due to ICP occurred in a previous pregnancy
  - Total serum bile acid concentration is ≥100 μmol/L
- Vaginal delivery may certainly be attempted in cholestasis of pregnancy. ICP is not an indication for elective cesarean section. Indications for cesarean are similar to other pregnancies.

Vitamin K for women with ICP
- As vitamin K is fat-soluble, women with fat malabsorption (as may happen in ICP) may develop vitamin K deficiency.
- There are no randomised controlled clinical trials that support or refute the use of vitamin K supplementation in the management of ICP.
- If the prothrombin time is prolonged due to vitamin K deficiency in a woman with ICP, the use of water-soluble vitamin K (menadiol) in doses of 5–10 mg daily is indicated (RCOG, 2011).
- Routine vitamin K must be offered to neonates in the usual way.

Postnatal follow-up

- ICP is not a contraindication for breastfeeding.
- Postnatal LFTs should be deferred for at least 10 days after delivery since LFTs may increase in the first 10 days of the puerperium.
- The mother should be educated regarding the chance of recurrence in a subsequent pregnancy.
- Contraception:
    - Estrogen–progestin contraceptives with low-dose estrogen may be prescribed to women with a history of ICP since it rarely results in recurrent cholestasis (Lindor and Lee, 2019). Liver function tests should be performed after three to six months of such contraception.
    - Progestin-only pills may be used for women who develop pruritus or cholestasis after using combined estrogen-containing contraceptives.

References

1. Abedin P, Weaver JB, Egginton E. 1999. Intrahepatic cholestasis of pregnancy: Prevalence and ethnic distribution. *Ethn Health*. 4:35.

2. Abu-Hayyeh S, Ovadia C, Lieu T et al. 2016. Prognostic and mechanistic potential of progesterone sulfates in intrahepatic cholestasis of pregnancy and pruritus gravidarum. *Hepatology*. 63:1287.

3. American College of Obstetricians and Gynecologists. 2017. ACOG Clinical Updates in Women's Health Care Summary. Liver disease: Reproductive considerations. *Obstet Gynecol*. 129:236.

4. Bacq Y, Sentilhes L, Reyes HB et al. 2012. Efficacy of ursodeoxycholic acid in treating intrahepatic cholestasis of pregnancy: A meta-analysis. *Gastroenterology*. 143:1492.

5. Chappell LC, Bell JL, Smith A et al. 2019. Ursodeoxycholic acid versus placebo in women with intrahepatic cholestasis of pregnancy (PITCHES): A randomised controlled trial. *Lancet*. 394(10201):849.

6. Dang A, Agarwal N, Bathla S, Sharma N, Balani S. 2010. Prevalence of liver disease in pregnancy and its outcome with emphasis on obstetric cholestasis: An Indian scenario. *J Obstet Gynaecol India*. 60(5):413–418.

7. Fisk NM, Storey GN. 1988. Fetal outcome in obstetric cholestasis. *Br J Obstet Gynaecol*. 95:1137.

8. Geenes V, Chambers J, Khurana R et al. 2015. Rifampicin in the treatment of severe intrahepatic cholestasis of pregnancy. *Eur J Obstet Gynecol Reprod Biol*. 189: 59–63.

9. Geenes V, Williamson C. 2015. Liver disease in pregnancy. *Best Pract Res Clin Obstet Gynaecol*. 29. 612–624.

10. Gurung V, Middleton P, Milan SJ, Hague W, Thornton JG. 2013. Interventions for treating cholestasis in pregnancy. *Cochrane Database Syst Rev*. Issue 6. Art. no.: CD000493.

11. Hay JE. 2008. Liver disease in pregnancy. *Hepatology*. 47(3):1067–76.

12. He J, Chen L, Liang C. 2011. Clinical Analysis of fetal death cases in intrahepatic cholestasis of pregnancy. *Zhonghua Fu Chan Ke Za Zhi*. 46(5); 333–7.

13. Kondrackiene J, Kupcinskas L. 2008. Intrahepatic cholestasis of pregnancy-current achievements and unsolved problems. *World J Gastroenterol*. 14:5781.

14. Lindor KD, Lee RH. 2019. Intrahepatic cholestasis of pregnancy. Lockwood CJ, Chopra S (Eds). *UpToDate*. Waltham, MA.

15. Ovadia C, Seed PT, Sklavounos A et al. 2019. Association of adverse perinatal outcomes of intrahepatic cholestasis of pregnancy with biochemical markers: Results of aggregate and individual patient data meta-analyses. *Lancet*. 393:899.

16. Pataia V, Dixon PH, Williamson C. 2017. Pregnancy and bile acid disorders. *Am J Physiol Gastrointest Liver Physiol*. 313:G1.

17. Puljic A, Kim E, Page J et al. 2015 The risk of infant and fetal death by each additional week of expectant management in intrahepatic cholestasis of pregnancy by gestational age. *Am J Obstet Gynecol*. 212:667.e1.

18. Royal College of Obstetricians and Gynaecologists. 2011. Obstetric cholestasis. Green-top Guideline No 43.

19. Zhang Y, Lu L, Victor DW et al. 2016. Ursodeoxycholic acid and S-adenosylmethionine for the treatment of intrahepatic cholestasis of pregnancy: A meta-analysis. *Hepat Mon*. 16:e38558.

20. Zimmerman P, Koskinen J, Vaalamo P et al. 1991. Doppler umbilical artery velocimetry in pregnancies complicated by intrahepatic cholestasis. *J Perinat Med*. 19, 351–355.

Chapter 53

Asthma in Pregnancy

INTRODUCTION

- Asthma is a chronic respiratory disease caused by persistent inflammation resulting in bronchial hyperreactivity, airway obstruction, and reduction of airflow.
- Asthma is a comorbidity often seen in pregnancy and is the commonest chronic disease to affect pregnant women.
- The prevalence of asthma in pregnancy has been reported to be between 4–8 per cent (Murphy et al., 2005). In India, 2 per cent of the adult population suffers from asthma (The Global Asthma Report, 2018).
- Asthma not only impacts maternal health, it is also associated with an increased risk of adverse perinatal outcomes.
- Optimising asthma management in pregnancy is important to protect the health of both mother and baby.

 Treating asthma with medications is safer for the mother and fetus than having poorly controlled asthma. Maintaining lung function is important to ensure oxygen supply to the fetus (NAEPP, 2012).

EFFECT OF PREGNANCY ON ASTHMA

- A seminal prospective study on the course of asthma in pregnancy (Schatz et al., 1988), found that the symptoms worsened in one-third of the group, improved in one-third and remained the same in another third.
- Acute exacerbations occur in 45 per cent of pregnant women with asthma. These exacerbations usually present between weeks 14 and 24 (Murphy et al., 2005).
- It is unusual to have an acute exacerbation during labour and delivery (Schatz et al., 1988).

 The risk and frequency of exacerbation of asthma depends on whether the mother had mild, moderate, or severe asthma prior to pregnancy. Women with severe asthma tend to have more serious exacerbations (Schatz et al., 2003).

EFFECT OF ASTHMA ON PREGNANCY

- Though asthma is associated with adverse outcomes in pregnancy, there is no reason to consider it a contraindication to pregnancy.
- Women with asthma are at greater risk for the following (Tata et al., 2007; Mendola, 2013.):
  - Miscarriage
  - Antepartum hemorrhage and postpartum hemorrhage

- Anemia
- Depression
- Preeclampsia
- Preterm birth
- Cesarean delivery

- Poor outcomes are usually associated with poorly controlled asthma. When asthma is not controlled, there may be repeated acute exacerbations that may result in maternal hypoxemia, hypocapnia, and alkalosis. This, in turn, can lead to impaired fetal oxygenation and uteroplacental blood flow resulting in fetal growth restriction.

MANAGEMENT OF ASTHMA IN PREGNANCY

Goals of management

The goals of management of asthma during pregnancy include the following:
- Prevention of chronic day and night symptoms
- Maintenance of optimal pulmonary function and normal activities
- Prevention of exacerbations with the use of medications that are safe for the mother and fetus
- Maintaining fetal oxygenation by preventing maternal hypoxia

Pharmacological management

- Pharmacological management in pregnancy is the same as that in non-pregnant adults. The medications used routinely have been shown to be safe in pregnancy.

> There is evidence to show that asthma tends to be undertreated in pregnancy, globally. This may be due to the woman's or practitioner's misplaced perception of the risk of drugs during pregnancy.

- Management involves a step-wise approach.
- **Theophylline (sustained-release)** has been used for years for the management of asthma in pregnant women. It may be used in women with mild, intermittent asthma (ACOG, 2008). Due to the risk of toxicity, serum levels should be maintained at 5–12 µg/mL.
- **Short-acting inhaled beta-adrenergic agonists (SABAs)** are recommended for quick relief of asthma symptoms. They have a good safety profile in pregnancy. Salbutamol is the SABA of choice in pregnancy and is used as an inhaler.
  - Mild-to-moderate symptoms
    - Two doses of inhaled salbutamol (two to six puffs) or nebulized salbutamol at 20-minute intervals
  - Severe exacerbation
    - Higher doses can be used for severe symptom exacerbation

> Women should be instructed to start therapy with a salbutamol inhaler if they have worsening symptoms such as coughing, chest tightness, dyspnea, or wheezing.

- **Low-dose inhaled corticosteroid** is recommended for women with persistent symptoms. It is the first-line therapy for persistent asthma during pregnancy. Currently, **budesonide** is the preferred inhaled corticosteroid for use during pregnancy (NAEPP Guidelines, 2012).
- **Leukotriene receptor antagonists**, e.g., montelukast, may also be considered as an alternative therapy. However, it is not considered a long-term control medication. Though there is not much data on its safety in pregnancy, it may be used in women who had responded favourably to it prior to pregnancy. Leukotriene receptor antagonists are useful in allergic asthma for prevention and maintenance therapy along with inhaled corticosteroids.
- **Oral/systemic glucocorticoids** are commonly used in pregnancy to treat acute exacerbations of asthma and rarely, for the control of severe asthma. Severe uncontrolled asthma may jeopardise both the mother and fetus. The benefits of oral steroids far outweigh the potential risks of using them. Oral glucocorticoids are strongly recommended for the management of severe asthma during pregnancy (Schatz and Weinberger, 2020).
- **Long-acting inhaled beta-adrenergic agonists (LABAs)** may be required in women with a persistent moderate asthma. **Salmeterol** has been found to be safe for use in pregnancy.

The step-wise approach to the management of asthma in pregnancy is detailed in Table 53.1.

Table 53.1 Step-wise management of asthma during pregnancy (adapted from NAEPP guidelines for managing asthma during pregnancy, 2012, and ACOG Practice Bulletin 90, 2008)

Category	Preferred management
Mild intermittent asthma	No daily maintenance therapy Inhaled salbutamol (SABA) as and when required
Mild persistent asthma	• *Preferred therapy:* Low-dose inhaled corticosteroid (budosenide) • *Alternative therapy:* Theophylline, montelukast
Moderate persistent asthma	• *Preferred therapy:* Low-dose inhaled corticosteroid + inhaled salmeterol (LABA) or medium-dose inhaled corticosteroid + inhaled salmeterol • *Alternative therapy:* Low-dose inhaled corticosteroid + montelukast or theophylline
Severe persistent asthma	• *Preferred therapy:* High-dose inhaled corticosteroid + salmeterol + oral corticosteroid (if needed) • *Alternative therapy:* High-dose inhaled corticosteroid + theophylline + oral corticosteroid (if needed)

LABA, long-acting inhaled beta-adrenergic agonist; *SABA*, short-acting inhaled beta-adrenergic agonist

Management of acute exacerbation of asthma in pregnancy

- Up to 45 per cent of pregnant women with asthma have moderate–severe exacerbations during pregnancy that require medical intervention (Murphy, 2015). Measurement of expiratory airflow with a peak flow meter (or spirometer) is the best method to objectively assess the severity of an asthma attack.
- Preventing exacerbations is important for avoiding adverse perinatal outcomes. Women with acute exacerbations of asthma in pregnancy are at risk for preterm labour and have a three-fold increase in the risk of having a low-birth-weight baby (Namazy et al., 2013).

- Preterm delivery is also associated with the use of oral steroids and severe asthma. This outcome might be a consequence of the following:
  - Maternal hypoxia
  - Maternal inflammation
  - Changes in uterine smooth muscle function
- Oral glucocorticoids are strongly recommended for the management of acute exacerbation during pregnancy (Schatz and Weinberger, 2020).
- Steroids are given to women with a poor response after one hour to treatment with a β_2-agonist in combination with ipratropium. In women who are already on chronic oral glucocorticoids, systemic steroids should be initiated with other medications.
- However, pregnant women who present with acute exacerbation are less likely to receive oral corticosteroids as compared to non-pregnant women (Hasegawa et al., 2015). **This represents sub-optimal treatment and increases the rate of recurrence**.
- The mother and the fetus should be monitored carefully during an episode of exacerbation.
- Oxygenation should be maintained by providing oxygen through a mask.
- Pharmacological management of an acute exacerbation is detailed in Table 53.2.

 Monitoring is done with continuous measurement of oxygen saturation by pulse oximetry. SpO_2 should be maintained at ≥95 per cent for the benefit of the mother and the fetus.

Table 53.2   Pharmacological management of acute exacerbation of asthma in pregnancy (adapted from NAEPP guidelines for managing asthma during pregnancy, 2012)

Drug	Dose
β_2-agonist bronchodilator (Salbutamol)	*Inhaler:* 4–8 puffs every 20 minutes up to 1 hour, then every 1–4 hours, as needed
	Nebuliser: (2.5 mg/3 mL), 2.5–5 mg every 20 minutes for 3 doses and then 2.5–5 mg every 1–4 hours, as needed
	Continuous nebulisation: 10–15 mg per hour
Ipratropium	*Nebuliser:* 500 μg every 20 minutes for 3 doses, then as needed; can be given simultaneously with β_2-agonist *Inhaler:* 4–8 inhalations every 20 minutes for 3 doses, then as needed
Systemic glucocorticoids	*Outpatient therapy:* Oral prednisone 40–60 mg per day in a single or divided dose
	Hospitalised women: Oral prednisone 40–80 mg daily in a single or divided dose, or Intravenous methylprednisolone 40–80 mg with tapering after recovery
	Life-threatening episode: Intravenous methylprednisolone, 60–80 mg every 6–12 hours, with tapering after recovery

EFFECT OF OBSTETRIC DRUGS ON ASTHMA

- Some medications that may be used during labour and delivery may have a deleterious effect on pre-existing asthma.
  - Carboprost (15-methyl prostaglandin F2α) may trigger bronchospasm and should be avoided for the following:
    - Termination of pregnancy
    - Control of postpartum hemorrhage

- Non-steroidal anti-inflammatory drugs such as ibuprofen may trigger asthma if used for postpartum pain relief.
- Indomethacin can induce bronchospasm in patients who are sensitive to aspirin.
- However, it is safe to use prostaglandin E_2 or prostaglandin E_1, which are bronchodilators and can be used for the following (ACOG, 2008):
  - Cervical ripening
  - Management of spontaneous or induced abortions
  - Management of postpartum hemorrhage

References

1. American College of Obstetricians and Gynecologists. 2008 (reaffirmed 2016). ACOG Practice Bulletin No. 90. Asthma in pregnancy. *Obstet Gynecol.* 111:457–64.
2. Hasegawa K, Cydulka RK, Sullivan AF, et al. 2015. Improved management of acute asthma among pregnant women presenting to the ED. *Chest.* 147(2):406-414.
3. Mendola P, Laughon SK, Männistö TI et al. 2013. Obstetric complications among US women with asthma. *Am J Obstet Gynecol.* 208:127.e1.
4. Murphy VE, Gibson P, Talbot PI, Clifton VL. 2005. Severe asthma exacerbations during pregnancy. *Obstet Gynecol.* 106:1046.
5. Murphy VE, Gibson PG, Smith R, Clifton VL. 2005. Asthma during pregnancy: Mechanisms and treatment implications. *Eur Respir J.* 25:731.
6. Murphy VE. 2015. Managing asthma in pregnancy. *Breathe (Sheff).* 11(4):258–267.
7. NAEPP. 2012. National Asthma Education and Prevention Program: Expert panel report III: Guidelines for the diagnosis and management of asthma. Bethesda, MD: National Heart, Lung, and Blood Institute.
8. Namazy JA, Murphy VE, Powell H et al. 2013. Effects of asthma severity, exacerbations and oral corticosteroids on perinatal outcomes. *Eur Respir J.* 41(5):1082–90.
9. Schatz M, Dombrowski MP, Wise R, Thom EA, Landon M, Mabie W et al. 2003. Asthma morbidity during pregnancy can be predicted by severity classification. *J Allergy Clin Immunol.* 112:283–8.
10. Schatz M, Harden K, Forsythe A et al. 1988. The course of asthma during pregnancy, post partum, and with successive pregnancies: A prospective analysis. *J Allergy Clin Immunol.* 81:509.
11. Schatz M, Weinberger SE. 2020. Management of asthma during pregnancy. Bochner BS, Lockwood CJ (Eds). *UpToDate.* Waltham, MA.
12. Tata LJ, Lewis SA, McKeever TM et al. 2007. A comprehensive analysis of adverse obstetric and pediatric complications in women with asthma. *Am J Respir Crit Care Med.* 175:991.
13. The Global Asthma Report 2018. Auckland, New Zealand: Global Asthma Network.

Index